·ǁ THE ǁ·
WHOLE BIRTH
C·A·T·A·L·O·G

A SOURCEBOOK FOR CHOICES IN CHILDBIRTH

Edited by

JANET ISAACS ASHFORD

Contributing Editors
   Priya Morganstern
   Susan Ritchie
   Mary Scott

Reviewed for Medical Accuracy and with a Foreword by Susan Rivard,
Licensed Midwife, Co-founder of The Seattle Midwifery School

THE CROSSING PRESS / Trumansburg, New York 14886

The grown-ups on the cover are participants in the Expectant
Parents' Class sponsored by the Tompkins County Health Department, New York, and taught by Susan Ritchie, a public
health nurse and a contributing editor to this Catalog. We
wish to thank her for her help in making this photograph
possible.

© 1983 Janet Isaacs Ashford
Book design by Janet Isaacs Ashford and Allison A. Platt
Typesetting by Martha J. Waters
Cover photograph by Pam Benham
Special thanks to Mary Extrom for assistance in production
Printed in the U.S.A.

NOTICE:

Library of Congress Cataloging in Publication Data

Ashford, Janet Isaacs, 1949-
    The whole birth catalog.

    Bibliography: p.
    Includes index.
    1. Childbirth--United States--Book reviews.
2. Maternal health services--United States--Directories.
3. Infants' supplies--United States--Catalogs.
I. Title.
RG525.A82   1983   618.2   83-838
ISBN 0-89594-108-2
ISBN 0-89594-107-4 (pbk.)

Foreword

Since the late 1960's, Stewart Brand has edited a series of publications called the Whole Earth Catalog. The purpose of the WEC is to serve as "an evaluation and access device. With it, the user should know better what is worth getting, and where and how to do the getting." Brand invited others to write similar books and Janet Ashford has both accepted and met that challenge. While the current edition of the Whole Earth Catalog has only two pages devoted to childbirth, the Whole Birth Catalog has over 300 pages filled with information on almost every imaginable aspect of birth. Whether you're a consumer trying to find the proper birth attendant, a professional thinking of starting a birth center, a grieving parent coping with a crib death, a lobbyist interested in changing your state's midwifery law, or just a person wondering what gift to give your next door neighbor's new baby, you're sure to find the information you need. That's what the Whole Birth Catalog is all about—helping people gain access to the resources, books, and organizations that can be of assistance for their particular situation.

This Catalog is an invaluable tool for every pregnant woman, couple, childbirth educator, and birth practitioner.

Thank you, Janet, for giving us such a complete resource on the subject of birth.

—Susan Rivard, Licensed Midwife, Co-founder of the
Seattle Midwifery School with Maureen Levy,
Assistant Midwife

Acknowledgements

I have learned about birth through giving birth, through attending other women's births, through talking with mothers, through reading, and through my work as editor of a childbirth newsletter. Many people have helped me with all these endeavors and I would like to thank them.

First of all, thanks to the members of my first "birth crew" in Illinois: Walt and Pat Innes, Penny and Bill Blough, Rick Cremer, Rick Starke, and Josephine Feltes, who had faith in my home birth plans and gave their support at an important time.

Many, many thanks to the women of Long Island Childbirth Alternatives, who encouraged me to publish Childbirth Alternatives Quarterly and the first, 16-page version of the Whole Birth Catalog. I would especially like to thank Nan Bunce and Ruth Longacre for being such good friends, and the other members of my second birth crew: Debby and Jim Ahrend, Kate and Tony LoPiccolo, and Sam Aronson, who took the photographs.

Heartfelt thanks to my contributing editors, who stepped in almost at the last minute to add sixty important pages to the Catalog. Susan Ritchie took a leave-of-absence from her job as a public health nurse to review materials and write introductions for the sections on Teenage Pregnancy, Outreach, Pregnancy after 30, and Family-Planning. Priya Morganstern spent many hours at the library gathering new material and writing introductions for the sections on Risks in Childbearing, Infants at Risk, and Stillbirth and Infant Death. My files on these difficult subjects were very thin and Priya filled them out in a very informative and compassionate way. Mary Scott found time in her busy life as the mother of a 5-year-old and 1-year-old to write many pages of reviews of the products and publications in the section on Baby and Child Care. Thank you all very much. Without your very high-quality and high-speed work, the Catalog would have been either sadly lacking or way behind schedule.

Thanks to Susan Rivard, who reviewed the book for medical accuracy. I thought long and hard about who should check the many obstetrical facts and figures in the Catalog and I decided that probably no one would be more qualified than an experienced, educated midwife. Susan checked each page of the manuscript and made many valuable comments and additions.

Thanks to Elaine Gill, my editor and publisher at the Crossing Press. At times when I was discouraged or stuck in my work, Elaine provided sympathy, encouragement, good advice, and money to pay for help.

Thanks to my babysitters, John Fitzgerald, Andy Morganthaler, Barbara Sipala, and Susan Hildenbrand, who really made it possible for me to work on the Catalog. And thanks to my neighbor, Marie Morganthaler, who stepped in on short notice to help out with typing the manuscript.

Thanks to my children, Rufus and Florence, for always being so cooperative and adaptable. They accept the fact that their mother is a person with a typewriter and they pay me the high compliment of imitating my efforts at writing, drawing, and making books. Thanks also to my parents, Jack and Alice Isaacs, who made me what I am and who have always encouraged and supported me.

My very special thanks go to my husband, Vic, whom I am very lucky to have met and married. Vic has always respected me as a person and supported my work both in art and writing. He acted as midwife for both our children's births and never disappointed my faith and trust in him. He has always let me be myself, never imposed any false notions of women's role on me, and has been a complete father and sharer in our family. Without Vic I would not be so happy, would not be able to work so well, and would have much less of interest to say.

Final thanks go to the many women and men who answered my queries for information for the Catalog. Your response created the book. The following people were especially helpful in providing information or answering questions by mail, in person, or on the phone.

Jan Alovus
Sandra Van Dam Anderson
Suzanne Arms
Jeannine Parvati Baker
Patricia Barki
Jamie Bolane
Riley Bostrom
Joan Bowen
Sally Branca
Jeanette Breen
Ronda Brooks
Barbara Charles
Estelle Cohen
Nancy Wainer Cohen
Theo Dawson

Cynthia Duffy
Jane Dwinell
Pat Edmonds
Rodger F. Ewy
Kitty Ernst
Cindy Feldman
Ed Feldman
Eileen Fitzgerald
Laurie Foster
Edine Frohman
Carole Gambrell
Doris Haire
Carol Halebian
Harriette Hartigan
Naomi Hoblin

Fran Hosken
Julie Hurlbut
Sandy Jamrog
Cheryl Jones
Jessica Lipnack
Ron Longacre
Rochelle Maucher
Lonnie Holtzman Morris
Judy Norsigian
Jo Oliver
Judy Palsgraf
Abby Pariser
Cheri Pies
Jane Pincus
Sharon Poidomani

Margaret Reid
Sue Roberts
Marcia Slatkin
Dianne Stamm
Norma Swenson
Katharine Tarr
Mary Ross Taylor
Maureen Turner
Katharine Warren
Rosemary Romberg Weiner
Rona Wenzel
Ariel Wilcox
Nancy Vaughn
Esther Zorn

Introduction

When I became pregnant with my first child in 1976, I decided early on that I wanted to have the baby at home. I had read enough to know that the hospital is an unpleasant place in which to give birth and as time went on I became convinced that it can also be an unsafe place. But in the beginning I didn't know much about childbirth or about how to manage a home birth so I went down to the small public library at the end of my street to see what I could learn. A few years before when I was learning to do silk-screening, an artist friend said to me, "Any fool can go to the library, read a book, and learn how to do it." I figured that this advice could be put to work on childbirth as well.

I read all the books on childbirth at the small library, checked out obstetrics and nursing textbooks from the community college library, ordered home birth and English midwifery books through the interlibrary loan system, and bought alternative birth books from our local progressive bookstore. I wrote away to all the home birth organizations listed in the backs of these books, ordered their materials, and soon had amassed quite a lot of knowledge, a batch of birth supplies, and a clear birth plan for myself. My son Rufus was born on December 4, 1976 after a very normal and painful eight hour labor, with my husband and friends in attendance. Everything happened exactly as it is described in the medical books and illustrations! I felt a wonderful sense of accomplishment in having achieved the birth I had set out to have, and I felt a sense of delight over the almost magical way in which words on paper can correspond to reality.

All of this, plus the daily care of my beautiful baby, might have been enough and I might have eventually left birth behind. But two things happened which led me in a different direction. First of all, some of the home birth manuals I had ordered didn't arrive until *after* the birth and not wanting to waste them, I read them anyway. Then I discovered that, secondly, I was still interested in birth. I kept going back to the library and looking out for the publication of new books. I began to join some of the childbirth organizations and read their newsletters. Many women who reach this stage decide to become midwives, but I didn't feel called in that direction. My overwhelming desire was simply to tell people how wonderful birth can be—how it can create love and affection, deepen marriage and friendships, build confidence and competence in women and communities. Why doesn't everyone have their babies at home?! Why do people troop dutifully into hospitals? I kept thinking about all the women in the country and how they could learn to take control of their own childbearing. I wanted to see women's births unfolding, without interference from anyone. I wanted everyone to know what I had learned.

My childbirth experience had been like a great bell sounding and it kept ringing in my mind. I began to write a book about it, which took the form of a journal of the pregnancy and birth. I got into the habit of writing everyday when my baby was asleep, and amazingly I was able to do *more* work than before I had a baby because now I was motivated about something exciting. Also, the back and forth between desk work and baby care was very refreshing and stimulating. When Rufus was about nine months old we moved from Illinois to Long Island and I met a group of women who were also interested in home birth. We started a group called Long Island Childbirth Alternatives (LICA) and I began publishing a newsletter for the group. I became even more systematic and intense in my information gathering and writing activities. I sent away for government publications on birth, subscribed to periodicals, got on mailing lists—all in order to present as much childbirth news as possible to my readers. I was especially interested in consumer efforts to make birth alternatives more available. Soon I had to start a filing system to keep track of all the material I was collecting.

The first Whole Birth Catalog came about as a fund-raising effort for LICA. It was part of our Pregnant Person's Packet of brochures and pamphlets on childbirth. I feel that it is very important for people to have consumer-oriented information on childbirth from a wide variety of sources. But many times parents don't know what's available or where to look. When I was gathering information for my son's birth, I had to start from scratch, for there was no single source which could refer me to all the information I needed. It's also important, when you're pregnant, to get what you need early and promptly. Women approaching their due date can't afford to wait weeks for manuals or birth supplies to arrive. I developed the idea of a Whole Birth Catalog in order to present parents with the best resources available, so that they wouldn't have to spend weeks and months ferreting things out of the library. When information is readily available, parents are in a better position to discover what kind of birth they want and how to achieve it.

The first Catalog was a 16-page booklet which included listings of national childbirth organizations and their Long Island affiliates, plus an article on the risks of labor drugs and a hospital birth checklist. The response to the booklet was good. By the end of 1980 we had sold about 500 packets *and* I had given birth to my second child at home, my daughter Florence, this time attended by my husband and my friends in LICA. Meanwhile the newsletter was gaining subscribers and I was exchanging information regularly with over 100 organizations and publications. I had finished my birth journal and tried to sell it to a publisher, but no one seemed interested in a personal birth story. So I decided to try a longer version of The Whole Birth Catalog, making plans for a 100-page edition. I hired a babysitter for two hours a day to help care for Rufus and Florrie, who were then 4½ and 1. I designed stationary, had form letters and fact sheets printed, and mailed them to about 2000 organizations, businesses, publishers, and individuals, soliciting information and review copies of materials.

By late summer the replies began pouring in. Every day my mailbox was packed with letters and 9 x 12 envelopes. I got letters from lay midwives and nurse-midwives; sample products from home businesses selling birth announcements, booties, toys, and T-shirts; copies of posters, pamphlets, booklets, brochures, tape cassettes, and film catalogs; childbirth preparation manuals; breastfeeding aids; artwork; birth stories; lists of publications, organizations, and services; statements of philosophy; and on and on. The mailman said, "Hey, get a bigger mailbox!" I became well acquainted with the UPS delivery man, who brought bags and boxes of review copies of books every day. I was amazed and delighted to find that the people "out there" were treating my project as seriously as I did.

During the Fall of 1981, amid massive amounts of filing and sorting, I began writing the first sections of the Catalog. I decided it was time to look for a publisher, so I prepared a "query" packet with samples of the Catalog and sent it to 48 publishers, about half big New York houses and half "small presses." The Crossing Press called within a week with an offer and after thinking about it for a few weeks, I decided to publish with them because I admire their reputation as a feminist-oriented and politically conscious small press. After we signed the contract I got five more positive responses (including two from major publishers) and found myself in the strange position of having to write tactful rejection letters to publishers.

Now the Catalog was really moving! I began working 7-8 hours a day on the project, hiring babysitters to fill the gaps between my children's naps and often working while they played (or whined) beside me. This period from December 1981 to August 1982 was the most intense working experience I've had. I literally slept, ate and lived the Catalog around the clock. Every day I reviewed books, wrote descriptions of organizations and programs, typed it all up, reduced it to size at the print shop down the street, and pasted up all these words and pictures onto 8½ x 11 sheets. I had dreams about fitting bits of information onto a page, pasting down pieces of fly-away paper over and over again. I thought about childbirth *all the time* and amazingly I never got tired of it. I was excited about the material I had gathered. The Catalog was beginning to take on a richness and diversity which was truly a pleasure to work with.

Of course, things didn't go entirely smoothly. By Spring I had fallen seriously behind schedule because the book kept getting bigger. Planned for 100 pages, then 200 pages, it was fast becoming 300. Elaine Gill at Crossing was very sympathetic and stepped in at this point to help. She advanced me some money to hire a typist (my nextdoor neighbor Marie did this job admirably) and to hire three of my best-qualified friends, Susan Ritchie, Priya Morganstern, and Mary Scott, to review and edit parts of the book. Also during the Spring my husband Vic got a new job at the Stanford Linear Accelerator Center and we happily made plans to move back to California, where we both were raised and where both our families live. But trying to finish the Catalog and arrange for moving in the Fall was not easy. I might have broken down under the weight of so many stressful events except that working on the Catalog was so compelling and rewarding. But many times I felt like Sisyphus; push, push, pushing on my rock of a book. I didn't let myself think about the end. I just kept pushing.

Now, finally, the Catalog is finished. What have I learned from the experience of writing it and what's in store for those of you who read and use the Catalog? Here are some of the ideas which have emerged from my work on this project:

* There is a vast living network of women across the country, working to reclaim birth and make it a better experience. These women are, for the most part, not working for money but out of a compelling desire to help each other and all of us. The Catalog is alive with their words and images.

* The science of childbearing has reached a potentially optimum point. If the valuable knowledge and techniques of scientific medicine could be combined with the art and science of midwifery, which respects women and provides one-to-one care, our childbearing experiences and birth statistics could be very good indeed. We have the knowledge and skill to make birthing almost perfect by providing individual, non-interventive midwifery care for the 95% of women who have normal pregnancies, and appropriate, proven high-risk physician care for the 5% who need special treatment. Unfortunately, the less-than-scientific practices of institutional obstetrics are misapplied to normal childbearing women, turning normal childbirth into a risky and stressful experience. This is the source of our whole problem.

* I hope that the next edition of the Whole Birth Catalog will be able to report that tremendous progress has been made since 1983. There is so much that I would like to include in future editions and I hope that as the Catalog is distributed, more and more people will share with me their resources and services. But will people still want to hear about consumer issues in childbirth in 1984? Will lay midwifery be legal or will it have been suppressed again? What will the cesarean-section rate be? 25%? 50%? 90%? How many drugs will the average woman consume during pregnancy and labor and how many subtle and not-so-subtle birth defects will result? Will home birth be effectively outlawed and hospital birth made compulsory? Will doctors and the state routinely be awarded temporary custody of the unborn child in order to perform "life-saving" procedures against the mother's will? Birth in America may be at a turning point and it is not clear which way it will go. I would like to believe that the efforts of women working for reform will win out, but I am sobered by the fact that the American medical establishment *did* succeed in outlawing midwifery at the turn of the century and has been in control of birth ever since. We will have to overcome a tremendously powerful economic and political force in order to regain birth for women. I don't know what will happen, but I am an optimist in practice. I keep working for childbirth reform and revolution, if only to set an example. We need more workers.

* The meaning and impact of childbirth resonate throughout life and art. Birth is a source of myth and religion; of great literature; of painting, sculpture, and new art forms; and makes possible tremendous personal growth and development in individuals and communities. And yet, our society does not recognize the new status and knowledge which mothers have gained through giving birth. I felt that as soon as I became a mother I became invisible in society. Men, especially, seemed to act as though birth did not exist. My husband's co-workers' ideal birth was one in which the father is late for the delivery because he's attending an important meeting. This conspiracy of silence and lack of recognition is deadening to the spirit and would have depressed me if not for the fact that most women who are mothers do understand and do acknowledge the importance of birth. But childbirth as a human act of significance must be brought into the public realm. Women should be praised and honored for their efforts in childbirth, just as athletes and adventurers are for their achievements. Questions concerning appro-

priate care for pregnancy and birth should receive consideration as important public health issues. The very shabby and disrespectful treatment of childbearing women by physicians and hospitals could not continue if birth were a public and much-celebrated rite of passage, of at least as much importance as marriage or school graduation. Birth must become universally honored and respected in society.

When I was pregnant with my first child, I went to a local obstetrician/gynecologist for prenatal care. A few weeks before my due date, I told him about my home birth plans. His first reaction was surprise, followed quickly by anger, and finally by resignation. He said, "It's really a pity that you have been *brain-washed by literature.*" I would like to dedicate this book to all the women who have written and spoken about childbirth, making it possible for me to achieve safe and satisfying births for my children. Long live women's rights in childbirth and long live *literature!*

How to Use this Catalog

By simply reading the many reviews, articles and excerpts in the Whole Birth Catalog, you will be taking a great step in educating yourself (or your clients) about childbirth and childbearing rights. But many of you will want to go further by ordering some of the materials listed here and by getting in touch with organizations. In doing this, you become part of the network which is working toward healthy childbearing. Here are some guidelines which will help you get the information you need *and* help the people you'll be contacting.

1. *Always include a self-addressed, stamped envelope (SASE)* with any request for information. This is especially important if you're writing to a non-profit organization or to a small, family business. By including a SASE you'll receive the information you need faster, which is important if you're pregnant and approaching a due date. Also, you'll relieve the financial burden on small childbirth groups, which usually rely on volunteer time and money to exist. A legal size envelope (4" x 9¼") and postage for one ounce, first class (currently that's $.20) will usually be sufficient.

2. *Write early.* If you're pregnant and seeking information to help in planning your birth, send for it right away! If you're really in a hurry it's a good idea to send an extra dollar or so with a request that your material be sent first class. Since many childbirth groups are operated by volunteers and often ship material by third or fourth class mail, response time can be very slow, sometimes from six to eight weeks. Businesses and publishers will usually be more prompt.

3. *Try to find materials locally.* If you're in doubt about which books or pamphlets to buy, or need them in a hurry, try to find them locally. Check out books at the library, then buy the ones you like at your local bookstore. Visit local health fairs, women's health centers, birth centers, etc. which feature displays of books and resources. Find a local childbirth educator or midwife who will share her personal library and resources. By looking for materials locally you'll be able to "try before you buy" *and* you'll be coming in contact with *people* who can help you.

4. *To find resource people and organizations in your own area,* use the referral services of the national organizations listed in the Catalog. We have not included a listing of every childbirth educator, midwife, and birth center in the country in this Catalog, but these names are available through the large, national childbirth organizations like the International Childbirth Education Association (ICEA), the Association for Psychoprophylaxis in Childbirth (ASPO), and the National Association of Parents and Professionals for Safe Alternatives in Childbirth (NAPSAC). Write directly for the name of the professionals or services you need (remember to include a SASE) or order a copy of the organization's membership directory, if available. When writing for referrals, it's useful to do the following:

A. Describe exactly what you're looking for (i.e. a local hospital with a good birthing room program, a midwife who attends home births, a childbirth class for vaginal birth after cesarean, the nearest free-standing birth center, etc.). Be specific in your request and you'll get a more specific answer.

B. Indicate in what major metropolitan area or region your home town is located. For instance, you might say, "North Aurora, Illinois is in Kane County, about fifty miles west of Chicago. Neighboring towns include Aurora, Batavia, Geneva, St. Charles, Naperville, and Downer's Grove." This information will help the person who answers your inquiry to find a local referral, even if nothing is available in your particular zip code or town.

C. If possible, include a donation (even one dollar will help) with every request for referrals.

5. *Become a member of childbirth organizations* whose philosophy you support and whose work you wish to further. Your membership dues and orders for products and publications help keep these groups alive. Even if you'll never attend a meeting or volunteer your time, help support childbearing rights by contributing your *money.* Many childbirth groups have federal tax-exempt status (this is usually stated on group literature) so your contribution will be tax-deductible.

6. *Consider volunteering your time, energy and ideas to the childbirth movement.* If you are happy with the goods and services you've received, consider becoming a *supplier* yourself. Get in touch with your local childbirth organizations and see what work needs to be done. You'll be passing along to others the gift of sharing that's been given to you.

7. *Expect prices to go up.* The prices listed here were compiled between July 1981 and August 1982. If you're ordering materials much later than that, it may be a good idea to request current price information or send 10 to 15% more money with your order.

8. *Expect addresses to change.* The childbirth movement is always changing. Some organizations fade away and others appear to take their place. Many small groups change their addresses as the volunteers who run them move from place to place. The addresses in this Catalog were current as of September 1982. If your letter to any group listed in this Catalog is returned as unforwardable, write to me. If I have the current address in my files, I will send it to you *if* you include a self-addressed, stamped envelope or postcard with your request. My address is listed in "Contributing to Future Editions."

9. *Don't send money or orders to me!* The Catalog does not function as a retail outlet. All materials should be ordered directly from the producer who is listed with the product, or from a book-order service.

Contributing to Future Editions

To gather the information for this first edition of the Whole Birth Catalog, I started with my own files and the materials collected during two years of publishing Childbirth Alternatives Quarterly and also sent out letters to over 2000 organizations, individuals, and businesses, beginning in July 1981. The response to this mailing was excellent and I received hundreds of replies and enough material to fill 300 pages of this Catalog. But even so, I know I have just scratched the surface. Undoubtedly, many worthwhile organizations and publications have been overlooked. In addition, many new books on childbirth have been published since this Catalog was completed and many new organizations and services are coming into being. It's exciting, and frustrating, trying to keep track of what's happening in the rapidly growing consumer health and childbirth movements. But I think it's very important to compile and review this material and make it available to as wide an audience as possible. Women and couples need consumer-oriented information on childbirth practices and options. The Crossing Press and I have committed ourselves to publishing an updated edition of the Whole Birth Catalog every 18-24 months, so long as there are enough sales and interest to warrant it. We hope that the Catalog will be a continuing resource and a forum for ideas from the childbirth movement. For those of you who are listed in this edition, we hope that the Catalog will serve a networking function, helping you to know about and get in touch with each other. And of course, we hope the Catalog will be a positive presentation of your ideas to the families of America. Please help us achieve these goals by sending your literature, reviews, news, stories, art work, and products for future editions of the Whole Birth Catalog. The guidelines listed below will help you in submitting materials.

Thank you all very much!

Janet Isaacs Ashford, editor

FOR ORGANIZATIONS, BUSINESSES AND PUBLISHERS

Please send the following:
1. Your name, address, telephone number, contact person.
2. A description of your services, activities, goals, etc. Please include a copy of your brochure or other literature.
3. A price list for any products, books, newsletters, etc. which you offer for sale. Include bulk rates, if available, and rates for postage.
4. A sample copy of any product or publication (book, newsletter, poster, teaching aid, etc.) which you would like to have considered for review in the Catalog.
5. If possible, a clear black and white photograph, preferably 8" x 10", of your product or publication cover.

FOR BOOK REVIEWERS

I wrote most of the reviews for this edition of the Catalog, but I would like future editions to reflect a wide variety of viewpoints and styles. If you are excited about a new book or think you have good insights to share about a book which is already listed in the Catalog, please send your review, along with a self-addressed, stamped envelope for its return. If your review is chosen for publication we will send you a simple contract to sign, a modest fee, and a copy of the Catalog in which your review appears. Please use the following guidelines for book reviews.

1. **Should the book be included in the Catalog?** Use the table of contents to see which subject areas are covered by the Catalog. Then ask yourself, "Does this book promote the readers's interest by helping her become self-sufficient and/or knowledgeable enough to make informed decisions about her own childbearing?" If so, it probably should be included.
2. **Reviewing the book.** It is not necessary to read every word, but look the book over and read enough to be able to answer the following questions:
   a. What is the book about?
   b. To what kind of reader is the book directed?
   c. Who is the author and what are her special qualifications/background/perspectives?
   d. How will the book be useful to readers?
   e. What special features does it have (illustrations, worksheets, bibliography, resource lists, etc.)?
   f. How is this book different from other books on the same subject?
3. **Writing the review.** Please type your review, double-spaced, and include the following:
   a. Title, author, publisher, price, etc., following the format of this Catalog.
   b. A one or two paragraph review (about 150 words) or longer if the book is of special merit.
   c. A few paragraphs from the book (1-5, depending upon the merit of the book) which you think give a fair impression of what the book is about, and which can also stand alone as containing useful information. **Important:** Don't type the book excerpts yourself. Send a photocopy of the relevant pages or a list of paragraph and page numbers. This will help reduce errors in transcription.
4. **General Guidelines.**
   a. Please keep a copy of your review.
   b. Don't send me a copy of the book. I will request a copy from the publisher if I decide to include it in the Catalog.
   c. If your review is very good, I may ask you to review other books and will send you review copies, okay?

FOR ARTISTS AND WRITERS

I would like to receive short features and articles, technical material (useful forms, lists, tables, etc.), art work, illustrations, photographs, personal birth stories, poetry and fiction from all readers: amateurs and professionals, parents and providers. Please type all submissions, double-spaced, and include an envelope with return postage. I would like to receive material on all topics covered in this edition of the Catalog and on important topics which you think should be covered in future editions. If your contribution is accepted for publication, you will receive a contract outlining our payment schedule and publishing terms and a copy of the Catalog in which your work appears.

1. **For factual material:** Please send informative short articles and descriptions of innovative programs or services in which you have been involved, either as a provider or a consumer.

2. **For birth stories, fiction, and poetry:** Please send work which describes your thoughts and experiences in giving birth, attending births, being pregnant, breastfeeding, etc. All experiences and points of view are welcome. I would especially like to receive birth stories collected by daughters from their mothers and grandmothers.

3. **For art work:** I would like to see art work in any medium which uses pregnancy or birth-related imagery or deals with women's health or child care. Please don't send your original art work, but send a good quality photocopy, photograph or print. Please include price information if your original work, or reproductions of it, is available by mail.

4. **For illustrations and photographs:** Please send childbirth-related drawings, cartoons, technical or medical illustrations, and photographs of pregnant and birthing women, their helpers and families, along with sufficient postage for safe return of your materials. (A Special Note to Photographers: In this edition of the Catalog I have included photographs of women giving birth in a normal, non-interventive way. I have purposefully avoided using photographs which show procedures which I believe are harmful or unnecessary for the normal childbearing woman. These kinds of procedures are, for the most part, illustrated with drawings. As a photographer, I decided that it would be unethical for me to take a picture or stand by without protest while a questionable procedure is being performed. Please keep this ethical concern in mind when submitting photographs.)

Please send all submissions to:
Janet Isaacs Ashford, editor
Whole Birth Catalog/Quarterly
Bin 62, S.L.A.C.
Stanford, CA 94305

If you are not able to contact me at the address above, send submissions to:
Whole Birth Catalog
c/o The Crossing Press
P.O. Box 640
Trumansburg, NY 14886
or call the Press at 607/387-6217 for my current address.

ABOUT CHILDBIRTH ALTERNATIVES QUARTERLY

CAQ is a 20-page quarterly newsletter which I edit and publish (see index for Catalog listing). The Quarterly will publish articles, reviews, and Catalog listing updates between editions of the Whole Birth Catalog. All materials received for the Catalog will be considered for review in the Quarterly also and the address for both is the same. CAQ is available for $10.00 a year or $3.00 for a sample issue.

ABOUT THE EDITOR

Janet Isaacs Ashford was born in Los Angeles in 1949. She studied music at the University of Southern California and received a bachelor's degree in psychology from the University of California at Los Angeles. Ms. Ashford has also studied art and has worked as a freelance artist and designer since 1974.

Ms. Ashford's interest in childbirth began in 1976 with the home birth of her first child and since 1979 she has been active as a consumer health advocate. Ms. Ashford was a co-founder and director of Long Island Childbirth Alternatives, a consumer organization which provides referrals and education for alternative childbirth. She is currently the editor and publisher of Childbirth Alternatives Quarterly, a newsletter devoted to issues in home birth, midwifery and maternal/child health.

Ms. Ashford lives in the San Francisco-Peninsula area with her husband, Vic, and her two children, Rufus and Florence, both born at home.

ABOUT THE CONTRIBUTING EDITORS

Priya Morganstern holds a bachelor of science degree in community health from the State University of New York and has studied midwifery at The Maternity Center in El Paso, Texas. She has been active in the childbirth movement for many years and is a co-founder of Long Island Childbirth Alternatives. Ms. Morganstern is presently working as a patient advocate at Bellevue Hospital in New York City and as a Gynecological Teaching Associate at North Shore University Hospital on Long Island. She plans to begin the nurse-midwifery program at Yale University in Fall 1983.

Susan Ritchie is a registered nurse and holds a master of science degree in nursing from Pace University in New York. Ms. Ritchie was a member of the Peace Corps, working in Colombia, South America on programs in nutrition and child development from 1972 to 1974. She is presently on Acting Supervising Public Health Nurse for Tompkins County, New York, where her work includes childbirth education and development of a new antepartum program with emphasis on prevention and outreach.

Mary Scott holds a master's degree in health services administration from the State University of New York at Stony Brook. Ms. Scott has toured the Far East as a musician with the U.S.O., worked as a consultant for the New York Consumer Affairs Council, helped to organize and set up two pre-schools, has done audio designing for local theater, and served as vice-president of her local Parent-Teacher Organization for the past two years. Ms. Scott is currently the director of Long Island Childbirth Alternatives and is the mother of two children, Tracy (6) and Morgan (2), born in the hospital and at home, respectively.

ABOUT THE MEDICAL REVIEWER

Susan Rivard is a Licensed Midwife who has attended over 150 home births since 1975. Ms. Rivard is a co-founder of the Seattle Midwifery School and was one of the first lay midwives to be licensed by the state of Washington. Ms. Rivard is the mother of three children, all born at home, and is currently attending home births through the Olympia Home Birth Service.

Contents

Being Pregnant

Pregnancy is a time of great change. Tremendous development is going on within the body of the unborn baby, within the mother's body, and within our minds and lives. As pregnancy progresses, mothers and fathers experience rapid physiological and psychological alteration and growth. The process of becoming parents and adjusting to a new role begins in pregnancy, producing changes in how we feel about ourselves, each other, our families, and society. At the same time, as we are living through a period of heightened experience and feeling, we are called upon to make important decisions and become informed about the medical care we receive. We are coming to realize, more and more, that our choices in childbirth will affect our families' health and happiness for a long time to come.

Information is a primary need of parents in pregnancy. To cope with the stresses and changes of pregnancy and childbirth, we need good information about how our bodies work. To choose the kind of maternity care which is best for us, we need information about the risks and benefits of different childbirth practices. Most people in our society are brought up knowing little about childbirth and are accustomed to giving over responsibility for birth to others. Both men and women are often ignorant and sometimes fearful about the normal functioning of women's bodies in pregnancy and childbirth. Because of our fears, lack of knowledge, embarrassment, or other strong feelings about this important life event, many of us are afraid to trust our own feelings and judgment, especially if they run counter to the advice of "experts." But experts don't always have the right answers. The standard practice of maternity care in our country is coming increasingly under question. Many parents want to make sure they have a childbirth experience which is both safe and personally satisfying to them.

Unfortunately, our society does not provide good support for experiencing pregnancy and childbirth in a healthy, humane, and unified way. No single community program or practitioner will provide us with all the information and guidance we need. Parents must adopt a "self-care" approach to learning and preparing for childbirth, drawing information from many sources. On the following pages you will find information on many of the concerns of pregnancy—fetal development, nutrition, drugs and other hazards, prenatal care, genetic testing, pregnancy after 30, exercise and comfort, sex in pregnancy, psychological adjustment, and expectant fathers. Both information itself and sources for finding more information are given. Hopefully, parents can also use the resources in this book to get in touch with other people who can provide help and emotional support—childbirth educators, midwives, and other parents who share their concerns. During pregnancy, both women and their partners are especially receptive to information and advice. You can use this special time to learn more about birth, develop positive attitudes, and form relationships with others in your community. Pregnancy can be an extremely life-enhancing and maturing experience. Taking it seriously and learning all we can is an important preparation for being strong parents.

Pregnancy and Childbirth, General Works

THE COMPLETE BOOK OF
PREGNANCY AND CHILDBIRTH
by Sheila Kitzinger
1981, 351 pages, Illus.

from
Knopf
201 E. 50th St.
New York, NY 10028
$14.95 hd

Sheila Kitzinger is a very experienced and prolific British writer and childbirth educator—the author of at least seven other books on childbirth and the mother of five children. Her widely-used "psychosexual" method of childbirth preparation encourages mothers to become aware of and "flow with" their emotions in pregnancy and labor. This new book is one of Kitzinger's best. Her exceptionally warm and knowledgeable advice is set in a beautifully produced book filled with photographs, drawings, and diagrams. The book covers everything from conception to the first weeks of the baby's life, always with the emphasis on the importance of choosing carefully the methods and place of birth.

"The modern technology of obstetrics, with its blinking lights and humming machinery, is reassuring for some women but alarms many others. There has been a technologi-

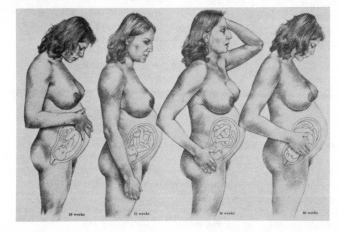

cal takeover of childbirth in recent years and women's bodies are now often regulated by space age technology and monitoring systems. As a result many mothers feel that it is not they, but the doctors who are having the baby.

"More and more women are deciding that they want to be active birthgivers rather than submit passively to delivery. To do this you need to prepare yourself well in advance with an understanding of how to adapt to the work being done by your uterus, using breathing, relaxation, change of position, massage and focused concentration to 'get in tune with' the contractions.

"Caring for the emotional aspects of birth is not a question of pampering or indulgent treatment of women. It is absolutely basic to the welding of the ties which bind human beings together in a family and families into the larger society. This is why I write not only about medical events, but about the quality of relationships important between people and the kind of society we want to create.

"Even though women all the world over have babies in much the same way, birth can be a vastly different experience for different women; just as, even though sexual intercourse involves certain mechanical and physiological processes which are the same everywhere, what people feel about it, exactly what they do and the meaning the total experience has for them, varies with the individual and the occasion. Childbirth is not primarily a medical process, but a psychosexual experience. It is not surprising that adaptive response to the stimuli it presents should be a matter of subtle and delicate working together of mind and body.

"To get the most out of the experience of being pregnant, you should insure that your body is in good condition. Remember that healthy activity can be pleasurable in itself as well as being an excellent preparation for labor. Sometimes books on pregnancy and even childbirth educators give the impression that childbirth is an athletic event for which you have to train like a marathon runner, a kind of examination for which you must study assiduously, or even an ordeal with which you are unlikely to cope but which will be quickly forgotten afterwards. No wonder expectant mothers become anxious! No mention is made of the excitement, joy and sheer pleasure that many women experience in childbirth."

RIGHT FROM THE START: Meeting the Challenges of Mothering Your Unborn and Newborn Baby
by Gail Brewer and Janice Greene
1981, 256 pages, Illus.

from
Rodale Press
33 East Minor Street
Emmaus, PA 18049
$11.95 paper

What's really best for mother and baby?—the many medical devices, drugs, and routines offered by today's maternity hospitals? or the closer-to-nature ways that served our foremothers for generations? Without rejecting appropriate technologies, Brewer and Greene make a strong case for a more natural approach to childbirth. Going right down the line, they examine each medical intervention and ask—is it really better? does it really serve the best interests of mother and child? Often the answer is No.

The focus throughout this book is on the mother/baby relationship, beginning at conception, and on how our common medical and child-rearing practices either foster or hinder a strong, loving bond. The authors examine prenatal care, nutrition, and birth practices and also take a close look at the care the baby receives during its first minutes of life, the hospital stay, intensive care, circumcision, breastfeeding , and caring for the baby at home. Always, when a decision must be made, they advise us to ask, "Does this practice/object/individual serve the urgent need my baby and I have to stay together?"

The book is arranged much like a workbook, with many useful tables, charts, action plans, and check-lists. There are many excellent photographs and an appendix which includes a guide to baby care products

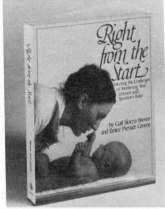

and practices, a list of organizations, a glossary, and a bibliography. Based on years of experience and concerned service to parents, this book represents much of the best the new childbirth movement has to offer.

"Almost every mother will tell you that she experiences feelings of attachment and commitment to her baby long before it's born. She thinks about the baby, she hopes for the baby. But until recently, her drive to provide direct care to her unborn child was dismissed as mere wishful thinking. There isn't much you can do until the baby's born, she was told. Babies are preordained by genetics, heredity, or pure luck to attain a certain length, weight, and completeness at birth, no matter

what the mother does during pregnancy, the experts agreed. A baby, they said, shares its mother's body for the first nine months of life, but emerges completely unaffected by that experience. The baby feels nothing, knows nothing, and can do nothing until separated from the mother. An unborn baby is a parasite.

"Happily, the more we learn about the processes of earliest human growth and development, the more we find that our maternal impulses have been right all along. The way we care for ourselves during pregnancy *is* our earliest mothering. And it has dramatic and lifelong impact on our well-being and that of our children. People working in the field of maternal and child health increasingly target maintaining or improving the mother's health during pregnancy as the key to better pregnancy outcomes for individuals and the country as a whole. They are quick to point out that the things that make the most difference—our diets, our exercise programs, our choices in medical care—are the things over which each of us exerts absolute control. Willingness to act on the new information we receive is a chief feature of good mothering during pregnancy. In the most direct way imaginable, our first job as new mothers is to take the best care of our own bodies. We and our babies are the beneficiaries of any improvements we are able to make."

BIRTH: Facts and Legends
by Caterine Milinaire
1974, 305 pages, Illus.

from
Harmony Books
419 Park Avenue South
New York, NY 10016
$12.95 hd
$ 6.95 pap

First published in 1974, this book is still in print and still very popular. Written by Caterine Milinaire, a fashion photographer, *Birth* is filled with the exuberance of a mother feeling the emotional intensity of her first birth. *Birth* is filled with lovely photographs of pregnant women and many charming drawings and illustrations. There are twenty personal birth stories, which describe a variety of birth experiences, including the author's own home birth. There is information on fetal development, exercise, herbs, nutrition, clothing, methods of childbirth, fathers, baby care, and a fascinating chapter on birth customs around the world. Above all, *Birth* conveys the sense of excitement and adventure which many women feel when their pregnancies are healthy and much wanted.

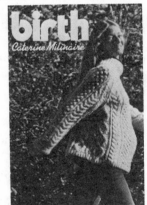

"10:54 A.M. THE SUN IS FLOWING INSIDE THE BEDROOM, BLASTING WITH VITAL RAYS A NEW HEAD. Push . . . episiotomy incision with my consent. Totally painless, the perineum is numbed by the baby's pressure. Push . . . the top of the head is out to the mouth and already screams. A reality sound, voice rendering concrete a long-awaited child. What a blessing to be a woman! What a magical gift! I cannot remember a more extraordinary burst of happiness in my life. Rapidly, the rest of the tiny body slips out. Alive in front of us, a long and thin little person, moonstone color, kicking and yelling, still circuited to me by a pale blue umbilical cord. Thank you!
'How is it?'
'Good, forceful, supernatural!' "

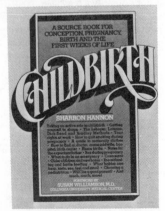

CHILDBIRTH: A Source Book for Conception, Pregnancy, Birth, and the First Weeks of Life.
by Sharron Hannon
1980, 248 pages, Illus.

from
M. Evans
216 E. 49th St.
New York, NY 10017
$9.95 paper

Women often learn about birth

the hard way, by having a childbirth experience which was not what they hoped it would be. This happened to Sharron Hannon and motivated her work on this book and her choice of a birthing center staffed by midwives for her next birth. *Childbirth* is an excellent resource for women who want to make sure they have a safe, family-centered childbirth without any last minute "surprises." The book includes book reviews, lots of lists, very good photographs of pregnancy and birth, and knowledgeable discussions of the many options available in childbirth.

"Given the fact that the choices you may make for the way you want to have your baby may not correspond to the options available, what can you do to increase the chances of having things your way? Here are several suggestions:
Be informed—Read as much as you can so you can present authoritative arguments supporting your point of view.
Know your rights—Do some home-

work on state health laws, hospital policies and so on, so you know which rules can be bent.
Keep records—Document everything and make an effort to get copies of your prenatal care and labor and delivery charts.
Write letters—If you can't get what you want, complain. Write to the administrator and the director of community relations at the hospital, the local medical society and the health department. Telling your story to the local newspaper may get results.

"Perhaps the best idea is to link up with others who share your concerns. There is a recognized and organized Childbirth Movement in this country and by joining it you can help not only yourself but others to achieve satisfying birth experiences. Because there is strength in numbers, most of the changes that have been accomplished, such as getting fathers into the delivery room, have come about through the efforts of various groups."

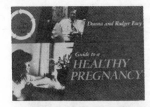
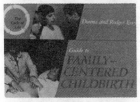
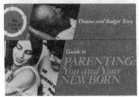

THE CYCLE OF LIFE:
Guide to a Healthy Pregnancy
Guide to Family-Centered Childbirth
Guide to Parenting: You and Your
Newborn
by Donna and Rodger Ewy
1982, 145-175 pages each, Illus.

from
Dutton Publishing Co.
2 Park Avenue
New York, NY 10016
$7.25 each, pap

This three-volume set of books presents the facts and important issues of pregnancy, birth, and parenting in a simple, straight-forward way. An attempt is made to play down the controversies currently raging in maternity care, while at the same time alerting parents to the important choices and decisions to be made. Each volume is generously illustrated with clear diagrams and drawings and excellent photographs, through which we are able to follow the same multi-racial group of couples from pregnancy through birth and into early parenting.

"The first responsibility you have is to obtain information on nutrition, fitness, and rest and relaxation. Your second responsibility is to choose a physician or birthing attendant who will give you early and personal prenatal care, whose philosophy is consistent with your own, who will take time to answer your questions, who cares about you as a person, who cares about your marriage, who cares about your baby, and who includes both of you in the visits. Third, you have the responsibility to find a prenatal class that will prepare you for pregnancy, childbirth, and early parenting. And, finally, you have the responsibility to surround yourselves with people who can give you the physical, emotional and psychological support you need for a healthy and happy pregnancy."

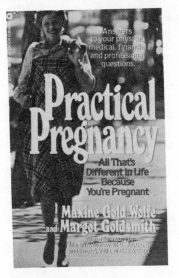

PRACTICAL PREGNANCY: All That's Different in Life Because You're Pregnant
by Maxine Wolfe and Margot Goldsmith
1980, 304 pages, Illus.

from
Warner Books
75 Rockefeller Plaza
New York, NY 10019
$12.95 hd
$ 5.95 pap.

Just about *everything* is covered in this book, from pregnancy tests to deciphering your health insurance coverage. The important medical aspects of pregnancy are discussed, but the unique feature of this book is its treatment of many practical concerns often left out of other books—what equipment and clothing will I need for the baby, how will pregnancy affect my make-up and grooming routines, what sort of maternity clothes should I have, what are my rights at my job? The authors found they were starting from scratch with their first pregnancies and set out to write the book they needed then.

"During pregnancy, while getting things ready for the baby, many women tackle major carpentry and painting projects. They may wallpaper, paint, and sand, or strip and refinish cribs, cradles, dressers, woodwork, floors, dressing tables, and toys. In so doing, they breathe in a variety of vapors, fumes, and dusts, and contact many chemicals that may be hazardous not only to their health but to their baby's as well."

PREGNANCY AND CHILDBIRTH:
The Complete Guide for a New Life
by Tracy Hotchner
1979, 689 pages

from
Avon Books
959 8th Avenue
New York, NY 10019
$6.95 pap.

Tracy Hotchner was a Los Angeles-based journalist when she researched this "consumer's guide" to childbirth. She wanted to gather together "every possible scrap of information" on childbirth in order to present the unbiased view she felt was lacking in other books. The result is an encyclopedic book which contains a great deal of useful information on virtually every aspect of birth. Hotchner presents the pros and cons of the many methods and procedures facing pregnant women today, hoping to help parents make up their own minds about how and where to give birth. I feel she sometimes goes too far in defending the drugs and devices used in modern obstetrics but on the whole her work has produced a book which respects

women and their right to make their own decisions.

"The consumer does have power in childbirth. Hospitals are profit-oriented institutions which must respond to what customers want or risk losing patients. Women are learning to ask for more, but they need to share the experiences of women who have already given birth. If the blame for the lack of information and the loneliness of childbirth in America is to be placed anywhere, the culprit is the wall of silence and isolation surrounding childbearing. Women can change existing choices in childbirth and encourage more options but they have to climb over that wall and ask for more."

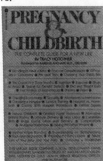

THE COMPLETE BOOK OF BIRTH:
From Grantly Dick-Read to Leboyer
—A Guide for Expectant Parents to
All Methods of Birth.
by Morton Walker, D.P.M., Bernice
Yaffee, R.N., and Parke H. Gray,
M.D.
1979, 316 pages, Illus.

from
Simon and Schuster
1230 Sixth Avenue
New York, NY 10020
$10.95 hd

This trio of health professionals from Stamford, Connecticut, has written a thoughtful and honest introduction to the many different kinds of maternity care available today. They are candid about the disadvantages of "non-participating" childbirth and present a reasonable discussion of controversial alternatives like home birth, lay midwives, acupuncture, and Leboyer birth. The book describes the differences among the Dick-Read, Lamaze, and Bradley methods of childbirth preparation and discusses prenatal yoga, hypnosis, birth centers, nurse-midwives, breastfeeding, bonding, cesarean section, and the common obstetrical interventions. An extensive set of appendices lists further reading, educational materials, and centers for childbirth education.

"Predictably, what intimidates some men at the outset of going into prepared childbirth classes is militant feminism. Their worry is that the techniques of unmedicated childbearing will in a way turn their wives more toward the women's liberation movement. Many husbands want no fires lit under their wives that will cause them to feel superior. They could not tolerate such an attitude. Consequently, a few men will feel suspicious of prepared childbirth classes and wonder if their women will be turned into those kinds of militant feminists.

"The various childbirth preparation techniques do raise a woman's realization of her own worth. Through having such a drugless experience, awake and aware, she comes to know that she is emotionally and physically tough. Such a realization may tend to threaten a lot of men.

"We suggest that attendance at childbirth preparation procedures should not scare you. Go ahead and find out if your male ego will be endangered. We know that it won't. Open your mind and grow as a couple from the experience. It is a worthwhile sharing—a labor of love."

Fetal Development

It is fascinating to think about what is going on inside a mother's body as her baby grows. Before this century, most people could only imagine how the embryo and fetus develop, though Leonardo DaVinci's illustration (on this page) is remarkably accurate. Now we are able to see inside the womb, mainly through drawings and photographs made of embryos and fetuses which were expelled prematurely, but also through photographs actually taken from within the living mother!

Being curious and learning about fetal growth and development is important in two ways. First, it helps us to realize how vulnerable the embryo and fetus are to poor diet and exposure to hazardous substances. The more we know about organ formation and development, the more careful we will be about our habits. Secondly, photographs and drawings can help us to visualize our unborn baby and contribute to the growing parent/infant bond which begins in pregnancy.

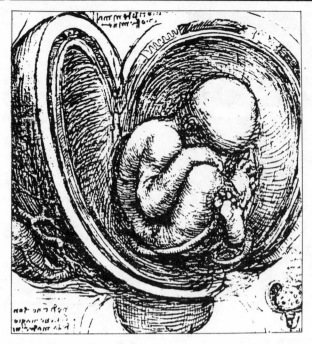

A CHILD IS BORN (Revised Edition)
by Axel Ingelman-Sundberg, Mirjam Furuhjelm, and Claes Wirsen
1977, 160 pages, Illus.

from
Delacorte Press
245 East 47th Street
New York, NY 10017
$11.95 hd

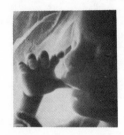

This lovely book was produced in Sweden and features the extraordinary photographs of embryos and fetuses taken by Lennart Nilsson. Interspersed with the story of fetal development, there are also many very charming photographs of what's going on "outside"—the mother's changing body, her prenatal visits, the father's role, the birth, and the new baby and family. It is especially nice to see that in Sweden, primarily women (with their smiling, empathetic faces) are in charge of prenatal care and delivery.

"Suck, grasp, and cling—these are the first necessary skills as one enters this world.

"Certain reflexes begin during the earliest fetal stage, as soon as the nerves have established connections with the developing muscles. Sucking and grasping reflexes are frequent. The legs kick and the arms wave. These reflexes increase in strength, and the impulse patterns of the nerves are gradually perfected. A thumb for comfort—yes, why not?

"The uterus is no silent, peaceful environment. The woman's pulse is constantly pounding; the placenta surges and murmurs; at times the woman moves abruptly, or speaks loudly."

THE FIRST NINE MONTHS OF LIFE
by Geraldine Lux Flanagan
1978, 96 pages, Illus.
(Published by Heinemann Medical Books, Ltd., London)

Distributed in the U.S. by
International Ideas Inc.
1627 Spruce Street
Philadelphia, PA 19103
$12.95 hd

This book was first published in England in 1963 and presents a very readable and literate overview of the science of embryology and what was then known about fetal development. It is illustrated with many black and white photographs of fetuses, including film sequences showing a fetus as young as seven weeks responding with motion to the stimulus of being stroked with a hair on its upper lip! There are also photographs showing the movements of babies born prematurely at six and seven months, demonstrating "the activities that are usually felt but not seen." Ms. Flanagan was for several years a science writer for *Life* magazine. Her prose is quite elegant and lends great dignity to her subject.

"We are the first generation to be able to have a clear picture of the course of our development from a single cell to an individual, active and responsive to our environment long before birth. We are also the first to know the full history of our earliest hours and days. The ripened human egg cell coming from the ovary was first seen in 1930. The union of the human parent cells, sperm and egg, was not observed until fourteen years later, in 1944. The events of our initial six days of life became known in the 1950's. Now in the 1960's we are finally beginning to decipher the intricate cell structures that shape our heredity."

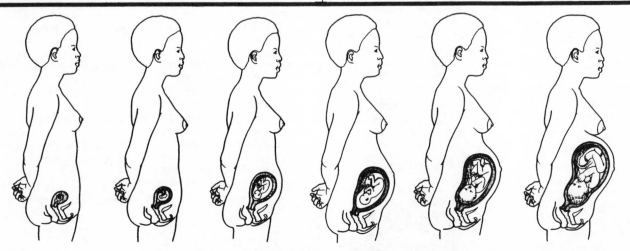

"The Development of the Pregnancy" from *The Childbirth Picture Book,* © 1981, 1982 Fran Hosken, drawings by Marcia L. Williams. Reprinted by permission.

DEVELOPMENT OF THE NORMAL HUMAN EMBRYO

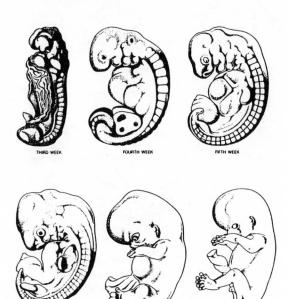

THIRD WEEK FOURTH WEEK FIFTH WEEK

SIXTH WEEK SEVENTH WEEK EIGHTH WEEK

Illustration reprinted from "The Thalidomide Syndrome" by Helen B. Taussig, (*Scientific American,* August, 1962). Available as a reprint for 60 cents each from W.H. Freeman and Co., 660 Market St., San Francisco, CA 94104

FROM CONCEPTION TO BIRTH:
The Drama of Life's Beginnings
by Roberts Rugh and Landrum B.
Shettles, M.D.
1971, 262 pages, Illus.

from
Harper and Row
10 East 53rd St.
New York, NY 10022
$19.95 hd.

The development of life, from the moment of conception (and even before, in the growth of the egg and sperm), is chronicled here in careful detail. Fine drawings and microscope photographs describe the processes of fertilization, cell division, implantation and embryonic development. Most startling, and sometimes a little frightening to look at, are the photographs, many in color, of human embryos and fetuses as they progress from strange, curled, fish-like beings to more human-looking small babies. In the early months of my first pregnancy, I had a great longing to know what the tiny fetus hidden deep inside me looked like. This book can help provide that "insight." Also included is an excellent, cautionary chapter on "Drugs, Disease, Radiation and the Fetus."

"During the first month after conception only the exceptional woman would be aware of the minute creature she is harboring. But in these 720 hours the embryo increases its size about 40-fold and its weight almost 3,000-fold. More remarkable than mere size or weight gain is the transformation of a single cell into an embryo with a head, a trunk, and the rudiments of organs, and the establishment of a close working association with the body of the mother. The embryo begins to form blood cells at seventeen days and a heart as early as eighteen days after the sperm invades the ovum. This embryonic heart, no more than a simple tube, starts a slow, irregular pulsation at 24 days which in one more week smooths into a rhythmic contraction and expansion. The heart eventually beats more than 100,000 times each day and will continue to do so, without interruption, for seventy, eighty, or maybe ninety years."

A BABY IS BORN: The Picture
Story of Everyman's Beginning
by the Maternity Center Association
1968, 64 pages, Illus.

from
Maternity Center Association
48 East 92nd Street
New York, NY 10028
$6.95 hd

First published in 1957 and now in its eleventh edition, A Baby is Born is an excellent graphic aid to understanding what is happening inside the pregnant woman's body. It includes the male and female reproductive anatomy, fertilization and fetal development, and the relation of the mother's organs to the growing uterus. It has two excellent series showing the baby moving through the birth canal in labor, both vertex (head first) and breech births. All the illustrations are in black and white, very detailed, and "easy" to look at, with a very good accompanying text. My three year old son very much enjoyed looking at this book while we awaited the birth of his sister.

"The family is the basic unit of human society. One of its functions is to pass life on from one generation to the next. When sperm and ovum unite, what follows in a woman's body, mind and feelings is only partly understood. Many of the questions which man has been asking about his beginnings for countless ages are still unanswered. But each year scientific investigations unravel more of the mystery of man's life before birth and suggest how it can be safeguarded . . . .

"The illustrations in this book are pictures of carefully prepared anatomical sculptures originally created for the Maternity Center Association by the famous doctor-sculptor team of Robert L. Dickinson and Abram Belskie who have achieved a feeling for life and growth unique in biological illustration."

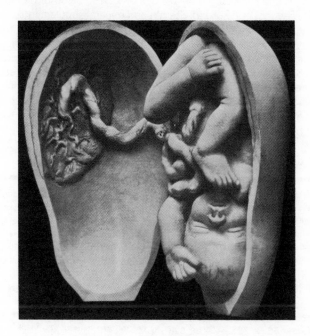

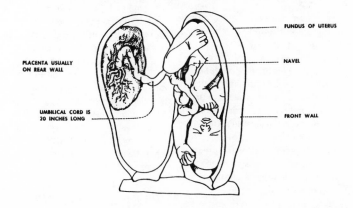

PLACENTA USUALLY
ON REAR WALL

UMBILICAL CORD IS
20 INCHES LONG

FUNDUS OF UTERUS

NAVEL

FRONT WALL

Nutrition in Pregnancy

Nutrition in pregnancy is a subject of some controversy and views have changed quite a lot in the last decade or so. Until quite recently, many obstetricians told pregnant women to restrict their calorie intake and weight gain and restrict their use of salt, under the false impression that these were related to the development of toxemia. The new, 1980 edition of *William's Obstetrics* now states that pregnant women should eat as much as they want, salt their food to taste, and gain at least twenty pounds during pregnancy. Unfortunately, many women still receive outdated advice on weight restriction from their doctors, and the medical profession as a whole still probably underestimates the role of nutrition in producing a healthy infant and mother. Most of the impetus for change has come from consumers and consumer organizations like SPUN (see this page).

Being advised to "eat as much as you like" is not helpful, of course, if your normal diet is poor. Women need to make sure that they gain their pregnancy weight by eating nutritious, wholesome foods. Pregnant women need adequate amounts of protein and essential vitamins and minerals and these are best provided by natural, unprocessed foods including milk, eggs, cheese, meats, whole grains, beans, fresh fruits, and vegetables. "Empty calorie" foods like candy, chips, and soda should be avoided or kept to an absolute minimum. The moderate use of vitamin and mineral supplements, including iron, is usually advised, but can't completely make up for a healthy diet. Teenagers, women who are underweight at the start of pregnancy, and women who've had two pregnancies close together need to be especially careful to get enough good food. Vegetarians need to be careful about getting adequate amounts of whole protein and may need to supplement their diets with Vitamin B12.

If you are pregnant or planning to be, now is the best time to develop healthy eating habits, the kind we should practice all our lives. Eating well in pregnancy is the first and most important gift you give your baby.

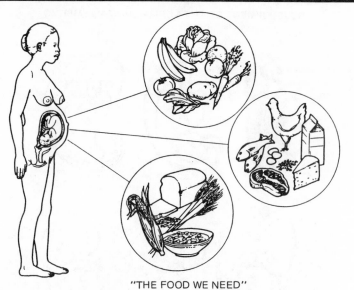

"THE FOOD WE NEED"

Illustration from *The Childbirth Picture Book*, ©1981, 1982 Fran Hosken, drawings by Marcia L. Williams. Available from Women's International Network (see index for listing). Reprinted by permission.

AS YOU EAT SO YOUR BABY GROWS: A Guide to Nutrition in Pregnancy
by Nikki Goldbeck
1980, 16 pages, Illus.

from
Ceres Press
P.O. Box 87
Woodstock, NY 12498
single copy $1.50 postpaid
bulk rates: 50 for $15., 100 for $26., 500 for $122.50

Nutrition may be the most important factor contributing to a healthy pregnancy, yet the subject is often neglected or given short shrift at prenatal visits. This handy booklet can help fill the gap. It provides basic information on dietary needs in pregnancy, including a discussion of protein (animal and vegetable sources), calcium, vitamins, iron, and salt. There are special tips for the pregnant teenager, a discussion of the importance of adequate weight gain, a daily diet guide, and sections on foods to avoid and food-related problems in pregnancy. Author Nikki

Goldbeck and her husband David have written several other books on food and nutrition (*The Supermarket Handbook, The Good Breakfast Book, Cooking What Comes Naturally*) and lecture frequently on these subjects.

"By using more non-animal sources of protein you will be able to fulfill this high protein requirement without overspending on the food budget, and at the same time limit the amount of saturated fat in your diet. Because many chemical residues including PCBs, PBBs, and dioxins are deposited in animal fat, limiting meat intake will also reduce the build-up of such chemicals in the pregnant woman's body. These chemicals are transferred through the placenta and breast milk, and until the effects on the newborn can be determined, pregnant women should make an extra effort to minimize their presence."

SOCIETY FOR THE PROTECTION OF THE UNBORN THROUGH NUTRITION (SPUN)

SPUN *was* a national educational organization founded in 1972 and dedicated to improving maternal and infant health by the establishment of scientific standards for nutrition management in standard prenatal care.

Unfortunately, while this *Catalog* was in production SPUN announced that it would cease operations as of September 1982, due to lack of money. In addition to holding seminars and providing direct nutrition counseling to women, SPUN published many excellent fact sheets and pamphlets on nutrition in pregnancy. Two of these are reproduced in this section (see "Nutrition Quiz" and "A Healthy Pregnancy Diet"). I was so sorry to see these materials go out of distribution that I made arrangements with SPUN to reprint a selection of their materials in a special issue of *Child-*

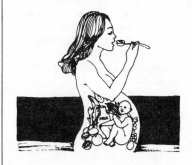

birth Alternatives Quarterly (see index for review). Included will be "Pregnant? and Want a Healthy Child?," "Professional's Flow Chart of Consequences of Prenatal Malnutrition" and others. Regular subscribers will receive this issue when it is published and others may order a single copy for $2.00. Bulk rates will be available. For more information contact: Childbirth Alternatives Quarterly, c/o Janet Isaacs Ashford, editor, Bin 62, S.L.A.C., Stanford, CA 94305.

Dr. Tom Brewer, author of *Metabolic Toxemia of Late Pregnancy* (new, revised edition, Keats Publishing, 1982) was on the board of directors of SPUN and contributed to many of its publications. Dr. Brewer and his wife, Gail Sforza Brewer (editor and co-author of *The Pregnancy-After-30 Workbook* and *Right From the Start,* both reviewed in this *Catalog*) continue their work in pregnancy nutrition through the: Nutrition Action Group, P.O. Box 124, Bedford Hills, NY 10507.

"Children born to inadequately nourished mothers of all socio-economic groups have been shown to have significantly higher rates of neurological dysfunction, mental retardation, motor incoordination and learning disabilities. In clinics and private offices where correct nutrition counseling is an essential feature of ongoing care during pregnancy, the incidence of metabolic toxemia of late pregnancy and prematurity/lowered birth weight (excellent indicators of maternal and infant health) are remarkably low."

—from SPUN literature

WHAT EVERY PREGNANT
WOMAN SHOULD KNOW: The
Truth About Diet and Drugs in
Pregnancy
by Gail Sforza Brewer with
Thomas Brewer, M.D.
1979, 239 pages

from
Penguin
625 Madison Avenue
New York, NY 10022
$3.50 pap.

Restricting weight gain, banning
salt, and using diuretics (drugs which
increase frequency of urination)—
these are the major hazards in prenatal care, according to Gail and Tom
Brewer. Dr. Brewer has spent many
years studying the development of
metabolic toxemia in pregnancy,
and he is convinced that the very
means often used to prevent it are in
fact the *cause*. And in addition to
jeopardizing the health of the mother, drugs and faulty diets can also
damage the baby and reduce its birth
weight. The Brewers are dedicated
advocates of a safer approach. They
have contributed much to the work
of SPUN (see page 6) and to the
pregnancy diet and nutrition quiz
reprinted in this section. Their book
carefully outlines the dangers of
weight and salt restriction and warns
women about accepting advice from
physicians who very probably have
had no formal training in nutrition.
Also included is an excellent selection of sample pregnancy menus and
recipes.

"As it stands now, most doctors
have never taken a course in applied
human nutrition. No medical school
in the United States requires such a
course of its students . . . .

"Doctors currently in training
need to learn about the protective
benefits of sound pregnancy nutrition. Just as important, doctors already practicing must also be educated and begin to apply the scientific
research in nutrition to routine prenatal care.

"In this they have much to learn
from ranchers, farmers and veterinar-
ians who are taught the importance
of breeding pregnant animals scientifically. They know exactly what con-
stitutes a healthful diet for a pregnant cow, sheep or horse. And they
enthusiastically put into practice
what they know. They have to.
Some cows are worth $5,000 apiece!
Is a pregnant woman as valuable as
a cow? . . ."

Circle the letter corresponding to the
correct answer:

1. **Pregnancy Creates A Nutritional
   Stress For:**
   a) Women under age 18.
   b) Women in poverty.
   c) Women who are pregnant for the
      first time.
   d) Every pregnant woman.

2. **Nausea or Vomiting in Early
   Pregnancy Is Best Helped By:**
   a) Following a liquid diet.
   b) Eating wheat crackers upon rising
      and six small meals a day.
   c) Not eating at all.
   d) Taking an antacid to settle the
      stomach.

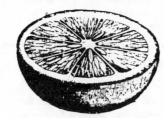

3. **A Pregnant Woman Should Cut
   Down On Her Salt Intake:**
   a) As soon as she knows she's preg-
      nant.
   b) If she gains too much weight.
   c) As soon as she has swelling of her
      hands or face.
   d) None of the above.

4. **Pregnancy Creates A Stress Because Of:**
   a) The development of the placenta
      and the baby, the expanded blood
      volume, and the increased demand
      on the liver.
   b) Additional weight gain.
   c) Inability to sleep well and other
      discomforts.
   d) Social adjustments.

5. **Complications During Pregnancy
   Are Least Likely To Occur When
   The Mother:**
   a) Follows her doctor's advice.
   b) Takes her prenatal vitamins reg-
      ularly.
   c) Eats a nutritious diet all through
      pregnancy.
   d) Gains at least 24 to 27 pounds.

6. **The Major Cause Of Low Birth
   Weight (Under 5½ Pounds) Is:**
   a) Inadequate diet during pregnancy.
   b) Small mother and/or father.
   c) Drinking alcoholic beverages
      during pregnancy.
   d) Smoking during pregnancy.

7. **Babies Weighing Under 5½
   Pounds At Birth Are Much
   More Likely To Have:**
   a) Deformities.

NUTRITION QUIZ

from SPUN (see page 6)
Reprinted with permission.

---

   b) Learning disability or hyper-
      activity.
   c) Cerebral palsy.
   d) All of the above.

8. **The Health Of Mothers And
   Their Unborn Babies Is Greatly
   Influenced By:**
   a) Fetal monitoring.
   b) Ultrasound (a device that deter-
      mines the size and position of
      the baby).
   c) Good nutrition during pregnancy.
   d) The mother's age.

9. **When A Pregnant Woman Gains
   Weight Rapidly, The Doctor
   Should:**
   a) Place her on a low-calorie diet.
   b) Ask her what she's been eating.
   c) Restrict her salt intake.
   d) All of the above.

10. **Some Women Cannot Tolerate
    Milk Because:**
    a) Many people over 18 cannot
       drink milk.
    b) They are of an ethnic group be-
       lieved to be unable to digest milk.
    c) Not drinking milk on a regular
       basis creates a lack of a substance
       that helps them digest milk.
    d) None of the above.

11. **Poor Nutrition During Pregnancy
    Can Cause:**
    a) Abruption of the placenta.
    b) Brain damage in the fetus.
    c) Long and difficult labor and
       delivery.
    d) All of the above.

12. **Diuretics (Water Pills) Taken
    During Pregnancy Can:**
    a) Drain the mother of nutrients
       needed to nourish her baby and
       can cause toxemia of pregnancy.
    b) Effectively treat swelling.
    c) Prevent high blood pressure.
    d) All of the above.

13. **Swelling Of The Hands And Face
    In Pregnancy May Be Caused By:**
    a) Gaining too much weight.
    b) Too much salt.
    c) Not enough protein or calories
       in the diet.
    d) All of the above.

14. **Most Cases Of Brain Damage In
    Babies Are Caused By:**
    a) Difficulties at the time of birth.
    b) Malnutrition during pregnancy.

   c) The genetic make-up of the
      parents.
   d) Unknown causes.

**Circle the following T(True) or F
(False):**

T F 15. The best diet for pregnan-
        cy is high in protein and
        low in calories.

T F 16. Vitamin A helps protect
        both the mother and her
        baby from severe infec-
        tions during pregnancy.

T F 17. Babies under 5½ pounds
        are the easiest to deliver.

T F 18. Two eggs and a quart of
        milk every day form the
        foundation of a good diet
        during pregnancy.

T F 19. A prenatal diet that is low
        in protein, calories, or
        salt can cause high blood
        pressure.

T F 20. In the United States, a
        course in applied nutrition
        is required for all medical
        students.

T F 21. Iron and vitamin pills pre-
        vent anemias during preg-
        nancy.

T F 22. The level of increased hor-
        monal activity during
        pregnancy is comparable
        to that of 100 birth con-
        trol pills a day.

T F 23. Mothers pregnant with
        twins should expect them
        to be born ahead of time
        and to weigh less than
        5½ pounds each.

T F 24. If a pregnant woman gets
        hypertension (high blood
        pressure) for the first
        time, she should reduce
        her salt intake.

T F 25. Except in rare cases, preg-
        nant women should not
        take any drugs.

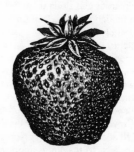

1)D 2)B 3)D 4)A 5)C
6)A 7)D 8)C 9)B 10)C
11)D 12)A 13)C 14)B 15)F
16)T 17)F 18)T 19)T 20)F
21)F 22)T 23)T 24)F 25)T

NUTRITION FOR THE CHILD-BEARING YEAR
by Jacqueline Gibson Gazella
1980, 173 pages, Illus.

from
Woodland Publishing Company
230 Manitoba Avenue
Wayzata, MN 55391
$8.95 pap.

Ms. Gazella is a certified nurse-midwife and a childbirth educator. Her book includes information on the importance of prenatal nutrition, essential nutrients, fetal hazards, the selection and preparation of food, nutrition during lactation, plus a listing of helpful resources and a bibliography. Included are complete menu plans for six weeks and 137 recipes.

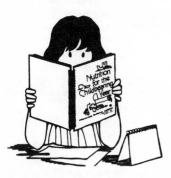

"Probably the most common fallacy about pregnancy nutrition is that one should limit weight gain to unwarranted levels. Adequate weight gain is essential to a good pregnancy outcome. It used to be thought that excess weight gain caused a condition called toxemia, characterized by increased blood pressure, inordinate swelling, and protein in the urine, and in the final states, convulsions. This concept was so widespread and accepted that care providers may still instruct you along these lines, even though the American College of Obstetricians and Gynecologists has explicitly stated that this is an incorrect concept. Studies have shown that increased weight gain does not have a causative effect on toxemia. To the contrary, there is a greater incidence of toxemia among underweight women who fail to gain weight adequately during pregnancy. The quality of the diet is important, however. Gaining weight on a sound diet consisting of the Basic Four is different from gaining weight on sugar, fat and white flour. Women with diets coded 'poor' or 'fair' have a high incidence of toxemia whereas women on diets coded 'good' or 'excellent' have a very low incidence of the disease."

WHEN FOOD IS LOVE
by Margot Edwards
1977, 4 pages

from
the pennypress
1100 23rd Avenue East
Seattle, WA 98112
single copy, 50 cents
bulk orders, $20. per 100

Part of the **Better Baby Series** (see index), this flyer provides good, concise information on our needs for protein, minerals, carbohydrates, fruits, and vegetables in pregnancy. There is also a section for vegetarians, advice on constipation, and a diet for breastfeeding.

"A pregnant woman needs to know that new medical views exist about weight gain and the use of table salt. There are more liberal attitudes toward both the use of salt and the pounds that you put on than there were a few years ago. Salt restriction is no longer considered necessary to prevent swelling. According to Dr. Tom Brewer, salt is necessary during pregnancy to maintain the larger blood volume needed to nourish the baby, and a gain of 25 to 30 pounds is insurance against the possibility of having a low birth weight baby. Your body build and tendency to put on weight will affect your rate of gain. Restrictive diets are not advisable at any time during pregnancy. According to one medical doctor, you should double the amount of protective foods—milk, eggs, fish, meat, leafy greens, whole grains, and legumes—and cut the sweets and pastry in half."

A HEALTHY PREGNANCY DIET
from SPUN (see page 6)

When you are pregnant, you need more of good quality foods than when you are not pregnant. To meet your own needs and those of your developing baby, you must have, *every day,* at least:

1. One quart (four glasses) of milk— any kind: whole milk, low fat, skim, powdered skim or buttermilk. If you do not like milk, you can substitute one cup of yoghurt for each cup of milk.

2. Two eggs.

3. Two servings of fish, shellfish, chicken or turkey, lean beef, veal, lamb, pork, liver, or kidney.

    Alternative combinations include:
    Rice with: beans, cheese, sesame seeds, milk
    Cornmeal with: beans, cheese, tofu, milk
    Beans with: rice, bulgar, cornmeal, wheat noodles, sesame seeds, milk
    Peanuts with: sunflower seeds, milk
    Whole wheat bread or noodles with: beans, cheese, peanut butter, tofu, milk

    For each serving of meat, you can substitute these quantities of cheese:

Brick	— 4 oz.
Camembert	— 6 oz.
Cheddar	— 3 oz.
Cottage	— 6 oz.
Longhorn	— 3 oz.
Muenster	— 4 oz.
Monterey Jack	— 4 oz.
Swiss	— 3 oz.

4. Two servings of fresh, green leafy vegetables: mustard, beet, collard, dandelion or turnip greens, spinach, lettuce, cabbage, broccoli, kale, Swiss chard.

5. Five servings of whole-grain breads, rolls, cereals, or pancakes: Wheatena, bran flakes, granola, shredded wheat, wheat germ, oatmeal, buckwheat or whole wheat pancakes, corn bread, corn tortillas, corn or bran or whole wheat muffins, waffles, brown rice.

6. Two choices from: a whole potato (any style), large green pepper, orange, grapefruit, lemon, lime, papaya, tomato (one piece of fruit or one large glass of juice)

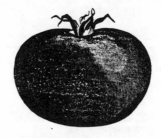

7. Three pats of margarine, vitamin A-enriched, or butter, or oil.

Also include in your diet:

8. A yellow-or orange-colored vegetable or fruit five times a week

9. Liver once a week, if you like it.

10. Table salt: SALT YOUR FOOD TO TASTE

11. Water: drink to thirst

It is not healthy for you and your unborn baby to go even 24 hours without good food!

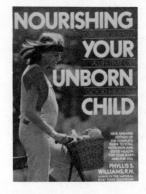

NOURISHING YOUR UNBORN CHILD
(Rev. Ed.)
by Phyllis S. Williams
1982, 288 pages

from
Avon Books
959 Eighth Avenue
New York, NY 10019
$4.95 pap.

This no-nonsense book, written by a pediatric nurse, describes the evolution of diet advice in our country and calls for a shift from the "negative"(telling women *not* to eat) to the "positive" (telling women *what* to eat). Also included are discussions of drug hazards and the effects of illness in pregnancy, and a large section of sample menus and recipes.

"Unless the *positive* is stressed throughout pregnancy—the foods that *must* be eaten to insure an adequate diet—nutritional deficiencies will continue. Perhaps we will find that when the nagging changes from 'Mrs. Doe, you've gained eight pounds this month—you've got to cut down,' to 'Mrs. Doe, have you been eating the way you are supposed to eat? Have you been eating plenty of milk, meat and fish, eggs and cheese, green and yellow vegetables, citrus fruits and whole grains every day?' then and only then will the problem be solved.

"A prescription for nutrition and nutrition training should be issued to every woman at the start of her pregnancy. Until the nation is retrained, the importance of following that prescription should be stressed and restressed at each visit. Each aspect of diet should be dealt with specifically. In the clinics, dietary evaluations should be carried out and foods which are needed *must* be made available to *every* poor pregnant woman along with training for their preparation and use. Only in this way will we be able to eliminate an important cause of learning problems, retardation, stunted growth, and poverty."

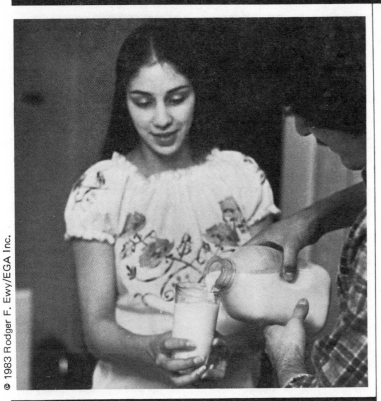

RECIPE FOR HEALTHY BABIES
by the March of Dimes
1980, 8-panel pamphlet

from
March of Dimes
1275 Mamoroneck
White Plains, NY 10506
single copy free

This pamphlet includes information on weight gain, helpful hints, a day's sample menu, and beautiful color photographs of foods in the four basic food groups. Unfolded to its full 8½ by 16-inch size, this pamphlet could be taped to the refrigerator as a colorful reminder to eat well during pregnancy.

VEGETARIAN PRENATAL NUTRITION AND HIGH PROTEIN RECIPES
by Margaret Nofziger
1977, 14 pages, Illus.

from
The Farm (see index)
The Book Publishing Company
156 Drakes Lane
Summertown, TN 38483
single copy free
(please include S.A.S.E.)

This pamphlet is excerpted from *The Farm Vegetarian Cookbook* It includes information on "Taking Care of Yourself While You're Pregnant" and sample recipes based on soybeans as the major source of protein.

"The Farm is a large longhair spiritual community of 1100 people in Tennessee... We are all complete vegetarians. Ours is a soy-based vegetarian diet....

"We have midwives who give prenatal care with nutrition instruction, and deliver our babies at home naturally.

"Here are our best high-protein recipes. This is what we eat and our babies are big and healthy.

"Good nutrition is the basis of a healthy body at any time. It is especially important that you are well-nourished during pregnancy, because you are also responsible for the good healthy body of another person. When the mother is well-nourished, there are fewer miscarriages, premature babies, and complications of pregnancy and delivery. A lot of new tissues are being formed and maintained during pregnancy, so naturally there is an increased need for all the essential nutrients."

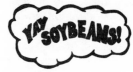

SOYBURGERS

Drain 5 cups of cooked soybeans through a colander or strainer. Mash the beans with a potato masher and add while mashing:

2 tsp. salt
3/4 - 1 cup whole wheat flour
1/2 tsp. pepper
2 tsp. garlic powder
2 tsp. oregano
1 tsp. basil
1 onion, finely chopped
1 green pepper, finely chopped
(optional) -----

Mix well. The batter should be quite stiff. To make patties, roll mix into a small ball, larger than a golf ball but smaller than a tennis ball. Then flatten the ball to 1/2 inch thick. Thin patties make better burgers because they stay crisp. Thick patties don't get done so well in the middle. Fry in a generous amount of oil so they'll be crisp. Makes 16 soyburgers.

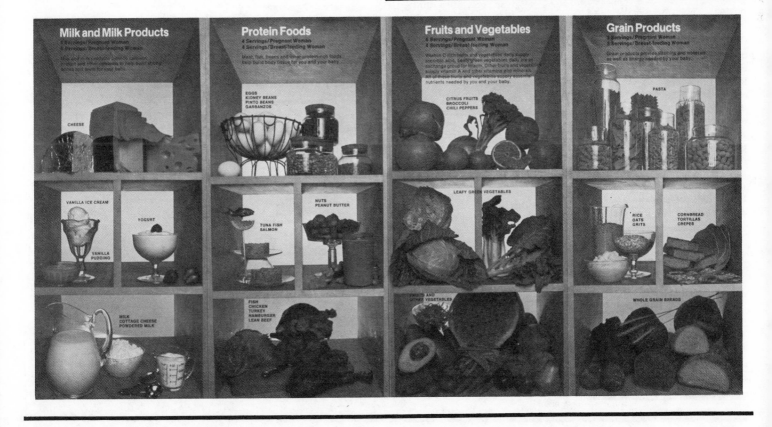

Drugs and Hazards

It is saddening to have to include a section on drugs and hazards in a book on childbirth. The world should be a safe place in which to grow a baby. Unfortunately, it is not. Most of the hazards described in the following pages are recent and man-made. They result from industrialization, environmental pollution, and also, significantly, from the medical profession and drug industries. Some hazards can be avoided, others cannot. We can control our own personal habits and use of dangerous substances like alcohol, caffeine, tobacco, and medical drugs and devices. It's not always possible, though, to control our exposure to hazards which have become imbedded in our environment and in the food chain. The drinking water, air, soil, and all the food we eat are contaminated to some degree. In fact, when thinking about what foods to eat for a healthy pregnancy, we have to consider not only their nutrient value, but their probable levels of contamination by pesticides, PCB's, etc. (For this reason, some people advise pregnant and lactating women to reduce their intake of animal products, especially those high in fat—whole milk, butter cheese, eggs, meat—since these are more likely to be contaminated than foods lower in the food chain.)

To make the uterine world a safer place for your baby right now, do what you can to reduce your own personal exposure to the drugs and hazards you can control. To make the world a safer place for yourself, your children, and future generations, join with others in political action to stop pollution and the promotion of unnecessary and harmful drugs.

HOW THE FDA DETERMINES THE "SAFETY" OF DRUGS—JUST HOW SAFE IS "SAFE"?
by Doris Haire
1980, 8 pages

from
American Foundation for Maternal and Child Health
30 Beekman Place
New York, NY 10022
$1.00

Doris Haire chairs the committee on Health Law and Regulation of the National Women's Health Network, which co-sponsored this report. She has worked for many years to help make childbirth safer for mothers and babies and her monograph, *The Cultural Warping of Childbirth* (see Index) is a classic in the literature. In this new report on the FDA, Ms. Haire sets out to let us know exactly how *inadequate* the regulations are which are supposed to protect us from adverse effects of drugs and medical devices. She points out that when the FDA says "safe" it does not mean "free from harm or injury" as dictionaries define the term, but safe in a very relative sense, based on the FDA's evaluation of the known or potential risks of a drug. "The Director of the FDA's Bureau of Drugs has confirmed in writing that the FDA does not guarantee the safety of any drug—not even those drugs which the FDA has officially approved as safe," says Haire.

What does this mean for pregnant women? It means that you cannot depend upon drug information supplied to you by the government, the manufacturer or your doctor. It means that you must assume that even drugs which are commonly considered "safe" may not be. It means that you can never take drugs during pregnancy, or during labor, with complete confidence that your baby will not be harmed. Any decision to use drugs must be considered very carefully. Is the benefit worth the possible risks? We should ask our doctor and druggist for as much information as they have, but evaluate it carefully and not consider it as absolutely accurate.

CARING FOR YOUR UNBORN CHILD
by Ronald Gots and Barbara Gots
1977, 276 pages, Illus.

from
Stein and Day
Scarborough House
Briarcliff Manor, NY 10510
$8.95 hd.

The authors of this book are both doctors and the parents together of two children. They are quite serious in their intent to educate women about the hazards of faulty diet and drug use in pregnancy, and quite aware of the limitations of much of the advice given on these subjects by physicians. *No drugs have been proven safe for childbearing women*—this alarm is sounded again and again throughout the book. And yet doctors continue to prescribe and women continue to consume prescription and over-the-counter drugs during pregnancy and labor, without knowing what the risks may be. Any woman who is concerned about giving birth to a healthy, perfect baby should read this book. She will learn how the baby grows and is nourished, what to eat, and how drugs, infections, and environmental hazards may affect her baby. There is also an excellent discussion of the risks of drugs used in labor and delivery and an appendix which lists the known or suspected adverse effects of over 100 common drugs.

"A great many drugs, viruses, poisons from the atmosphere, and chemical food additives can pass into the baby as readily as foods and gases—something we have learned quite recently. Scientists used to believe that there was a so-called 'placental barrier'—a kind of an armed fortress that differentiated between good things and bad, letting the good things pass while barring the bad ones. It is true that some substances are destroyed by the placenta and that others are unable to get through. But many things that we would like to keep out slip through easily. For those drugs and chemicals that have been studied, the 'placental barrier' is more like a wide-holed sieve: the vast majority pass effortlessly into the baby. As we will see later, many of these intruders are staunch fetal enemies."

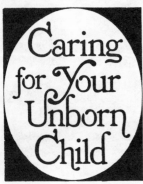

TO MEN

When we speak of drug hazards and birth defects, we are usually speaking to women, who carry the developing fetus in their bodies for nine months. But men should know that the drugs and environmental or workplace hazards which damage the fetus can also damage sperm. If you are planning to father a child, you need to think about your own drug habits and history of exposure to chemicals at work.

Smoking tobacco and marijuana and heavy use of alcohol have been linked to human sperm damage. In the workplace, Kepone, Sevin, and DBCP (all pesticides), lead, anesthetic nitrous oxide, and radiation are all linked to sperm damage. In some industries women of childbearing age are barred from jobs involving the use of these substances. But evidence is mounting that sperm are just as vulnerable to damage as women's ova or the fetus. So men also need to be protected from exposure to hazardous substances.

Sperm damage can lead to a low sperm count, infertility, and an increase in miscarriages and birth defects. For more information see the sections on Environmental and Workplace Hazards.

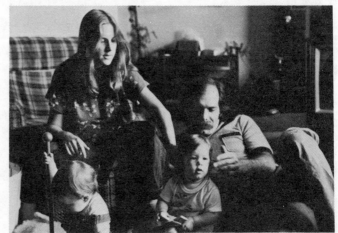

J.I.A.

MOTHERING YOUR UNBORN BABY
By David W. Smith, M.D.
1979, 97 pages, Illus.

from
W.B. Saunders Co.
West Washington Square
Philadelphia, PA 19105
$6.95 pap.

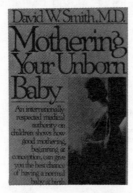

David Smith is a professor of pediatrics at the University of Washington School of Medicine and director of the School's Dysmorphology Unit (study of the abnormal development of form). Many of the children he sees in his work suffer from developmental problems which resulted not from genetics but from environmental factors in pregnancy which could have been prevented. "It is the environmental ones which I am most loath to see. I cannot escape that feeling 'if only this woman had known, this child would not have this problem.' " In this book he sets out to explain the normal processes of pregnancy and fetal development and show how deficiencies in diet, use of drugs, illnesses, radiation, hyperthermia (high body heat), and other factors can cause them to go awry. His discussion is illuminated by many fine drawings, including sketches of the characteristic patterns of facial malformation associated with specific, harmful drugs.

"In order to provide good mothering from conception, it is obviously best to have a planned pregnancy. With an unplanned pregnancy, you may not know that you are pregnant until the developing baby is three to seven weeks old. You may have already passed through the most critical period of directly mothering your unborn baby before you are aware that you are pregnant. During this time you may have been to a celebration such as a New Year's party and taken more alcoholic drinks than than you would have if you had a planned pregnancy—and were more consciously mothering the unborn baby . . . ."

This black and white poster (17" x 22") is available free from the Dept. of Health and Human Services, Public Health Service, Food and Drug Administration, 5600 Fishers Lane, Rockville, MD 20857. Request HHS Publication No. 80-3096.

DRUGS AND PREGNANCY
by Pauline Postotnik
1978, 4 pages
(HHS Pub. No (FDA) 80-3083)

WHEN THE BABY'S LIFE IS SO MUCH YOUR OWN . . .
by Margaret Morrison
1979, 4 pages
(HHS Pub. No. (FDA) 79-1057)

from
Dept. of Health and Human Services
Public Health Service
Food and Drug Administration
5600 Fishers Lane
Rockville, MD 20857
single copy free

These two pamphlets are both reprints of articles from *FDA Consumer,* a publication of the Food and Drug Administration. They contain essentially the same material on the importance of avoiding unnecessary drugs, x-rays, and other procedures during pregnancy. The FDA knows only too well that most drugs and procedures used in childbearing "have not been tested specifically for safety during human pregnancy."

These articles caution against the use of sex hormones (estrogens and progestin), tetracycline antibiotics, barbiturates, amphetamines, and tranquilizers, live vaccines, alcohol, tobacco, caffeine, diuretics, anesthetics, elective induction of labor, Demerol, and electronic fetal monitoring.

"Whatever else you do during pregnancy, few things are quite as important to your unborn child as the proper use of medicines or drugs. Many drugs can be taken safely during pregnancy. But some cannot. No medicine of any kind should be taken except as you are advised by your physician—and this includes over-the-counter drugs for such minor ills as colds, coughs, nervousness, insomnia, and so forth. Science does not know everything yet about the effects of drugs on the unborn child, so the best rule is to use medicine only when absolutely necessary, and always under a doctor's instruction."

from *When the Baby's Life is So Much Your Own.*

DRUGS IN PREGNANCY

Many commonly used drugs, both over-the-counter drugs and prescription drugs, can cause birth defects or other adverse effects to the fetus or the mother. Some of these drugs are listed below along with their known or suspected effects. For more information on the use and abuse of drugs in pregnancy, see the other resources listed in this section. In pregnancy, the best policy is to take *no* drugs at all.

Alcohol in excess (miscarriage, stillbirth, brain and heart defects, cleft palate, lower birth weight)
Amphetamines (heart defects, blood malformations)
Antihistamines (various anomalies)
Aspirin (miscarriage, fetal hemorrhage, postpartum hemorrhage)
Barbiturates (addiction in fetus)
Birth Control Pills (anomalous genitalia, limb defects, cancer)
Caffeine in excess (cleft palate)
Certain Herbs (cohosh, pennyroyal, mugwort, tansy, slippery elm may cause miscarriage)
Phenobarbital (a sedative used for morning sickness, may cause neonatal bleeding)
Quinine (limb defects, congenital deafness, thrombocytopenia)
Radioactive Iodine (from nuclear fallout, may cause hypothyroidism)
Steroid Hormones (androgens, progestins, estrogens may cause masculinization of the fetus)
Streptomycin (congenital deafness)
Sulfonamides (kernicterus, a form of jaundice)
Tetracycline antibiotics (congenital cataract, inhibition of bone growth, staining of deciduous teeth)
Tobacco Smoking (miscarriage, stillbirth, prematurity, abruptio placenta, placenta previa, Rh disease, heart malformations, sudden infant death syndrome, low birth weight, shorter stature)
Tranquilizers (Valium, Librium, Miltown, Equinil may cause cleft lip or palate and various other anomalies)
Vaccinations (various anomalies)
Vitamin A (in excess can cause eye damage and cleft palate)
Vitamin C (in excess of about 1 gram a day can cause neonatal scurvy)
Vitamin D (in excess can cause mental retardation, supravalvar syndrome)
Vitamin K (in excess can cause kernicterus and hemolysis)
X-rays (leukemia)
Miscellaneous toxic substances (automobile exhaust and the fumes from lead paint, cleaning fluid, contact cement, lacquer thinner, benzene, oven cleaner, and some household glues can cause various anomalies)

WOMEN AND SMOKING
by Jane E. Brody and Richard
Enquist
1972, 24 pages, Illus.

from
Public Affairs Pamphlets
381 Park Avenue South
New York, NY 10016
single copy, 50 cents
request bulk rates and catalog

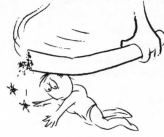

Jane Brody writes the "Personal
Health" column for the New York
Times. In this pamphlet she and her
husband, Richard Enquist, present
the facts on smoking in plain language including the effects of smoking in pregnancy and on children.

"Doctors have often observed
that smoking mothers tend to have
smaller babies than do nonsmoking
mothers, and careful scientific studies both in the United States and in
other countries have borne out this
observation. On the average, babies
born to smoking mothers weigh five
to eight ounces less than those borne
by women who abstain from smoking
during pregnancy. The smaller babies, as a rule, have more difficulty
getting a good start in life than those
of normal birthweight, and indeed
the babies of smoking mothers have
been found to be more likely to die
within the first year of life."

CLEARING THE AIR: A Guide to
Quitting Smoking
Office of Cancer Communications
1981, 36 pages

from
Office of Cancer Communications
National Cancer Institute
Bethesda, MD 20205

"There is no one magic way for
everybody to quit smoking. But
there are a great many effective ways.
If at first you don't succeed, quit
and quit again!" This booklet lists
many of the effective ways to quit
smoking.

New evidence from the United
States Collaborative Perinatal Project
indicates that smoking has negative
effects on pregnancy even when wom-
en quit smoking *before* becoming
pregnant. Dr. Richard Naeye, head
pathologist for the study, advises
women who plan to have children to
give up smoking as early as possible
before conception. For more information contact the National Institutes of Health, Div. of Public Information, Bethesda, MD 20205.

NO SMOKING: FETAL GROWTH
IN PROGRESS
by the International Childbirth
Education Association (ICEA)
8½ x 11-inch sign, blue lettering on
white card

from
ICEA Bookcenter (see index)
P.O. Box 20048
Minneapolis, MN 55420
single copy, 25 cents
request bulk rates

Put this sign up at home or at work to remind yourself and others that
cigarette smoke, even second-hand smoke, is not good for your health
or that of your unborn baby.

NO SMOKING
Fetal Growth
in Progress

ALCOHOL, TOBACCO, CAFFEINE
AND PREGNANCY
by Mary Ann Holtz
1981, pamphlet

from
Do It Now Foundation
P.O. Box 5115
Phoenix, AZ 85010
20 cents each plus 50 cents minimum postage
bulk rates available

This simply written pamphlet is
designed for reading levels of 8th
grade and up and is one of a series

SMOKING FOR TWO: Cigarettes
and Pregnancy
by Peter A. Fried and Harry Oxorn
1980, 146 pages

from
The Free Press
A Division of Macmillan Publishing
866 Third Avenue
New York, NY 10022
$10.95 hd.

Fried and Oxorn consider many
of the aspects of pregnancy and
smoking, including the effects of
second-hand smoke, constituents of
cigarette smoke, and the effects of
smoking on maternal weight gain,
the placenta, complications of pregnancy, birth weight, fetal growth
and prematurity, the effects of smoking on the newborn, breastfeeding
and smoking, and long-term effects.

THE PREGNANT SMOKER:
Hazards to Fetal and Maternal
Health
Edited by Susan McKay
1978, 8 pages

from
ICEA Bookcenter
P.O. Box 20048
Minneapolis, MN 55420
$1.00 plus 60 cents postage

This Fall/Winter 1978 issue of
ICEA Review provides an introduction, recommendations, commentary, and abstracts of nine journal
articles on the effects of smoking
during pregnancy.

"Those who work in prenatal
programs can today assess their own
settings and actions. For example
... is there follow-up on smoking
behavior throughout the pregnancy
or is the question only raised at that
all-encompassing initial prenatal
visit? Are antismoking activities undermined by the presence of ash
trays in offices or by staff who
smoke? Is there room on the medical chart to record amounts smoked
along with monthly weight gain and
blood pressure?"

of publications on drugs, alcohol,
and health published by Do It Now
Foundation.

"Mothers who smoke greatly increase their chances of complications
in pregnancy, including those that
can bring on pre-term birth. Nearly
14 percent of all pre-term births in
the U.S. may be caused by maternal
smoking. Complications of pregnancy can include placental damage,
bleeding, premature rupture of membranes and pre-term delivery, all of
which increases the risk of fetal or
infant death."

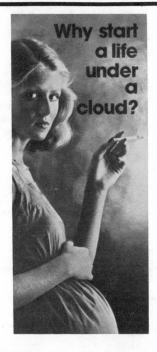

WHY START A LIFE UNDER A
CLOUD?
by the American Cancer Society
1979, brochure

from
American Cancer Society
777 Third Avenue
New York, NY 10017
single copy free
request bulk rates

Whenever I see a pregnant woman smoking a cigarette in a supermarket or restaurant, I want to walk
right up to her and tell her to stop!
Usually I don't. But maybe we
should all carry a few extra copies
of this flyer to give to smoking
mothers.

"If you're pregnant or planning
a family, here are three good reasons to quit smoking now.
1. Smoking retards the growth
of your baby in your womb.
2. Smoking increases the incidence of infant mortality.
3. Your family needs a healthy
mother."

SHOULD I DRINK?
by The National Institute on Alcohol Abuse and Alcoholism
1980, brochure
DHHS Pub. No. (ADM) 80-919

from
National Institute on Alcohol Abuse and Alcoholism
5600 Fishers Lane
Rockville, MD 20857
single copy free

This fold-out brochure features minority women, simple language and diagrams to explain why alcohol is harmful to the developing fetus. The NIAAA publishes alcohol re-lated pamphlets, books, posters, and other materials which are distributed free in single copies or in bulk by the

National Clearinghouse for Alcohol Information
Box 2345
Rockville, MD 20852

Publications available include:
Should I Drink?
Alcohol and Your Unborn Baby
My Baby Will Be Strong (poster)
Alcohol as a Risk Factor in Pregnancy
Fetal Alcohol Syndrome and Teratogenic Effects of Alcohol

Should I drink?

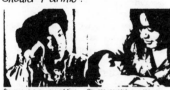

Pregnancy is a very special time. You wonder at times if your baby will be normal.
You can increase your chances of having a healthy baby.

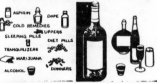

Be extremely careful about taking drugs. They can hurt your baby.
You may not think of alcohol as a drug because it is so popular.

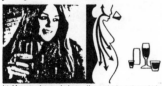

What happens when you drink wine with a meal, beer while watching TV or whiskey at a party?
You are taking a drug which slows down your brain and body actions.

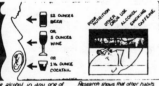

The alcohol in any one of these drinks can harm your baby.
Research shows that other habits can harm your baby. Together these can cause greater risks.

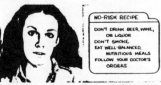

NO-RISK RECIPE
DON'T DRINK BEER, WINE, OR LIQUOR
DON'T SMOKE.
EAT WELL-BALANCED, NUTRITIOUS MEALS
FOLLOW YOUR DOCTOR'S ORDERS

What should you do about drinking during your pregnancy?
This is your safest approach.

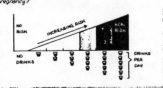

As you increase the number of drinks per day, you
also increase the risk to your unborn baby.

→ MUSCLE DISEASE
→ HEART DISEASE
→ LIVER DISEASE

Heavy drinking over a period of time can contribute to serious problems in your body.
Alcohol may also cause serious problems in your baby's development.

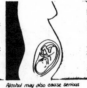

PLACENTA

The alcohol you drink quickly flows from you to your baby in the same concentration.
Because it is still growing, your baby's delicate system is more easily damaged than yours.

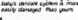

EFFECTS OF ALCOHOL:
MENTAL RETARDATION
SHORTER HEIGHT, LIGHTER WEIGHT
SMALL HEAD
FACE DEFORMITIES
HEART DEFECTS
JOINT/LIMB PROBLEMS
NERVOUSNESS, JUMPINESS
POOR CONDITION

Alcohol can cause one or more birth defects in your baby which cannot be changed.

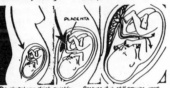

Don't switch to other drugs. Check with your doctor before taking any drugs.
Stop and think about ways other than alcohol to celebrate or relax during pregnancy.

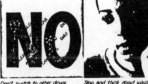

Do something special to take care of yourself.
• Take a long walk.
• Talk to a friend.
• Listen to music.

ALCOHOLICS ANONYMOUS
LOCAL WOMEN'S CENTERS AND SUPPORT GROUPS
COUNSELING PROGRAMS
YOUR OWN DOCTOR
WOMEN FOR SOBRIETY

If you need to, get outside help.
Most of these services can be found in your telephone directory.

When you drink, your UNBORN BABY does, too!

ALCOHOL AND YOUR UNBORN BABY
by the National Institute on Alcohol Abuse and Alcoholism
1979, brochure
DHHS Pub. No. (ADM) 80-521

from
National Clearinghouse for Alcohol Information
Box 2345
Rockville, MD 20852
single copy free

More sophisticated than *Should I Drink?*, this pamphlet discusses the risks of alcohol and the current un-certainty about whether a "safe" level of alcohol consumption exists.

"Pregnancy changes your life in some important ways, and you're bound to feel some stress during this period. For various reasons, some women experience more anxiety and depression than usual during preg-nancy. In any case, there may be times when a few friendly drinks will seem like a good antidote to whatever is troubling you. At those times, stop and try to think of other ways you might handle your feelings.

"First, make sure you are clear about just what is bothering you. Is there any specific action you could take to improve the situation? Or would simply talking about your feel-ings to someone close to you help? Sometimes a long walk, some relax-ing music, or some kind of creative outlet can do a lot to relieve stress. Have you ever tried meditation? Pounding a pillow to vent frus-tration? Writing out your feelings? You may be surprised at how effective some of these alternatives to alcohol can be."

PREGNANT? BEFORE YOU DRINK, THINK . . .
by the March of Dimes
1979, brochure

from
March of Dimes
Division of Public Health Education
Box 2000
White Plains, NY 10602
single copy free

According to the U.S. Depart-ment of Health and Human Services, alcohol-related birth defects rank third in producing mental retarda-tion (after Down's syndrome and Spina Bifida). This March of Dimes pamphlet describes the symptoms of the alcohol-related birth defects known as fetal alcohol syndrome.

"Growth deficiency is one of the most prominent symptoms. Affected babies are abnormally small at birth, especially in head size. Unlike many small newborns, these youngsters never catch up to normal growth.

"Most affected youngsters have small brains and show degrees of mental deficiency. Many are jittery and poorly coordinated, and have short attention spans and behavioral problems. Evidence to date shows that their IQs do not improve with age."

DRUGS, ALCOHOL AND PREGNANCY
by Christina Dye
1981, 20 pages, Illus.

from
Do It Now Foundation
P.O. Box 5115
Phoenix, AZ 85010
75 cents each plus 50 cents minimum postage
bulk rates available

This booklet covers the hazards of "recreational drugs" like alcohol, marijuana, narcotics, hallucinogens, etc., prescription drugs, over-the-counter drugs, tobacco, caffeine, vi-tamins in excess, and food additives. Also included are sections on drugs and lactation, and a bibliography.

"Alcohol poses the greatest dan-ger to the fetus during the first three months of pregnancy. Unfortunate-ly, this is also the period during which many women are unaware that they are pregnant. If you are plan-ning a child, don't drink. If you dis-cover that you are pregnant, don't just reduce your drinking, stop com-pletely! Also be aware of the alco-holic content of many other sub-stances and over-the-counter medica-tions. Your baby's worth it."

X-RAYS

X-rays were first hailed as a major medical advance. We now know that the use of x-radiation poses potential risks, especially in the development of cancer, and x-rays must be used with caution. In fact, over-exposure to medical x-rays is now a major public health problem. This affects pregnant women in several ways.

First, some studies have shown that x-ray exposure *before* pregnancy can increase the chance of neoplasia (the formation of benign and malignant tumors) in the children of mothers who are exposed. In fact, the results of one study showed that the effects of preconception radiation were greater than the effects of x-rays during pregnancy. This means that young women who plan to have children some day must be very careful to limit their x-ray exposure to the absolute minimum.

Secondly, several studies have shown a link between prenatal x-ray exposure and the development of childhood cancers like leukemia. In addition, x-ray exposure during pregnancy can cause microcephaly ("small brain"), skeletal malformations, and mental retardation.

Prenatal exposure includes the use of x-ray pelvimetry, which is used quite commonly to determine the size of the pelvis when there is a question of difficult labor or possible cephalopelvic disproportion. However, in a publication of the Bureau of Radiological Health, dated January, 1980, the authors cite a recommendation adopted by the Pelvimetry Panel of the Department of Health, Education, and Welfare in 1978: "In appreciation of the potential risks of radiation received by the embryo or fetus during pregnancy, x-ray pelvimetry has been selected for review of its utilization in the practice of obstetrics. The panel has carefully reviewed and analyzed this procedure. No benefit to patient or physician is discernable in the studies reviewed by the panel. Therefore, this procedure [x-ray pelvimetry] should not be considered as 'usual and customary' in the practice of obstetrics."

As with all other medical devices and drugs, the fact that x-rays are approved for use by the FDA does not mean that they are necessarily safe. If your physician suggests the use of an x-ray at any time either before or during pregnancy, insist on your right to a full discussion of the risks and benefits of the procedure in your particular case, including a discussion of the alternatives to x-rays. In considering the use of x-ray pelvimetry during labor, it would be a good idea to discuss your doctor's policies *before* labor begins, since during labor it is difficult to concentrate on decisions about medical procedures.

For more information on x-rays, see the resources listed below.

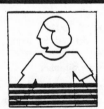

X-RAYS, PREGNANCY AND YOU
by the Food and Drug Administration
1980, brochure

from
Department of Health and Human Services
Public Health Service
Food and Drug Administration
Rockville, MD 20857
HSS Pub. No. (FDA) 79-8087
single copy free

A great deal of the radiation exposure received by Americans comes from medical x-rays, many of which are unnecessary. X-radiation during pregnancy has been linked with the development of leukemia. The cells of the rapidly developing fetus are especially vulnerable to damage, particularly in the first months of pregnancy. This brochure is co-sponsored by the FDA, The American College of Obstetricians and Gynecologists, and the American College of Radiology. Like many publications sponsored by professional medical organizations, it is reserved about describing the hazards of radiation, but the message is still clear—x-rays should be used with caution, if at all.

PRECONCEPTION RADIATION, INTRAUTERINE DIAGNOSTIC RADIATION, AND CHILDHOOD NEOPLASIA
by Patricia H. Shiono, et. al.
Journal of the National Cancer Institute
Volume 65, No. 4, October 1980

The abstract of this paper states, "Generally, the data were consistent with increased risk of malignant neoplasms among children of women exposed to X-rays before and during pregnancy, with a somewhat higher relative risk estimate for preconception exposure." The paper contains a list of 28 further medical references.

INFECTIOUS DISEASES

Certain infectious diseases can cause birth defects, miscarriage, or problems at birth. Pregnant women should be especially careful to guard their health through proper nutrition and rest and by avoiding contact with people who are sick. This may be difficult for mothers of other small children, who often bring home infections. But most colds and mild infections are not harmful in pregnancy.

RUBELLA

Rubella, or "German measles," is a mild virus disease characterized by a low-grade fever, whole-body rash, and swollen lymph glands. The disease does little harm to adults and children but can cause devastating damage to a fetus, especially during the first three months of pregnancy. Birth defects caused by rubella include deafness, and defects of the eyes, cardiovascular system and central nervous system.

In 1969 a vaccine against rubella was licensed and health personnel now recommend that all children be vaccinated to prevent their infecting susceptible pregnant women. If you had rubella as a child, you will probably be immune as an adult, but because the disease is so mild women often don't know if they've had it. Women who are planning to have children should have a blood test to determine whether they are immune. If you are not immune, you should have a rubella vaccination at least three months *before* becoming pregnant. Pregnant women should not be vaccinated, as the vaccine may harm the fetus.

HERPES

Herpes Simplex virus (Type II) has become a venereal disease of epidemic proportions. If you get a primary (first time) infection of genital herpes during pregnancy it can cause birth defects, including microcephaly (small brain), microphthalmia (small eyeballs), or retinal dysplasia. So, it's very important not to expose yourself to herpes through sexual contact with possibly infected partners during pregnancy. Once you've had genital herpes, the infection can recur spontaneously and women often have recurrences during pregnancy. This type of infection does not harm the fetus unless there is an active infection, with lesions (sores) in the genital area at the time of delivery. Then the baby can become infected as it passes through the birth canal and runs a very high risk of blindness, severe brain damage, and death. In these cases, a cesarean-section is recommended to protect the baby. There is no cure for herpes. Fortunately, though, cases of active herpes infection at delivery are fairly rare.

INFLUENZA

Severe "flu" infections, especially when they progress to pneumonia, can cause miscarriage or premature birth.

VENEREAL DISEASE

Gonorrhea and syphillis infections should be treated during pregnancy. Gonorrhea can infect the baby's eyes as it is born and cause blindness. Syphills during pregnancy can cause late miscarriage, fetal death, birth defects, and congenital syphilis in the infant.

TOXOPLASMOSIS

Toxoplasmosis is an animal disease which is passed to human beings through contact with the feces on infected cats or by eating raw or rare meat. It is a mild disease in a pregnant women but can cause serious birth defects in the fetus. Pregnant women should be careful to avoid contact with cat litter (especially if the cat runs free in filelds where it may contact infected mice) and should never eat uncooked meat.

Other diseases which can cause problems during or after pregnancy include smallpox, common red measles, chickenpox, hepatitis, mumps, malaria, polio, tuberculosis, and typhoid fever. Women should consult their care provider if they think they've been exposed to these diseases.

RESOURCES

Can A Mother's Illness Harm Her Unborn Baby?
Report on Rubella Vaccine
Booklets available free from
The American College of Obstetricians and Gynecologists
600 Maryland Ave., SW, Suite 200
Washington, DC 20024

Rubella (14 page booklet)
DHHS Pub. No. (HSA) 80-5225
from
Public Health Service
Office for Maternal and Child Health
Rockville, MD 20857

Herpes Simplex Virus and Pregnancy
(from the October, 1979 issue of
The Helper Newsletter)
$2.00 from
HELP/ASHA
260 Sheridan Ave.
Palo Alto, CA 94306

Preventing Birth Defects Caused By Rubella
Venereal Disease Hurts You and Unborn Babies
free from
March of Dimes
Box 2000
White Plains, NY 10602

CAFFEINE

Caffeine, the stimulant drug found in coffee, tea, cocoa, and cola drinks, has recently come under scrutiny as a possible cause of birth defects. A large, well-controlled study commissioned by the FDA has shown adverse effects on bone and skeletal development in rats, at doses equivalent to what pregnant women might consume. In March, 1980, the Center for Science in the Public Interest held a press conference to ask the Food and Drug Administration to require warning labels on coffee, tea, and over-the-counter drugs containing caffeine. At the same time it announced the establishment of a Caffeine-Birth Defects Clearinghouse to gather information on the effects of caffeine on human offspring.

In September, 1980, FDA Commissioner Jere Goyan made a public statement on the possible dangers of caffeine to unborn children. He said, "So while further evidence is being gathered on the possible relationship between caffeine and birth defects, a prudent and protective mother-to-be will want to put caffeine on her list of unnecessary substances which she should avoid. The old saying that a pregnant woman is 'eating for two' has a special meaning in regard to caffeine."

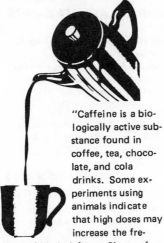

"Caffeine is a biologically active substance found in coffee, tea, chocolate, and cola drinks. Some experiments using animals indicate that high doses may increase the frequency of birth defects. Since caffeine intake may have consequences for the fetus, pregnant women who reduce the amount of these liquids containing caffeine may avoid possible harm for their babies."

from DATA: Drugs, Alcohol, Tobacco Abuse During Pregnancy. Available free from the March of Dimes, Box 2000, White Plains, New York 10602.

CSPI's Caffeine Birth Defects Clearinghouse was conducted during 1980-81 to "gather data from women who had consumed large amounts of caffeinated products during pregnancy and gave birth to a child with birth defects." Results were published in the June 27, 1981 issue of *The Lancet,* suggesting a link between high coffee consumption (8 to 25 six-ounce cups) and defects of the hands and feet, including ectrodactyly ("split hands"). For further information contact:

Center for Science in the Public Interest
1755 S Street, NW
Washington, DC 20009
202/332-9110

MORE RESOURCES

The following books contain information on avoiding birth defects through careful attention to nutrition, prenatal care, and avoiding drugs and other environmental hazards.

BUILDING BETTER BABIES: Preconception Planning for Healthier Children
by Daniel Elam
1980, 149 pages, illus.

from
Celestial Arts
231 Adrian Road
Millbrae, CA 94030
$6.95 pap.

LIFE BEFORE BIRTH (Revised Edition)
by Ashley Montagu
1977, 248 pages, Illus.

from
Signet
1301 Avenue of the Americas
New York, NY 10021
$2.25 pap.

IS MY BABY ALL RIGHT?: A Guide to Birth Defects
by Virginia Apgar and Joan Beck
1972, 492 pages, Illus.

from
Trident Press (Simon and Schuster)
1230 Sixth Avenue
New York, NY 10020
out of print

BENDECTIN

Bendectin, manufactured by Richardson-Merrel, is a drug used to treat "morning sickness," the nausea often experienced in early pregnancy. Over the past 20 years, the drug has been used by an estimated 30 million women around the world. However, reports that Bendectin might cause birth defects led to government hearings in September of 1980. The Fertility and Maternal Health Drugs Advisory Committee of the U.S. Food and Drug Administration reviewed the available scientific studies on Bendectin and concluded that the data currently available did not prove a link between Bendectin and birth defects but that "residual uncertainty" about the drug's safety warranted further studies and changes in the drug's package label. The proposed new package insert would warn that Bendectin be used only for "significant nausea and vomiting" which is unresponsive to non-drug treatment.

ASSOCIATION OF BENDECTIN CHILDREN
Betty Mekdeci, President
3201 E. Crystal Lake Avenue
Orlando, FL 32806

Betty Mekdeci's son, David, was born with arm and chest deformities which she believes were caused by Bendectin. As part of her campaign to gather information on the drug, Ms. Mekdeci would like to hear from other parents of children with deformities whose mothers took Bendectin during pregnancy.

THE BENDECTIN COVER-UP
by Mark Dowie and Carolyn Marshall
1980, 8 pages

from
Mother Jones Reprint Service
625 Third Street
San Francisco, CA 94107
Two copies (minimum order), $1.00 plus 35 cents postage
Additional copies 50 cents each.
Request bulk rates.

Investigative reporters Dowie and Marshall believe that Richardson-Merrel and the FDA have withheld information showing that Bendectin causes birth defects in animals. Their report, which appeared in the November, 1980, issue of *Mother Jones* magazine, traces the development and approval of Bendectin, in their words, "a modern-day horror story of corporate and bureaucratic irresponsibility."

The common discomforts of pregnancy, like morning sickness, can be remedied or at least made more bearable by changes in diet, posture, and by other non-drug means. Mothers should also be comforted by the reassurance that these uncomfortable feelings are fairly common, nothing to worry about, and will pass. For information on natural remedies in pregnancy, see the index.

HANDBOOK FOR PRESCRIBING MEDICATIONS DURING PREGNANCY
by Richard L. Berkowitz, M.D.
Donald R. Coustan, M.D., and
Tara K. Mochizuki, Pharm. D.
1981, 257 pages

from
Little, Brown and Co.
34 Beacon St.
Boston, MA 02106
$11.95 pap.

This handbook is designed to help doctors decide which drugs might be safe to use in pregnancy and labor. Its value for mothers may be somewhat different—reading through the "adverse effects" section for several common drugs, I began to wonder whether the benefits of any drug are really worth the risks. Pregnant women who consult this handbook before taking a drug prescribed by their doctor may decide that whatever symptoms they are suffering (nausea, headache, runny nose, etc.) are preferable to the side effects and possible damage to the baby caused by the remedy. To this end, the handbook is well-organized and very accessible for lay people. I am not terribly familiar with the chemical names of common drugs, but it was easy to look things up by using the "Generic and Trade Name Index" and the "Drug Classification Index."

Each drug entry includes a discussion of "special considerations in pregnancy" as well as information on indications, dosage, adverse effects, mechanism of action, absorption and biotransformation, and references. Included are common drugs like aspirin, Tylenol, alcohol, tobacco, caffeine, antihistamines, penicillins, diuretics, laxatives, cough medicines, antacids, tranquilizers, and also drugs commonly used in labor, including Nisentil, Demerol, and Pitocin.

ENVIRONMENTAL AND WORKPLACE HAZARDS

REPRODUCTIVE HAZARDS FACTPACK
Women's Occupational Health Resource Center
48 pages

from
Women's Occupational Health Resource Center
Columbia University
School of Public Health
60 Haven Avenue, B-1
New York, NY 10032
$3.00 plus $1.00 postage

This FACTPACK is made up of back issues of *WOHRC News,* fact-sheets, and other journal articles and reprints covering the effects of toxic agents on reproduction, "The Pregnancy Discrimination Act," genetic testing by industry and its effects on hiring practices, and references on reproductive hazards in the workplace Women's Occupational Health Resource Center (WOHRC) also produces many other publications and factpacks on women's health and work and publishes a bimonthly newsletter. Memberships are $6. a year for students/low income, $12. for professionals, and $25. for libraries and institutions. Request a copy of their Publications List.

"One million American women in their prime child-bearing years work under conditions which could damage their ability to bear healthy children. A few of them have been sterilized in order to keep their jobs; many of them may be faced with the same kind of choice . . . . The fact is that there are many, many reproductive hazards in the workplace. Many of these can affect the ability of male as well as female workers to have healthy children. Some hazards can even spread into the home where they can harm growing children."

—from *Fact Sheet on Reproductive Health in the Workplace,* 1979
WOHRC

WOMEN'S WORK, WOMEN'S HEALTH: Myths and Realities
by Jeanne Mager Stellman
1977, 262 pages, Illus.

from
Pantheon Books
A Division of Random House
201 East 50th Street
New York, NY 10022
$12.95 hd.

Women's Work, Women's Health contains a chapter on "Work, Reproduction, and Health" which discus-

REPRODUCTIVE HAZARDS AT WORK
4 pages, Illus.

from
MassCOSH
718 Huntington Avenue
Boston, MA 02115
15 cents plus self-addressed, stamped envelope
request complete publications list

Massachusetts Coalition for Occupational Safety and Health (MassCOSH) is one of many state organizations which provide information and assistance to help win better health and safety conditions in the workplace. To find out about similar organizations in your area, contact a local labor union and ask for information on worker health and safety.

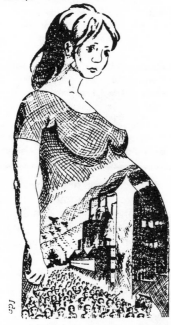

ses patterns of employment in pregnancy, the biology of reproduction including mutations and the function of the placenta, reproductive and environmental hazards, the effects of pregnancy on women's ability to work, and the role of men in producing birth defects. Included as an appendix is an extensive listing (30 pages) of "Health Hazards in Selected Women's Occupations," including chemicals and physical hazards. Author Jeanne Stellman is Executive Director of the Women's Occupational Health Resource Center.

The book is also available in paperback for $5.95 plus $1.00 postage from the Women's Occupational Health Resource Center, see listing on this page.

GUIDELINES ON PREGNANCY AND WORK
by the American College of Obstetricians and Gynecologists
1977, 73 pages, Illus.

from
Superintendent of Documents
Government Printing Office
Washington, DC 20402
$2.75
GPO Stock No. 017-033-00-279-5

This research report was prepared by the American College of Obstetricians and Gynecologists (ACOG) under contract to NIOSH. (National Institute for Occupational Safety and Health). It is intended primarily for physicians, but will be useful for consumers too. It provides recommendations for providing care to pregnant workers, describes environmental hazards, and outlines how particular job factors may affect pregnancy.

"While the focus of this document is the work environment, it must be emphasized that the woman's activities and exposures at home and in the community are also important. These should be examined and considered as carefully as her work exposures because they may involve greater levels of physical activity or more hazardous environmental exposures than those of the job."

WHITE PAPER ON THE IMPACT OF HAZARDOUS SUBSTANCES UPON INFERTILITY AMONG MEN IN THE UNITED STATES AND BIRTH DEFECTS
by Erik Jansson
1980, 20 pages

from
Friends of the Earth
530 7th Street, SE
Washington, DC 20002
$2.00

Erik Jansson is a research associate for Friends of the Earth, an organization which lobbies for environmental safety. Mr. Jansson has done a great deal of work on the subject of low sperm count and male sterility caused by exposure to hazardous substances in the environment, especially pesticides, which have worked their way into the food chain. His White Paper describes how the sperm counts of American men have declined sharply during the past 30 years and postulates that because sperm production is so sensitive to environmental damage, men may now be responsible for most (perhaps up to 83%) of birth defects.

COEVOLUTION QUARTERLY GENETIC TOXICITY ISSUE
No. 21, Spring 1979
featuring
"Human Harm to Human DNA"
by Stewart Brand
"Herbicides: A Faustian Bargain"
by Carol Van Strum
"A Guide to Worrying Intelligently About Having a Baby" by Susan Stern

from
CoEvolution Quarterly
P.O. Box 428
Sausalito, CA 94966
$3.00 for each back issue

CoEvolution Quarterly is the "ongoing" *Whole Earth Catalog,* edited by Stewart Brand. Issue No. 21 was devoted to genetic toxicity, with 39 pages of articles and reviews. The authors discuss the increasing problem of birth defects and cancers caused by harmful chemicals like environmental pollutants, workplace hazards, and drugs. Advice is given on personal action (reducing your own exposure to hazards) and political action to help do something about the poisoning of our earth. Warning: this issue contains photographs of babies with birth defects which are extremely difficult to look at. Stewart Brand suggests that these babies should replace the traditional skull and cross-bones as symbols of "lethal human folly."

". . . if you hear that something is a mutagen, it is probably also a carcinogen. And vice versa. They both can be called 'genotoxic.'"

"Lay off items that appear to cause cancer—cigarettes, hair dyes, nitrites in meats (that's one I've just dropped thanks to all this), unnecessary x-rays, unnecessary anesthetics, chronic alcohol or drug use, pesticides, herbicides, moldy nuts, charred meat or fish, too much fat, food additives generally, medical drugs generally including birth control pills, aerosol cans, cleaning agents with benzene or chlorinated compounds (carbon tetrachloride, trichlorethylene, etc.), asbestos insulation, wallboard, etc., and whatever else turns up on the endangering list.

"If you're pregnant, take this list quadruply seriously.

"As for political action, the usual: research, bitch, organize, boycott, demonstrate, publicize, vote, help, and thank."

—from "Human Harm to Human DNA"

THE NEW PREGNANCY: The Active Woman's Guide to Work, Legal Rights, Health Care, Travel, Sports, Dress, Sex, and Emotional Well-Being.
by Susan Lichtendorf and Phyllis Gillis
1979, 311 pages

from
Random House
201 East 50th St.
New York, NY 10022
$10.95 hd

Bantam (1981)
666 Fifth Ave.
New York, NY 10019
$2.95 pap.

This book is especially geared to the many women who work outside the home during pregnancy. It covers the laws which protect pregnant women from discrimination in employment, the problem of environmental hazards at work, health insurance and maternity benefits, and how to file a complaint. There are excellent chapters on "Taking Charge of Your Medical Care," and on sports, travel, health, beauty, emotional well-being, and sex, all with the emphasis on making pregnancy "an integral part of your life."

"If you are concerned about occupational hazards, it is especially important that *you* take the initiative and discuss your medical concerns about your job, first with your physician and then, if necessary, with your employer .... Be as honest and complete as possible, because your physician *can* suggest modifications in your job activities. Tell him exactly what you do, what your hours are, whether you have slack time and rest periods, what the pace is. Describe your working environment, everything from the accessibility of clean bathrooms to the noise level, amount of vibration and airborne dusts at work, and, of course, specific chemicals you are in contact with. If you do not know what they are, ask your employer what hazardous substances you may have been exposed to. You have a right to this information ...."

Pregnancy Discrimination Act

The Pregnancy Discrimination Act (an amendment to Title VII of the 1964 Civil Rights Act) went into effect on April 29, 1979. It prohibits discrimination against women employees on the basis of pregnancy, childbirth and related medical conditions. Specifically, the Act provides the following protections:

1. Women cannot be fired or refused a job or promotion because they are pregnant.

2. If a woman takes a maternity leave, she is entitled to her old job back, without loss of seniority, on the same basis as other employees who are disabled or take sick leave.

3. If a woman is unable to work because of pregnancy, she is entitled to sick leave and disability payments on the same basis as other employees.

4. Employer health insurance plans must include coverage for pregnancy-related conditions.

In general, employers are required to treat pregnancy and childbirth as they do any other health-related conditions of their employees, so that women do not suffer unfair discrimination because of their sex and reproductive capacity.

WORKING POSITION PAPER ON WOMEN AND OCCUPATIONAL HEALTH, 4 pages

from
National Women's Health Network
224 Seventh St., SE
Washington, DC 20003

NWHN is a consumer advocacy group devoted exclusively to the concerns of women and health (see index). The Network has identified occupational and environmental health as priority issues and their *Working Position Paper* outlines the major issues and concerns involved.

JOURNAL OF OCCUPATIONAL MEDICINE
American Occupational Medical Association
150 N. Wacker Drive
Chicago, IL 60606
312/782-2166
$25.00 a year

Reprints of *Journal* articles on reproduction and pregnancy (mutagenicity, women in industry, genetic monitoring) are available for 60 cents each. Request a copy of Journal of Occupational Medicine's publications list.

HAZARDS AT WORK

The following chemical and physical hazards have been linked with reproductive damage in animals and humans, including sterility, miscarriage, stillbirth, birth defects, and childhood disease. These hazards effect both men and women.

Alcohol
Alkylating Agents
Anesthetic Gases
Arsenic
Benzene
Cadmium
Carbon Disulfide
Carbon Monoxide
Carbon Tetrachloride
Chlorinated Hydrocarbons
Chloroprene
Diethylstibesterol (DES)
Dimethyl Sulfoxide
Dioxin (Agent Orange)
Elevated Carbon Dioxide
Elevated Temperatures
Ethylene Oxide
Hair Dyes

Infectious Agents
　rubella virus
　cytomegalovirus
　herpes virus hominis
　toxoplasma
　syphilis
Ionizing Radiation
Lead
Manganese
Microwaves
Nickel
Organic Mercury Compounds
Organophosphate Pesticides
　Dibromochloropropane
　Kepone
　DDT
　DBCP
　Carbaryl
　DDVP
　Malathion
Polychlorinated Biphenyls (PCB's)
Tris (flame retardant)
Vinyl Chloride
X-irradiation

—source, Women's Occupational Health Resource Center

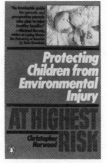

AT HIGHEST RISK: Environmental Hazards to Young and Unborn Children
by Christopher Norwood
1980, 280 pages

from
Penguin (1981)
625 Madison Ave.
New York, NY 10022
$4.95 pap.

Toxic substances are literally pouring into our environment and are causing birth defects and cancers in increasing numbers. So says Christopher Norwood, who is a science journalist, and has based this book on an investigative look at the recent literature on hazards of lead, x-rays, asbestos, fluorescent light, smoking, DES, birth control pills, aspirin, anesthesia, pesticides, microwaves, food additives, and many other substances. The author describes many of the environmental disasters which appear with increasing frequency in the headlines of our newspapers—high rates of miscarriage, Agent Orange in Vietnam and 2,4,5-T herbicide spraying in Oregon, air pollution and smog, PCB's in breast milk, polluted drinking water, Love Canal, noise pollution, and birth defects among operating room personnel. Norwood discusses the limitations of drug testing and regulation and expresses serious reservations about the use of amniocentesis and selective abortion as a "solution" to the problem of environmentally caused birth defects. The author includes chapters on hyperactivity, prenatally caused cancer, the overuse of radiation, and hazards in the workplace. A final chapter is devoted to the hazards and high infant mortality associated with American hospital birth and obstetricians' overuse of drugs and procedures.

"... It is hard to think of any other work environment that presents a more intense melange of known hazards to the fetus than hospitals; they are not only strewn with chemicals, anesthetic gases, radiation equipment, and sonar machines, but they are also a gathering place for sick people who may be carriers of any number of biological organisms—the rubella, mumps, herpes, and influenza viruses, the typhoid bacillus, syphilis spirochete, and malaria protozoa, to name but some—known to injure the fetus. It is also hard to think of another working environment as systematically organized, not just to put women in low-paying positions, but to put them in the positions that involve the most intense hazardous exposures."

Prenatal Care

A healthy woman with a normal pregnancy will probably deliver a healthy baby without complications whether she has received prenatal care or not. So why is prenatal care important? Mainly, to find out whether the mother has any health problems which will affect the pregnancy, and to make sure that the pregnancy does progress normally. For the five percent or less of pregnancies with problems, prenatal care can help detect and remedy them before they deteriorate into life-threatening conditions. For the ninety-five percent or so of pregnancies which are normal, prenatal care is more a form of "monitoring" and can provide a good opportunity for the mother and her care provider to get to know each other before the birth. In a typical physician practice, prenatal care involves an initial exam and health history-taking, followed by regular visits to check certain signs and symptoms like weight gain, blood pressure, presence of sugar or protein in the urine, and the size, position, and heart beat of the fetus. One complaint about obstetricians has been that they rarely go beyond this minimum physical care. Women often do not feel comfortable discussing personal or "trivial" concerns with a male doctor. Physician care is also quite expensive. Midwife care is a good alternative for many women. Midwives usually provide nutrition counseling, can provide sympathetic help in dealing with the discomforts and emotional adjustments of pregnancy, and encourage their clients to become actively involved in preparation and planning for the birth.

CHOOSING A CARE PROVIDER

One of the most important decisions to be made early in pregnancy is your choice of a medical care provider—the person who will monitor your health in pregnancy and assist you in labor and delivery. In this country most babies are delivered by obstetricians (in Europe, midwives handle most deliveries), so it is sometimes difficult to find alternative attendants. But there are many different kinds of care available. You may choose an obstetrician/gynecologist in private solo or group practice, a family-practice physician or general practitioner who specializes in childbirth, or a clinic setting where you may be cared for by doctors, nurse-midwives, and nurse-practitioners. Certified nurse-midwives (CNM's) are becoming increasingly available and popular. CNM's practice in hospitals, birthing centers, and at home deliveries. Lay midwives are making a strong comeback, providing assistance at home births. Their licensing and legal status varies from state to state. There are also a variety of lay "birth attendants" available, who may have less training than a midwife, but some experience and skill in attending births.

To find a birth attendant, you can consult your local medical society, childbirth advocacy group, women's health organizations, your friends or childbirth educator or local La Leche League leader (see the sections on Alternative Childbirth, Home Birth, Midwives, Birthing Centers, etc. for more information).

Whatever kind of care you choose, it's a good idea to approach medical care providers as you would any professional offering a service. In other words, "shop around" and use your rights and power as a consumer to get the care you want. Arrange for consultation visits and ask questions. If you are not happy with your care giver, look for another one.

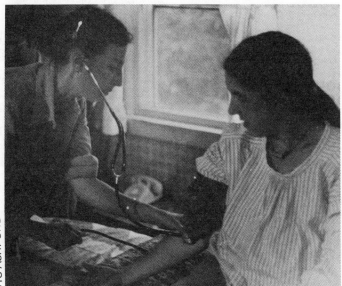

VIC ASHFORD

QUESTIONS TO ASK

Pertinent questions to ask a physician include:

1. Do you view birth as a normal, healthy process?
2. Are you comfortable working with informed, knowledgeable parents?
3. What are your feelings about family-centered birth?
4. Do you encourage your patients to attend childbirth education classes? Have you attended a course yourself?
5. Do you encourage the participation of the father in prenatal visits, labor, and delivery?
6. Do you provide counseling in nutrition and drug use in pregnancy?
7. What medical interventions do you commonly use? (Enema, shaving, IV, pitocin induction or augmentation, electronic fetal monitoring, ultrasound, episiotomy). What are their risks and benefits?
8. What drugs do you commonly use for labor and delivery and what are their risks and benefits?
9. Are you experienced in the vaginal delivery of twins and breech babies?
10. What percentage of your patients require a cesarean section?
11. Do you encourage parent/infant bonding and breastfeeding?
12. What is your fee? What arrangements for payment are available?

Questions to ask a midwife or birth attendant include:

1. What is your training and background?
2. How many births have you attended as primary care giver?
3. Will you provide full prenatal care services and refer to other professionals when necessary?
4. Are you skilled in monitoring the progress of normal labor and in detecting any abnormalities?
5. What arrangements do you have for medical back-up and transfer if necessary?
6. Can you deal with medical emergencies (control of bleeding, resusitation of infant, etc.)?
7. What equipment do you routinely use at birth?
8. What is your fee? What arrangements for payment are available?

HEARTBEAT

Just yesterday
I had a sweet surprise
Lying on the doctor's table
He said, Lady, please close your eyes
And then what did I hear
It was my little baby's heart
Beating soft and clear

Oh, I've had so many dreams
Of this new life soon to be
But dreams are all I've had
'Till the truth came pulsing through
    me
That now deep within me you'll find
There's another little heart
Doing doubletime with mine

* * *

Now when I think of me
I have to think of two
That second heart that beats within
Is my own life's rhythm renewed
Oh, I can't tell you how fine
It was to hear my baby's heart
For the very first time.

from *Nine Months: Songs of Pregnancy and Birth*, by Linda Arnold, on Ariel Records (see index)

THE DOPPLER STETHOSCOPE

Many physicians (and some midwives) are now using Doppler stethoscopes (sometimes called a Doptone) to listen to fetal heart tones during pregnancy. It is important to know that the Doppler is an ultrasound device (ultrasound is also used in genetic testing [see index] and for electronic fetal monitoring [see index]). These devices are generally described as "safe" by the people who use them, but in fact, the effects of ultrasound exposure on human beings, especially the developing fetus, are not clearly known. Two reasons why the Doppler is so popular with practitioners are: 1.) It is quicker and more convenient to use than the conventional fetoscope, and 2.) Heart tones can be detected earlier in pregnancy. However, these "benefits" should be weighed carefully against the possible risks of ultrasound. A thoughtful article on the safety of Doppler ultrasound appears in the Winter/Spring 1981 issue of *The Practicing Midwife* (available from The Farm, 156 Drakes Lane, Summertown, TN 38483). *The Practicing Midwife* offers the following guidelines for the use of Doppler ultrasound:

"1. Avoid use during the first trimester, except when medically indicated...

2. Avoid use for extended period....

3. Use an instrument with the lowest possible power output...."

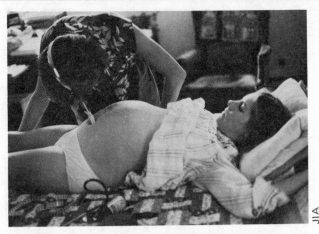

DOING YOUR OWN PRENATAL CARE

When we depend on a doctor to listen for the baby's heart beat and wait passively for his announcement that the baby is "alive," we can feel almost that the doctor causes the baby to be alive and that his or her skill in listening is crucial to the baby's life. If women can learn to use the stethoscope themselves, perhaps they can release more feelings of competence and control in their situation. There is no reason why a woman should not use her own skill and tools to keep in touch with the reality of her healthy pregnancy. Then she can go to her prenatal visits with more confidence in herself as a working partner in the health care team, and with more confidence that the doctor will not tell her much that she doesn't already know.

During my first pregnancy I went to an obstetrician for prenatal care. I observed what he and his nurses did at each visit and decided it was pretty simple and something I could learn to do myself. So, during by second pregnancy I did my own prenatal care and gave birth at home, without once seeing a doctor. I bought or borrowed equipment and supplies and read obstetrics and midwifery texts to learn techniques. My pregnancy progressed normally, so my husband and I felt confident about going-it alone. I cannot recommend this course for everyone but it worked well for us.

I kept a prenatal record for myself, similar to the one used by my doctor. Parents who are seeing a doctor or midwife for care might also want to follow along at home with their own exams and record-keeping (see *A Wandering Journal*, opposite). We found that regular "auscultation and palpation" (listening to and feeling the baby) was fun and helped put us in close touch with the realities of pregnancy.

The following tools and supplies are needed for prenatal care and can be purchased from department stores, medical supply stores, or from mailorder supply services (see index).

Scale — For recording weight gain, which should be adequate (20-40 lbs.) but steady. A sudden, large gain could signal the development of toxemia.

Blood Pressure Cuff (Sphygmomanometer) — Blood pressure is measured regularly during pregnancy to establish a norm for each woman. A sudden rise could signal the development of toxemia. Chronic high blood pressure can also be a problem during pregnancy.

Urine Reagent Strips — These test for protein or glucose (sugar) in the urine, to help confirm a suspected case of toxemia. Protein in the urine can also be a sign of a bladder infection; sugar in the urine is monitored to check for the development of gestational diabetes.

Fetoscope — This is a stethoscope specially adapted for listening to the baby's heart beat through the mother's abdominal wall. Several types are available, including the horn type used more commonly in Europe and the type with ear pieces and an attached forehead piece to help amplify sounds. Heart tones taken during pregnancy establish a norm for each baby (from 120 to 160 beats per minute), and during labor monitoring of heart tones is done to check for fetal distress.

Hands — Use your hands to gently palpate the mother's abdomen. In the later months of pregnancy, you should be able to feel the contours of the baby's head, back, and "small parts." Your midwife or doctor will probably palpate at each prenatal visit. Ask her or him to show you how.

WANDERING JOURNAL

In Denmark, women receiving prenatal care carry a "wandering journal" with them to each visit with midwife or doctor. This is their prenatal record. Unlike American mothers, who often never see their own medical records, Danish women watch as their chart is filled in and each notation is explained to them. This kind of patient participation and sharing of knowledge helps Denmark to achieve one of the lowest infant mortality rates in the world (in 1972 Denmark ranked 6th from the best while the U.S. ranked 16th).

To help you participate more fully in your own prenatal care (or even to aid you in doing your own care, if you choose that option), you might like to use the prenatal care chart which is included in this section, or a similar one. Fill it in with your midwife or doctor's assistance and bring it with you to each prenatal visit, filling in details of weight, blood pressure, etc., at the same time they are recorded on your office record.

Consult an obstetrics or midwifery textbook (these are available through your local library or check the section on Medical Reference [see index]) to learn the meaning of any unfamiliar terms.

PRENATAL AND BIRTHING RECORD FORMS
by Ina May Gaskin
6 pages

from
The Practicing Midwife/The Farm
156 Drakes Lane
Summertown, TN 38483
sample set free
bulk rates $5. for 25, $8. for 50

Designed for midwives, these forms can also help parents keep clear medical records of pregnancy and birth, as a supplement to their prenatal care.

QUESTIONS FOR MIDWIVES: Interviewing a Prospective Birth Attendant
by Rosemary Wiener
4 pages

from
Rosemary Wiener
6294 Mission Road
Everson, WA 98247
single copy 15 cents plus self-
    addressed stamped envelope
50 copies for $6.00
100 copies for $11.00

This flyer is especially geared for couples who are considering home birth and looking for a qualified birth attendant.

NAME _____ AGE _____ HEIGHT _____ WEIGHT _____

ADDRESS _____ PARITY _____ GRAVID _____

PHONE _____ LMP _____ EDC _____

DATE CARE BEGUN: _____ BLOOD TYPE _____ RH _____ FATHER _____

MEDICAL HISTORY (CIRCLE)

ASTHMA TUBERCULOSIS RESPIRATORY DISEASE RHEUMATIC FEVER HEART TROUBLE
HIGH BLOOD PRESSURE PHLEBITIS VARICOSE VEINS ULCERS HEPATITIS PELVIC INFECTION
ANEMIA ALLERGIES HERPES CANCER GERMAN MEASLES DIABETES THYROID PROBLEMS
EPILEPSY BLADDER INFECTION KIDNEY DISEASE

CURRENTLY ON MEDICATION? _____
PAST SURGERY _____
FAMILY HISTORY _____
TOBACCO _____ ALCOHOL _____ OTHER DRUGS _____ WORKPLACE EXPOSURES _____

PHYSICAL EXAMINATION—GENERAL

SKIN _____ ENT. (EARS) _____ BREASTS _____
HAIR _____ EYES _____ ABDOMEN _____
TEETH _____ HEART _____ EXTREMITIES _____
THYROID _____ LUNGS _____ REFLEXES _____

GYNECOLOGICAL EXAM

VULVA _____ CERVIX _____ VAGINAL SMEAR _____ ANUS _____
PERINEUM _____ CORPUS _____ CYSTOCELE _____
VAGINA _____ ADNEXA _____ PAP SMEAR _____ RECTOCELE _____

Diagonal Conjugate _____ Shape/sacrum _____ Coccyx _____ Pubic Arch _____ Ischial Spines _____

MENSTRUAL HISTORY

Onset _____ Interval between Periods _____ days Duration _____ days

OBSTETRICAL HISTORY

NUMBER OF PREGNANCIES _____ MISCARRIAGES _____ ABORTIONS _____

PREVIOUS BIRTHS

Date _____ Weeks Gestation _____ Duration of Labor/Spontaneous? _____ Type of Delivery _____ Anesthesia? _____ Presentation Sex/Weight _____ Complications _____

PROBLEMS WITH PREVIOUS PREGNANCIES (CIRCLE)

MORNING SICKNESS VOMITING BLADDER INFECTION VARICOSE VEINS KIDNEY PROBLEMS PROTEINURIA
GLUCOSE IN URINE PRE-ECLAMPSIA ECLAMPSIA HIGH BLOOD PRESSURE ANEMIA SPOTTING OR BLEEDING
VAGINAL INFECTIONS EDEMA PREMATURITY

DRUGS OR TREATMENTS

PRESENT PREGNANCY

HEMATOCRIT _____ URINALYSIS _____
HEMOGLOBIN _____ SEROLOGY _____
RH TITRE _____ SYPHILIS _____
RUBELLA TITER _____ GONORRHEA _____

DATE															
WEEKS GESTATION															
FUNDAL HEIGHT															
WEIGHT															
BLOOD PRESSURE															
URINE SUGAR															
URINE PROTEIN															
FETAL HEART TONES															
PRESENTATION															
NOTES															

PRENATAL CARE
by the American Medical Association and the American College of Obstetricians and Gynecologists
1978, 26 pages, Illus.

from
American Medical Association
Order Department
P.O. Box 821
Monroe, WI 53566
single copy free
request bulk rates

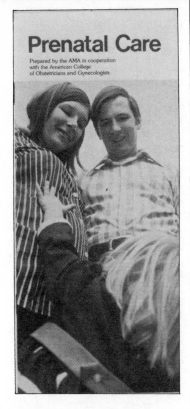

This pamphlet is useful because it lets you know just what the American Medical Association (AMA) and the American College of Obstetricians and Gynecologists (ACOG) think about prenatal care and childbirth. It contains good advice on nutrition and drugs to avoid in pregnancy, but it also contains the standard medical profession "line" on anesthetics ("[your doctor] is the best judge of your needs because he knows your medical history and condition") and home delivery ("labor and delivery present potential hazards to both the mother and baby. These hazards require safety standards that can be provided only in a hospital, not at home.").

"Most women need some pain relief even though they may have had prepared childbirth classes. The main type of pain relievers are analgesics, general anesthetics, and local and regional anesthetics. An analgesic deadens pain and is used during early labor. Since this type of pain killer enters the woman's blood stream, it works its way through the placenta to the baby. The doctor must be careful not to give the anesthetic too early because it could slow or stop labor and not to give too much because it may discourage respiration of the baby."

TAKE CARE OF YOURSELF
by the Association for Retarded Citizens
brochure

from
Association for Retarded Citizens
2709 Avenue E East
Arlington, TX 76011
1-25 copies free
bulk rates $5. for 100

Only about one quarter of the cases of mental retardation are hereditary. The majority are caused by factors in pregnancy and childbirth and are preventable. This brochure lists the things you can do during pregnancy and before to help prevent mental retardation.

"If you think you have venereal disease, seek treatment immediately. Damage to the unborn baby's heart, skeleton, nervous system and brain can be caused by VD—the result can be a mentally retarded child."

ARE YOU POSITIVE ABOUT YOUR RH BLOOD FACTOR?
by the March of Dimes
1979, pamphlet

from
March of Dimes
Division of Public Health Information
Box 2000
White Plains, NY 10602
single copy free
request bulk rates

If a woman with Rh-negative blood conceives a child with an Rh-positive man, the baby could have Rh-positive blood. If the mother's and baby's blood should mix during pregnancy or delivery, the mother's body would produce antibodies which could harm her next baby if it were also Rh-positive. This pamphlet describes the Rh-factor and Rh blood disease and explains why it is important for women to have their blood tested for Rh factor in pregnancy.

"Before 1968, Rh blood disease caused death or severe birth defects in 10,000 American babies each year. That year, a vaccine—Rh immune globulin—was licensed which protects against the disease. Despite the vaccine's availability, Rh blood disease has not disappeared. Its frequency has been reduced, but one out of five American women who needs the vaccine does not get it. This places 90,000 women needlessly at risk, and results in 7,000 infants born each year with Rh blood disease. The March of Dimes, whose mission is prevention of birth defects, wants every couple to know that Rh blood disease usually can be prevented by giving the vaccine to the woman with Rh negative blood within 72 hours after the birth of a baby with Rh positive blood. The same is true after a miscarriage, or abortion."

ABOUT OFFICE "HAND-OUTS"

Many drug companies, formula manufacturers and other businesses produce pamphlets and brochures on pregnancy and childbirth and these are often distributed free in doctors' offices and clinics. It is important to "consider the source" when reading this material because although these pamphlets often contain useful illustrations and are accurate in their description of the basic physiology of birth, most present current medical opinion and practice as "givens" rather than the subjects of much debate. Many ideas are presented without mention of alternatives. In addition, doctors and clinics often use pamphlet "hand-outs" in order to save time spent on explaining facts about childbirth to their patients. Knowing this, companies produce pamphlets geared toward producing a pliant and cooperative patient, not one who will question her doctor's advice. In some cases, the pamphlets also hope to produce a customer for whatever is being sold—infant formula, hospital-based maternity care, baby food, drugs, etc. So, go ahead and read whatever material is offered . . . but do so with a healthy skepticism.

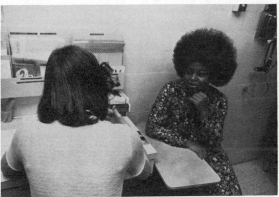

PRENATAL CARE
by Marion Slatin
1973, 70 pages, Illus.
HHS Pub. No (OCD) 75-17

from
Dept. of Health and Human Services
Office of Child Development
Children's Bureau
Washington, DC 20201
single copy free

Prenatal Care was first published in 1913 and was revised in 1962 and again in 1973. It is still available from the government but contains significantly outdated and false information on many important topics in pregnancy, including the use of caffeine, alcohol, restriction of salt intake, safety of birth control pills, and the safety of hospital delivery. There is much good information in this booklet and it could be a useful resource if it were updated to reflect more current thinking. I suggest that concerned readers review this publication and write to the Children's Bureau requesting that this booklet be either revised or discontinued.

Genetic Testing

Genetic testing, like many advances in medical science, may be a mixed blessing. On the one hand, prenatal diagnosis and selective abortion makes it possible for genetically "high risk" couples to go through a pregnancy with more confidence that their baby will be normal. But as genetic testing becomes more readily available, there will be more and more pressure on low—and moderate—risk women to undergo procedures which may be harmful to the healthy fetus. Many obstetrical procedures, which were originally developed for high-risk patients, have ended up being promoted as routine for all mothers. Pressures will no doubt increase to make genetic testing a normal part of prenatal care for all pregnant women. Unfortunately, the procedures which are used or are being developed (amniocentesis, ultrasound, fetoscopy) have definite risks and the practice of exposing all fetuses to these procedures may create more problems than it detects. Parents need to realize that the medical profession and medically-related industries have a financial interest in promoting and selling obstetrical services and products. This may sometimes run counter to the best interests of the mother and fetus. It is wise to get as much information as possible about the risks and benefits of any medical procedure before making a decision.

The whole question of genetic testing becomes moot, of course, unless women have access to safe, legal abortions. Without the possibility of abortion, high-risk couples are once again put in the position of facing sometimes a 50/50 chance of producing a seriously defective child with each pregnancy. Efforts to make abortion illegal seriously threaten the right of couples to use genetic testing and counseling to plan their families, and impose an arbitrary restriction on what should be a deeply private and personal decision and responsibility. For more information on abortion, see the index.

GENETIC COUNSELING: LEARNING WHAT TO EXPECT
by Judith Willis
1980, 3 pages, Illus.

from
Department of Health and Human Services
Public Health Service
Food and Drug Administration
Office of Public Affairs
5600 Fishers Lane
Rockville, MD 20857
(request HHS Pub No. (FDA) 81-9006
single copy free

This article is reprinted from the September 1980 issue of *FDA Consumer.* It describes briefly the fetal abnormalities most commonly detected by prenatal testing, including sickle cell anemia, Tay-Sachs disease, phenylketonuria (PKU), Down's syndrome, hemophilia, thalassemia, and neural tube defects, followed by a description of the available testing methods—amniocentesis, ultrasound, alpha-feto-protein testing (restricted to pilot programs approved by FDA) and fetoscopy and placental aspiration (both considered experimental). Risks associated with these methods are discussed.

"Genetic counseling can actually start before the couple marries, for knowing that their pairing may result in a child with an inherited disorder can make a difference in the couple's decisions about marriage and childbearing. Some inherited disorders are carried by the mother and passed on almost exclusively to male children. These disorders are known as X-linked recessive disorders, and include color blindness, hemophilia, and childhood muscular dystrophy. They are called X-linked recessive because they are carried on the X sex chromosome of the mother.

"Other inherited disorders—known as autosomal recessive—are inherited only if both parents carry the gene for it. Even then, the chances are only one in four that each offspring will have the disease. Years ago, knowing that such a disease existed in the families of two people planning to marry might have been enough to call off the wedding. But today, carrier tests for these genetic disorders often rule out one or both partners as carriers."

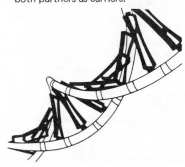

KNOW YOUR GENES
by Aubrey Milunsky
1977, 335 pages, Illus.

from
Houghton Mifflin
2 Park Street
Boston, MA 02107
$9.95

The main concern of *Know Your Genes* is to prevent the birth of children with birth defects through the education of prospective parents. To that end, it provides a great deal of information which will be useful to parents, whether or not they decide to undergo genetic testing. The book is written in lay terms, without footnotes or references, and discusses a wide range of subjects, including types of genetic defects, gene mutation, environmental effects, racial and ethnic factors, effects of incest or rape, common superstitions, causes of mental retardation, hazards in pregnancy, artificial insemination, amniocentesis, abortion dilemmas, heredity and cancer, treating genetic disease, intelligence, selecting for baby's sex, twins, and medical treatment (or non-treatment) for defective babies. In each area Dr. Milunsky presents the medical facts *and* the difficult moral, ethical, and legal questions which are often involved. On the negative side, Dr. Milunsky does not acknowledge or discuss the safety questions about ultrasound. He is also somewhat unsympathetic toward parents who decide not to avail themselves of indicated genetic testing or abortion of a defective fetus.

"Amniocentesis is of course a minor surgical procedure and as such requires prior consent. In agreeing to undergo the procedure (as would be the case for elective abortion), the physician is required to inform the patient carefully about the very small risks of the test. In addition, both he and the laboratory doing the studies should ensure that the couple involved know that the removed cells may not grow in the laboratory in 5 to 10 percent of cases, that a second or even third amniocentesis may be needed, that the answers provided are not 100 percent guaranteed, and that *other* genetic disorders or birth defects will *not* be excluded by the test . . . "

NATIONAL CLEARINGHOUSE FOR HUMAN GENETIC DISEASES
805 15th Street, NW, Suite 500
Washington, DC 20005
202/842-7617

The Clearinghouse was established in October, 1978, by the Department of Health and Human Services (then the Department of Health, Education and Welfare), under the "National Genetic Diseases Act." This act, which became law in April, 1976, provides for the Secretary of HHS to "develop information and educational materials to persons providing health care, to teachers and students, and to the public in general in order to rapidly make available the latest advances in the testing, diagnosis, counseling and treatment of individuals respecting genetic diseases." The Clearinghouse provides services and publications to both lay and professional people.

HUMAN GENETICS: Informational and Educational Materials
Vol. I, No. 1 (DHHS Pub. No. (HSA) 79-5132
Supplement No. 2 (DHHS Pub. No (HSA) 80-5136
Single copies free

These two catalogs are about 175 pages each and provide resource listings for books, brochures, pamphlets, journal articles, book chapters, and audio-visual materials on human genetics.

CLINICAL GENETIC SERVICE CENTERS: A National Listing
1980, 117 pages

from
National Clearinghouse for Human Genetic Diseases
P.O. Box 28612
Washington, DC 20005
single copy free

This directory lists institutions in the United States (arranged by state) which provide services in clinical genetics (including diagnosis and treatment), genetic counseling, prenatal diagnosis, cytogenetics (study of the chromosomal basis of heredity), and biochemical genetics. Also included is a listing of federally-funded programs in hemophilia and sickle cell anemia.

NEURAL TUBE DEFECT SCREENING

Neural tube defects result when the neural tube, which contains what will later become the brain and spinal cord, fails to fuse completely in the first month of pregnancy. Spina bifida and anencephaly are neural tube defects.

A new screening program has been developed to detect neural tube defects during pregnancy. A blood sample drawn from the mother in her 16th to 18th week of pregnancy is tested for levels of AFP. Higher than usual levels can mean that the woman is carrying twins or that the fetus has a neural tube defect. If the first blood test shows elevated levels, a second blood test is done, followed by ultrasound and amniocentesis to rule out twins or a mistake in estimating gestational age. If a neural tube defect is diagnosed, the mother may decide to have an abortion or make plans for special medical assistance when the baby is born. It is estimated that neural tube defects occur in about one out of every 1000 births.

The screening is currently restricted to FDA approved pilot programs which provide the follow-up procedures of ultrasound and amniocentesis and provide genetic counseling. Pharmaceutical companies are vigorously lobbying, however, for regulations which would allow unrestricted sale and use of the blood test by any doctor or lab. Critics claim that without the assurance of follow-up testing and counseling, healthy fetuses might be aborted unnecessarily. In August, 1979, Dr. Sidney Wolfe and Robert Leflar of the Public Citizen Health Research Group wrote the following to then Secretary of HEW, Patricia Harris: "If the testing process is carried out in carefully controlled prenatal diagnosis programs, such as the successful pilot projects on Long Island and in the Boston area, the tests should prove beneficial. However, if the testing process is not closely controlled, the likely result will be that many women, although they and their husbands want children and the pregnancies are in fact perfectly normal, will have unnecessary abortions because of unwarranted fears of a birth defect—fears generated by false-positive test results. In addition, many normal fetuses may be unnecessarily harmed by expanded use of a procedure (amniocentesis) that is part of the testing process. In fact, the number of normal pregnancies harmed by an uncontrolled testing program might well exceed the number of neural tube defects detected." The FDA held hearings on the matter in January, 1981, and proposed to restrict the marketing of AFP test kits until the agency can determine what restrictions, if any, are necessary.

MATERNAL SERUM ALPHA-FETOPROTEIN: Issues in the Prenatal Screening and Diagnosis of Neural Tube Defects.
Barbara Gastel, et al., eds.
1980, 201 pages

from
Department of Health and Human Services
National Center for Health Care Technology
5600 Fishers Lane
Rockville, MD 20857

This publication presents the proceedings of a conference held by the National Center for Health Care Technology and the Food and Drug Administration in July, 1980. Participants included physicians and scientists involved in alpha-fetoprotein (AFP) testing, pediatricians and specialists in birth defects, consumer advocates, and parents of affected children. The conference addressed the medical and scientific background of AFP testing, ethical, legal, economic and social perspectives, and issues in the implementation of AFP screening.

"American women have grown increasingly skeptical of medical 'breakthroughs.' Experience has taught them that today's medical marvel may be tomorrow's tragedy . . . built-in economic incentives exist for industry to promote, and health-care providers to perform, routine AFP screening—for reasons unrelated to benefits to society or to the mother as an individual."

—Doris Haire in *Maternal Serum Alpha-Fetoprotein.*

THE CPK TEST: For the Detection of Female Carriers of Duchenne Muscular Dystrophy
1980, brochure

from
Muscular Dystrophy Association
810 Seventh Avenue
New York, NY 10019
free

This brochure describes Duchenne muscular dystrophy and how female carriers are detected.

MARCH OF DIMES

MARCH OF DIMES
P.O. Box 2000
White Plains, NY 10602

The March of Dimes provides many publications and resources on birth defects. A selection of their pamphlets (with order numbers) is listed below. The March of Dimes also provides a national listing of genetic counselors. Write for a copy of their publications list or for more information. Publications are available free in single copies or in bulk for distribution in packets, classes or clinics.

GENETIC COUNSELING
22 pages, Illus. (9-0022)

Genetic counseling is a relatively new scientific specialty which involves determining whether or not a couple is likely to produce a child with a birth defect and what can be done to reduce the risk. This booklet explains what genetic counseling is and why it may be needed, describes the actions of genes and chromosomes, differentiates between genetic and environmentally-caused birth defects and suggests that families keep a medical record of all infections, medications, and X-rays, which may also cause birth defects. Dominant, recessive, X-linked, and multifactorial inheritance are explained, accompanied by clear diagrams. Testing for carriers of genetic defects and prenatal diagnosis by amniocentesis are explained.

"When risks are stated in percentages or fractions, parents unfamiliar with genetic mechanisms often interpret them incorrectly.

"For example, those with one child affected by a disorder due to recessive inheritance may think that a 25 percent—or one-in-four—risk means that the next three offspring are not endangered. *This is not true.*

"The risk of genetic disease is the same for every child of the same mother and father."

"Women with a history of Duchenne muscular dystrophy in their families should take the CPK test . . . . Since there is a 50 percent risk that male children of carriers will develop Duchenne muscular dystrophy, some parents decide to adopt children rather than raise children of their own. Testing and counseling of all suspected carriers could substantially reduce the future incidence of this type of muscular dystrophy."

TAY-SACHS DISEASE (9-0100)

Describes Tay-Sachs disease, how to detect carriers, and prevention through prenatal diagnosis and counseling.

"Victims are primarily descendents of Central and Eastern European (Ashkenazi) Jews, although members of any group may inherit the disease. Some 90% of American Jews are of Ashkenazi origin . . . Voluntary screening by young men and women of Jewish heritage to learn if they are carriers, prenatal diagnosis, and genetic counseling are methods now being used in efforts to prevent this disease."

SICKLE CELL ANEMIA (9-0001)

Describes sickle cell disease, who is at risk, and why testing for the trait is important.

"In the United States, most cases of sickle cell anemia occur among Afro-Americans. About one in ten carries the gene which may cause the disorder in offspring if two gene carriers marry."

THALASSEMIA: A Birth Defect (9-0041)

Describes thalassemia (Cooley's anemia), how carriers are detected, and how affected babies are diagnosed.

"Thalassemia is one of the most common of the inherited diseases of the blood yet few people have ever heard of it. In the United States some 2,500 people are hospitalized every year for treatment of this disease. Many of these individuals trace their ancestry to the Mediterranean region. Most are of Italian or Greek descent."

FOR FURTHER READING

The Future of Motherhood by Jessie Bernard (Dial, 1974)

Prenatal Diagnosis and Selective Abortion by Harry Harris (Harvard University Press, 1975)

The Genetic Connection by David Hendin and Joan Marks (Signet, 1979)

Genetic Disorders and the Fetus: Diagnosis, Prevention, and Treatment by Aubrey Milunsky, ed. (Plenum Press, 1979)

Altered Destinies: Lives Changed by Genetic Flaws by William Stockton (Doubleday, 1979)

ULTRASOUND

RESEARCH IN ULTRASOUND BIOEFFECTS: A Public Health View
by Melvin E. Stratmeyer, Ph.D.
1980, 12 pages, Illus.

from
BIRTH
Reprints
110 El Camino
Berkeley, CA 94705
$1.50 for single copies

Dr. Stratmeyer is a research scientist at the Bureau of Radiological Health of the U.S. Food and Drug Administration, where he is investigating the biological effects of ultrasound exposure. In this paper he reviews what is currently known about the safety of ultrasound, based on human and animal studies. He describes the bioeffects which have been observed in animal studies. These include: developmental, hematologic, vascular, neurologic, behavioral, immunologic, and genetic effects. Dr. Stratmeyer concludes that current studies are not sufficient to determine whether the use of ultrasound in pregnancy is safe or effective and that more studies are needed. Numerous tables and a list of 25 references are included.

"I . . . assume that you have all heard that ultrasound is safe and effective. This assumption of safety and effectiveness is based primarily on clinical impressions . . . . Although clinical impressions do have some value, we really cannot make decisions based on clinical impressions . . . . At the present time, we cannot take what we know about exposed human populations and say that ultrasound is safe or unsafe."

PROCEEDINGS OF A SYMPOSIUM ON BIOLOGICAL EFFECTS AND CHARACTERISTICS OF ULTRA-SOUND SOURCES
HSS Pub. No. (FDA) 78-8048

from
Food and Drug Administration
2600 Fishers Lane
Rockville, MD 20852
single copy free

This collection of scientific papers is quite technical and covers the effects of fetal exposure to ultrasound as well as questions of instrumentation and technique. Professionals and others may find the publication useful as a source of references, statistics, and researchers to contact. Even though ultrasound is approved for use by the FDA, many serious questions exist about its long-term safety for the baby. Contributors to this Symposium stress the lack of adequate research and information on the safety of ultrasound use in pregnancy.

"It can be stated generally that the data on many of the effects of ultrasound is, at best, inconclusive. However, in public health protection, unlike the situation in law, inconclusive evidence cannot be construed as presumable innocence. From a public health point of view, any ultrasound-induced effect that reasonably might represent a potential health hazard, even in selected individuals, must be thoroughly investigated. Until more information is available on such effects, a definitive assessment of the potential risk will not be possible."

—Melvin E. Stratmeyer

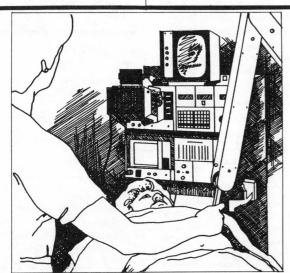

Illustration of an ultrasound examination (above) is from *Seeing With Sound,* a free brochure from the American College of Radiology, 20 N. Wacker Drive, Chicago, IL 60606.

AMNIOCENTESIS

AMNIOCENTESIS FOR PRENATAL CHROMOSOMAL DIAGNOSIS
1980, 40 pages, Illus.

from
Center for Disease Control
Attn: Chronic Diseases Division
Bureau of Epidemiology
Atlanta, GA 30333
single copy free

This booklet uses drawings, photographs, and a very simple text to describe the risk of Down's syndrome, what Down's syndrome is, the procedure for amniocentesis (photos show each step), the mild and serious risks, and the interpretation of results.

CONSENSUS: Antenatal Diagnosis brochure

from
Office for Medical Applications of Research
National Institutes of Health
Building 1, Room 216
Bethesda, MD 20205
single copy free

This brochure summarizes the consensus reached by the Consensus Development Conference on Antenatal Diagnosis held in 1979 by the National Institutes of Health.

NATIONAL GENETICS FOUNDATION, INC.
555 West 57th Street
New York, NY 10019
212/586-5800

The National Genetics Foundation is "a nonprofit voluntary health agency which coordinates a Network of 54 genetic counseling and treatment centers in the United States and Canada. The Foundation acts as a Clearinghouse for the Network, and can refer an individual, a family, or an entire kindred to the center most appropriate for the diagnosis or treatment of a specific genetic problem."

The foundation provides five informative brochures on genetic counseling:

* *How Genetic Disease Can Affect You and Your Family*
* *Can Genetic Counseling Help You?*
* *Genetic Counseling and Treatment Network*
* *For the Concerned Couple Planning a Family*
* *Should You Consider Amniocentesis?*

The first three are available in bulk for $5. per 100 and the last two for postage and handling charges only. Single copies are available free with a self-addressed, stamped envelope.

GENETIC AMNIOCENTESIS
by Fritz Fuchs
1980, 7 pages, Illus.

from
Scientific American Offprints
W.H. Freeman & Co.
660 Market Street
San Francisco, CA 94104
single copy 60 cents
request bulk rates

This article first appeared in the June, 1980, issue of *Scientific American* magazine. Like most articles in this excellent publication, it is geared to the educated reader or student with some background in science, but is written in lay terms without technological jargon. Dr. Fuchs describes in detail the procedure for amniocentesis, and the kinds of disorders which can be detected, including sex-linked disorders (like hemophilia), chromosomal abnormalities (like Down's syndrome), and inborn errors of metabolism (Tay-Sachs disease). Alpha-fetoprotein testing for neural tube defects is also discussed. The major risks of amniocentesis are described and weighed against the risks of bearing a defective child. The present availability of genetic testing, its legal implications, and future are also presented.

"The advantage of prenatal diagnosis is clear. Among the numerous fetal abnormalities that can now be detected, many lead to debilitating disease and many cause death at an early age. Others cause mental retardation so severe that it precludes a normal life. For most of the abnormalities no treatment now exists, but if they can be detected early in gestation, the pregnancy can be ended. Even those prospective parents who do not consider the termination of a pregnancy acceptable may think it important to know the diagnosis so that they can prepare for the birth of an affected infant. Moreover, a large proportion of parents who know themselves to be at risk of bearing a child with a genetic disease no doubt would never undertake a pregnancy if prenatal diagnosis were not available, or would choose abortion automatically if a pregnancy occurred."

For information about amniocentesis and ultrasound, plus other tests done to determine fetal well-being during and just prior to labor, see *Obstetric Tests and Technology* by Margot Edwards and Penny Simkin (see index).

Should You Have An Amniocentesis?

Amniocentesis is a procedure in which amniotic fluid is removed, the fetal cells grown in culture and then analyzed to determine whether the fetus suffers from any of the genetic defects which currently can be detected in this way. If the fetus is affected, the parents can decide to have an abortion.

If you know you are the carrier of a genetic defect like hemophilia or Tay-Sachs disease, the decision to undergo amniocentesis may be fairly easy, since your chances of having a defective child are very high (25% or more). In this case, you are considered to be in a high-risk group. Before the availability of prenatal diagnosis and selective abortion, many couples in this group were afraid to have children at all.

More difficult is the decision to have an amniocentesis based on the mother's age alone. For women at age 40, the risk of having a Down's syndrome child is about 1 percent or equal to the risk of complications from the procedure itself. After age 40 the risk of Down's syndrome rises sharply to a rate of about 8.5 percent or 1 in 12 at age 49 (see graph). Women over 40 are considered to be at moderate risk.

For women between 35 and 40 the decision is most difficult. The risks of the procedure are estimated at 1 to 2 percent and can mean the loss of a healthy fetus. These risks must be balanced against the somewhat smaller risk of having a Down's syndrome child, which ranges from about .25 percent (1 in 400) at age 35 to 1 percent (1 in 100) at age 40. Amniocentesis is generally termed a "safe" procedure. It is, however, a minor surgical procedure for which informed consent, often in writing, is required. Risks of the procedure include:

1.) Amniotic fluid embolism
2.) Maternal hemorrhage
3.) Maternal infection
4.) Induced labor or miscarriage
5.) Abruptio placentae
6.) Puncture of the mother's bladder or intestine
7.) Rh isoimmunization
8.) Fetal death
9.) Amnionitis
10.) Fetal injury caused by the needle
11.) Fetal hemorrhage
12.) Rupture of membranes

An additional risk involves the use of an ultrasound scan, usually done to locate the fetus and placenta before inserting the needle. Ultrasound has never been proven safe and animal studies indicate a wide range of adverse effects (see index).

A difficult personal decision must be made. For some women the thought of miscarrying a healthy baby is unacceptable and these women may decide not to undergo amniocentesis even if they are at risk. Likewise, women for whom abortion is unacceptable may decide not to have the procedure, since they would not act on its results anyway. For others the thought of giving birth to a defective baby is far more devastating than the possible loss or damage of a normal baby. There is no easy answer, and these difficult decisions are bound to increase as more and more women delay childbearing into their 30's.

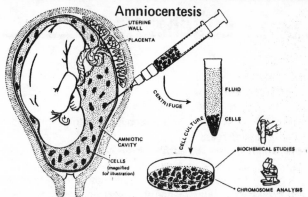

Illustration of the amniocentesis procedure from *The New Human Genetics* published in April, 1981, by the National Institutes of Health, Bethesda, MD 20205. "Cells shed by the growing fetus are cultured from a sample of amniotic fluid, withdrawn from the expectant mother's uterus by means of a hypodermic needle. The cells are then tested for biochemical or chromosomal defects. Some 80 serious genetic diseases, including Down's syndrome, can now be detected prenatally in this way."

An excellent discussion of "Prenatal Diagnosis and the Unwanted Abortion" appears in *When Pregnancy Fails: Families Coping with Miscarriage, Stillbirth, and Infant Death* by Susan Borg and Judith Lasker [(Beacon, 1981) see index].

FACTS ABOUT DOWN'S SYNDROME FOR WOMEN OVER 35
1979, 16 pages, Illus.

from
National Institute of Child Health and Human Development
Office of Research Reporting
National Institutes of Health
Bethesda, MD 20205
single copy free

This booklet uses a question-and-answer format and illustrations of chromosomes to explain Down's syndrome, including the outlook for Down's syndrome children (degree of mental retardation, related medical problems, life expectancy) and the three kinds of Down's syndrome (Trisomy 21, the most common, Translocation, and Mosaicism). A table shows how the risk of Down's syndrome increases with maternal age, rising sharply from about 1 in 900 at age 30 to 1 in 105 at age 40. Women are advised to take good care of their health in pregnancy and to consider genetic counseling if they are over 35 or have a family history of Down's syndrome. A glossary of terms is included.

Incidence of Down's Syndrome by Maternal Age
Based on Griffith, G.W. (1973)

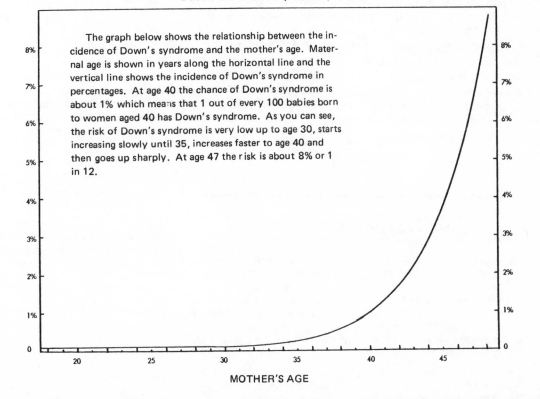

The graph below shows the relationship between the incidence of Down's syndrome and the mother's age. Maternal age is shown in years along the horizontal line and the vertical line shows the incidence of Down's syndrome in percentages. At age 40 the chance of Down's syndrome is about 1% which means that 1 out of every 100 babies born to women aged 40 has Down's syndrome. As you can see, the risk of Down's syndrome is very low up to age 30, starts increasing slowly until 35, increases faster to age 40 and then goes up sharply. At age 47 the risk is about 8% or 1 in 12.

MOTHER'S AGE

Risks in Childbearing

Priya Morganstern, editor

The term "high risk," commonly used in obstetrics, is problematic for the following reasons:

1) *All risk judgments are subjective.* While certain conditions certainly do necessitate closer attention and/or caution, ultimately "risk" depends on the mother's physical and emotional condition, the health professional's knowledge and experience, and whether the condition is being treated and/or whether it has improved. The effects of psychological or spiritual strength should not be ignored.

2) *Risks change over time.* According to many books, the *history* of certain transient conditions (that have passed) would still categorize a woman as high risk. If a woman has a history of "small-for-gestational-age" baby, yet the current pregnancy is progressing with good fundal height growth, it is not clear what purpose is served in giving her a high risk label. If a woman was pre-eclamptic in a previous pregnancy, but has prevented it this time with conscientious diet habits and/or supplements, many practitioners would not consider her "at risk."

3) *Risks are relative.* Frequently, it is not a condition *per se* which determines risk but the *severity* of the condition. That is a judgment in and of itself.

4) *What is the opposite of "high risk"?* If a pregnancy is not high risk, is it low risk? No risk? This is not merely a game in semantics; our language directly affects our beliefs and perspectives. I do not believe that pregnancy should be perceived in terms of risk, however relative. The word *risk* implies a certain stigma and this can affect self-image and outcome. In effect, a "high risk" label may become self-fulfilling.

5) *Too many of us are "high risk."* The factors which determine risk have—in the medical profession—gotten out of hand. One recently published book declares simply that 25% of all pregnancies in the U.S. are high risk!! When percentages become that high, the term "high risk" begins to lose its meaning.

It is hoped that the resources in this section will help inform women who are significantly at risk during pregnancy, and help others to evaluate the risk judgments which may be made by their medical care providers. There is other related information regarding twins, cesarean births, Vaginal Birth After Cesarean (VBAC), and pregnancy over thirty elsewhere in the book. Please check the index.

(PM)

RISK FACTOR ASSESSMENT

The Oregon Midwifery Council has developed an excellent "risk factor assessment" table for use by lay midwives. The table assigns a risk factor number of 1-5 (for example, emotional stress is accorded a rating of "1" and abruptio placenta a rating of "5"). Midwives are advised not to attend a home birth where the combined risk total is 5 or above. The table was published in Vol. 4, No. 16 of OMC's newsletter, *Birthing.* For back issues contact Pat Edmonds, editor, at 3839 Pacific Avenue, No. 189, Forest Grove, OR 97116. (JIA)

RISK FACTORS

For this list we have combined the recommendations of several respected lay midwives concerning the risks which would contraindicate (indicate against) a home birth, or which would require some treatment or attention before a home birth could be recommended. Nurse-midwives would also probably consider these factors to rule out giving birth in a free-standing birth center or hospital 'birthing room' unless the problem can be resolved. Remember that the conditions listed here are not equal in severity or seriousness and the presence of a single risk factor from this list may not necessitate 'high risk' treatment. This list is intended as a guideline to help parents understand what is meant by the term 'risk' in childbirth. Your doctor or midwife will want to know whether you have had or now have any of these conditions. Screening for these risk factors is one of the most important parts of prenatal care. With appropriate medical care, the outlook for pregnant women with risk factors can be improved.

(JIA)

Diabetes Mellitus or Gestational Diabetes
Chronic Hypertension (high blood pressure)
Sickle Cell Anemia
Epilepsy
Renal Disease
Heart Disease
Hypothyroidism
Hyperthyroidism
Maternal age under 17
Previous Cesarean-section
Grand Multiparity (6 or more babies)
Previous Hard-to-control Postpartum Hemorrhage
Incompetent Cervix
Rh Sensitization (Iso-immunization)
Narcotic Addiction
Alcoholic Mother
Very Poorly Nourished Mother
Excessive Cigarette Smoking
Rubella Infection during Pregnancy
Untreated Venereal Disease (Syphilis or Gonorrhea)
Active Herpes Infection at Time of Birth
Severe Anemia
Eclampsia or Pre-eclampsia (Toxemia of pregnancy)
Polyhydramnios (too much amniotic fluid)
Multiple Pregnancy (twins or more)
Vaginal Bleeding in 2nd or 3rd trimester of pregnancy (more than just "spotting")
Abnormal Fetal Heart Tones
Placenta Previa (placenta implanted over cervix)
Abnormal Uterine Growth
Abnormal Presentation (Breech or Transverse lie)
Premature Rupture of Membranes (24 hours before labor)
Premature Labor (three weeks before due date)
Postmature Labor (two weeks after due date)
Abruptio Placenta (premature separation of placenta)

THE CHILD BEFORE BIRTH
by Linda Ferrill Annis
1978, 194 pages, Illus.

from
Cornell University Press
124 Roberts Place
Ithaca, NY 14850
$12.50 hd

The Child Before Birth provides a general introduction to prenatal development and factors which may influence the unborn child. Although there are many books written on the subject (some of which are reviewed in this *Catalog*), Ms. Annis's book seems to cover more of the influencing factors that are potentially negative. In this light, the book becomes a source of information on conditions that predispose a pregnancy to higher risk.

The book covers a wide range of factors in a brief but concise form. Annis frequently refers to scientific studies; her style is clear, non-judgmental and academic. The chapters on prenatal nutrition, maternal characteristics and experiences, and drugs and disease are particularly relevant.

The last chapter, "Every Child's Right to be Normal," was a bit disappointing. Annis discusses pre-maturity, genetics, amniocentesis, sex determination, and abortion, but never really deals with the difficult moral question of whether a child *does* have the right to be born normal. But for purely factual information, the book is fine.   (PM)

"Rubella's threat to the developing child is strongest in the first three months of pregnancy. During the first four weeks after conception, the chance of defects is about 50 percent, diminishing to 17 percent in the third month and to almost zero after the third or fourth month (Rhodes, 1961). Miscarriage, too, may occur if rubella is contracted during the first three months of pregnancy. It is generally agreed that there is a one out of three chance that a defective child will be born if the mother contracts rubella during the first four months of pregnancy, and, because the chances for a normal birth are so poor, many authorities feel justified in ending the pregnancy. If maternal rubella occurs after the fourth month and especially during the last trimester of pregnancy, the child does not appear to be harmed in any way except for the fact that the infant shows the rash of rubella. Babies born with the rash of rubella, of course, promptly start a German measles epidemic in the neonatal nursery."

HAVING TWINS
by Elizabeth Noble
1980, 240 pages, Illus.

from
Houghton Mifflin Co.
2 Park Street
Boston, MA 02107
$14.95 hd., $7.95 pap.

Elizabeth Noble is a physical therapist who specializes in obstetrics and gynecology, and is the author of the classic *Essential Exercises for the Childbearing Year.* In *Having Twins* , Noble has done a beautiful job of exploring the cultural, social, emotional, and physiological aspects of twins. The book is a joy to look at and to read. While acknowledging and describing the known risks of twin pregnancy and birth, she maintains that through good prenatal care most of the risk can be reduced or eliminated. By interviewing many mothers who successfully carried normal birthweight babies to term, Noble presents their experience and advice.

Noble discusses our fascination with multiple birth, how twins are formed, and who is most likely to have twins. She covers detection of twins, and parent's emotions while awaiting the birth. The most significant portion of the book, however, deals with how to prevent prematurity and low-birth-weight babies—the major causes of higher perinatal mortality rates in multiple births. Excellent nutrition and prenatal care can alleviate these problems in twins (as they do for singletons), and Noble outlines exactly what to do.

Noble also discusses comfort in pregnancy, labor and birth, dealing with problems, caring for twins, and special features of twinship. In addition, the book contains quotations from twins, or parents of twins, in the border on every page. Those quotations, in a sense, are the heart of the book; it is through them that we can share the wonder, doubt, difficulties and pleasures that are part of a twin birth. Noble's book definitely lets us know that for most parents, twins—however difficult or unexpected—are a special blessing.
(PM)

'' *'The Best Prenatal Care* is what you give yourself' is an important maxim. The medical profession really just measures, monitors, and manages any complications that may arise. Only you can make the daily commitment to a good diet, exercise, rest, relaxation, and education about pregnancy and birth. The best time to start such a program is even before conception, but it is never too late to change one's habits for the better. The greatest demands on the body occur after the fifth month, by which time it is certainly possible to diagnose a multiple pregnancy. A mother can only know to eat for three if she knows she is carrying two.

"Important issues are often forgotten in the doctor's office. It is helpful to write down a list of questions for your physician to answer at each prenatal visit. As we saw in Chapter 4, women often believe they are carrying twins, but the idea may be rejected by the obstetrician. Do not hesitate to get a second opinion or to insist on an ultrasound scan if you are reasonably sure your suspicions are correct. Some doctors just don't like to admit that their patients know something they don't. Ultrasound, as was explained in Chapter 4, is not always reliable; it may show twins when there are actually triplets.

"While most health care providers and consumers would consider twins a contraindication for home birth, home delivery of twins does happen. Often, the twins are undiagnosed and the second baby is usually delivered without mishap. Twins are routinely delivered at home at The Farm, an alternative lifestyle community in Tennessee. Ina May Gaskin, author of *Spiritual Midwifery,* explains that the usual 7 or 8-pound birth weights are due to the quality of prenatal care and nutrition. To date only one twin labor, out of more than ten, has required transfer to the hospital, and no Caesarean deliveries have been necessary."

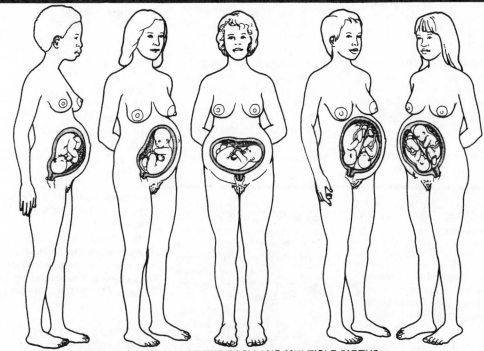

UNUSUAL POSITIONS OF THE BABY AND MULTIPLE BIRTHS
Illustration from *The Childbirth Picture Book,* © 1981, 1982 Fran Hosken, drawings by Marcia L. Williams, available from Women's International Network (see index for listing). The illustration shows (from left) a normal head-down presentation, breech presentation, transverse lie, identical twins (sharing a placenta), and fraternal twins (with two placentas).

SAFEGUARDING YOUR HEART DURING PREGNANCY
14 pages, Illus.

from
American Heart Association
7320 Greenville Avenue
Dallas, TX 75231
single copies free

This is a short, concise booklet for women with any history of heart disease—whether it be a congenital defect or due to an infection such as rheumatic fever. The book discusses the increased stress placed on even a normal heart during pregnancy, and the special problems that it may pose to a woman with heart disease. The booklet explains what the doctor will look for and test for, and general recommendations that he or she will make for health and comfort during pregnancy. It also includes information on anesthetics and medications likely to be used during labor and delivery, and stresses that a "natural childbirth" is preferable.

The American Heart Association is composed of health professionals, scientists and lay people. It endeavors to support research, education and community programs in order to reduce death and disability due to heart disease. Write to them for further information. (PM)

"If you have a history of heart disease, heart murmur, or rheumatic fever, and want to have a baby, it is important for you to go to your family doctor before you become pregnant to talk about your health, to plan for your pregnancy, and to consider what may be involved in caring for your child later.

"Your family doctor can help you go through pregnancy and childbirth without undue risk, and to stay healthy during the months following delivery. He knows you best and knows your history. And he can help you to seek and obtain any special advice needed from a heart specialist, internist, or obstetrician. Usually the family doctor is better able to care for your everyday needs during pregnancy and to coordinate any special tests that may be necessary. He can also suggest special services that are available in your community to help you before, during, and after pregnancy."

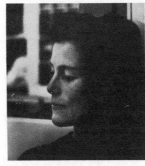

LIFE DANCE
by Nell Dorr and Covington Hardee
1975, 75 pages, Illus.

from
Alleluia Press
Box 103
Allendale, NJ 07401
$9.75 pap.

This very moving and unusual book is a photo essay by famed natural-light photographer Nell Dorr of the pregnancy and family life of her friend, Joan Chappell Hardee. Joan was afflicted with polio at the age of 21 and died in 1974 at the age of 47. But during the period of her disability and partial paralysis, she gave birth to five of her six children. Joan wrote the text for this book which documents the birth of her last child. (JIA)

"Of all the intangible forces—with such tangible results—in making the human being whole and happy, love is the prime one. There are many kinds of love: love of children, of husband and wife, of close family and friends, and for many of us, love of God. Soon after we met, my husband said to me, 'I think I might not have fallen in love with you if your arms had not been paralyzed.' Every living person has different needs and desires to be fulfilled by other people, but that which is common to us all is the need to be loved. When I first was paralyzed, I thought I was no longer of any value and therefore not worth loving. How woefully wrong I was, and selfish, to start from that point of view. I found through love, and because of love, that one is filled with love not by the taking but by the giving. One gives and gives of love and eventually one is filled with it. Love is the most healing force in the world, and I am certain that discovering how to love deeply was the most effective way to learn to live with myself and polio."

GIVING BIRTH
by John Hare and Elizabeth Kay Soloman
1981, 4 pages

from
American Diabetes Association, Inc.
2 Park Avenue
New York, NY 10016
single copies free

Giving Birth is a brief but very informative booklet for the diabetic woman. Both Hare and Soloman work with the Joslin Diabetes Clinic in Boston, and have a realistic, down-to-earth attitude regarding pregnancy with diabetes. They point out that the mortality rate for infants of diabetic mothers has dropped considerably and is now very close to the infant mortality rate of the general population. They stress that the key to this success is diabetic control, with the mother's blood sugar carefully controlled from the moment of conception—or preferably, before.

The booklet breaks pregnancy down into its trimesters, and describes the special needs of the diabetic mother over time. It is nice that the authors not only discuss the medical aspects of pregnancy, but also its anxieties and joys.

When writing to the association to obtain this booklet, also request their short bibliography of lay and professional articles regarding diabetes and pregnancy. (PM)

RESOURCES FOR HANDICAPPED MOTHERS
(information supplied by Jeanette Breen)

HUMAN SCIENCES PRESS
72 Fifth Avenue
New York, NY 10011
publishes booklets about pregnancy and the disabled, including paraplegia

NATIONAL HEALTH INFORMATION CLEARINGHOUSE
P.O. Box 1133
Washington, D.C. 20013
800/336-4797
for information, write or call toll free.

PEOPLE TO PEOPLE COMMITTEE FOR THE HANDICAPPED
Suite 1130
1575 I St. N.W. 4th Floor
Washington, D.C. 20005
publishes the *Directory of Organizations Interested in the Handicapped 1980-1981.* (1980, 55 pages), available for $3.00

DISABLED LIVING FOUNDATION
346 Kensington High Street
London WI48NS
England
publishes *Early Years,* and *Motherhood: How to Cope.* Both are about mothers with physical handicaps.

CHILDBIRTH EDUCATION ASSOCIATION
P.O. Box 1609
Springfield VA 22151
Provides childbirth education classes for deaf couples and a teaching manual in Braille.

SPECIAL PUBLICATIONS LIST
1978, 6 pages

from
LaLeche League
9616 Minneapolis Avenue
Franklin Park, IL 60131
free

This publication lists books and other materials available from La Leche League in Braille, on cassette, on reel-to-reel tape, or in large type. The list itself is available in Braille for $3.00. Subjects include breastfeeding, pregnancy and childbirth, child care and the family, nutrition, and resources for the professional. Also listed are resources available from the Library of Congress and Recordings for the Blind.

DRUG DEPENDENCY IN PREGNANCY: Clinical Management of Mother and Child
1979, 109 pages

from
Alcohol, Drug Abuse, and Mental Health Administration
5600 Fishers Lane (Room 6C-02)
Rockville, MD 20857
free

This highly detailed publication is actually a short nursing text. It describes the complications arising when mothers are addicted to psycho-tropic and other kinds of drugs. The authors discuss the prevalence and classification of drug use, the pharmacologic effects on mother and infant, and the clinical management of the drug-dependent woman during pregnancy. They describe the management of labor and delivery, care of the newborn, and the continuing care for the mother and infant.

Each chapter has been well thought out and reflects a deep understanding of the problems presented by drug-dependent mothers. There is a great deal of compassion shown these women by the authors of the book. (PM)

Miscarriage

Priya Morganstern, editor

A miscarriage is the unintended ending of a pregnancy before the fetus can survive on its own. Called a "spontaneous abortion" in the medical literature, it occurs surprisingly frequently: fifteen to twenty percent of all conceptions are miscarried. Given this frequency, it is surprising how little understanding there is of the causes, and more importantly, the emotional issues involved. In most cases, the grief that results from a miscarriage is belittled. "It's nothing to cry about." "It's all for the best." "You can always have another baby." Parents are frequently surprised by the depth of their sorrow and may find little support from friends or family who expect them to "get over it quickly." In one sense, this is understandable; the baby was really only known to its parents. As one author put it, for friends and family there "is no object of grief." Even those who are normally very supportive and compassionate can underestimate the loss felt by parents. Doctors are often less than sympathetic with parents' emotional reactions and medical terms like "fetal wastage" and "habitual aborter" can be cruel. Probably we all need to become more sensitive toward those who have suffered a miscarriage. Important lessons are: 1) Friends or family of a couple who have miscarried should be willing to listen. Many parents have said that they wanted desperately to talk about the miscarriage, but no one wanted to listen. 2) Those who miscarry should not try to deny their grief but allow themselves a time of mourning and seek help and support if they need it. 3) Medical professionals need to practice compassion in dealing with their patients who miscarry a pregnancy. (PM)

COPING WITH A MISCARRIAGE
by Hank Pizer and Christine O'Brien Palinski
1980, 179 pages

from
Dial Press
1 Dag Hammarskjold Plaza
New York, NY 10017
$10.95 hd.

Coping with a Miscarriage was written by a woman who, after a normal first pregnancy and birth, went on to have three miscarriages within the next two years. During that time Ms. Palinski experienced fear, doubt, and confusion. Mostly, however, she was frustrated with the lack of available information on miscarriage. She also became aware of a "silence" which surrounds miscarriage and found it almost unbelievable that it occurs in fifteen to twenty percent of all pregnancies. Why hadn't she heard more about it? After her three miscarriages, she did finally carry a child to term and decided then and there to put into book form all the information that she had accumulated over the years.

The book that she wrote with Hank Pizer (a medical writer and physician's assistant) is very complete and clearly written. Some of the topics covered include: basic physiology of conception, implantation and pregnancy; genetics and its relevance to spontaneous abortion; other causes of miscarriage; and

medical interventions to predict or prevent miscarriages (of which she clearly notes their controversial nature). The second half of the book deals with the emotional issues, specifically dealing first with mothers, then fathers, and then the reactions of others. She also discusses normal pregnancy after miscarriage and its special aspects, both physical and emotional. The book also features a glossary, references, and concise summaries at the end of each chapter. (PM)

"There is no reason to change your exercise or work patterns in order to prevent a recurrence of your spontaneous abortion problem. However, if your work exposes you to chemicals, you may want to be more cautious. No scientific proof demonstrates that you can dislodge a developing embryo by moving. This is true of sexual intercourse as well as work and exercise."

PREGNANCY AFTERMATH HOTLINE
4742 North Sheffield Avenue
Milwaukee, WI 53211
414/445-2131

A 24-hour hotline staffed by trained volunteers, designed especially for women who have just gone through a miscarriage, abortion, or have relinquished a baby for adoption.

LETTER TO A CHILD NEVER BORN
by Oriana Fallaci
1976, 114 pages

from
Simon and Schuster
630 Fifth Avenue
New York, NY 10020
$6.95 hd

Letter to a Child Never Born is a beautiful, anguished monologue between a woman and her unborn child. Oriana Fallaci, a prizewinning Italian journalist and writer, has struck at a raw and sensitive nerve: ambivalence and doubt regarding an unplanned pregnancy. While intellectually the women she describes is very removed and cautious about the child she has decided to bear, emotionally she has merged with the child more than she ever expected. The book is an amazing journey through time, it is a monologue not only with her unborn child, but ultimately also with the woman's conscience. The book is brilliant in its exploration of anger, resentment, love and acceptance as we follow the woman accepting motherhood, yet feeling deprived by it too. When the woman miscarries early in the pregnancy, she experiences a depth of grief she hadn't expected. She had truly created a relationship with this child, albeit an agonizingly ambivalent one. (PM)

Oriana Fallaci's *Letter to a Child Never Born* details the psychological journey of a pregnant woman prior to a miscarriage. At first ambivalent, later protective, at last in grief, the woman "talks" to the fetus about herself, the place of women in society, and her perspective on the parenting process. Through this conversation a bond between the woman and the fetus develops which is as real to her as any between two living beings. Two sources of anger for this woman are the "father" and the doctors, neither of whom provides enough support through her sad experience.

This book is ethereal, mystical, political, angry, sad, and difficult—in other words, it is like any woman's emotions during a short, unexpected pregnancy interrupted by a long, drawn-out miscarriage. It would be very hard to read during a miscarriage, but enriching afterwards. (Abby Pariser)

"Last night I knew you existed: a drop of life escaped from nothingness. I was lying, my eyes wide open in the darkness, and all at once I was certain you were there. You existed.

...Now I am locked in fear that soaks my face, my hair, my thoughts. I am lost in it .... It is fear of you, of the circumstance that has wrenched you out of nothingness to attach yourself to my body. I was never eager to welcome you, even though I've known for some time that you might exist someday. In that sense I have long awaited you. But still I've always asked myself the terrible question: What if you don't want to be born? What if some day you were to cry out to reproach me: 'Who asked you to bring me into the world, why did you bring me into it, why?' Life is such an effort, Child. It's a war that is renewed each day, and its moments of joy are brief parentheses for which you pay a cruel price. How can I know that it wouldn't be better to throw you away? How can I tell that you wouldn't rather be returned to the silence? You cannot speak to me; your drop of life is only a cluster of cells that has scarcely begun. Perhaps it's not even life, only the mere possibility of life ....

"I'm not one to be frightened by the sight of blood. To be a woman is a schooling in blood: every month we pay odious homage to it. But when I saw that tiny spot on the pillow, my eyes clouded, and my legs shook. I fell into panic, then despair, and I cursed myself. I accused myself of every sort of negligence toward you, you who couldn't protect yourself, couldn't rebel, so small and defenseless and at the mercy of all my caprices and irresponsibility. It wasn't even red, that spot. It was pink, a light pink. Nevertheless it was more than enough to transmit your message, to announce that perhaps you were dying. I seized the pillow and ran."

FOR MORE INFORMATION

WHEN PREGNANCY FAILS: Families Coping with Miscarriage, Stillbirth, and Infant Death
by Susan Borg and Judith Lasker
1981, Beacon Press

AFTER A LOSS IN PREGNANCY: Help for Families Affected by a Miscarriage, a Stillbirth or the Loss of a Newborn.
by Nancy Berezin
1982, Simon and Schuster

Both books are reviewed in the section on Infant Death.

Exercise and Comfort

Most childbirth educators feel that the average woman can give birth without training for it "like an athlete," but that regular exercise does have an important place in pregnancy because it can help us learn to relax, increase general feelings of well-being, and make us more aware of our bodies and the muscles involved in labor.

In fact, most people concerned with health seem to agree that regular exercise is a good idea for everyone, all through life. Exercise can help prevent health problems, keep our weight at a proper level, and help our bodies function more efficiently. Women who are accustomed to daily exercise are usually encouraged to continue during pregnancy, as long as their activity doesn't involve a risk or falls or other injuries. Women who have not exercised before are generally encouraged to begin moderate exercise during pregnancy, the earlier the better. It is not clear whether significant changes can be made in muscle tone and strength during a few weeks of exercising prior to giving birth, but certainly the other benefits of exercise (relaxation, well-being, pleasure, body awareness) will be felt. Exercise and good body mechanics will also help relieve or prevent some of the common discomforts of pregnancy.

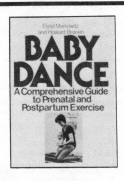

BABY DANCE: A Comprehensive Guide to Prenatal and Postpartum Exercises
by Elysa Markowitz and Howard Brainen
1980, 252 pages, Illus.

from
Prentice-Hall, Inc.
Englewood Cliffs, NJ 07632
$12.95 hd

Baby Dance provides "gentle flowing exercises" (beautifully illustrated with photographs) for the whole childbearing year and beyond. They cover: preparing for birth both physically and mentally, helping muscles recover after childbirth, and exercises to do with your new baby. This in itself would be enough, but *Baby Dance* provides much more, making it almost a comprehensive book on childbirth preparation. Also included are: an excellent chapter on comfort tips and natural remedies in pregnancy; detailed information on labor coaching and support; a look at the anatomy of pregnancy and labor; two very beautiful and graphic photo essays of birth (the author's home birth and an in-hospital "alternative birth center" birth); and special sec-

tion on post-partum information and exercises for cesarean mothers. Elysa Markowitz is a childbirth educator and dancer who emphasizes movement therapy, dance, and yoga in her work."

"As you exercise, remember:
* Respect your body. Warm up slowly and build up the number of repetitions gradually.
* Exercise gently. Avoid strain or stress. If you feel any pain, stop! Relax. Do some breathing exercises.
* Limit the time you spend lying flat on your back. During the last three months of pregnancy, do not lie on your back for more than five minutes. If you feel dizzy or lightheaded, roll over to your side and bend your knees. Breathe gently.
* Avoid exercises that cramp or suddenly shorten your lower back muscles, like the 'blow' in yoga.
* Sit up and lie down slowly. Avoid doing sit-ups, and don't use your abdominal muscles when lowering your back to the floor. To raise or lower your body, roll over onto your side and let your arms do the work.
* Avoid bouncing. (It will not effectively stretch muscles.) Relax slowly and gently into stretches.
* Never do *double* leg lifts. These can strain your lower back.
* Avoid exercises that cramp the space for your uterus and constrict your breathing—for example, putting your legs over your head or being upside down.
* Exercise on a surface that is firm and supportive—grass, carpet, or foam mat (½ inch thick).
* Remember to breathe with all your movements!"

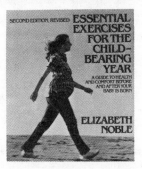

ESSENTIAL EXERCISES FOR THE CHILDBEARING YEAR: A Guide to Health and Comfort Before and After Your Baby is Born (Second Edition, Revised)
by Elizabeth Noble
1982, 177 pages, Illus.

from
Houghton Mifflin Company
2 Park Street
Boston, MA 02107
$13.95 hd.
$ 6.95 pap.

Elizabeth Noble is an Australian-trained physical therapist who has worked hard to introduce the idea of physical training as a regular and important part of pregnancy and prenatal care. Her book begins with an explanation of why "pregnancy creates a special need for exercise" and goes on to discuss in detail the structure and function of the pelvic floor (the muscles which support the pelvic organs), the abdominal muscles, posture and comfort, relaxation, breathing, and the special needs of cesarean mothers. Beneficial exercises and

body mechanics (as well as harmful positions to avoid) are clearly described and illustrated with simple line drawings. In her preface to the second edition, Doris Haire points out the new material on labor and delivery which emphasizes the importance of being able to sit, stand, and move about during labor and the need to *avoid* controlled breathing patterns and prolonged breath-holding pushing during labor. Both have adverse effects on the circulation and blood-oxygen supply to the fetus. A useful summary of pre- and post-natal exercises appears at the back of the book along with a list of recommended reading and resources.

"Exercise will provide significant benefits not only throughout the maternity cycle but for the rest of your life as well. During the birth, however, additional expenditure of voluntary muscles is often not needed—the uterus works by itself to ensure that the baby is born with or without your contribution. Training for this event, then, is more for coordination and relaxation than for maternal physical exertion....

'Walking, swimming, and bicycling are enjoyable activities that not only provide excellent general exercise but bring you into the fresh air and sunshine. Done regularly, they combine many of the desirable features of prenatal exercise planning: to strengthen muscles, build up endurance, improve circulation and respiration, adapt to increasing weight and changing balance."

YOUR BABY, YOUR BODY: Fitness During Pregnancy
by Carol Stahmann Dilfer
1977, 149 pages, Illus.

from
Crown Publishers
1 Park Avenue
New York, NY 10016
$8.95 hd.
$5.95 pap.

Carol Dilfer was living in Germany during her first pregnancy and discovered that vigorous exercise is a normal part of prenatal care for European women. After returning to the U.S., she began teaching a Prenatal/Postpartum Fitness Program, upon which this book is based. Dilfer argues that regular exercise will prevent pregnant women from getting too fat ("You can avoid becoming one of tomorrow's dumpy young mothers") and recommends that weight gain be limited to about 24 pounds. This advice may put vanity above the health of the baby how-

ever, if it encourages women to try to limit their weight gain in pregnancy. Dilfer also feels that regular exercise will make for an easier labor and delivery, and faster recovery, claims which are also open to debate.

The women who "model" for the book's illustrations were chosen from Dilfer's classes; I like what she says about them:

"I chose to include several women as models because I wanted to illustrate how very different women's bodies can look and still be beautiful. I have become aware, over the years, of how discontented most of us are with our bodies. I suppose a big part of that comes from the cultural indoctrination that says that in order for a woman's body to be considered beautiful it must be lean, long-legged, and big-breasted. But I think that all -the women who modeled for my book have beautiful bodies. And, as you can see, they are very different ...."

EXERCISES FOR PREGNANT WOMEN & NEW MOTHERS
Tape Cassette and Wall Chart

from
BABES (Bay Area Birth Education Supplies)
c/o Deanna Sollid
59 Berens Drive
Kentfield, CA 94904

Cassette and Wall Chart* $12.95
Wall Chart*   5.00
Cassette   10.00
* Add $1.25 shipping charge
California residents add 6% sales tax

"A cassette and wall chart brings you this exercise program that includes warmup stretches and exercises for flexibility, coordination, and strengthening of muscles usually weakened during pregnancy."

TEACHING PRENATAL EXERCISE: PART II - EXERCISES TO THINK TWICE ABOUT
by Pamela Shrock, Penny Simkin, and Madeleine H. Shearer
(*Birth and the Family Journal*, Vol. 8:3, Fall 1981)

Reprints available from:
Penny Simkin
1100 23rd Avenue East
Seattle, WA 98112
request price information

These three women are all registered physical therapists and experienced childbirth educators. They have doubts about some of the exercises being taught in prenatal classes and illustrated in manuals and books. This article discusses some of the exercises which may be harmful and calls for more research on the subject.

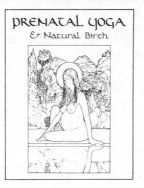

PRENATAL YOGA AND NATURAL BIRTH
by Jeannine O'Brien Medvin
1974, 64 pages, Illus.

from
Freestone Innerprizes
P.O. Box 398
Monroe, UT 84754
$5.00 pap.
plus $1.00 postage

One of the first books to emanate from the California childbirth counterculture in the early 70's (the most well known is probably *Birth*

Book by Raven Lang [see index]), *Prenatal Yoga* is lovingly produced and bears the mystically idiosyncratic stamp of its author throughout. The pages feature decorative borders, calligraphy, clean black line drawings, and good photographs. In the text, Jeannine speaks of becoming pregnant while studying yoga in India and seeking to combine her life as a "yogini" with her new life as a mother. Her descriptions of the various yoga stretches and postures illustrated in the book are interlaced with meditations on the feelings and moods of pregnancy. Jeannine is also the author (under her new name, Jeannine Parvati) of *Hygieia: A Woman's Herbal* (see index).

"Discipline is very much needed during pregnancy, not only from the ritual aspect, but to prepare for the great discipline required in caring for a baby. You can choose daily whether to do prenatal yoga or not—but you *have* to 'do' a baby every day."

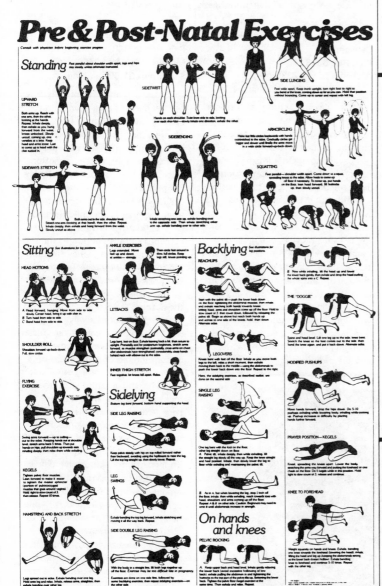

POSITIVE PREGNANCY THROUGH YOGA
by Sylvia Klein Olkin
1981, 240 pages, Illus.

from
Prentice-Hall
Englewood Cliffs, NJ 07632
$14.95 hd.
$ 7.95 pap.

This book seeks to integrate pregnancy with the yogic way of life. Sylvia Olkin has developed her ideas through the teaching of prenatal yoga classes. Her advice is always gentle and well-tuned to the psychic and physical needs of pregnant women. There is an illustrated selection of "asanas" or yoga positions, which have been adapted to the pregnant figure. Included is a special "Salute to the Child" series to replace the "Sun Salutation" which is physically inappropriate for pregnancy. In addition, there are good chapters on breathing and relaxation, nutrition,

moods in pregnancy, and making love. Especially useful is the section on "Natural Aids for Some Common Pregnancy Complaints," which shows how dietary changes, exercise, postures, and other simple remedies (a hot bath, a cold compress) can replace the drugs often used to relieve symptoms. There is also a complete section on labor, birth, and preparation for breastfeeding.

"Even if you feel lazy, practice your asanas as often as you can. The asanas within this book all stimulate and activate your inner energy to flow smoothly and freely along your inner passageways. That is why they are called asanas and not calisthenics. The asanas will help you to become calm and flexible while energizing you physically. One of my students remarked that she was very lazy and really did not want to practice, but she always felt better both mentally and physically after she did."

... maidens should harden their bodies with exercise of running, wrestling, throw the bar, and casting the dart, to the end that the fruit wherewith they might afterward be conceived, taking nourishment of a strong and lusty body, should shoot out and spread the better: and that they by gathering strength thus by exercises, should more easily away with the pains of child bearing ...

Plutarch (Greece, 46?-?120 A.D.)
from the *Lycurgus* (North trans.)

KEGELS

The "Kegel" exercise is recommended by many practitioners to help strengthen and increase awareness of the muscles around the vagina. It is done by tightening these muscles, holding for a count of ten, and letting go. The muscles involved are the anal sphincter, the meatal sphincter, and the pubococcygeus; you get to know where they are by practicing trying to stop and start the flow of urine when you're on the toilet. Some people suggest that women practice "Kegels" many times a day (up to 100 times). Benefits have not been "proven" but are thought to include: improved muscle tone; increased blood flow to the area; improved control of urination; increased sexual pleasure and awareness; improved ability to respond to coaching and relax the pelvic floor during labor and delivery.

PELVIC TILT
and
PELVIC ROCK

The "pelvic rock" and "pelvic tilt" appear to be the exercises most consistently recommended by childbirth educators. They help ease low back pain and improve posture. When standing, the pelvic tilt is done simply by tucking the buttocks under. You can feel your abdominal and lower back muscles tensing to hold this posture. Reminding yourself to maintain this posture throughout the day while standing and walking will strengthen these muscles which support the weight of the growing uterus. The pelvic rock is done on all fours. On your hands and knees, alternately arch your back like a cat and then relax. The posture helps relieve low back pain in pregnancy and during labor.

LEARNING TO RELAX: A Programmed Instruction Booklet for the General Public, but especially: Pregnant Mothers
by Mary Kirkpatrick, Virginia Tate and Diane Johnston
1980, 22 pages, Illus.

from
American Society for Psychoprophylaxis in Obstetrics
1411 K Street, NW, Suite 200
Washington, DC 20005
$1.50
bulk rates available

This booklet uses extremely simple language and humorous cartoon drawings to teach pregnant

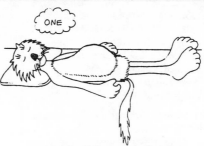

women about stress and relaxation. A pretest tests knowledge of the health effects of stress. Part I describes stress itself, including a listing of 42 stressful life events. Part II describes simple relaxation techniques including quiet breathing, and tensing and relaxing muscles

THE RELAXATION RESPONSE
by Herbert Benson
1976, 222 pages, Illus.

from
Avon Books
959 Eighth Avenue
New York, NY 10019
$2.95 pap.

Many childbirth educators and parents have found the simple meditation techniques described in this book to be very applicable and useful in promoting relaxation during pregnancy and labor.
"You will learn that evoking the Relaxation Response is extremely simple if you follow a very short set of instructions which incorporate four essential elements: 1) a quiet environment; 2) a mental device such as a word or a phrase which should be repeated in a specific fashion over and over again; 3) the adoption of a passive attitude which is perhaps the most important of the elements; and 4) a comfortable position. Your appropriate practice of these four elements for ten to twenty minutes once or twice daily should markedly enhance your well-being."

RELAXATION TAPES FOR CHILDBIRTH . . . AND AFTER
by Rae K. Grad
Set of three 2-sided tapes, 12-15 minutes each, with explanation sheet

from
Alliance for Perinatal Research and Services
P.O. Box 6358
Alexandria, VA 22306
$18.00 plus $1.00 shipping per set

The relaxation strategies provided in these tapes are set to classical music and include progressive relaxation, controlled relaxation, auto-genic training, mental imagery, meditation, and the relaxation response. They are recommended for practice in childbirth classes and for pregnant women/couples to use at home.
"Relaxation is a skill. As in learning to ride a bicycle, one must be taught strategies and then must practice. Those living or working in the childbirth field know how important relaxation skills are for so many reasons: pregnancy discomforts, coping with labor, postpartum recovery, nursing anxieties, colic frustrations, changing family relationships . . . and on and on."

while lying down.

"1. Be sure and get a quiet environment.
2. Maintain a passive attitude. Block all the thoughts of the job, home, children, from your mind. Pretend you're in a "bubble" all alone.
3. Get in a comfortable position.
4. Concentrate on a focal point or one object. Choose a spot or scene and do not let your eyes wander, or close your eyes and do not vary.
5. Breathe in and out, slowly and deeply, and say 'one' silently on exhalation. This repetitive mental device assists in the relaxation response."

MATERNAL STRESS AND PREGNANCY OUTCOME
Susan McKay, editor
ICEA REVIEW, Vol. 4, No. 1
April 1980, 8 pages

from
ICEA Bookcenter
P.O. Box 20048
Minneapolis, MN 55420
$1.50 plus $1.00 shipping

Stress and anxiety are considered normal parts of pregnancy, but some studies have shown that high levels of stress may be related to obstetric problems, including pre-eclampsia, premature labor, and dysfunctional labor. This reprint of ICEA Review is a publication of the International Childbirth Education Association, intended mainly for childbirth educators and other professionals. It provides an introduction to the subject of stress in pregnancy (including the role played by catecholamines) and abstracts nine journal articles on the subject. In the commentary, the authors are careful to point out that studies cannot always show whether anxiety "causes" an obstetric problem or whether some other underlying factor is the cause of both the stress and the complication.
"The utilization of stress management procedures such as biofeedback, exercise programs, meditation, relaxation techniques, and other self-awareness therapies can be useful therapies during pregnancy. An important intervention strategy is to provide the opportunity for each pregnant woman to ventilate her concerns to caring individuals—perhaps to her birth attendant, in a discussion group for pregnant women, or with a counselor, psychologist, or psychiatrist. Research findings indicate that conscious knowledge and expression of anxiety has beneficial effects upon pregnancy and labor outcome."

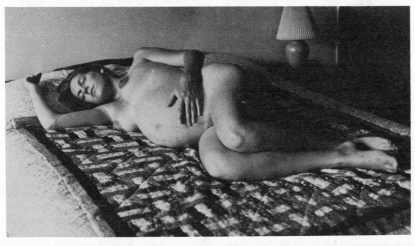

COMMON COMPLAINTS AND SIMPLE, SAFE REMEDIES

SYMPTOM/CAUSE	REMEDIES	THINGS TO AVOID
Swollen Feet/Ankles: Weight of uterus and decreased efficiency of veins which return blood from the legs can cause swelling; aggravated by prolonged standing or hot weather.	Elevate feet frequently, exercise to improve circulation, wear loose-fitting clothing and shoes, drink plenty of fluid for natural diuretic effect.	Avoid diuretics (water pills).
Leg Cramps: Caused by nerve compression, inadequate calcium, poor circulation.	Increase calcium in diet, assure adequate salt intake, elevate legs to prevent cramps, stretch calf by pointing heel (not toe) to relieve cramp, apply heat or use massage on affected muscle.	Avoid too much phosphorus in diet, may need to limit milk intake.
Hemorrhoids: pregnancy hormones relax smooth muscle of veins, causing vasocongestion; may be aggravated by straining over bowel movements.	Elevate feet and relax pelvic floor when having a bowel movement; drink plenty of fluids; eat "roughage" (whole grains, fruits, vegetables); assume knee-chest position to relieve pain; apply cold compresses with witch hazel; try hot sitz bath.	Avoid straining and pushing too hard when having a bowel movement. Avoid developing constipation or diarrhea.
Backache: Caused by strain of increased uterine weight on back muscles; aggravated by poor posture.	Use good posture, rest with weight off back, wear flat-heeled shoes, sleep on a firm mattress, try pelvic rock exercise.	Avoid high-heeled shoes, fatigue.
Shortness of breath: Caused by pressure of enlarging uterus on diaphragm and lungs.	Maintain good posture, sit up straight, sleep with upper body propped up.	Avoid anemia, stop or decrease smoking, avoid over-exertion.
Heartburn: Enlarging uterus presses on stomach, forcing stomach fluids back up into esophagus.	Eat several small meals instead of three large ones; sit up straight, elevate rib cage; sleep with upper body propped up; sip milk or hot tea.	Avoid antacids; check with health care provider before use. Avoid greasy, spicy food. Avoid coffee and alcohol.
Varicose Veins: Pregnancy hormones decrease efficiency of venous return from the legs; aggravated by enlarging uterus.	Elevate legs frequently, use support stockings, walk daily.	Avoid prolonged standing, avoid sitting with crossed legs, avoid constrictive clothing or garters.
Constipation: Progesterone relaxes smooth muscle of gut making it less efficient; intestines compressed by enlarging uterus.	Increase roughage by eating raw fruit, vegetables, and grains; take a daily walk, drink lots of water; eat prunes; raise feet on foot stool and relax pelvic floor when on the toilet.	Avoid laxatives, mineral oil, and enemas.
Nausea: many pregnant women experience some nausea ("morning sickness") during the first 3-4 months of pregnancy. May be caused by hormonal changes and/or emotional factors.	Increase intake of Vitamin B6, eat 4-6 small meals a day, drink peppermint tea, munch on dry toast or crackers before getting up in the morning; ginger ale can help but avoid caffeine-containing soft drinks.	Avoid cigarette smoking; greasy, spicy food; avoid either an empty stomach or an over-full stomach. Especially, *avoid Bendectin,* a medication commonly prescribed for morning sickness. It may cause birth defects (see index).
Insomnia: It's often hard to sleep in the last months of pregnancy because of difficulty in getting comfortable, frequency of urination, worries, and fetal movement.	Take a hot bath, drink hot milk or soothing herb teas (peppermint, chamomile) at bedtime, use relaxation techniques, exercise daily, increase intake of B vitamins, use massage, avoid coffee and caffeine drinks, use extra pillows to help get comfortable in bed.	Avoid sleeping pills and tranquilizers.
Mild Headache: may be caused by emotional tension or eye strain. Fluid retention may affect your prescription for eye glasses or contact lenses, causing eye strain. Be sure to report prolonged or severe headache to your health care provider.	Use neck roll exercise, relaxation techniques, soothing herb teas (peppermint, chamomile), alternate hot and cold showers, neck massage.	Avoid aspirin or other medications, avoid coffee, alcohol, and MSG (monosodium glutamate).
Bladder Infections: may be caused by a pre-existing asymptomatic infection or by catheterization at delivery.	Drink lots of water and acidic fruit juices, especially cranberry juice. Increase Vitamin C; pay strict attention to hygiene; wear cotton underwear; consult your care provider if symptoms persist to avoid development into kidney infection.	Avoid underwear or pants which are too tight or made of synthetic "non-breathing" materials. Avoid drinking coffee or black tea. Avoid catheterization, if possible.
Yeast Infections: may be more common in pregnancy; altered natural balance of vaginal organisms.	Use plain yogurt or acidophyllus capsules in vagina to restore pH balance.	Avoid excessive sugar or refined flour products in diet. Avoid antibiotics, if possible, which alter balance of bacteria in vagina.

DANGER SIGNS IN PREGNANCY

The following danger signs should be reported immediately to your midwife or doctor. Don't be afraid to call at night or after hours if your symptoms are severe. If you have no care provider, call the nearest hospital emergency room and report your symptoms.

1. Vaginal bleeding
2. Swelling of the face or fingers
3. Severe or continuous headache
4. Double vision, blurring, dimming
5. Unusual or severe abdominal pain
6. Persistent vomiting
7. Chills or fever
8. Pain when urinating
9. Leaking fluid (not mucus) from the vagina
10. Absence of fetal movement

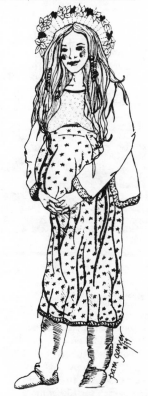

HERBS

Many women are now using and recommending herbs for the common complaints of pregnancy and childbirth and for health care in general (see index). Herb teas can be a good replacement for coffee and caffeine-containing teas and soft drinks, but it's important to know that herbs can also contain chemically active substances which may be harmful. (For instance, the herbs which have traditionally been used to induce an abortion—cohosh, pennyroyal, mugwort, tansy, slippery elm—can cause miscarriage.) Be sure you are certain about the properties of any herb you use. Consult your library if you are not certain.

SAFE NATURAL REMEDIES FOR DISCOMFORTS OF PREGNANCY

by the Over-the-Counter Committee of the Coalition for the Medical Rights of Women
1981, 30 pages, Illus.

from
Coalition for the Medical Rights of Women
1638-B Haight Street
San Francisco, CA 94117
$1.50
bulk rates available
also available in Spanish

We are used to taking medicine whenever we are sick or have aches and pains, and for many women that habit continues into pregnancy. But

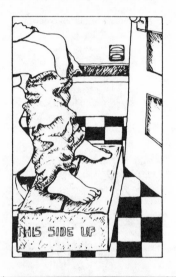

most drugs cross the placenta to reach the unborn baby and some may cause birth defects. Because the government does not adequately test drugs, we can't be sure which drugs are safe. *Safe Natural Remedies* provides a much-needed alternative. It lists tips for prevention, useful remedies, possible choices of medicines, and medicines not to be used for the most common discomforts of pregnancy. These include: nausea and vomiting, fatigue, headache, stuffy nose and allergies, heartburn, leg cramps, constipation, varicose veins and hemorrhoids, backache, difficulty sleeping, and edema (swelling). There is also a good introduction to drugs and pregnancy, a description of the Kegel exercise, and information on additional hazards like cigarettes, alcohol, and caffeine. The booklet is easy to read and enlivened by very charming, funny illustrations.

Hemorrhoids:
* Try not to become constipated. Using laxatives too often will make hemorrhoids worse (see 'Constipation').
* Try not to sit on the toilet for long periods of time, or strain while having bowel movements. If you push too hard, it may increase your chances of getting hemorrhoids or varicose veins. Putting your feet up on a stool may help to relieve strain.
* Doing 'Kegels' regularly helps prevent (and control) hemorrhoids. . . .

PROMATT SUPPORT SYSTEM
Pregnancy Mattress
Model No. 778, size 74" x 30" x 6"

from
Altrex Corporation
14712 Franklin Avenue, Suite H
Tustin, CA 92680
$79.95

The ProMatt is basically a mattress with a hole in it, that is, there is a depression in the surface of the mattress to help pregnant women sleep more comfortably (see illustration). The manufacturer claims that use of the ProMatt (you place it right on top of your own bed) can eliminate many of the discomforts of late pregnancy, including: backache, leg cramps, swelling of the extremities, and frequent urination at night. The product is new and I don't know anyone yet who has used the ProMatt, but it sounds like an idea worth investigating. Request a free brochure from Altrex.

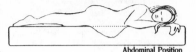

Abdominal Position

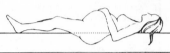

Supine Position

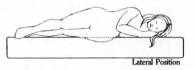

Lateral Position

IF YOU'RE PREGNANT . . . Safety Belts Will Protect You and Your Unborn Child
poster, 14" x 20"

from
Minnesota Department of Public Safety
Office of Public Information
318 Transportation Bldg.
St. Paul, MN 55155
single copy free

Only about 12% of Americans regularly use seat belts when they drive. That is a shocking statistic, especially when so many studies have shown that seat belts can save lives (see index for section on car safety seats for infants and children). The Minnesota Department of Public Safety has put out a poster showing pregnant women the right way to buckle-up. If your family doesn't use seat belts regularly, please start now. It could protect you from serious injury or death.

COMFORT DURING PREGNANCY
Maternity Center Association
Illustrated 6-panel leaflet

from
Maternity Center Association
48 East 92nd Street
New York, NY 10028
25 cents single copy
15 cents each for 10-99 copies
10 cents each for 100 or more

This leaflet is adapted from MCA's longer booklet, *Preparation for Childbearing* (see index). It illustrates comfortable positions for resting, standing with correct posture, lifting objects, and reaching. The

leaflet is available in both English and Spanish. Specify which you'd like when ordering.

"Everyday work and play activities continue during pregnancy, but the type of activity should be varied throughout the day. Frequent change of position is recommended to avoid circulatory congestion and continued pressure on nerves and veins. Periods of activity in general should be of shorter duration."

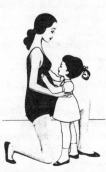

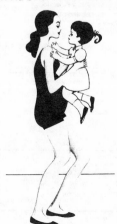

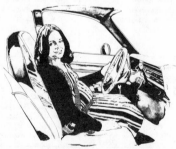

NEWBORN BEAUTY: A Complete Beauty, Health, and Energy Guide to the Nine Months of Pregnancy and the Nine Months After
by Wende Devlin Gates and Gail McFarland Meckel
1981, 352 pages, illus.

from
Bantam Books (1981)
666 Fifth Avenue
New York, NY 10019
$10.95 pap.

The way women feel about their personal appearance has changed in the past years. The women's movement has shown us that standards of beauty which emphasize the woman as an "object" are not always healthy for our minds or our bodies (hair dyes can damage our hair and cause cancer, make-up can cause allergic reactions, over-zealous dieting or thinness is bad for our health, high-heel shoes cause muscle shortening and injury, etc.). Though women have shifted to more "natural" definitions of beauty in recent years, we do still want to look attractive and it's hard to know sometimes whether this impulse is "vanity" or a positive desire for health and pride in ourselves. The authors of *Newborn Beauty* definitely believe the latter: "With fewer babies being born today, there seems to be a new pride in preg-

nancy—and this 'pregnant and proud' attitude is important. If you feel you're looking your best, you will act and feel your best and people will respond to you accordingly." Their book provides advice on caring for hair and skin in pregnancy and after, nutrition, exercise, clothing, and sex—all geared to helping pregnant women and new mothers be both attractive and healthy. The book is illustrated with photographs of professional models as they go through pregnancy, birth, and life with their new babies.

"At no time in your working life is it more important to look well—dressed and attractive than during your pregnancy. Whether you plan to stop working indefinitely when the baby comes or you expect to return to work six weeks after the baby's birth, the image you project during your pregnancy should be as poised and professional as ever. There are plenty of people—co-workers and competitors—who will imagine you've dropped out of competition by 'fulfilling your biological destiny.' You don't want to give them any ammunition."

GREAT EXPECTATIONS: How to Make 30 Easy, Fast, Sexy, Cheerful Maternity Outfits That Let You Feel Like a Woman As Well As A Mother-to-be.
by Leigh Adams and Lynda Madaras
1980, 169 pages, Illus.

from
Houghton Mifflin Company
2 Park Street
Boston, MA 02107
$7.95 pap.

Pregnant bellies should not be hidden under "tentlike constructions" or "little-girlish" designs, say authors Adams and Madaras. Their book presents patterns and instructions for making dresses, robes, pants, skirts, tops, and capes that flow easily over the belly, sometimes emphasizing it and sometimes baring it altogether (as with their halter tops combined with below-the-belly pants and skirts). Their clothing designs are attractive and look easy to make. Sewing experience will be helpful, but there is a lengthy introduction to techniques for beginners. Most designs can be worn after pregnancy, though not all will accomodate breastfeeding.

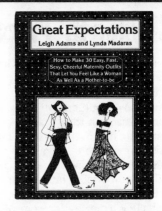

There is an especially interesting collection of designs to make from unusual materials like scarves, pillowcases, bed sheets, towels, and tablecloths. I saw a lot of nice ideas I'd like to try for my regular, non-pregnant wardrobe.

"Why do we attempt to hide pregnancy and clothe the obviously sexually experienced woman as if she were a little girl? The answer to this question probably lies in murky Oedipal depths and in our cultural embarrassment about sexuality . . . ."

A YEAR OF BEAUTY AND EXERCISE FOR THE PREGNANT WOMAN
by Judi McMahon and Zia Odell
1981, 224 pages, Illus.

from
Lippincott and Crowell
c/o Harper and Row
10 East 53rd Street
New York, NY 10022
$12.95 hd.

This book is an upbeat collection of "home remedies, psychological tips, fashion helps, and nutritional advice," plus exercises and beauty tips for the pregnant woman. The author (McMahon) is a fashion and beauty editor and she uses an emphasis on beauty and health to create a general attitude of "taking control" of pregnancy. The book is organized in a month-by-month format, but the advice is headlined in bold face letters so readers can easily skim through and pick and choose among the offerings. The use of midwives and unmedicated deliveries are strongly emphasized as options. There is a lovely personal foreword by Doris Haire in which she describes her very successful natural childbirth experience (". . . I felt as if I had given birth to the sun.")

"This is the ideal time to develop new and more healthful habits if you haven't already done so. For instance, you might begin to limit your

intake of foods and drinks that can have harmful side effects during pregnancy. Some of these we have already mentioned—alcohol, cigarettes, and certain prescription drugs. Remember, you're not giving up anything, you're getting rid of something you can always replace with a superior, far more life-giving force of energy. Doubtful? Try it and you'll see."

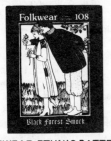

FOLKWEAR ETHNIC PATTERNS
c/o Ethnic Accessories
Box 250
Forestville, CA 95436

Folkwear patterns feature ethnic designs from the Middle East, the Far East, Europe, and North and South America, as well as a new line of "antique" 19th century clothing. Many of these designs are suitable for pregnancy. I made the Black Forest Smock in a man's size and it was a mainstay of my wardrobe during pregnancy. Each pattern is printed on heavy reuseable paper and includes all sizes. Also available is a pattern for children featuring six folk garments in sizes ranging from newborn to age four. Prices average $4. to $5. per pattern. Send $1.50 for a copy of complete catalog.

MOTHERS WORK
P.O. Box 40121
Philadelphia, PA 19106
request mail-order catalog

Mothers Work was started by an "executive mother" to sell maternity clothes to business and professional women who want to maintain a professional-looking appearance during pregnancy. The mail-order catalog features jumper-and-blazer suit combinations, dresses, blouses, casual jeans and a "postpartum" skirt, all in a choice of fabrics including wool gabardine, poly-linen, and cotton. Prices range from $34. to $180.

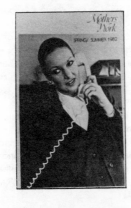

MOTHERCARE-BY-MAIL
P.O. Box 3881
New York, NY 10017
request free catalog

Mothercare is a British company with stores in Europe and America (listed in their catalog) and a mail-order service. Their catalog features a good selection of moderately priced maternity clothing and includes: nursing and maternity bras, support girdles, slips, panties, pantyhose, nightgowns for pregnancy and nursing, maternity pants, blouses, swim suits, dresses, and jumpers. There is also a full line of clothing for infants and small children, plus baby carriers, car safety seats, strollers and buggies, cribs, high chairs, bedding, bath and feeding accessories, and toys.

Childbirth Preparation

Ideas about how the pain of labor should be dealt with and experienced have changed in the last 150 years. During the 19th century, birth was often seen as a time of suffering for women. Birth was plagued by conditions which made it very much more dangerous for women than it is today. Advances in public health (immunization, sanitation, improved nutrition, birth control, etc.) and medical advances (improved technique for cesarean section, antisepsis, anesthesia, forceps deliveries, etc.) have radically lowered the maternal and infant mortality rates in our century.

Early feminists originally welcomed the use of anethesia for birth, seeing it as a remedy for women's suffering in childbirth. Queen Victoria was the first prominent woman to accept chloroform for the delivery of her eighth child in 1853. This helped to silence opposition from religious leaders and others who felt that women must not be spared the "curse of Eve." The use of anesthesia and hospitalization for birth spread rapidly in America, and by the 1940's virtually all births were managed in this way. But by this time also, women began to be dissatisfied with the new way of birth. Some began to feel that they had paid too high a price for being relieved of consciousness during birth. The greatly reduced dangers of childbearing may have played a part in women's increasing confidence that birth could become something joyous and fulfilling. Women began hearing from their European sisters of births which were "ecstatic." Popular psychologists began calling for a return to conscious birth, claiming that the pains of labor help to instill the maternal instinct. Women who were completely anesthetized for birth sometimes felt as though they had not given birth at all, feeling both removed from the experience and disinterested in the baby. Some women suffered bad psychological reactions to the use of drugs in labor (especially to medications like the "Twilight Sleep" combination of morphine and scopolamine, an amnesic). The resurgence of interest in the "feminine mystique" documented by Betty Friedan defined motherhood as woman's chief occupation and crowning glory. With improved methods of birth control, women were able to plan their pregnancies. Children were "wanted" and women began to worry about the mounting evidence showing that obstetrical medications are harmful to babies.

THE DICK-READ METHOD

Into this cultural climate came the first American publication of Grantly Dick-Read's *Childbirth Without Fear,* in 1944. Dick-Read, a British obstetrician, had come to believe that fear is the greatest cause of pain in childbirth. He felt that education, combined with exercise and breathing techniques, could eliminate pain. Dick-Read also emphasized motherhood as the ultimate fulfillment for women. His stress on religion, femininity, and "passive" acceptance of the forces of labor corresponded with American ideals at the time. In addition, his idea that the husband should provide emotional support for his wife in labor corresponded with the American stress on "togetherness" in marriage. Natural childbirth was seen as a way of strengthening middle class marriages. The husband, not female relatives and friends, was the only significant other person to be admitted to the delivery room. Some also began to see natural childbirth as part of a Christian way of life: a moral action which could be taken to safeguard the baby's health. The sexual aspect of birth also began to be stressed. Women were advised to expect a "climax" with delivery and analogies were made between the responses of women in sexual intercourse and in undrugged childbirth.

For all of these reasons, natural childbirth was warmly accepted by many American women, but the medical establishment was not happy to accommodate this new way of birth. A backlash against the demand for natural childbirth soon developed. Doctors began recounting stories of women who had tried to achieve natural childbirth and "failed," leading to serious psychological consequences like postpartum depression. Indeed, many women did feel that if they experienced pain in labor they had failed at the method and had failed, in fact, to be true women. Dick-Read's method relied heavily on education and the intellectual lessening of fear to relieve pain, but this did not always succeed. Furthermore, his method was compromised by the American hospital way of birth, which continued to be alienating (compared with the home deliveries which Dick-Read attended) and continued to insist on forceps deliveries and local anesthesia for routine episiotomies. Eventually the Dick-Read method became less popular and was replaced by the Lamaze method.

Dick-Read's work continues to be a major source of information and inspiration for women who want more control over their childbearing experiences, however. Over the years since it was first introduced, and probably also in response to the success of the Lamaze method, proponents and teachers of the Dick-Read method have incorporated new principles into their teaching. Dick-Read teachers today are, like many childbirth educators, eclectic in their approach, adapting their classes to the particular needs of their students and the childbirth situation in their area.

To learn more about how methods of childbirth preparation have grown and changed, read the introductions to the sections on the Lamaze, Bradley, and Kitzinger methods, which follow.

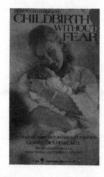

CHILDBIRTH WITHOUT FEAR: The Principles and Practice of Natural Childbirth (Revised 4th edition) by Grantly Dick-Read 1978, 420 pages, Illus.

from
Harper and Row
10 East 53rd Street
New York, NY 10022
$4.95 pap.

Early on in *Childbirth Without Fear,* Grantly Dick-Read tells the story of attending an English woman in labor in her poor home in Whitechapel. Despite the poverty of her surroundings, the woman gave birth normally, without fuss, and refused Dick-Read's offer of chloroform. When asked why, the woman said: "It didn't hurt. It wasn't meant to, was it, doctor?" That remark made Dr. Dick-Read "see the light" and begin the thinking and writing which ultimately led to his theory of "Natural Childbirth." Dick-Read became convinced that, indeed, childbirth is not *meant* to hurt, and determined that fear, based on ignorance, is the major source of pain in childbirth.

In *Childbirth Without Fear,* he elaborates his theory much in the manner of a "philosophy of childbirth." He discusses the history of childbirth, the anatomy and physiology of labor, the basis of pain and factors which aggravate it. He describes the centuries-old imagery and mental conditioning which have surrounded birth with fears of pain and injury. He then offers his alternative, describing the hazards of universal use of anesthesia. Dick-Read shows how good diet, education, exercise, healthy attitudes, and relaxation will enable most women to give birth comfortably without anesthesia. He includes chapters on emergency childbirth, breastfeeding and rooming-in, and the husband's participation in birth.

So much has changed in childbirth in the past 40 years, that *Childbirth Without Fear* is almost only of historical interest. One drawback of the book, for some, is its strong emphasis on religious and spiritual aspects of birth and motherhood itself. Dick-Read saw childbirth as a woman's crowning achievement, and is deeply romantic in his conception of the mother as a source of all goodness in society. The book does provide essential, factual information, however, about the physiology and conduct of normal labor, and includes useful guidelines and exercises for childbirth preparation.

"Superstition, civilization and culture have brought influences to bear upon the minds of women which have introduced justifiable fears and anxieties concerning labor. The more cultured the races of the earth have become, so much the more positive have they been in pronouncing childbirth to be a painful and dangerous ordeal.

"Thus fear and anticipation of pain have given rise to natural protective tensions in the body, and such tensions are not of the mind only, for the mechanism of the protective action by the body includes muscle tension. Unfortunately, the natural tension produced by fear influences those muscles which close the womb and oppose the dilatation of the birth canal during labor. Therefore fear inhibits, that is to say, gives rise to resistance at the outlet of the womb, when in the normal state those muscles should be relaxed and free from tension. This resistance gives rise to pain because the uterus is supplied with sensitive nerve endings which record pain arising from excessive tension. Therefore, fear, tension and pain are three evils opposed to the natural design which have been con-

cerned with preparation for attendance at childbirth. If fear, tension and pain go hand in hand, then it must be necessary to relieve tension and to overcome fear in order to eliminate pain. The implementation of my theory demonstrates the methods by which fear may be overcome, tension may be eliminated and replaced by physical and mental relaxation."

"Prejudice denies women their wish to be calm and courageously composed. The consciousness of the purposeful physical sensations, and the emotional reactions to those sensations, is denied the modern wife. She is deprived of the full reward of childbirth, which is the realization of her achievement in the birth of her child. Too many never know the deep glory of a woman's pride as the hungry child ceases its demanding whimper and draws the ready nipple to itself and snuggles in the soft satisfying security of its mother's breast. Is this sensuous, sentimental or scientific? I hope it's all three—intense and uninhibited—for if there is one thing I have ever envied woman, it is that perfect peace and detached happiness she demonstrates in her movement, breathing and facial expression when her baby lies contented and semi-conscious at her breast. Can our male science willingly disregard these female experiences because it can never share them!"

PREPARATION FOR CHILDBIRTH: Handbook for Use in Exercise Classes for Expectant Parents (7th Revision)
by Mabel Lum Fitzhugh
1980, 32 pages, Illus.

from
Margaret B. Farley, publisher
21 Santa Margarita Drive
San Rafael, CA 94901
$2.50 pap., bulk rates available
$3.00 for Instructor's Manual
(no bulk rates)

Mabel Lum Fitzhugh was trained and worked as an architect and became a physical therapist after being widowed during the depression. Her handbook, "Mrs. Fitzhugh's Blue Book," was first published in 1955 and is still a useful tool. Minor revisions were made in 1973 and 1980. *Preparation for Childbirth* is based on Dick-Read's teaching. It includes exercises and techniques for relaxation, breathing, posture, preventing constipation and hemorrhoids, strengthening the pelvic floor and abdominal muscles, and breastfeeding. There are also sections on instructions for fathers, emergency delivery, an outline of labor and delivery

(adapted from Niles Newton), and a well updated list of suggested reading. Included with each handbook is a large, fold-out "Daily Exercise Check-Off Chart." The instructor's Manual includes an additional 16 pages of class outlines for an 8-lesson series of childbirth preparation classes.

"Learning how to relax is like learning how to play a violin. Practice faithfully, day by day becoming more proficient until suddenly you realize the beauty and harmony of your efforts. So if you will practice regularly these simple stretching and sighing exercises, you may find before long that you are really relaxed and at peace in your mind and in your body as well. Your worries and fears may evaporate, since when the body is relaxed, there is no thought in your conscious mind—it can relax also."

MIDWEST PARENTCRAFT CENTER
627 Beaver Road
Glenview, IL 60025

The Midwest Parentcraft Center is directed by Margaret Gamper, RN, who has been teaching her "Gamper Method" of childbirth preparation, based on Dick-Read, since 1946. The Center certifies teachers in the Gamper/Dick-Read method and provides classes for parents.

The Gamper/Dick-Read method emphasizes that "sensitivity to inner body changes enhances the mother's ability to cooperate with events during labor." Classes provide information on the importance of good nutrition, body mechanics and exercise, breathing and relaxation techniques, and preparation for breastfeeding and baby care. The breathing and relaxation techniques taught are flexible and designed to "conform to the natural pattern of the mother in order not to burden her with still another adjustment problem." The mother learns to apply these techniques not only to labor, but to other situations in her life which cause tension. Couples attend classes together and the father is expected to become closely involved in preparing for and participating in the birth.

The Center regularly sponsors conferences to provide certification and education for childbirth educators, nurses, and others interested in maternity care. In addition, the

READ NATURAL CHILDBIRTH FOUNDATION, INC.
1300 S. Eliseo Drive, Suite 102
Greenbrae, CA 94904
415/461-2277 or 456-3143
Kendra Downey, Corresponding Secretary

The Read Natural Childbirth Foundation was started by Margaret Farley over 20 years ago to help promote the teaching of Dick-Read and the exercises developed by physical therapist Mabel Lum Fitzhugh (see this page). Ms. Farley and her associates are still teaching Dick-Read classes for parents in Marin County, California, but unfortunately have decided they cannot certify teachers outside their area at this time. However, the Foundation will answer inquiries about Dick-Read's philosophy and methods. They have produced a film about natural labor and birth, *A Time to be Born* (16 mm, color, sound, 30 minutes), which is available from the Foundation for purchase or rental. Write for price information.

Center publishes a quarterly newsletter, *Heir-Raising News,* which is available to the general public for $6.00 a year. Contact the Center for referrals to Gamper/Dick-Read teachers in your area.

PREPARATION FOR THE HEIR MINDED
by Margaret Gamper
1971
$3.50 plus 75 cents postage
40% discount for 24 or more

Gamper's booklet, now in its 8th printing, is used as a class manual for the Gamper/Dick-Read method.

BARTUSCH LABOR & BIRTH CHARTS
Set of 6 color charts, 20" x 30" each, laminated on poster board
Includes 12-page instruction booklet
$30.00 per set

Excellent, clear charts show the processes of labor and delivery, with a full-sized, cut-out baby. Developed by the Midwest Parentcraft Center and executed by artist Nelle Bartusch.

CHILDREN MAKE LOVE VISIBLE
16 mm color film
$25. for film rental
request purchase information

Film follows a couple through pregnancy, prenatal classes, and an unmedicated delivery, using the Gamper method.

A WAY TO NATURAL CHILDBIRTH: A Manual for Physiotherapists and Parents-to-Be (Third Edition)
by Helen Heardman
revised and re-edited by Maria Ebner
1973, 100 pages, Illus.

from
Churchill Livingstone
19 W. 44th Street
New York, NY 10036
$3.25 pap.

Helen Heardman was an English physiotherapist who developed an exercise and childbirth preparation program to accompany Grantly Dick-Read's philosophy of natural childbirth. *A Way to Natural Childbirth* was first published in 1948 and has been revised twice since then. It provides a basic outline of exercises and relaxation techniques for labor, a description of the events of normal labor and the postpartum period, tips for breastfeeding, and a section of personal comments from mothers who have used the method.

THE LAMAZE METHOD

The Lamaze method is the most well-known and widely used method of prepared childbirth in our country, so much so that when couples are asked about their plans for natural childbirth, many will simply answer, "We're going to have Lamaze." The method is named after Dr. Fernand Lamaze, a French obstetrician who based his "psychoprophylactic method" on the work being done in Russia in applying Pavlov's theories of the conditioned response to the prevention of pain in childbirth.

Briefly, the Lamaze method employs what it sometimes called the "gate theory" of sensation. Lamaze felt that by concentrating on specific distracting stimuli during labor (like breathing in a controlled way, or staring at a "spot" or focal point), women could block the transmission of pain messages from the uterus to the brain. The assumption is that the brain can receive only one kind of stimulation at a time, and pain messages cannot get past the "gate" if other messages are competing.

The Lamaze method was introduced in the United States largely through the efforts of Elisabeth Bing, who helped to found the American Society for Psychoprophylaxis in Obstetrics (ASPO) in 1960. Her book, *Six Practical Lessons for an Easier Childbirth*, contains a basic outline of the Lamaze method as it is taught by ASPO-certified instructors. Since its introduction the Lamaze method has evolved to incorporate additional elements, such as the participation of a partner as a labor "coach." Lamaze courses today may vary in content and emphasis from teacher to teacher, though the basic principle remains the use of breathing patterns to block sensations of pain.

There are several reasons why the Lamaze method has been so popular and successful in the U.S. In the first place, Lamaze himself was careful to present his ideas as being based on scientific theories and methods, steering clear of the emphasis on "natural" and "spiritual" which characterizes the work of Grantly Dick-Read (see index). This fits in well with the secular reverence for science in our society. Secondly, as Silvia Feldman has pointed out (see index), the Lamaze method enables women to "be in control" during birth in a way that fits in with our American notions of rational, stoic adult behavior. For these reasons, and also because the Lamaze method as practiced in the U.S. does not forbid the use of drugs, it has gained

acceptance from obstetricians. ASPO-Lamaze teachers are more likely to have a nursing background than teachers of other methods, and they tend to be somewhat more medically oriented. ASPO courses are often taught in a hospital setting, where students are less likely to receive the kind of consumer-oriented information which private teachers offer. These factors have also made the method more acceptable to doctors, hospitals, and parents who do not wish to question medical authority.

On the positive side, the Lamaze method and its advocates are largely responsible for introducing the concept of unmedicated hospital birth in our country, and proponents have worked hard to achieve acceptance for their goals in the medical community. On the negative side, critics of the Lamaze method point out that it does not stress enough the goal of a totally unmedicated delivery. Most Lamaze literature points out that accepting medication does not mean "failure," and Lamaze patients often do accept drugs which enable them to be awake for delivery. The harmful side effects on the baby are often underemphasized, in order to spare the mother a painful labor. Recently, some critics have also pointed out that the strenuous, prolonged pushing efforts which are taught for the expulsion phase of labor are in fact physiologically harmful to the baby. Lamaze teaching is being modified to reflect this concern.

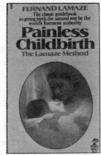

PAINLESS CHILDBIRTH
by Fernand Lamaze
1977, 191 pages, Illus.

from
Pocket Books
1230 Avenue of the Americas
New York, NY 10020
$2.75 pap.

Dr. Lamaze describes his observation of the psychoprophylactic ("psychological prevention") method in Russia and his application of it in France. He discusses the physiology of pain and describes the "scientific" method for abolishing it through the use of controlled breathing and relaxation. Included is the series of lectures which he gave to his own patients.

"Pain and childbirth have for so long been associated in the mind of the human race, and have for so long concurred, that they had become synonymous. The normal uterine contraction so necessary for the active progress of labor is mistaken for pain to such an extent that the word 'pain' is taken to mean both . . . The result is a typical conditioned reflex in which the normal painless contraction has become the signal for the occurrence of pain. The characteristic of this reflex is not that it has been acquired by experience, but above all by 'common knowledge'—in other words by the influence of speech."

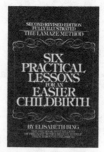

SIX PRACTICAL LESSONS FOR AN EASIER CHILDBIRTH
by Elisabeth Bing
1981, 176 pages, Illus.

from
Bantam Books
666 Fifth Avenue
New York, NY 10019
$2.95 pap.

Elisabeth Bing is a registered physical therapist who helped to found ASPO (see opposite page) and has been teaching the Lamaze method of childbirth preparation for twenty years. *Six Easy Lessons* was originally published in the 60's and contains the same material which Ms. Bing provided to students in her classes. The book can be used as an adjunct to classes or as a course of home study for couples who are not able to attend a Lamaze class.

"Our goal throughout these lessons—in addition to understanding what happens during childbirth and learning various exercises to prepare our bodies—will be to recondition ourselves and to create a new center of concentration, thereby causing the awareness of pain to become peripheral. We have found that this is possible not just by looking at an outside object, but by concentrating on a very special activity of our own.

"This special activity consists of active and difficult techniques of breathing, which will demand a great amount of concentrated effort. We use different breathing techniques because our breathing is so closely connected with all our activities, whether physical or emotional . . . .

"You will learn to change your breathing deliberately during labor, adjusting it to the changing characteristics of the uterine contractions. This will demand an enormous concentrated effort on your part. Not a concentration on pain, but a concentration on your own activity in synchronizing your respiration to the signals that you receive from the uterus. This strenuous activity will create a new center of concentration in the brain, thereby causing the painful sensations during labor to become peripheral, to reduce their intensity. And at the same time, you will learn to relax your body in such a way that you will allow the uterus to work under optimum conditions."

THANK YOU, DR. LAMAZE: A Mother's Experiences in Painless Childbirth (revised edition)
by Marjorie Karmel
1981, 192 pages

from
Harper and Row
10 East 53rd Street
New York, NY 10022
$10.95 hd.

This book, first published in 1959, really introduced the Lamaze method to Americans. Marjorie Karmel describes her own experience of giving birth in France with Dr. Lamaze, and her later efforts to find a doctor in New York who would help her give birth to her next child in the same way.

"My mother was thoroughly incredulous when I told her about the Pavlov method, and my experience. But when I really went into it, she admitted there might be something to it. Then, for the first time in our

lives, we discussed the subject of childbirth. And for the first time I realized why she had never spoken of it before. My recollection that my father had once mentioned finding her alone in a pool of blood was substantiated. And other details, no less horrifying, were added. This had all happened in one of the best hospitals in the capital of the United States not so very long ago. She looked back on her experience with childbirth as an ordeal that had been necessary, but certainly not as something to talk about. I couldn't help marveling at the difference between her feelings and mine. I was thankful that her fundamental tact had kept me from being conditioned in a way that might have been difficult to overcome, and I was even more thankful that a series of happy chances had led me to Dr. Lamaze and an experience that I would be proud and happy to tell my children."

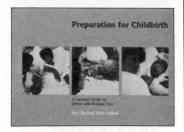

PREPARATION FOR CHILD-BIRTH: A Lamaze Guide (revised second edition)
by Donna and Rodger Ewy
1976, 112 pages, Illus.

from
Pruett Publishing Company
3235 Prairie Avenue
Boulder, CO 80301
$5.95 pap.

This basic guide provides an introduction to the Lamaze method and clear, simple information on the anatomy and physiology of pregnancy and birth, relaxation and breathing techniques, instructions for fathers, and the course of normal labor and delivery. Included are parent's birth reports and excellent photographs of birth

"Tensing during childbirth is a natural response to the tensing of the uterus. However, tension not only causes exhaustion, oxygen depletion, and a lower pain threshold, but actually prolongs labor physiologically. The hormone that causes your uterus to contract is oxytocin. Adrenaline, the hormone that accompanies the tension-fear-pain syndrome, actually inhibits the effects of oxytocin and makes your contractions less effective. So remember, the more you tense up during labor, the longer will be your labor. The more you relax, the shorter will be your labor.

"The goal of the Lamaze method is a 'healthy baby,' not childbirth without anesthetics. Every doctor knows that the adult dosage of anesthetics given to the mother passes through the placenta in full dosage and can be harmful to the baby. On the other hand, at times (i.e., long labor, prolonged transition, complications, C-sections, lazy uterus, or fetal distress) analgesics and anesthetics are needed to produce a healthy baby."

"... remember, the more you tense up during labor, the longer will be your labor. The more you relax, the shorter will be your labor."

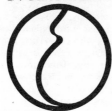

AMERICAN SOCIETY FOR PSYCHOPROPHYLAXIS IN OBSTETRICS

AMERICAN SOCIETY FOR
PSYCHOPROPHYLAXIS IN
OBSTETRICS
1411 K Street, NW, Suite 200
Washington, DC 20005
202/783-7050

The American Society for Psychoprophylaxis in Obstetrics (ASPO) was founded in 1960 in New York City, largely through the efforts of Marjorie Karmel and Elisabeth Bing (see opposite page). It was originally a society of physicians supported by volunteer lay people, who worked hard to introduce and promote acceptance of the Lamaze method (and fathers in the delivery room) by American obstetricians and hospitals. ASPO soon began certifying instructors to teach Lamaze preparation classes for parents. The Society was reorganized to comprise three coalitions—physicians, professionals (mostly childbirth educators), and parents—each with equal board representation and voting power. Headquarters were moved to Washington, DC, where ASPO now operates as a national, non-profit organization.

"Lamaze prepared childbirth offers prospective parents a way to experience the miracle of birth with dignity and confidence, and gives them the chance to share their baby's first moments of life together."

The majority of ASPO's current members belong to the Professional Coalition and are ASPO-certified childbirth educators (A.C.C.E.'s), most with backgrounds in nursing or physical therapy. Most of ASPO's publications and services are geared to this group, but parents will also find these resources very useful.

ASPO

MEMBERSHIP
Physician	$45.
Professional	$30.
Parent: Single	$10.
Couple	$15.

Memberships are tax-deductible and include a subscription to *Genesis,* publication discounts, mailings and other member benefits. For more information on ASPO classes, services, etc., contact ASPO.

MEMBERSHIP DIRECTORY: Lists names and addresses of physicians and teachers who are members of ASPO. (Parents are listed by name only.) Parents can use the directory to locate a Lamaze teacher or supportive physician in their area.

ANNUAL CONVENTION: The 1981 Convention was held in Arlington, Virginia, and featured seminars on obstetric drugs, preparation for parenting, sexuality, breastfeeding, childbirth education for the handicapped, and many other topics. Some seminars qualify for continuing education credits for physicians and nurses. In addition, continuing education workshops are held throughout the year in various locations.

PUBLICATION SERVICE: ASPO members can order ASPO publications and other books on childbirth and child care by mail-order, often at a discount. Several ASPO publications (*Cesarean Childbirth, Learning to Relax,* and *Medication Chart*) are reviewed in other sections of this *Catalog.* See index for page numbers.

GENESIS: ASPO publishes a bimonthly magazine for members, which provides articles on obstetrics, teaching, and parenting plus legislative updates, news of chapters and member groups, letters, and book and film reviews. *Genesis* recently changed its format and is now a very professionally-produced 32-page magazine, printed in two colors.

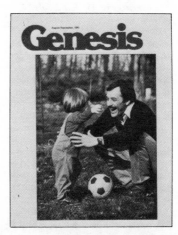

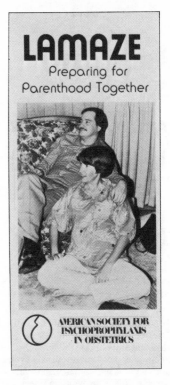

LAMAZE PARENT PAK: The Parent Pak is available free to members and is designed as a hand-out for Lamaze class members. The one I received included ASPO brochures, a reprint from *Parent's Magazine,* and booklets on childbirth, breastfeeding, and parenting produced by manufacturers of infant formula, baby food, baby products, and disposable diapers. The material came in a large plastic bag with handles and imprinted with the ASPO logo. It could easily be used as a Lamaze "goodie bag" to carry labor supplies to the hospital.

FILMS: *Nan's Class,* produced in 1977, follows the members of a Lamaze class as they go through preparation for birth and birth itself, including one cesarean. Class members are multi-racial and include five couples and one single mother. All deliveries take place in the hospital. The film shows the important role of the labor coach, and also shows the amount of routine hospital intervention which even well-prepared Lamaze students receive. *Fathers,* ASPO's newest film, features interviews with fathers and author Henry Biller (*Father Power*), sharing their personal feelings about pregnancy and birth, nurturing, "masculine" roles, work vs. home life, and other concerns.

MOTHERS ARE PEOPLE, TOO: A program of support/discussion groups for postpartum mothers, led by ASPO certified "MAPT" trainers.

THE BRADLEY METHOD

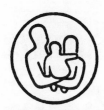

AMERICAN ACADEMY of HUSBAND-COACHED CHILDBIRTH®

AMERICAN ACADEMY OF HUS-
BAND-COACHED CHILDBIRTH
P.O. Box 5224
Sherman Oaks, CA 91413
213/788-6662
Marjie and Jay Hathaway, directors

The Bradley Method as taught by
the American Academy of Husband-
Coached Childbirth, emphasizes
"true natural childbirth" which
means giving birth without any drugs.
Unlike the ASPO-Lamaze method,
the emphasis is on avoiding drugs
completely, rather than simply minimizing their use or using drugs which
permit the mother to be awake during delivery. Another difference is
that the Bradley Method prepares
women to experience the "intensity
and pleasure" of birth by using deep
relaxation and "tuning in" to the
body's sensations during labor, rather than using distracting breathing
techniques. The Bradley Method is
particularly well suited for couples
who are planning to give birth in a
birth center or at home or who plan
to labor without obstetrical intervention. Classes are usually very consumer-oriented and are often taught by
a husband and wife team.

The Academy trains teachers in
the Bradley Method (regular teacher
training workshops are held throughout the country) and refers parents
to the certified Bradley teacher nearest them (write for a National Directory). The Academy also sells books,
buttons, and T-shirt transfers. Write
for more information.

**TO PREPARE FOR A JOYOUS
BIRTH**

1. Read *Husband-Coached Child-
birth* by Robert A. Bradley, M.D.
(Harper and Row, Third edition
1981) and *Exercises for True Natural
Childbirth* by Rhonda Hartman,
AAHCC (Harper and Row 1975). . . .
These books will help you learn the
basic information so that YOU CAN
MAKE WISE INFORMED CHOICES!
2. Seek out your nearest Bradley
Method instructor . . . .

3. Choose the place for your
baby's birth carefully. If you choose
a hospital or birth center, be sure it
has a high rate of UNMEDICATED
births, and a LOW cesarean section
rate. If you choose to give birth at
home, be sure to check-out the training and back-up of your birth attendant. Check the feelings of your chosen attendants about BIRTH rather
than delivery, also check out their
attitudes on husband participation
and other support people YOU may
choose to invite to your birth. Is
the Bradley Method supported?
DON'T BE AFRAID TO ASK QUES-
TIONS . . . NOW, so you will have
time to make other arrangements,
should their answers not meet your
expectations. It is important to
know what the policies are IN AD-
VANCE, so you will not be surprised
during labor.
4. Get a list of doctors who are
on the staff of a supportive hospital
and interview them. Evaluate the
doctor's views and decide if they are
compatible with your own. If not,
KEEP LOOKING and politely tell
the doctor why. This is important
for home birth couples as well.
5. Check with your local La
Leche League, Red Cross or other
groups, these people are often supportive and helpful.
6. See childbirth movies. . . .
7. TRAIN, STUDY, PREPARE
and QUESTION EVERYTHING.
The husband really needs to coach
during pregnancy so the mother is
prepared. During labor he plays the
key supportive role. DO NOT UN-
DERESTIMATE THE HUSBAND-
COACH ROLE.
8. Start now taking care of your
baby by eating lots of good food
(protein is vital) and avoid unnecessary drugs, and be sure you are getting plenty of salt. The nutrition is
THE MOST IMPORTANT FACTOR
IN A HEALTHY PREGNANCY!!!
9. Have a beautiful Husband-
Coached Childbirth!! Congratula-
tions and Happy Birth-Day!"
—from AAHCC National
Directory, July 1981

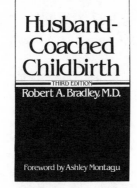

Husband-Coached Childbirth
THIRD EDITION
Robert A. Bradley, M.D.
Foreword by Ashley Montagu

HUSBAND-COACHED CHILD-
BIRTH (third edition)
by Robert A. Bradley
1981, 256 pages, Illus.

from
Harper and Row
10 East 53rd Street
New York, NY 10022
$9.95 hd.

Dr. Bradley's book is seriously
marred, I feel, by its sexist attitudes
and a writing style which is casual to
the point of being flippant. (Giving
advice to fathers on the psychology
of pregnant women, he says: "Let's
face a fact: they're nuttier than a
fruitcake!") Apart from this, the
content of the book is very sound
and a radical departure from the Lamaze approach. Dr. Bradley's
avowed goal is a totally unmedicated
delivery for the ninety-four percent
of women whose labors are normal.
In a chapter, "It's Not Nice to Fool
Mother Nature," Bradley argues that
any intervention in the natural birth
process introduces risks. He elaborates specifically on problems which
are caused by the typical hospital
procedures and drugs. These include:
the ill effects of labor medication on
babies, problems with establishing
breastfeeding, harmful separation of
babies in the newborn nursery, pro-
longation of labor, increased maternal risks, and postpartum depression.
Dr. Bradley grew up in a farm
town and saw many animal births as
a child. As an obstetrician he wondered why women could not give
birth as "peacefully and joyfully."
His elaboration of how labor and delivery should be conducted is based
in great part on an attempt to imitate
the natural birthing behavior of other
mammals. He outlines the basic
needs of animal mothers as follows:
1. The need for darkness and
solitude.
2. The need for quiet.
3. The need for physical comfort.
4. The need for physical relaxation.
5. The need for controlled
breathing.
6. The need for closed eyes and
the appearance of sleep.
By withdrawing to a secure, private and comfortable place, and being able to relax completely, Bradley
feels that women will be able to give
birth without drugs or the breathing
techniques and other "odd activities"
advocated by Lamaze. Curiously, in
attempting to adapt his theory to human mothers, Bradley rules out home
birth as an alternative to the brightly
lit, unprivate, unrelaxing hospital environment. Disagreeing with Ashley
Montagu, whose preface argues for
home birth, Bradley feels that the
small risk in childbirth requires all
mothers to give birth in a hospital
where medical emergency equipment
and staff are available. Instead, he
advocates bringing the "home environment" into the hospital, and sees
the participation of the husband in
labor and delivery as crucial to this
goal. This brings us to the title, *Husband-Coached Childbirth.* The husband's main role in the Bradley method is to help his wife achieve the
sense of peace, security, and relaxation she needs to give birth naturally
in the hospital. He does this by helping her achieve the six conditions
listed above. The husband is also encouraged to take an active role in his
wife's preparation for childbirth, becoming attuned to her needs, habits,
and responses both physically and
psychologically.

Bradley goes on to advocate the
squatting position for delivery and
encourages mothers to suckle their
babies immediately, on the delivery
table. He reports that his natural
childbirth mothers often feel so well
after delivery that they walk back to
their rooms from the delivery room,
with the baby in their arms. Bradley
advocates early discharge, and no routine separation of mothers and infants during the hospital stay. Unfortunately, Bradley devotes a whole
chapter to explaining why an episiotomy is necessary for most women.

"Other methods of childbirth
state that 'a little medication won't
hurt anything.' Natural-childbirth
principles state proudly that our firm
goal is totally unmedicated pregnancy,
labor, and birth. We do not want
our pregnant women taking any form
of drugs in any doses at all during
pregnancy. . . . We do not want our
mothers in labor accepting drugs of
any kind unless they have a complication wherein the risk of the medication is less than the risk of complication—and these are to be decided by
your doctor and are rare indeed!

"First-stage labor in animals was
briefly described as sleep imitation.
Although they were not asleep, they
looked like it and were positioned as
in sleep. It behooves you as a husband, then, to have a good idea of
how your big-tummied wife *positions*
herself at home in her own bed while
asleep. During the last few months
of pregnancy you should make careful observations of her position in
bed, the relationship of her arms, legs,
etc., when she is deeply asleep. Try
not to awaken her as you come in
late from that long poker party with
the boys, and carefully study her
while she sleeps. She then presents
the identical picture we want you as
a labor coach to help her assume now
in the hospital, by your careful guidance during her uterine contractions.
This same position that she selected
at home as being the most comfortable for her should be repeated at
this stage of labor."

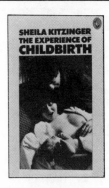

THE KITZINGER METHOD

At last!—a childbirth "method" which was developed by and bears the name of a woman—Sheila Kitzinger. One cannot help but notice how the field of obstetrics is strewn with the names of men (Heger, Chadwick, Leopold, DeLee, Kegel, Duncan, Schultz, Montgomery, Fallopius, Dick-Read, Lamaze, Bradley, Leboyer) who have staked out their territories and layed claim to small bits of woman's anatomy and psyche.

Sheila Kitzinger is a British social anthropologist, the mother of five children, and has been teaching, lecturing, and writing about childbirth and childbirth education since the late 1950's. Her "psychosexual" method is not, in fact, taught as a separate method. There is no "Kitzinger" organization or certified "Kitzinger" teachers. But Kitzinger's ideas have been taken up and used by many teachers and parents and worked into the other methods of childbirth preparation.

Kitzinger brings her background in social anthropology and psychoanalytic theory to bear on the childbirth experience. She is interested in how our personal attitudes about birth and our bodies, learned from our families and our society, influence how we give birth. She is also concerned with the social context of birth and how women communicate and negotiate with the people who are helping them in birth (the obstetrician, the midwife, the nurses, etc.). Kitzinger is especially interested in the psychological aspects of childbearing. She focuses attention on birth as a sexual experience; she discusses sex in pregnancy and how sexual adjustment may be related to women's acceptance of the sensations and events of labor and birth. She is concerned with pregnancy as a developmental "crisis" in a woman's life, looking at both women's common concerns and feelings and at the importance of the mother/daughter relationship.

The foundations of Kitzinger's physical preparation for birth are, once again, relaxation, breathing, and the use of comfortable positions for labor. But Kitzinger provides one of the richest, most complex elaborations of these fundamentals to be found in the literature. She uses a variety of methods for teaching the art of deep relaxation, including "centering," "touch relaxation" (learning to "let go" when your partner lightly touches a body part which has become tense), and massage. She also uses fantasy and mental imagery to develop body and sensory awareness. Regulated breathing rhythms are taught as an aid to relaxation and body awareness, not as a means of "distraction." Walking, standing, sitting, and an all-fours position are encouraged for labor comfort.

In reading Kitzinger's work I am impressed by the warmth and depth of her understanding of birth. Men truly are at a disadvantage in attempting to describe the complex and overlapping emotional and physical aspects of an event they have never experienced. I find much in the writing of Dick-Read, Lamaze, and Bradley to be idealized and oversimplified, while Kitzinger's work is much more realistic. It is really like a pulling-together of the life-time learning of a wise and experienced mother.

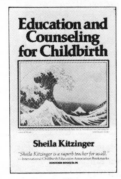

THE EXPERIENCE OF CHILD-BIRTH (4th Edition)
by Sheila Kitzinger
1981, 335 pages, Illus.

from
Penguin Books
625 Madison Avenue
New York, NY 10022
$3.95 pap.

The first edition of this classic book was published in 1962 and it has been revised regularly since then. Kitzinger introduces the concept of "childbirth with joy" by describing the contributions of Dick-Read and Lamaze and the important role of relaxation and emotions in childbirth. She describes the physical process of pregnancy and provides an excellent chapter on the psychology of pregnancy. She then outlines her method for "learning harmony in labor" with the emphasis on adapting to the stresses of labor through relaxation, breathing, and relaxing the birth outlet. There is a chapter for fathers on how they can best help their partners in pregnancy, birth and after the baby is born. The chapter on "Drugs in Labour" stresses the importance of fully informing women about the disadvantages, both to them and their babies, of drug use in labor. Kitzinger then explains the course of normal labor, birth and the postpartum period, describing how mothers and fathers commonly react. This section includes many first-person comments from her students. Appendices include "Preparing for the Birth at home," items to include in a "hospital labour kit," and cesarean birth.

"The experience of bearing a child is central to a woman's life. Years after the baby has been born she remembers acutely the details of her labour and her feelings as the child was delivered. One can speak to any grandmother about birth and almost immediately she will begin to talk about her own labours. It is unlikely that any experience in a man's life is comparably vivid.

"There is a strange unconscious neuro-muscular association between the vagina and the mouth. The pads of flesh at either side of the vagina are even called *labia* (lips). Our earliest experiences of erotic delight are centered in our mouths and lips and associated with pleasurable feeding. Even when our eroticism has developed to full genital maturity we retain a pleasure in stimulation of the surfaces of the lips and tongue, which are still sensitive to touch: we enjoy kissing; some smoke; others chew gum or sweets or chocolates. We never entirely outgrow our early infantile mouth-centeredness.

"When a woman proves tense in the region of the pelvic floor she can often be helped to relax by teaching her how to relax her mouth and jaw. If one then asks her to get the same feeling of looseness in the area of the vagina she can do it with far less difficulty. But if she starts tightening up her mouth, she finds that she is automatically tightening up the pelvic floor too.

"The second stage is that of the expulsion of the baby . . . . Women often enjoy it, and the pleasure it brings is similar to the simple delight in defecation that one can witness in a small child, and is a reminder of once vigorous infantile pleasures which have often been repressed in the adult and have become taboo—which may in itself threaten the inhibited woman's composure. When the bearing-down reflex is fully established, the urge to push is compelling and irresistible. Some women are horrified at the intensity of the desire to bear down. 'It is,' as one mother commented afterwards, 'a very primitive sort of urge. I was astonished that it was so strong.' Women who have been inadequately prepared for the passion they feel welling up in them in labour may try to escape from the sensations. They panic and grip themselves in pain, resisting the urge with all their might."

EDUCATION AND COUNSELING FOR CHILDBIRTH
by Sheila Kitzinger
1979, 303 pages

from
Schocken Books
200 Madison Avenue
New York, NY 10016
$6.95 pap.

The content of this book is very similar to that of *The Experience of Childbirth* except that it is directed to childbirth teachers rather than to parents. Included is practical information on how to teach and organize classes, with attention paid to the importance of language in teaching an and with a chapter on teaching "underprivileged women." Kitzinger presents her methods and exercises for relaxation and breathing, and her ideas on the psychology of pregnancy, the father's role, and support in labor. An excellent final chapter provides information for teachers on parenting, the "fourth trimester," postpartum depression, and helping women who have experienced a miscarriage or stillbirth.

The emphasis throughout is on how teachers can help parents meet the challenge of "the normal life crisis of having a baby." Some sections of the book may be helpful for parents, too, for sometimes the advice given to teachers is more honest and straightforward. The chapters on how the childbirth teacher can provide support in labor are especially enlightening in this regard.

"More than one teacher uses the phraseology of equipping oneself with techniques as *weapons* for labour, and the birth as *B-Day*, thereby implying that childbirth is a battle which has to be won, rather than a natural process. I always remember my own doctor examining me in late pregnancy, finding twins, and remarking 'I think I can feel two heads' rather than suggesting that she thought there were two *babies* there. A physiotherapist friend who is an antenatal teacher recalls with horror that she used to talk about the fetal head 'hitting' the perineum in the second stage.

"Use words which avoid negative suggestion, and select those which reinforce a positive image of the healthy human body in childbirth..."

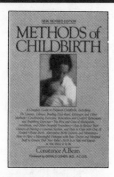

METHODS OF CHILDBIRTH
(New, Revised Edition)
by Constance A. Bean
1982, 254 pages, Illus.

from
Doubleday/Dolphin
245 Park Avenue
New York, NY 10017
$7.95 pap.

"This book is ten years old, but it is still one of the most useful books available on consumer-oriented preparation for childbirth." That's how I began my first review of this book, but while I was writing, Constance Bean published her new, revised edition of *Methods of Childbirth,* which is even better than the first and reflects the many changes which have occurred in the last ten years.

As in the first edition, Bean describes the basic anatomy and physiology of pregnancy, labor and birth. She explains the different methods of prepared childbirth, noting the differences between the Dick-Read, Lamaze and Kitzinger methods and this time also including the Bradley and Leboyer methods and the special characteristics of home birth preparation classes. Bean explains what to expect from a childbirth preparation class and instructor and thoroughly describes the relaxation and physical conditioning exercises and breathing patterns which are usually taught.

Bean's chapter on labor drugs provides a good introduction to the history and rationale for anesthesia in childbirth and carefully describes the medications used during labor (including narcotics, tranquilizers and amnesics) and anesthesia for the birth itself (including local, regional and general anesthesia). Bean stresses that all childbirth drugs cross the placenta and reach the baby, that childbirth drugs have never been proven safe for use with women and babies, and that use of drugs often leads to other interventions (for instance, the use of forceps).

The three chapters devoted to explaining hospital procedures for labor, delivery and after-delivery describe in detail the "advantages and (mostly) disadvantages of the current technology." Bean explains the history of hospitalization for birth and provides very useful descriptions of the most common hospital interventions, including artificial rupture of the membranes, induced labor, admission procedures, electronic fetal monitoring, intravenous fluids, use of Pitocin to speed up labor, episiotomy, cord clamping, routine infant suctioning, silver nitrate, and more. She also includes information on rooming-in, bonding, and how to get a good start at breastfeeding.

New to this edition is a complete chapter on Cesarean section, reflecting the phenomenal rise in C-section rates in the past ten years. Bean describes some reasons for the increase, how obstetric interventions can lead to cesarean, and how to prevent cesareans. Another new chapter describes home birth, alternative birth centers, and midwives and includes an excellent discussion of the good safety record of home birth and midwifery.

The final chapter, "Patient Rights, Parent Choices," is perhaps the most important. It is unfortunate, but true, that parents must be extremely well-prepared and informed of their legal rights as parents, in order to avoid unwanted intervention in the hospital. Bean discusses physician attitudes toward consumers and advises parents to actively plan for their birth. Planning includes choosing the place for birth, choosing an obstetrician or midwife, and writing an "optimum birth letter" to the hospital, outlining requests. Bean explains the important concept of informed consent and reminds parents that a person has the right to refuse any medical treatment. A glossary and list of useful organizations is included at the end of the book.

Without doubt, Constance Bean is an experienced and strong patient advocate and though she is always tactful and low-key in style, she doesn't hesitate to state the disadvantages of modern obstetric drugs and procedures. She is also very candid in describing the limitations and biases of medical professionals and hospital systems. Ms. Bean has observed many births and has participated in the childbirth consumer movement for many years. Parents will find her descriptions and advice very valuable.

"The technology can be life-saving This statement is made frequently, and it is true. Needed in certain circumstances are ways to start labor, to give fluids to incapacitated women, to give blood, to monitor the baby, and to remove the baby surgically.

"However when they are used without adequate standards or cause, normal labors may be altered in ways that require further intervention. Risks, including that of surgery, are increased subtly. Amidst the web of labor procedures this may not be clearly perceived by the hospital staff, who are caught up with the immediacy of daily tasks and responsibilities. Therefore, leadership in this area can often best come from outside the institution. Inside the hospital, there is no one (with the possible exception of midwives, and their professional position is still in many instances precarious) with the responsibility of overseeing a patient's total situation and minimizing unnecessary risks. However, individual couples, if they have the knowledge, can alter this pattern."

"Often, hospital-sponsored classes, with notable exceptions, are taught by a labor and delivery-room nurse untrained in education for childbirth and with the responsibility of explaining what the hospital does, not what it *should* do, and not the pros and cons of any procedure. Therefore, hospital-sponsored classes can tend to encourage patients to accept what is currently done, making no pretense of addressing controversial issues or the sensitive area of patients' rights."

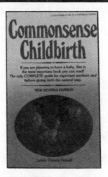

COMMONSENSE CHILDBIRTH
(Revised Edition)
by Lester Hazell
1976, 281 pages, Illus.

from
Berkley Publishing
200 Madison Avenue
New York, NY 10016
$2.25 pap.

Lester Hazell's first birth was a "nightmare." Drugs, hospital procedures, and mismanagement created a very unhappy experience. In response, Ms. Hazell joined a local group of women who were working to promote the natural childbirth practices of Grantly Dick-Read. She trained as a childbirth educator, began teaching students, and had a much better experience giving birth to her second child in a hospital with her husband present for the first time. Her third child was born at home and that was the best experience of all. *Commonsense Childbirth,* first published in 1969, grew out of these experiences: "As time moved along, I felt the need to reach more people than I could by teaching prenatal classes. Birth in America is still swathed in mystery, and since the process is relatively simple and women can be easily taught how to respond to it, it seemed that a commonsense labor 'cookbook' was in order. As I went along, some of the anger and irritation I feel at our society which makes difficult a perfectly normal process has crept in, and I've left it there. The 'cookbook' has become something of a polemic, but it is a polemic which is based on more than a decade of solid experience wading through the quagmire of American birth practices."

Hazell begins by describing and comparing a medicated hospital delivery, an unmedicated hospital delivery, and a home birth, emphasizing that "the choice is yours." She goes on to give advice on pregnancy, nutrition, and choosing a doctor. She describes the process of labor and delivery in detail, including an excellent section on "What Does It Feel Like to Have a Baby?" Hazell also covers childbirth drugs, home birth, breastfeeding, dealing with complications, sexuality in childbearing, emergency childbirth, and answers frequently asked questions about birth.

"Here we should talk about the important subject of pain. I find that it is one of the major fears surrounding childbirth in the United States. Women ask themselves consciously or unconsciously: 'Will I be able to stand the pain?'

"Although I have been told that there is such a thing as painless childbirth, I have never seen a case myself. On the other hand neither have I ever seen a prepared woman who was stymied by pain, and I have never seen an upset, unprepared one who didn't respond to quiet, confident coaching that showed *her* what to do, instead of doing something to her or for her.

"What does the bearing-down reflex feel like? Everyone has experienced this to some degree. It is very like the pushing of a bowel movement, only more sustained and more demanding. It is far easier *not* to push when one is having a bowel movement than when one is having a baby. However, the second-stage contractions are not, as a rule, painful. In fact, they are very satisfying. You may be surprised at the noises you make. So may your family. One husband had been told to wait in the hall outside the delivery room. A sudden cry from his wife brought him on the run. She looked surprised to see him, and when he said he was worried by her cry, she said, 'Oh, that! That was just a war whoop! I'm fine.' Most of the noises of second stage are comparable to those of a stevedore exerting himself. Because of the fact that you need to close your throat in order to push, sometimes this leads to your vocal cords being involved, and they do make noise. However, this usually sounds louder to you than to anyone else. (Comparably, a firm grunt is recommended at the beginning of exertion in karate.)"

CHOICES IN CHILDBIRTH
by Silvia Feldman
1979, 267 pages, Illus.

from
Grosset and Dunlap
51 Madison Avenue
New York, NY 10010
$8.95

In her introduction, Dr. Feldman points out that maternity care experts today have separated into two sharply divided and increasingly hostile camps—those who advocate "aggressive medical management" for birth and those who advocate less technological, more family-centered alternatives. The expectant mother is often caught in the middle, receiving conflicting advice from doctors, educators, and books. *Choices in Childbirth* can help women sort out the controversy and take an active role in making the important decisions which Feldman feels are crucial to a satisfying birth experience. "As a psychotherapist and marriage counselor, and mother of three girls, I have known for a long time how important a good childbirth is for a happy family life," says Feldman. She emphasizes that pregnant women are responsible adults who should not be shielded from "unpleasant facts" about the way childbirth is handled.

Feldman suggests three major guidelines for women as they begin to learn about childbirth: first, become aware of your own feelings about birth, since the choices you make should serve your own emotional needs; second, become fully informed about your options in childbirth, including what's available in your community both in and outside of the "system"; third, get involved in community groups and support systems which can provide for your needs both in birth and as a new parent. Feldman has organized the book to explore each of these guidelines in depth.

Part One, "Becoming Aware," discusses our cultural ignorance about birth and compares conventional American practices with birth in other cultures and in the "countermovement." Part Two, "Mapping Your Own Route," provides an excellent introduction to prenatal care, preparing for childbirth, the hospital experience, cesarean birth, childbirth drugs, the different methods of natural childbirth training, and breastfeeding. Part Three, "Getting Involved," explains how to use community groups and resources to find the birthing setting, attendant and services you want, and discusses bonding, siblings at birth, midwives, Leboyer-birth, birth centers, and home birth. The book concludes with "After the Baby Comes," which stresses the importance of postpartum support for parents.

Two features of Feldman's book are especially unique and useful. First of all, she discusses the different methods of childbirth preparation in terms of the way they suit the specific emotional needs and temperament of the mother. For instance, she feels that "Lamaze" may be the best approach for women who value self-control and acceptance of medical authority, whereas the Bradley method may be better for women who feel confident about a freer, more permissive approach. This way of evaluating methods is more useful, I think, than just comparing breathing techniques and exercises.

Secondly, Feldman's book is also unique in presenting the concept of the Mother's Center, which she helped pioneer on Long Island. The model Mother's Center in Hicksville, New York, began as a place for women to meet to discuss their delivery experiences, and quickly grew to include peer-facilitated discussion groups in childbirth preparation, many aspects of baby and child care, and parenting. Feldman believes strongly that groups led by "experts" can exploit dependency rather than encourage reliance on personal strength. She prefers the Mother's Center approach of training mothers to provide support services for their peers.

For more information on Mother's Centers, see index.

"The Lamaze method is popular in this country because Americans value self-control, mastery of experience, and acceptance of the doctor's authority. Lamaze training gives a woman the tools she needs to succeed in the most socially acceptable manner possible. She is kept fully occupied with exercises and breathing, so she isn't likely to be overwhelmed by her feelings. She learns to distract herself from the physical sensations rather than become engulfed by them. She is expected to behave as a rational adult at all times.

"Unfortunately, rationality is oversteemed in our culture. Many women ask for painkillers, even anesthesia, so they can continue to behave in the approved rational way, which bolsters their self-image of being grown-up and sensible. In my view, a little less emphasis on self-control and a little more expression of real feelings wouldn't hurt the childbirth situation a bit. However, if you tend to be a sensible, conforming, brave person—and you like yourself that way—a Lamaze delivery is a definite possibility. Many women do feel more comfortable with this kind of prepared childbirth than with any other. For a later delivery, when you're more experienced and self-confident and less concerned with others' opinion of you, a more permissive method and a freer atmosphere may be your choice."

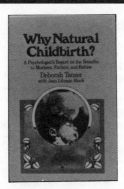

WHY NATURAL CHILDBIRTH?:
A Psychologist's Report on the Benefits to Mothers, Fathers, and Babies
by Deborah Tanzer
with Jean Libman Block
1976, 289 pages

from
Schocken Books
200 Madison Avenue
New York, NY 10016
$5.50 pap.

As a doctoral student in psychology at Brandeis University, Deborah Tanzer became interested in the controversy over "natural" versus "conventional" childbirth, especially the claims of psychological benefit being made for natural childbirth. At that time, Dr. Abraham Maslow chaired the psychology department at Brandeis, and Tanzer wondered whether or not natural childbirth might be a "peak experience" of the type Maslow was describing. Her doctoral thesis examining natural childbirth was originally presented in 1967 and later published as *Why Natural Childbirth?* in 1972. It is based on a five-year study of pregnant women, divided into "choosers" and "non-choosers" of natural childbirth. Tanzer found that, indeed, women who had natural childbirth did accrue "important psychological benefits." She says, "During pregnancy, the attitudes toward pregnancy of the women taking the natural childbirth course changed far more positively than those of the other women. During childbirth, women using the natural method had a more positive subjective experience, especially in late labor and delivery when it was possible for them to participate actively in the birth process by breathing and pushing. Another benefit for the natural childbirth women was a tendency toward reduction in pain. Finally, after the baby was born, natural childbirth women generally had more positive views of themselves."

Tanzer explains her research carefully. She first presents a history of childbirth practices. She points out the risks in using drugs for pain relief. She discusses the psychology of childbirth and disputes the claims made by some obstetricians that women who choose natural childbirth are "masochistic," "castrating," "neurotic," or otherwise suffering from personality disorders. She describes how the experience of pregnancy, labor, birth, and pain was different for the two groups, and includes many comments from the mothers themselves. There are also two chapters on the important role of fathers in birth and the benefits for both partners when fathers participate in labor and birth. Tanzer concludes by arguing for increased acceptance of natural childbirth methods by the medical profession, citing both medical and psychological benefits for the mother, father, and baby.

"My study revealed clearly the enhanced sense of self felt by many of the women in the natural childbirth group. It seems logical that this sense of mastery generated at a crucial time could carry over beyond the childbirth situation. I strongly suspect that once a woman has experienced her own ability to cope with birth, she is better prepared to handle many later situations, including the care of her child . . . .

"To stress the ability of a woman to derive enduring strength from a successful delivery by no means relegates her to a child-bearing role as the core of her existence. On the contrary, it honors the full potential of the female person. Whether she bears a child or children as her primary life work or as one facet of her life, each woman has the right to her sense of triumph. And to let that triumph carry over to other aspects of her daily life.

"Whether she bears a child or children as her primary life work or as one facet of her life, each woman has the right to her sense of triumph. And to let that triumph carry over to other aspects of her daily life."

"By sharing the birth process with her husband, the natural childbirth woman experiences other important effects: the rapture which we have noted, the healthier perception of the world and the healthier feeling about herself. And we should recall, peak-experiences occurred only to those who had their husband present. This is no slight benefit, since as Dr. Maslow has noted about the peak-experience, '. . . so many people find this so great and high an experience that it justifies not only itself but even living itself. Peak-experiences can make life worthwhile by their occasional occurrence. They give meaning to life itself. They prove it to be worthwhile.' "

MATERNITY CENTER ASSOCIATION

MATERNITY CENTER ASSO-
CIATION
48 East 92nd Street
New York, NY 10028
212/369-7300
Ruth Watson Lubic, CNM, General
Director
Martin Kelly, Director of Public In-
formation

The Maternity Center Association (MCA) was founded in 1918 by
a group of women and physicians
who were concerned about the lack
of prenatal care available to women
in New York City. At that time, the
United States had one of the highest
maternal death rates of any developed nation, ranking 17th from the
best. Childbirth was the second
leading cause of death among wom-
en aged 15 to 45, after tuberculosis.
MCA set up a network of prenatal
clinics. The success achieved led to
acceptance and use of these services
by hospitals and public institutions.
Prenatal care is now the standard
for maternity care in our country.
In her foreword to a recent MCA
publication, current president, Mrs.
Philip W. Farley said, "This beginning is a perfect illustration of the
way the Association has functioned
ever since. Our role as a voluntary
agency, independently supported by
our members, has been to serve as a
bellwether, developing and launch-
ing demonstration programs for
which we saw a public health need
and which public institutions were
either unable or unwilling to undertake. This has been true of prenatal
care, comprehensive maternity services, parent education, nurse-midwifery, prepared childbirth, and
family-centered maternity care."
In 1931, MCA began training
public health nurses in midwifery,
creating the modern day, American
nurse-midwife. MCA-trained midwives provided a home birth service,
delivering babies among poor people in the New York area. In 1958,
the home birth service was ended
and the nurse-midwife training program taken up by Kings County Hospital in Brooklyn, which continues
to use nurse-midwives for a large
number of deliveries, with excellent
results.
In 1947, MCA sponsored the
first American tour by natural childbirth proponent, Grantly Dick-Read
(see index) and began incorporating
his principles into their classes for
expectant parents.
During the 1970's MCA became
aware of the growing public disenchantment with traditional hospital
maternity services. They were
alarmed by the number of parents
who were turning to unsupervised
home births. A compromise was
sought and the result was the establishment, in 1975, of the MCA Child-

bearing Center in New York City,
the country's first free-standing birth
center. At the Center nurse-midwives handle normal deliveries,
backed up by a health team of obstetricians, pediatricians, and other
professionals. In 1981 MCA received a large grant to promote the
development of other birth centers
around the country.
Summing up the Association's
activities, director of public information, Martin Kelly, writes, "Devoted
to the improvement of maternity
care, the Association maintains a
childbearing center for low-risk families; conducts classes on pregnancy,
childbearing and baby care for expectant mothers and fathers; responds to requests for information
on childbearing and family life problems from parents, community agencies, city and state health departments, and the communications
media; conducts conferences and
seminars on maternity care for doctors, nurses, nurse-midwives, and
other interested professionals; conducts parent-education institutes for
nurses who teach expectant parent
classes; and sponsors research to investigate problems in maternity and
infant care and to help resolve
them."
MCA's excellent publications are
used by parents and professionals
throughout the 50 states and in 82
other countries. Some of the Center's most popular publications are
described below. For a complete
ordering and price list, request a
copy of "Publications and Teaching
Aids" from MCA.
Also consult the index for reviews of MCA's *A Baby is Born* and
The Birth Atlas, and see section on
Birth Centers.

PSYCHOLOGICAL ANALGESIA:
Natural Childbirth and Psychoprophylaxis
by Ruth Watson Lubic and Eunice
K. M. Ernst
1975, 16 pages

$.50 for single copies
.40 @ for 10-99
.35 @ for 100 or more

In this "review of the history and
major methods of prepared childbirth," Lubic and Ernst note the public interest and demand for natural
childbirth and relative lack of interest
and acknowledgement for the subject
among medical professionals. They
review and compare the major
methods and discuss the importance
of environment and personnel (father,
nurse, midwife) in making natural
methods successful. A design for
prepared childbirth classes includes
an outline for course content.

PREPARATION FOR CHILD-
BEARING (4th Edition)
1973, 48 pages, Illus.

$1.00 for single copies
.80 @ for 10-99 copies
.60 @ for 100 or more

This booklet is simply written
and well illustrated to provide essential information on childbirth preparation and comfort measures to a
wide audience of women. "Comfort in Pregnancy" covers posture
and body mechanics, relaxation
and breathing, comfort measures
and exercises, and advice for expectant fathers. "Participation in Labor" describes the process of normal
labor, provides controlled breathing
patterns for labor and delivery, instructions for the father/coach in
labor, and an extremely useful chart
of labor which outlines physical
signs, support measures, and breathing patterns for each of seven stages
of labor. "The Postpartum Period"
covers postpartum comfort and recovery, muscle toning, advice for new
fathers, and how to hold and lift a
new baby. A listing of additional
reading and resources is included.

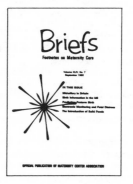

BRIEFS: Footnotes on Maternity
Care

Published by
Charles B. Slack, Inc.
6900 Grove Road
Thorofare, NJ 08086
$6.00 a year (10 issues)

Briefs is a small monthly (except
July and August) digest which provides reports on issues in maternal
and child health, based on abstracts
and reviews of current medical literature. Issues are 16-pages long and
usually contain four to seven reports
each. *Briefs* is an extremely useful
resource for professionals and parents
who want to keep up with developments in obstetric practice, maternity services, breastfeeding, infant
care and other topics in birth and
public health. *Briefs* is the official
publication of the Maternity Center
Association but should be ordered
directly from the publisher, above.

ICEA

INTERNATIONAL CHILDBIRTH
EDUCATION ASSOCIATION
(ICEA)
P.O. Box 20048
Minneapolis, MN 55420
612/854-8660

ICEA was founded in 1960 by a
group of parents and professionals interested in promoting education for
childbirth. The Association serves as
a network, binding together childbirth educators, parents, physicians,
midwives, nurses, physical therapists,
and nutritionists. They can join
ICEA both as individuals and as members of participating member groups.
Within ICEA, members and member
groups are autonomous, "establishing
their own policies and creating their
own programs. There are no membership requirements for individuals
other than a commitment to family-
centered maternity care and the philosophy of "freedom of choice based
on knowledge of alternatives." ICEA
is a non-profit, volunteer organization. In 1981, it had over 13,000
members.
The concept of Family-Centered
Maternity Care (FCMC) is one of the
important contributions of ICEA.
ICEA literature describes FCMC as
"an individualized and flexible program that offers choices to the entire
childbearing family in a warmly supportive environment. It is respectful
of the family's needs and rights before, during and after childbirth. It
strengthens family bonds by encouraging shared and informed participation in all aspects of the birth process within the bounds of medical
safety. FCMC is based on scientific
evidence from medicine, sociology,
psychology, nursing, midwifery, nutrition and other fields." What this
means, in practice, is an emphasis on
childbirth preparation, informed consent to medical procedures, avoidance
of unnecessary intervention, father's
participation in labor and birth, use
of alternative settings for birth, use of
midwives, opportunities for parent/
infant bonding, rooming-in for mothers and infants, and encouragement
of breastfeeding.
Childbirth preparation classes
are provided by individual teachers
and groups who are members of
ICEA.
ICEA has recently revised its
teacher-certification program with
the development of the *ICEA Teacher
Certification Packet* in September
1982. The packet contains all the
descriptive material, evaluation, veri-
fication and application forms needed for completing the program. Included are study guides which provide objectives for study and refer-

ICEA, cont'd

ences to specific texts. Applicants are required to obtain contact hours, observe births, complete an approved teaching series, and pass an exam. Packets are available for $38. (plus $5.00 for air mail) from ICEA headquarters. Parents who would like to take classes taught by an ICEA-certified teacher can consult the Membership Directory or request local referrals from the main office. Many Lamaze, Bradley and Dick-Read teachers are also members of ICEA.

ICEA serves as a valuable resource for its members by providing publications and teaching materials, a book service, numerous committees, regional coordinators, conferences and meetings, member group services, and access to medical and professional consultants. A selection of these many services is listed below.

MEMBERSHIP

$15. a year for individual members

$35. for contributing professionals

Membership includes four issues of *ICEA News,* the opportunity to subscribe to other member periodicals, member discounts at ICEA Bookcenter, news of conferences, conventions, etc., election and voting privileges, use of ICEA resource services, and a listing in and one copy of the annual Membership Directory.

Write to ICEA for a membership application. Organizations and groups can also apply for Group Membership.

PERIODICALS

ICEA News

This 12-page quarterly newsletter is the official publication of ICEA. It provides short articles and updates on ICEA activities and reports on "research, legislation and community action on childbirth issues." Included are international and regional reports, letters, book reviews, resources, and a national calendar. Subscriptions are available to non-members for $5. a year. ICEA also publishes *ICEA Review* (review of research), *ICEA Forum* (the newsletter for groups) and *ICEA Sharing* (the newsletter for teachers). All are pub-

lished three times a year and subscriptions are available for $3. each only at the time of beginning or renewing membership.

ICEA BOOKCENTER

The Bookcenter regularly publishes *Bookmarks,* a catalog which includes an annotated listing of over 400 books and pamphlets available by mail from ICEA, plus short book reviews of new books. Topics include childbirth preparation, pregnancy and birth, teenage pregnancy, family planning, cesarean birth, home birth and alternatives, breastfeeding, fathers, parenthood, infant and child care and health, women's health, professional reference, sex education, and nutrition. All ICEA publications are also available through the Bookcenter. Service is very prompt (within 1 to 2 weeks), an important consideration for pregnant parents. Request a free copy of Bookmarks from ICEA main office.

PUBLICATIONS

ICEA has published many excellent booklets, guides, and pamphlets on a variety of topics. Write to ICEA for a complete listing of publications and prices. Bulk rates are available for all ICEA publications.

"ICEA promotes educational programs to assist expectant parents in preparing for childbirth, breastfeeding, and parenting. ICEA further promotes the recognition of the rights of expectant parents to be involved in their health care planning and to become aware of health care options."

PARENTS' GUIDE TO THE CHILD-BEARING YEAR (7th edition)
by Peg Beals
1980, 84 pages, Illus.
$3.50 pap.

This guide was first published in 1974 and is one of ICEA's best sellers. It is a basic introduction to prepared childbirth and is used by teachers and parents as a class manual. Chapters provide information on physical fitness (nutrition, drugs to avoid, exercise and posture), conscious release (relaxation techniques), controlled breathing patterns, second stage of labor (the 1980 edition contains new information on maternal position for labor), comfort measures for labor, the hospital birth experience (including a useful chart of labor progress and participation), and family life education.

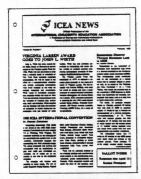

MORE CHILDBIRTH PREPARATION ORGANIZATIONS

NATIONAL ASSOCIATION OF CHILDBIRTH EDUCATION, INC.
3940 Eleventh Street
Riverside, CA 92501
714/686-0422

National Association of Childbirth Education (NACE) is the new name of the Childbirth Without Pain Education League, which was originally founded in 1964. The acronym, NACE, is pronounced NAH-say and means "is born, budding, springing forth" in Spanish. NACE is a nonprofit, volunteer organization which trains and certifies teachers in the Pavlov/Lamaze method of childbirth preparation. It also provides teachers with ongoing support and education services. NACE teachers are not required to have a medical background and often are mothers who have experienced a prepared childbirth. NACE emphasizes the importance of breastfeeding and does require its teachers to have breastfed for at least six months. NACE teachers offer childbirth preparation classes around the country; a Correspondence Class for women in isolated areas is also available. Parents are encouraged to "make informed responsible choices concerning birth alternatives, procedures, breastfeeding, nutrition, family participation, infant and child care, and family planning." Contact NACE for information on becoming a teacher or for referrals to NACE classes in your area.

FOCAL POINT—NACE's 8-page, bimonthly newsletter provides teachers with information on teaching techniques and updates on maternity care. It is available to non-members for $6.00 a year.

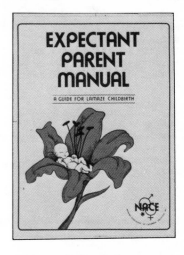

EXPECTANT PARENTS MANUAL:
A Guide for Lamaze Childbirth
by NACE
1981, 98 pages, Illus.
$6.00 plus 75 cents postage
bulk rates are available

The NACE Manual is excellent. It covers the usual material on anatomy, nutrition, and Lamaze techniques, but also includes very helpful information and checklists on choosing your medical care, doctor discussion points, variations on labor and birth (coping with back labor, breech presentation, hospital procedures), the side effects of labor drugs, and "working with the sensations of labor." The approach is realistic and very consumer-oriented.

The manual is also available in Spanish ("El Cuidado Prenatal y Preparacion Para El Parto: Guia Completa") for the same price.

SAFE BIRTHING INFORMATION NETWORK
Route 1, Box 27
Blackfoot, ID 83221

Safe Birthing Information Network (SBIN) was founded in 1980 by childbirth educators Joyce Hull and Terry Ann Denning to promote childbirth education to prepare parents for "a *safe* birth in *any* setting." SBIN has designed a Parent Modular Series of seven lectures with accompanying hand-outs, reading assignments, and pre-lecture questions. SBIN also provides training for childbirth educators, labor monitresses, and "family health workers." It publishes a quarterly journal and a monthly update. Write for more information.

CHILDBIRTH WITHOUT PAIN EDUCATION ASSOCIATION
20134 Snowden
Detroit, MI 48235

This group promotes and teaches the Psychoprophylactic Method of Painless Childbirth.

PREPARING EXPECTANT PARENTS (PEP)
c/o Mary Kay Woodward
350 S. Willow, Sp. 40
Rialto, CA 92376

This organization trains and certifies teachers and provides classes in the Lamaze method of childbirth preparation.

CHOOSING A CHILDBIRTH EDUCATOR

FINDING A CHILDBIRTH EDUCATOR

To find a childbirth educator in your area, write to the national organizations listed in this section. They can give you referrals to teachers who are members of these groups. You can also ask for referrals from your doctor or midwife, your local hospital, women's centers and health clinics, or from your local representative of La Leche League. To find a teacher who emphasizes alternative methods of childbirth, contact the national organizations listed under home birth, and NAPSAC (see index).

CHOOSING A CHILDBIRTH EDUCATOR

Childbirth teachers have an important role to play in educating parents for birth. Their attitudes and methods can make a real difference in how a couple experiences childbirth. It is wise to choose a childbirth teacher as carefully as you choose your doctor or midwife. Look around for a teacher whose philosophy and feelings about birth are compatible with yours. Ask her for the names of some former students and talk to these people about whether or not the classes were helpful to them in achieving their own goals in childbirth.

SOME QUESTIONS TO ASK

1. What is your background and training? (Some people feel more comfortable with a nurse, others with a lay teacher.)

2. What has been your personal experience with childbirth and breastfeeding?

3. What method(s) of childbirth preparation do you teach?

4. What topics are covered in addition to labor and delivery? (Nutrition, body mechanics, emotional concerns of pregnancy, preparation for parenting and breastfeeding.)

5. How many classes do you offer, when do they start, what times are they available? Do you offer an "early bird" series for early pregnancy? Do you offer refresher courses?

6. What class materials do you use? Will films and slides be shown? Do students receive a class manual? Do you maintain a lending library of books on childbirth and parenting?

7. What is your average class size? Will I be able to receive individual attention?

8. Do classes include time for personal discussion and exercise practice?

9. Are fathers included in the classes? (Some classes, especially Bradley classes, are taught by a husband/wife team.)

10. Do you emphasize the goal of a totally un-medicated birth? What percentage of your students have medication for their births?

11. Do you provide information on the risks and benefits of common labor drugs and hospital procedures?

12. Do you emphasize cesarean prevention? What percentage of your students have had a cesarean birth?

13. Are you familiar with the services and natural childbirth philosophy of local area hospitals and doctors?

14. Can you refer me to alternative childbirth services? (Midwives, birth centers, home birth services.)

15. Will you be able to serve as a labor coach? Is there an additional fee for this service?

16. What is your class fee and what arrangements are available for payment?

HOSPITAL VS. INDEPENDENT

Many hospitals and clinics offer childbirth education classes for their maternity patients. These are usually taught by a nurse, who may or may not be certified as a childbirth educator. Often, hospital courses are geared to preparing couples to accept routine hospital procedures. Information on the risks of drugs and procedures is often not given. You will probably receive more consumer-oriented information from a class taught by an independent childbirth educator, who offers classes in her home, or at a local women's center, church or YWCA. Remember, you do not have to take a hospital class in order to have a tour of the maternity floor or to have the father admitted to the labor and delivery rooms.

"You will probably receive more consumer-oriented information from a class taught by an independent childbirth educator . . ."

LICENSED VS. UNLICENSED

At the present time childbirth educators are not licensed or regulated by the states in any way (doctors, midwives, nurses, and other health care professionals are licensed and their practice is regulated by state law). The organizations which train childbirth educators are independent, non-governmental bodies whose authority to "certify" childbirth educators is self-declared and rests upon their own reputations as viable consumer organizations. The teaching of information about childbirth is considered to fall under the protection of the first amendment right of free speech. Lay people are able to teach childbirth education, just as lay people teach woodworking, yoga, and dance. Even though medical information is presented, no medical services or procedures requiring a license to perform are offered by childbirth educators.

In 1978, the Nurses' Association of the American College of Obstetricians and Gynecologists (NAACOG) issued a Technical Bulletin on *Preparation for Parenthood,* which defined the childbirth educator as a "licensed professional nurse" and stated, "Ideally, the childbirth educator functions within the institution in which the birth experience occurs and helps the parents to be more comfortable with the hospital and its illness conditions." This caused quite a furor among independent and non-nurse teachers, who felt that NAACOG (and its parent organization, American College of Obstetricians and Gynecologists [ACOG]) was making a bid to restrict the teaching of childbirth classes to ACOG-approved nurses. Some feared that legislation would be initiated to license and regulate childbirth educators. Licensing which would restrict childbirth education to classes taught by nurses in hospital settings would have a great impact on the kind of childbirth information available to the public. Access to consumer-oriented information on the hazards of childbirth drugs and routine hospital procedures would be severely limited.

The Association for Childbirth at Home, International (ACHI), is a group which certifies teachers to provide childbirth education classes especially geared to preparation for home birth. In 1980 it was charged with consumer fraud by the Attorney General's office in Illinois, even though no consumer complaints had been received. An extensive list of ACHI's records was subpoenaed, including the names and addresses of all parents who had ever taken ACHI classes. ACHI refused to honor the subpoena and the case is still being fought out in the courts. At issue is the right of independent organizations to provide consumers with information about birth and childbirth practices. President Tonya Brooks feels that a defeat for ACHI could give impetus to a drive by the medical profession to "control the source and type of medical information provided to parents about childbirth."

The Spring, Summer, and Fall 1980 issues of *BIRTH* (formerly *Birth and the Family Journal*) included editorials on "The Childbirth Educator: Certified to Represent the Hospital or the Parents?" and featured contributions from ten nurse and non-nurse educators. Editor Madeleine Shearer said: "We should remember that NAACOG is the only nurses' organization that exists under the direct financing and control of a physician professional group—the ACOG. As with the present special training programs of NAACOG, a major goal is to train nurses to be willing and able to carry out hospital revenue-generating and public relations programs. NAACOG nurses will not be trained to represent the parents. They will represent the hospital to the parents and socialize the parents to accept gratefully—or gracefully—whatever procedures the hospital staff deem necessary . . . . The strength of present childbirth educator certification programs lies in raising the new teachers' consciousness of their roles as parents' representatives in childbirth. Present certification and subsequent continuing education fosters the childbirth educator's ability to evaluate procedures from the viewpoints of parents, and to help parents cope with or avoid hospital practices that are exclusively for the training or convenience of the hospital staff, are labor saving or simply 'billable.' "

In 1981, NAACOG issued a new booklet of *Guidelines for Childbirth Education.* The requirement that teachers be nurses has been dropped. NAACOG now states, "that childbirth educators represent a variety of backgrounds . . . that the most valid approach would be to identify competencies for practice, rather than to specify credentials for entry into practice."

In a time when so many medical practices are coming under question, when the cesarean rate is soaring, and when the U.S. still ranks behind most of Western Europe and Japan in infant mortality, I feel that the continued existence of independent childbirth education is the best insurance parents have of receiving consumer-oriented information about childbirth which represents their own best interests.

TEACHING AIDS FOR CHILDBIRTH EDUCATION

DIRECTORY OF INSTRUCTIONAL MATERIALS IN CHILDBIRTH AND NEW PARENT EDUCATION
by Pamela Shrock, et. al.
1982, 144 pages, Illus.

from
BIRTH
110 El Camino Real
Berkeley, CA 94705
$5.00

Lists brochures, pamphlets, flyers, etc., many free from pharmaceutical companies and other businesses, as well as organizations, publications, and periodicals.

CHILDBIRTH EDUCATION INFORMATION SHEETS

from
Rosemary Romberg Wiener
6294 Mission Road
Everson, WA 98247
$5.50 Sample Packet

Sample packet includes one each of 19 "sheets" (some have more than one page) on topics in childbirth including emergency childbirth, silver nitrate, expulsion, established labor, transition, birth choices, back labor, induced labor and cesarean birth, and more. Available in single copies or in bulk.

CHILDBIRTH EDUCATOR
352 Evelyn Street
Paramus, NJ 07652
Free to instructors of childbirth and baby care classes
$10.00 a year to others

This new magazine for childbirth educators is published by *American Baby* and features responsible, consumer-oriented articles on birth and birth practices, interspersed with advertisements for diapers, toys, cosmetics, drugs, books, and infant formula.

AVERY PUBLISHING GROUP, INC.
89 Baldwin Terrace
Wayne, NJ 07470

Avery specializes in publishing handbooks which have been prepared by local childbirth groups. Titles include:
Handbook in Prepared Childbirth by Boston Association for Childbirth Education
Our Baby . . . Our Birth by Childbirth Education Association of Tulsa
Pregnancy to Parenthood: Your Guide to Prepared Childbirth by CEA of Jacksonville, Florida

Avery handbooks can be used as class manuals and represent a range of approaches from traditional to alternative. Request a complete list.

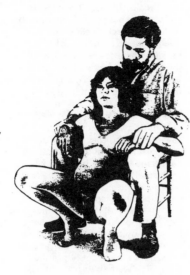

CHILDBIRTH GRAPHICS, LTD.
P.O. Box 17025
Irondequoit Post Office
Rochester, NY 14617

Excellent source for illustrations of topics in childbirth, including obstetrical procedures, anatomy and physiology of labor, labor support, alternative childbirth, etc. Available as large posters or as color slides. Also provides additional teaching materials, models, and books. Write for free catalog.

THE PENNYPRESS
1100 23rd Avenue East
Seattle, WA 98112
206/325-5098
free catalog

The Pennypress produces the *Better Babies Series* of pamphlets and several other books on childbirth.

The *Better Babies* pamphlets are excellent and each one is reviewed separately in this *Catalog* (see the index). The pamphlets are available for $.50 each or $2.75 for a sample pack of one of each. Bulk rates are available for use in childbirth classes, clinics, and hospitals.

SIT'N SNOOZE
Bean Bag Pillow

from
Sandy Schurdell
21321 Beachwood Drive
Rocky River, OH 44116
$1.50 pattern
$20.00 kit
$30.00 ready made

Light weight bag filled with styrofoam pellets, with muslin liner and denim cover. Can be used to make an "expectant mom" more comfortable at home and in childbirth classes.

LAMAZE GOODIE BAG
Kits Unlimited
P.O. Box 223
Agoura, CA 91301
$10. plus $2.00 postage

A clear plastic tote bag which contains 15 items to aid in prepared childbirth (lotion, sour pop, bootie socks, pad and pencils, focal point, etc.). Teachers should request information on bulk rates.

Audio-Visuals

AUDIOVISUALS ABOUT BIRTH AND FAMILY LIFE, 1970-1980
by Doreen Shanteau
1981, 124 pages

from
ICEA Bookcenter
P.O. Box 20048
Minneapolis, MN 55420
$10.00 plus $1.25 postage
bulk rates available

Excellent annotated listing of films and slides on all aspects of birth, arranged by subject, with good indexes.

CINEMA MEDICA
2335 W. Foster Ave.
Chicago, IL 60625
312/784-7686 in Illinois
800/621-5147 toll free

Excellent selection of films describing "some of the changes taking place in and out of the hospital with regard to childbirth, prenatal nutrition, infant feeding, family planning, and social issues in medicine." Includes the classic film *Primum Non Nocere* (above all do no harm).

BIRTHIN' SHIRTS
Stacy McCullough
P.O. Box 6304
Huntington Beach, CA 92646

T-shirts available in six different designs, including "Birth is a Team Effort!", "Resist the Urge," "Kegel, Kegel, Kegel." Cotton/polyester knit in Maternity cut or ladies' french cut T-shirt. Bulk rates are available. Request free literature.

EDUCATIONAL GRAPHIC AIDS, INC.
1315 Norwood Avenue
Boulder, CO 80302
303/449-8049

Donna and Rodger Ewy, authors of several books on childbirth, direct this firm which produces slides, filmstrips, and audio cassettes on pregnancy, childbirth, parenting, and family planning. Request their catalog.

ARTEMIS ASSOCIATES
P.O. Box 3147
Stamford, CT 06905

Harriette Hartigan, midwife and photographer, produces scripted slide sets, art prints, post cards, and calendars reflecting "the emotional, spiritual, social and psychological dimensions of pregnancy, childbirth, new baby life and family bonding." Slide sets include a birth of twins, cesarean birth, use of hands in labor support, siblings at birth, and the history of childbirth in illustrations. Request a catalog.

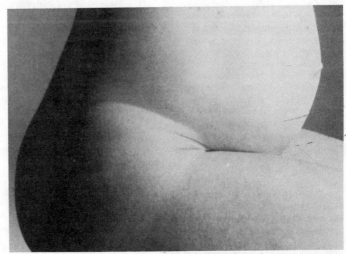

© 1983 Artemis/Harriette Hartigan

Psychology of Pregnancy

Our feelings about birth and our bodies come to the surface as never before during pregnancy. Thinking about ourselves and how we will experience and accomplish the events to come is one of the great tasks of this period. Especially for women in their first pregnancy, great changes are taking place in the psyche. Also, we are forming a picture of and relationship with the growing fetus, so that by the time the baby is born we are already, so to speak, "acquainted" and attached. The psychological change we experience is affected by our social environment and expectations, our culture, our own personality and life situation, and by the physical realities of our pregnancy and birth. Because so many forces are converging, pregnancy can be a particularly rich time in our lives. Many pregnant women dream more frequently and more vividly. We may have more daydreams and fantasies, more doubts and fears, more moments of elation. Keeping a journal or expressing our feelings in any of the arts can be especially rewarding during pregnancy, both to chronicle and "save" this special time and to help us become even more aware of our feelings. The hours of labor and delivery and the many days afterward of intensive new baby care will try our psychic resources to the limit. Pregnancy is a good time to become aware of our truest feelings, of our limitations and strengths, to acknowledge, accept, discover, work through, change, and grow toward the work ahead.

PREGNANCY: The Psychological Experience
by Arthur D. Colman and Libby L. Colman
1971, 179 pages

from
Continuum Books
The Seabury Press
815 Second Avenue
New York, NY 10017
$7.95

It's hard to imagine that pregnancy was once considered a static period, with no "content" of its own, a time of "passive waiting." That's how authors Arthur and Libby Colman had thought about it, until they became pregnant for the first time and were motivated by their own experience to start thinking about the psychology of pregnancy. They established a weekly discussion group for women in their first pregnancies, to talk about the changes in their bodies and feelings. They discovered that pregnant couples, including themselves, are acutely interested in their inner lives. They asked women to record their dreams in pregnancy, and found that the dreams followed similar patterns—dreams in early pregnancy often involved water and fish, perhaps indicating an identification between the mother and her fetus; dreams later in pregnancy often involved having a baby and then "losing" it, forgetting to feed it, neglecting it. The Colemans describe the major psychological landmarks in the journey from conception to birth and also describe the psychology of the process of labor and delivery, stressing that "each woman entered the labor room with a *psychological* task to carry out. She often saw this task as only slightly less important than the safe exodus of the baby." There is a long chapter on the expectant father, emphasizing the "pervasive changes of both a physical and psychological nature which affect him during pregnancy."

I read this book during my first pregnancy, five years ago, and found it extremely useful. I was encouraged to keep a journal, record my dreams, and take my own changing thoughts and feelings seriously. As described in the book, I did experience tremendous psychological change (I literally transformed myself from a girl to a mother in a few short months) and I was glad to have the insights the Colmans provide.

"The increased importance of obsessions, phobias, and dreams in the mental state of pregnant women is often both embarrassing and alien to them. Such matters are generally brought up only when someone is under great psychological pressure. Invariably, in the discussion group, the other women responded with shared emotions and relieved feelings. Perhaps those most memorable moments in the group were the few occasions when one of the women, obviously terribly anxious, would mention a 'peculiar thought' that she was having, or the particularly frightening dream that she had had 'a month ago' and then, with obvious relief, other women would admit to similar experiences. Some of the more secure women seemed able to give themselves over to the dreams and fantasies, not as an escape, but as a way of capturing the potential richness of their new inner life."

A PREGNANCY DREAM

I dream I am swimming in a large, enclosed pool. The edges of the pool are bounded by walls, with no ledge or deck to climb out on. There is an exit, an area off to the far left, where the water passes through a wide archway into an unseen, lighted space. The enclosure itself is dark. The water is black and lightly waving and shining. There are seals as large as myself swimming in the water with me. One of them brushes up against me and I feel its skin slither past. I am naked and I feel the bulk and weight of the seal's body against mine as it swims past me again. It occurs to me that I am in labor and that the motion of the seal is part of the movement of labor. I try to push a baby out by bearing down with my stomach muscles, but nothing happens. It is time to get out of the pool. The water is warm. If I get out, will I shiver and be cold? I do not remember.

I find myself walking down a corridor in a large, quiet building. I am shown into a room which is like a motel room, containing a bed, a dresser, a chair, and with a sliding glass door which opens onto a small balcony. Everything in the room is white; the walls, the rug, the bedspread, the drapes, the furniture. It looks very neat and clean and impersonal. I am alone. This is where I am to have my baby. I look out of the glass doors and see the rest of the building curving around; a giant, multi-storied, crescent-shaped structure. Below I see the ground, a partly enclosed garden area devoid of trees or bushes, with slightly undulating landscaped mounds and pathways. The ground is covered with a shallow, uniform layer of unmarked snow. It is very cold outside but warm inside, even though the white room looks chilly. I am wearing only a light cloth tunic, open at the back, but I do not feel cold. After a time some men dressed in white come. They try to take me down the hall, grabbing my wrists. I resist. I lock myself into the room alone. If I must give birth in this place, at least I will do it by myself. I imagine what a burst of color the birth of the baby will be in this room of solid white.

—a dream recorded at the end of the third month of pregnancy J.I.A.

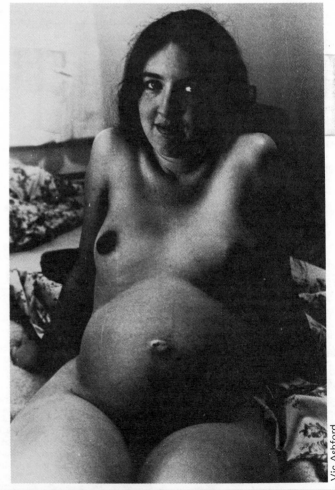

Vic Ashford

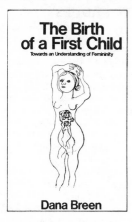

THE BIRTH OF A FIRST CHILD:
Towards An Understanding of Femininity
by Dana Breen
1979, 262 pages, Illus.

from
Tavistock Publications, publisher
Methuen Inc., distributer
733 Third Avenue
New York, NY 10017
$11.95 pap.

Dr. Breen, a psychologist, reports on her study of how pregnancy changes a woman's "self-concept," based on extensive interviews with a group of women pregnant for the first time. She describes her research methods and aims in simple language and gives a good overview of current "points of view" on the psychology of pregnancy. Dr. Breen speaks extensively on the psychological and social characteristics of the women who adjusted well to motherhood as opposed to those of the mothers who had difficulty. She is sensitive in her rendering of the lives and experiences of the women she studied. Her book is further illuminated by very nice drawings by artist Nan Lurie and many insightful quotes from authors and the mothers under-study. The emphasis in this book is on understanding the processes of femininity in a biological sense, especially where this conflicts with our cultural stereotypes of femininity.

"Most striking . . . was the fact that the women who went through the experience of having a child with least difficulties, were those women who were able to feel themselves to be active, not only after the birth of the baby but also during pregnancy. Such a sense of initiation and activity is one which has often been denied women in our culture.

"In sum, those women who are most adjusted to childbearing are those who are less enslaved by the experience, have more differentiated, more open appraisals of themselves and other people, do not aspire to be the perfect selfless mother. . . and do not experience themselves as passive, the cultural stereotype of femininity."

PREGNANT ARTIST AS A MOTHER TO BE
Laura Shechter
Pencil drawing, 10 1/2" x 13 1/8"
1973

Artist Laura Shechter has provided this commentary on her drawing:

"The iconography of the *Pregnant Artist as a Mother to Be* is this: I am pregnant and sitting next to a still life (I am a still life painter and rarely paint figures). In the drawing I am presented with equal importance as the still life. That is saying something about roles—the mother versus the painter. The long hall represents the birth canal and probably I was most interested in that part of the drawing. The cube that I am holding in my hand is a symbol for the skull that painters (males) hold in 17th and 18th century self portraits. In the drawing I am not wearing pregnancy clothes. Recently a friend who saw the drawing remarked about how heavy I looked. I didn't like that."

(See index for listing of another of Laura's paintings.)

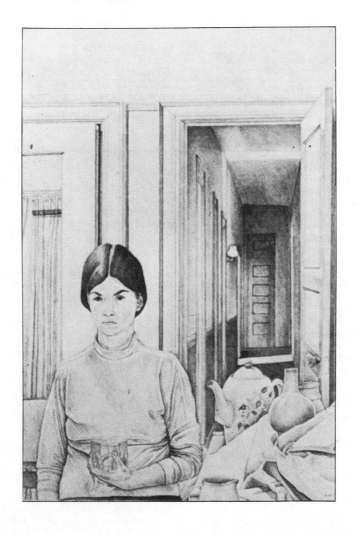

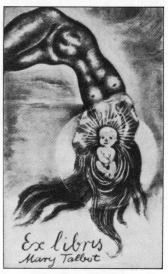

from *A Treasury of Bookplates from the Renaissance to the Present*, Dover Publications, 1977.

COMMON FEELINGS AND CHANGES

FIRST TRIMESTER

Joy at proof of fertility
Freedom from contraception and fear of pregnancy
Lessened sexual desire from nausea and fatigue
Fear of miscarriage

SECOND TRIMESTER

Nausea, fatigue, and fear of miscarriage usually end
Pleasure in increased breast size
Increased interest in sex, masturbation, possibly with guilt feelings
Enjoying woman's new shape
Ambivalence about woman's changing body

THIRD TRIMESTER

Adapting to large belly
Lessening desire and interest in sex
Increased awkwardness, uncomfortableness
Feeling big and less attractive sexually, conflict between commercial definition of "sexy" and reality of pregnancy
Focussing more on the coming baby
Increased fetal activity during intercourse

C.O.P.E.

C.O.P.E.
37 Clarendon Street
Boston, MA 02116
617/357-5588

Coping with the Overall Pregnancy/Parenting Experience (C.O.P.E.) is a non-profit organization which provides individual counseling and support groups for parents in Massachusetts. In addition, C.O.P.E. staff travel throughout New England providing consultation, in-service education, and program development services to institutions and groups which are interested in implementing similar services.

A paper which describes C.O.P.E.'s program (*The COPE Story: A Service to Pregnant and Postpartum Women,* by Margaret Finnerty Turner and Martha H. Izzi) appears as Chapter 8 in *The Woman Patient,* Vol. I (1978, Plenum Publishing, Notman and Nadelson, eds.) and reprints are available for $1.00 each from C.O.P.E. The paper describes COPE's support group model and provides an outline of the emotional "stages" of pregnancy and the postpartum period. A useful list of references is also included.

COPE is currently involved in a pilot program at Newton Wellesley Hospital offering a 2-session "Parenting Preparation Program" which provides an opportunity for parents to learn about and discuss their emotional changes in pregnancy. A male/female teaching team encourages participation by both fathers and mothers. COPE hopes to provide a model for other hospitals for incorporating parenting preparation into their regular childbirth preparation classes. "[parenting preparation] is an attempt to reach prospective parents in their pregnancy and help them prepare for the changes in their lives (role, relationships, etc.) that are inherent in the transition to parenthood. We try to address the complex emotional issues involved in becoming a parent and encourage them to begin acknowledging them before their baby is born. We are hoping to have these issues addressed as part of childbirth education programs, so that we may involve both men and women (using a male/female teaching team) as they prepare for the birth of their child."

COPE has also initiated a "Work in Family Management" systems program to help encourage business and industry to provide services to help working parents cope with the dual demands of work and family (day care at the work place, flexible work times, etc.).

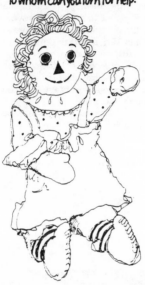

You're going to have a baby. Or your child has just been born.

Suddenly, you have feelings, questions, choices, decisions, you never faced before. And you've never felt more alone.

To whom can you turn for help.

"An important COPE innovation was using mixed groups of pregnant women and new mothers. The new mothers often find great pleasure in sharing their new knowledge and experiences, while pregnant women pose poignant questions that new mothers might be reluctant to ask of one another. Many pregnant women also welcome the opportunity to offer the new mother babysitting services, often holding a new baby for the first time.

"COPE groups, such as pregnant women/new mothers, have been conducted for five years, involving over 600 women. Our experiences contradict an historically strong cultural bias that unveiling emotional issues among pregnant women could lead to serious consequences for the unborn child. Instead, they are a vehicle for positive transition into parenthood . . ."

—from *The COPE Story*

For more information on pregnancy support groups see the index under Postpartum Adjustment and Mothers' Centers.

PREGNANCY SUPPORT GROUPS

Unfortunately, there is no formal or established group or network providing pregnancy support group services nationwide. Women will need to actively seek out whatever programs exist in their own communities. La Leche League, childbirth educators, and women's organizations are likely sources of information. Ask around among your friends. Women can also establish discussion groups on their own with the members of their childbirth preparation class, or place an ad in their local newspaper. Groups needn't have a "leader." Just getting together for refreshments and informal talk can be very helpful in breaking through the isolation which many pregnant women and new mothers feel. But groups may also want to consult some of the books available on "consciousness-raising" and group therapy techniques for ideas on facilitating discussion. Also—don't forget the fathers. Discussion groups for fathers only and for couples together can be very important in bringing men into the pregnancy experience and recognizing their needs during this time (for more information see index under Expectant Fathers).

"During my first pregnancy in 1971, I happened to be visiting the Free Clinic one day when a notice about the forming of a pregnancy rap group caught my eye. Six of us met and continued to meet throughout our pregnancies, supporting and sharing each other's fantasies, hopes and fears. Not realizing the isolation of pregnant women in our culture, it was only later that I realized the significance of that support group. Going through our pregnancies together bonded all of us and our children. Without a particular structure in mind, we continued to meet weekly, as each of us had our baby. Oh, what a blessing! We became involved in each birth tale, agonized over our body changes, supported each other's first breastfeeding attempts and went through the postpartum adjustment together. As we continued to meet, we gradually decided to leave all six babies with two of the women for an hour at a time. Lo and behold, slowly the men started to share the child care, and we organized our first playgroup, eventually meeting four mornings a week, always two parents at a time. This group lasted for five years, finally splitting up when the children went on to public school."

—Ruth Longacre

THE WORLD OF THE UNBORN:
Nurturing Your Child Before Birth
by Leni Schwartz
1980, 310 pages

from
Richard Marek Publishers
200 Madison Avenue
New York, NY 10016
$12.95 hd

Psychologist Leni Schwartz believes that people are affected by and can remember their own birth. Her own experience with "rebirthing" under LSD led to her interest in working with pregnant couples. In this book she describes how pregnancy discussion groups can help parents become aware of their feelings about pregnancy and the developing fetus. Included are specific exercises and group activities designed to help explore emotions concerning ambivalence, dependency, attachment with the baby, self-image, sexuality, becoming a parent, communicating as a couple, and preparing for birth. Noting that pregnancy discussion groups are not very widely available, Schwartz offers guidelines for parents on setting up their own groups. She concludes with a description of her ideal "family-centered birth house," a wholistic model for care during pregnancy, birth and the postpartum period.

"Pregnancy, especially the first time, is a profound and often overwhelming experience for most women. All that they know and trust about themselves and their lives is called into question—daily, in fact, many times each day for nine months! In turn, her partner is sharing her concerns, as well as having to cope with his own changes. How can this period of profound physiological and psychological change be made easier? Is it simply a passage to be endured in isolation, hoping for the best, or can acknowledgment of the distinct stages of pregnancy as current research now defines them give insights that place the transitional crisis in manageable perspective? Even further, could talking about these feelings, fears and hopes with other pregnant couples provide a sustaining foundation on which to develop as parents of a new family? . . . Based on my experience with pregnant couples in the groups I have led, there is still an urgent need for such workshops, as a complement to the recent resurgence of interest in making the delivery itself more 'natural' for both mother and child."

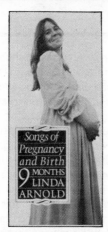

NINE MONTHS: Songs of Pregnancy and Birth
Words and Music by Linda Arnold
Album or stereo cassette

from
Ariel Records
Box 2999
Santa Cruz, CA 95062
$6.98 postpaid
Ten or more, $4.98 each, including shipping

This music is gorgeous—both in sound and spirit. It made me cry the first time I heard it and the "surprise" at the end of Side 2 brings tears to my eyes still. Linda Arnold has written fourteen songs which cover the range of concerns and emotions women feel in pregnancy. Her lyrics are very informed and strong and the music is beautifully melodic and subtle, very reminiscent of Joni Mitchell in her early days. Linda's clear alto voice is always perfectly controlled and expressive and her rich guitar accompaniment gives a great softness and intimacy to the sound. The album is soothing, thoughtful, and very professionally produced. I cannot think of a lovelier gift for a pregnant or newly-delivered mother.

"The songs on *Nine Months* celebrate the process of pregnancy and birth. They're meant to open hearts to the rich and challenging experience which birth is. My husband and I produced the record ourselves and have been distributing it under a label named after our daughter, Ariel."
—Linda Arnold

DAVID, WE'RE PREGNANT!:
101 Cartoons for Expecting Parents
by Lynn Johnston
1981, 107 pages, Illus.

from
Meadowbrook Press
18318 Minnetonka Blvd.
Deephaven, MN 55391
$2.95 pap.

I suppose that it isn't necessary to be pregnant to fully appreciate this book, but this book may be necessary to fully appreciate being pregnant. It simply is not possible to go through nine months of pregnancy without needing a sense of humor, and Lynn Johnston's cartoons can come to the rescue when all else fails. Johnston is poignant and funny about all the common events of pregnancy, but always

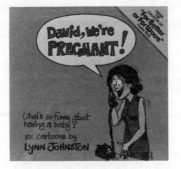

sympathetically and never in a way that makes fun of pregnant parents. Treat yourself (and I am referring to *both* partners) to a copy when you reach one of those crisis points during the pregnancy. I'm happy to be reading it now, in my ninth month . . . .
(review by Sue Roberts)

THE PREGNANT WOMAN'S JOURNAL
by Susan and John Hopkins
1978, 56 pages, Illus.

from
Universe Books
381 Park Avenue South
New York, NY 10016
$4.95 pap.

This spiral-bound book is like a desk calendar in format and is illustrated with twelve lovely "mother and child" paintings by artist Mary Cassatt (1845-1926). The authors have included notes on maternal and fetal development for each month, as well as information on nutrition, recommended reading, exercise, relaxation, preparation for childbirth, and the postpartum period up to

baby's third month. There is room in the calendar pages to write a brief journal entry each day.

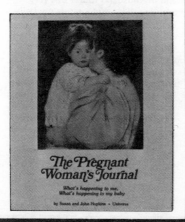

WITH CHILD: A Diary of Motherhood
by Phyllis Chesler
1979, 288 pages

from
T.Y. Crowell
521 Fifth Avenue
New York, NY 10017
$9.95 hd.

Phyllis Chesler is a well-known feminist, psychologist, and author of the influential book, *Women and Madness.* At the age of 37, with an established career as a writer, lecturer, and teacher, Chesler decided to have a baby. This book is based on her diary record of the pregnancy, birth and first year of her son's life (he was born in 1977). It contains expressions of doubt, fear, surprise, determination, hope, joy, disappointment, fatigue, ambivalence, need, wondering, selfishness, love, distress, trust, and mistrust. Chesler quizzes all the mothers she knows, trying to find out what it will be like and how she will manage. She makes clear how unprepared most of us are for motherhood and how little we know about the day-to-day experience of caring for a child.

This book is, I believe, the first and only journal of pregnancy in print. It may be useful to women who can relate to the fast-paced, New York City professional life which Chesler lives. I found three aspects of the book to be especially striking: first, that Chesler complains so much (about her mother, about her husband, about everything!), secondly, that some of her feminist friends were no longer friendly upon hearing of the pregnancy, and thirdly, that Chesler, with all her resources, knowledge, and intelligence, was still not able to have the kind of birth experience she wanted (she received Demerol without her knowledge or consent, Pitocin to speed the labor, an episiotomy, etc.).

"Chicago. Today I was interviewed on television. The nearly all-female audience thrilled and embarrassed me by wanting to know more about my pregnancy than about my ideas or books.
"One woman asked me if 'this' meant I wouldn't write any more books.
" 'Do you think that "working" mothers should work at motherhood only?' I ask her.
"She did. This belief frightens me. So many women have sacrificed themselves to it. So many women feel that all mothers must do the same.
"Why don't I just deliver at home with a midwife in attendance? With a physician on call? Because I don't know any physician who'll do it. Because I can't stop my life to search for one. Because I want Frederic.
"Because I'm afraid. If enough women supported me, with personal

experience, with specific information about home birth, I'd probably do it that way. But I know so few pregnant women, so few new mothers to give me names of private midwives. I know *no one.*"

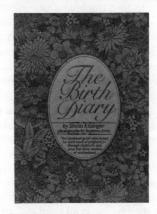

THE BIRTH DIARY
by Sheila Kitzinger, photographs by Suzanne Arms
1980, 160 pages, Illus.

from
Grosset and Dunlap
51 Madison Avenue
New York, NY 10010
$7.95 pap.

What a fine culmination of efforts—from the original concept, text, and photographs right down to the cover design and typography! Kitzinger and Arms have created a personal diary for women, to take them through pregnancy and into motherhood. The text covers fetal development, physiology, and consumerism month by month, as well as the personal fears, excitements, and apprehensions of the pregnant woman. Kitzinger writes, as always, with her characteristic understanding of women. Suzanne Arms' photographs are a perfect complement. Her sensitivity to her subject seems to emanate from a combination of professional talent and feminine awareness. Blank pages are included so that women can make their own notations. *The Birth Diary* is just the right thing for those of us who vow to keep a diary in pregnancy but never muster up the discipline.
(Review by Sue Roberts)

"Thirty Weeks. Now the life of the mind sometimes seems to exist independently of everything that is going on outside the body and surges with all the feelings aroused by the baby inside, the pressure, the tightenings of the uterus and the blood pulsing through the pelvic organs. You find yourself waiting for the baby's movements, however faint, and it is hard to concentrate on the external world. For many women it is as if they are having a two-way conversation, one with the world outside and the people around them and the other with the baby inside them."

Sex in Pregnancy

Different cultures have different ideas about the role of sex during pregnancy. Some make it taboo altogether. Others feel that frequent intercourse is necessary in pregnancy, believing that semen helps to feed the fetus. Our culture has been reluctant to discuss this subject openly until fairly recently (to date, there is just one book available on the subject, though most of the new general books on childbirth now include sections on sex in pregnancy), but we do place a high value on sex. Sex during pregnancy is seen as an important factor in maintaining an affectionate and close relationship. Generally, the burden of proof falls on those who would prohibit sex during pregnancy, though certain obstetrical conditions like threatened miscarriage or premature labor may warrant abstinence. Needs and desires may vary greatly, though, from couple to couple and will probably also change as the pregnancy progresses. Certainly the personal preferences and feelings of each partner need to be respected. Medical advice on sex during pregnancy has been fairly consistent for the past fifty years or so. Physicians generally advise that intercourse is all right except in cases where there is a possibility of miscarriage or premature labor, and except during the last four to six weeks. However, there is little solid evidence on the validity of this advice and studies have been contradictory.

The physiology of intercourse, pregnancy, childbirth, and lactation are closely linked. In fact, sexuality can be said to encompass all of these things. The same hormone, oxytocin, is responsible for mediating orgasm, labor contractions, and the "let-down" reflex in breastfeeding. Couples will notice many interrelations: for instance, stimulation of the nipples will cause the uterus to contract and the breast to "let-down" or eject milk and lead to sexual arousal. Stimulation of the clitoris and orgasm will cause a strong, tonic uterine contraction during pregnancy; during breastfeeding it may cause milk to come spurting out; during labor, sexual stimulation (kissing, nipple play, stimulating the clitoris) can increase the strength and frequency of contractions and speed the labor along. During pregnancy there is an increase in vascularity (blood supply) in the pelvic area, including the genitals, and this can lead to an increase in the woman's sexual sensitivity, interest, and arousal. The threshold for orgasm may be lower and because the resolution phase after orgasm may be less complete, some women are multiorgasmic for the first time during pregnancy. Some authors feel there is a relationship between sexual adjustment and the ability to give birth easily and with pleasure. Exploring your body, masturbating, and enjoying orgasm can all be very good preparations for childbirth. Labor and delivery involve very strong sensations in the genital area, especially during second stage, when the baby is moving through the vagina. Learning to relax and enjoy sexual feelings can help when it's time to let the baby "flow out."

Most couples want to and do continue making love during pregnancy. But many have questions about how their sexual feelings may change in pregnancy, how intercourse might affect the pregnancy, and how long intercourse can be continued. For help, consult the resources in this section and talk with your midwife or childbirth educator. As the woman's abdomen becomes larger, alternative positions for intercourse may be more comfortable. Couples can try woman-on-top, lying side by side, or rear-entry positions. Alternatives to penis-in-vagina sex are fine during pregnancy (kissing, hugging, massage, mutual masturbation, oral sex, etc.) and can be used if intercourse becomes awkward, especially in the later months. However, couples who enjoy oral sex must be very careful not to blow air into the vagina, since this can cause a fatal air embolism (an air bubble which passes into the mother's blood stream and blocks a blood vessel).

MAKING LOVE DURING
PREGNANCY
by Elisabeth Bing and Libby Colman
1977, 166 pages, Illus.

from
Bantam Books
666 Fifth Avenue
New York, NY 10019
$6.95 pap.

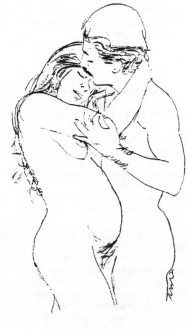

Elisabeth Bing is a long-time advocate of prepared childbirth and the author of several books on the Lamaze method. Libby Colman is a psychologist and coauthor of *Pregnancy: The Psychological Experience* (see index). Their ground-breakbreaking book on sex during pregnancy is based on their own experience and research and on questionnaires returned by 200-300 couples. They describe the characteristic aspects of sex in each of the three trimesters of pregnancy and during the postpartum period and include many personal comments from couples, which are for the most part very positive. There are also very nice, soft drawings showing a pregnant couple making love, which illustrate the variety of positions that can be used. In their introduction, the authors note that most of the people who responded to their inquiries were happily married and enjoyed sexual activity. Thus, reading account after account of happy, fulfilling sex during pregnancy may be a little overwhelming for women who are single, or unhappily married, or unhappily pregnant, or for whom sex is not a central element in life.

"As my body changed in shape, I feared I'd be less attractive to my husband, but this proved to be quite false, both of us taking great pleasure in my new shape. I became very conscious of my shape and loved it, and my husband found this very arousing. He would caress my belly as if it were a new erogenous zone.

"I found my sexual desires heightened after my fourth month of pregnancy and continued until the end of my eighth month. My orgasms were stronger and longer than usual. My husband was not always available when I desired him. I found myself indulging in and enjoying masturbation more than I care to admit.

"Sometimes after orgasm I had an almost painful uterine contraction—which went away almost immediately—so I would think I was bringing on labor—but so far, it hasn't worked, which is too bad because I'm two days past my due date and am anxious to have my baby.

"Men and women undergo profound personal, interpersonal, and social changes during pregnancy and the postpartum period. Lovers must add the roles of partner and parent to the way they interact with each other. They will never be the same again, alone, together, or in the eyes of the world. They may have to work hard to stay in touch with these changes in themselves and in their partner. Parenthood makes a shared life more complicated, but it also carries with it the potential to make life together more meaningful as lovemaking goes beyond caring for each other and spreads out to embrace the family unit."

SEX AND PREGNANCY COMPLICATIONS

Parents are often told that it is all right to have intercourse during the first six months of pregnancy, but the question of whether sex is safe in the last trimester has always been an area of doubt. Professionals have increasingly advised that intercourse is safe right up to the onset of labor (but not if the membranes have ruptured) provided that the woman has no history of obstetrical problems.

In November, 1979, a study published in the *New England Journal of Medicine* suggested that sexual intercourse during the last month of pregnancy is associated with an increased rate of amniotic fluid infection ("Coitus and associated amniotic fluid infections," Naeye, R.L. *N Engl J Med* 301 (22): 1198-1200, 29 November 1979). The rate of infection was 156 per 1000 among women who had intercourse one or more times a week in the last month, as opposed to 117 per 1000 when no intercourse was reported. Of the babies who were affected, 11.0% from the "coitus group" died and 2.4% of the "non-coitus group" died. This study was widely reported in the media and alarmed many parents. Childbirth educators and health professionals were left feeling unsure about what advice to give pregnant couples.

Many questions were raised about the validity of the study, which was based on data collected between 1959 and 1966. Dr. Naeye, director of the study, bases his diagnosis of amniotic fluid infection on the presence of acute inflammation indicated by neutrophils (white blood cells which combat infection) in the subchorionic plate of the placenta. However, in an editorial accompanying the *Journal* article, Dr. Arthur Herbst, of the University of Chicago, indicated that as many as 30% of all placentas show neutrophil infiltration, without infection or morbidity in the majority. This may be part of the normal "degeneration" of the placenta.

A study published in *Lancet* in July 1981 ("Should coitus late in pregnancy be discouraged?" Mills, J.L., et. al. *Lancet* 2(8235):136-38, 18 July 1981) considered this question again (based on data collected from 1974 to 1976) and discovered no relation at all between intercourse late in pregnancy and differences in pregnancy outcome, including premature labor or rupture of membranes, low birth-weight, and perinatal death. However, all women who would have been advised not to have intercourse in the last trimester (almost 38%) because of obstetrical problems were excluded from the study. These problems included multiple pregnancy (twins), hypertension, uterine scar, history of premature birth, stillbirth, miscarriage, or third trimester bleeding. So this study did not show whether or not that group of women would be adversely affected by intercourse.

Dr. Naeye's most recent paper appears to confirm his original report, but this time includes results from a preliminary study showing that using condoms during intercourse can reduce the risk of infection to the levels of "non-coitus" groups. Parents may now be advised to use condoms during the last trimester and attention to hygiene (clean hands and genitals) has also been mentioned by childbirth educators as a possible preventive measure.

SEX DURING PREGNANCY
by Sheila Kitzinger
1979, 4 pages

from
the pennypress
1100 23rd Avenue East
Seattle, WA 98112
single copy 50 cents
bulk rate, $20. per 100

Briefly and succinctly, Sheila Kitzinger discusses the most important aspects of sex during pregnancy—how the ban on sex got started, cultural attitudes about abstinence, fears about harming the baby, how sexuality can prepare us for birth, women's feelings about their bodies and partners, and the adaptation of love-making techniques to the changes of pregnancy. This pamphlet is part of the *Better Babies Series* (see index).

"So spontaneous, affectionate and gentle lovemaking plays its part in helping a woman to relax—and to know what release is like. Women starting a training course for childbirth often wonder if they can relax, and think there must be a special sort of athletic neuro-muscular control—different from anything else—which they have to achieve in labor. In fact if one is really relaxed in childbirth it is very much like the complete release from tension and the luxurious warmth and peace after happily making love. The expression a man sees on a woman's face after a satisfying orgasm is in fact similar to that on the face of one who is enjoying her labor—glowing skin, flushed cheeks and shining eyes, damp and untidy hair, and a sense of deep contentment. Coitus and childbirth create their own sanctuaries from the cares and horrors of the surrounding world."

BIBLIOGRAPHY ON PREGNANCY/CHILDBIRTH/BREAST-FEEDING AND SEXUALITY

from
Sex Information and Education Council (SIECUS)
80 Fifth Avenue, Suite 801
New York, NY 10011
$.90 plus $.50 postage
Order code No. 195

This bibliography contains 18 citations of literature on sexuality and reproduction compiled in September/October 1980. The 1967 Sex Information and Education Council (SIECUS) Study Guide on *Sex Relations During Pregnancy and the Post-Delivery Period* is no longer in print. Write to SIECUS for a complete list of their current publications.

SEX DURING PREGNANCY
Rosemary Cogan, editor
1982, 8 pages
(Spring, 1982 issue of *ICEA Review*)

from
ICEA Bookcenter
P.O. Box 20048
Minneapolis, MN 55420
$1.50 back issue copies

This issue of ICEA's professional review newsletter is devoted to exploring issues in sex in pregnancy.

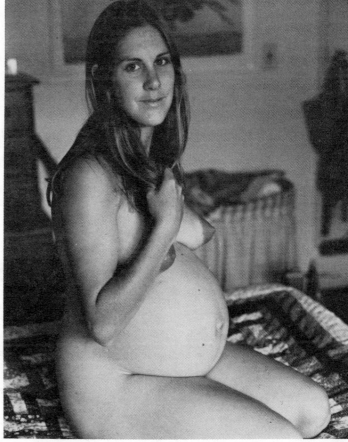

JIA

he kissed me and now I am someone else;
    someone
else in the pulse that repeats the pulse of my
own veins and in the breath that mingles with
    my
breath. Now my belly is as noble as my heart.

Gabriela Mistral (1889-1957)
"He Kissed Me" from *Desolacion,* 1922

Expectant Fathers

"Human fatherhood is a social invention," Margaret Mead has said. And truly, after conception the man has no biologically-defined or necessary role to play in pregnancy and early infant care. In many ways, the first year of a baby's life is a continuation of its life in the womb, with continued close contact with the mother and breastfeeding being vital to human survival. By contrast, in some other animal species, the male actually carries and incubates the young in his own body, after the eggs have been produced by the female and fertilized. But human fathers must "invent" their fatherhood, devising roles and activities. This is often difficult in our culture, in which there is little social support or acknowledgment of the needs or contributions of fathers. ". . . it appears that the American male's parental role is almost limited to impregnation, paying bills nine months later, and then magically appearing again as a role model for adolescent boys," say authors Phillips and Anzalone (from *Fathering: Participation in Labor and Birth*, see index). But changing ideas about sex roles are altering the way men feel about their identities as fathers. As women are questioning the feminine role expectations which define motherhood as their primary activity and source of fulfillment, so men are questioning the definition of masculinity which has denied them access to the intimacy and satisfaction of caring for babies and children in a primary way.

But where are men to turn for information and role models for the new fathering? Many men feel underserved and left out by the books and classes on childbirth which concentrate on the woman's feelings and experiences. Most childbirth educators and nurses are women, and men often don't feel comfortable discussing personal concerns with them. And though most obstetricians are men, fathers don't expect to discuss their own feelings and needs with their wife's doctor. Pregnancy discussion groups have worked well for women (see index) and may be a good idea for men as well. Or just informal talk with other expectant and new fathers can help.

In this section there are reviews of books devoted exclusively to expectant fathers. In addition, most of the books on pregnancy and childbirth, especially the newer ones, contain sections for fathers. Especially good is "The Expectant Father's Experience" in *Pregnancy: The Psychological Experience* by Arthur and Libby Colman (see index).

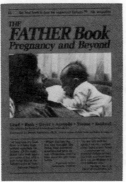

THE FATHER BOOK: Pregnancy and Beyond
by The Alliance for Perinatal Research and Services
1981, 263 pages, Illus.

Published by
Acropolis Books Ltd.
2400 17th Street, NW
Washington, DC 20009
$17.50 hd., $8.95 pap.

Also available from
The Alliance for Perinatal Research and Services
P.O. Box 6358
Alexandria, VA 22306
$15.25 hd., $7.60 pap. plus $1.00 per book for postage

This excellent book for fathers is written by six women (a neonatal psychologist, a counselor, an immunologist, a nurse-midwife, nurses, and health and childbirth educators) who make up the Alliance for Perinatal Research and Services. Their book is based on their own experience as parents, research, and interviews with fathers. *The Father Book* provides information on the importance of fathers' involvement in choices in birth care, the history of men's participation in (or exclusion from) birth, attending childbirth classes together, learning how to be a labor "coach," dealing with the unexpected, the first days and months with baby, sexual adjust-

ments, and changing trends in fathers' role in the family. The authors' lucid explanations are interspersed throughout with very good first-person accounts of fathers' experiences culled from the interviews. Personal birth stories are presented from a variety of settings: hospital delivery rooms, birthing rooms, and home birth. The chapter on labor and birth is very specific about ways the father can help his partner in labor, and will be helpful for both first-time fathers and mothers who are facing this unknown experience. Also included is an appendix, prepared by a lawyer, which covers the current legal status of the father's right to be present at the birth of his child.

"Many women become paranoid and discouraged during transition. They feel they are not making progress, that labor will never end, and so on. Often it is during transition that the woman who planned an unmedicated delivery feels she can no longer cope without medication. Her expressions of anger, pain, unhappiness, and resignation will frighten you. No one likes to stand by while another person is in pain, especially if that person is someone he loves. Try to calm down. After all, you knew this might happen. As terrible as you feel, take some comfort in the fact that these terrible feelings are signals from your heart and your mind. You will have to help her make the right decision at a most difficult time. Does your partner really want anesthesia? Does she really want to lose the sensations associated with birth? Will she regret, in the days and months to come, not feeling or seeing the birth of her baby? Do you know what your partner really wants?

"If you find yourself in this very difficult situation, pause for a moment while you collect yourself. Then say to her, 'Let's try to make it through one more contraction.'. . .'"

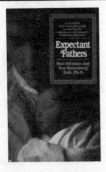

EXPECTANT FATHERS
by Sam Bittman and Sue Rosenberg Zalk
1979
from
E.P. Dutton
2 Park Avenue
New York, NY 10016
$12.95 hd.

I like this book because co-author Sam Bittman and his wife gave birth at home; Bittman speaks in his preface of how planning for the birth

helped him deal with being pregnant in a concrete way: "Having agreed to enter a home-birth training course, we made the decision to *take control* of the pregnancy and the birth too. I had a role. I was still very frightened, but now I was learning how to prepare myself for having something coherent and responsible to do." But all fathers will find this book useful. It is based on the authors' work with Expectant Fathers' Groups, interviews and questionnaires. My husband especially liked the fact that negative feelings and worries were expressed, often in the father's own words. *Expectant Fathers* discusses the emotional (and physical) reactions of fathers to pregnancy and many other important issues including reactions when getting pregnant is difficult, forming a relationship with the unborn baby, developing a "role" as a father, the father's relationship with the obstetrician and prenatal care, meeting the mother's needs for emotional support, actively preparing for the

baby's birth, sex during pregnancy, thinking about your own father and childhood, conflicts between being a father and being a "man," participating in labor and birth, and early days as a new family. A set of Appendices provide a summary of the fathers' questionnaire responses and additional information on home birth.

"Classes in prepared childbirth over the past several years have boomed into popularity. Men who would have sooner registered for an evening class in needlepoint are now enthusiastically enrolling in the so-called Lamaze courses for what is now referred to as the 'husband-coached birth.'. . . These classes have done much to bring men into an area previously forbidden them and deserve great praise.

"Objectively viewed, however,

most classes only prepare an expectant father for assisting in and becoming involved in a *single day* in the life of his family. [in a recent study] the investigators found no evidence that the classes helped to give a stronger sense of belonging. Rather, they speculated that the exposure to the physiology and anatomy of pregnancy, labor, and delivery tended to alienate men, since it pointed up the physical differences and their natural exclusion from the routine of the prenatal family triad. The men in the study reported that while the Lamaze classes were very interesting and informative so far as preparing them for the day of labor and birth, they did nothing whatever to prepare them for what was to come after. In other words, a man's presence at conception and then again at birth does not a father make."

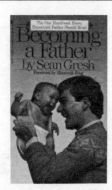

BECOMING A FATHER: A Handbook for Expectant Fathers
by Sean Gresh
1980, 144 pages

from
Butterick Publishing
708 Third Avenue
New York, NY 10017
$12.95 hd.

Sean Gresh started thinking about this book when his wife became pregnant with their first child. His research and reading on the issues of fatherhood is presented in parallel with his own experiences, including excerpts from his diary and a long personal account of the labor and birth of his daughter. His book is fairly short (about 120 pages of large print text) and covers most of the important issues without going into a lot of detail. Topics include the psychological and physical changes of father and mother in pregnancy, sex in pregnancy, the costs of having a baby, planning for the birth, birth options, participating in delivery, and fathers and newborns. Included are several useful tables and a listing of all local member groups of ICEA (International Childbirth Education Association) and ASPO (American Society for Psychoprophylaxis in Obstetrics).

"Describing how he had done a turnabout when his wife became pregnant, John Clift said, 'I felt myself becoming more like a woman.' He felt pressured into being more nurturing—more caring, more giving, more supportive—because his wife needed this help. At first, he viewed his behavior as womanly or feminine, but later he accepted it as part of him, concluding that there indeed was a strong nurturant side of every man.

"You too may feel uncomfortable at first if you find your wife needs extra support. By being more nurturant, you are going against the culture, though not against nature. . . ."

EXPECTANT FATHER'S "SHOWER"

The February, 1982 issue of *Ms.* magazine features several articles on fathers, including the story of a father-to-be's "shower," ("Charlie's Shower—Celebrating the Expectant Father" by Ned O'Malia). Charlie's friends organized a men-only, surprise potluck supper at which they ate, drank beer, talked, watched Charlie open his presents, and offered their best advice on being a father. Everyone had a good time." . . . with a light, loving humor not associated with traditional male advice and counsel, the other fathers told Charlie about everything from the first day alone with a new child, to the first bath, to different types of fatherly fears." Afterwards, several fathers spoke of wanting to organize a shower for others. "One man spoke for all when he said: 'We were *lucky* to be part of this.' "

COMMON CONCERNS OF EXPECTANT FATHERS

Discovery and acceptance of pregnancy
Pride in pregnancy as proof of virility
Memories of being a child, of one's own father
Concerns about making enough money
Experiencing sympathetic "symptoms" of pregnancy
Envy or jealousy of wife's reproductive powers
Rivalry with the fetus
Concerns about sexuality
Ambivalence about wife's changing body
Rivalry with male obstetrician
Engaging in "super-masculine" activities
Reaction to wife's increased introspection
Losing wife's complete attention and support, having to "mother" her
Forming a relationship with the unborn baby
Feelings about feeling the baby move
Development of nurturant or "female" feelings in self
Conflicts with grandparents-to-be
Concerns about the sex of the child
Strong feelings about breastfeeding, positive or negative
Efforts to become a "new person" by changing appearance or dress
Surge in creative activities, hobbies
Wondering what the baby will be like, what baby care will be like
Concerns about living space, needing more room, furniture, etc.
Wanting to escape, leave the relationship
Tensions and restlessness in the last weeks
Concerns about getting to the hospital on time
Worry about being able to recognize when true labor begins
Anxiety about the hospital environment, what will happen, how to act
Fears for the physical safety of mother and baby
Concerns about participating in labor and birth

Someone's gonna have to explain it to me
I'm not sure what it means
My baby's feeling funny in the morning
She's having trouble gettin' into her jeans.
Her waistline seems to be expanding
Although she never feels like eating a thing
I guess we'll reach some understanding
When we see what the future will bring. . .

Baby's feeling funny in the morning
She says she's got a lot on her mind
Nature didn't give her any warning
Now she's gonna have to leave her wild
    ways behind.
She says she doesn't care if she never spends
Another night running loose on the town—
She's gonna be a mother.
Take a look in my eyes and tell me, brother
If I look like I'm ready. . .

"Ready or Not" by Jackson Browne
(Benchmark Music/ASCAP) from *For Everyman*,
© 1973 WB Music Corp. All rights reserved.
Used by permission.

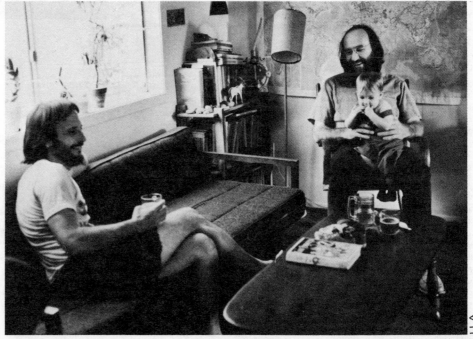

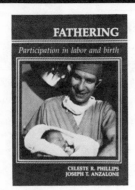

FATHERING: Participation in Labor and Birth
by Celeste R. Phillips and Joseph T. Anzalone
1978, 151 pages, Illus.

from
C.V. Mosby Company
11830 Westline Industrial Drive
St. Louis, MO 63141
$9.50 pap.

Phillips and Anzalone (a nurse and an obstetrician, respectively) have written this book primarily for medical people and teachers to help them understand and encourage fathers' participation in labor and birth, specifically, fathers in the delivery room.. But fathers will find the book very helpful too. The first chapter provides a masterfully simple introduction to a complex subject—the historical and changing role of the father and men's involvement with childbirth. Dr. Anzalone provides a unique chapter on his own experiences as an obstetrician with fathers in the delivery room. In his opinion, *active* participation (not passive watching) by the father in the birth process creates a stronger family unit. He provides reassurance for many of the common fears fathers have about attending the birth ("Why am I needed?" "But I'll be nervous!" "Won't it be bloody?" "What if

something goes wrong?"). The authors discuss the concept of family-centered maternity care, describing in detail the Alternative Birth Center program, which can best meet the needs of all members of the family. In the final two chapters we can read "a collection of intimacies about birth experiences"; stories told by the fathers themselves, right after birth and years later. The book is illustrated throughout with photographs of fathers with their babies.

"So finally the doctor said, 'Well, Dorothy one last push and the baby will be out.' Dorothy just couldn't believe it and she said 'Oh, is that right?' She was exhausted and elated at the same time. Then she gave the one last big push, and this baby came out—just a little girl, a red little girl, and a tiny little girl. I couldn't believe how tiny she was because Dorothy was so big, and so as the doctor had her out and handed her to the nurse, he said one of the most unbelievable things I had ever heard. He said, 'Oh! there's another one in there.' And so we had twin girls!. . .

"And it was a complete surprise but a good surprise. I have to say I saw those girls come out, and I saw them cut the umbilical cords, I saw them wash them up, put them on oxygen, and I was right there. I have to say it was a smoother transition when we took them home because I was in the delivery room—because I was there all the time. It was consistent for me to take them home, and to help there. I was less hesitant and fearful in helping than I was when I took my son home. I don't know if I feel any closer to them than I do to my son, but there was more of a consistent transition when I got home because I was with them. I was there, and also I got to hold them in the hospital, and that made a real difference."

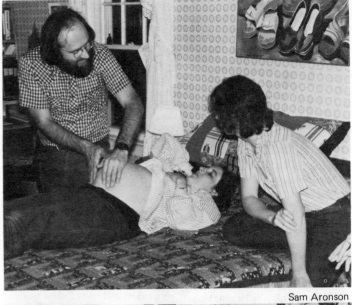

Sam Aronson

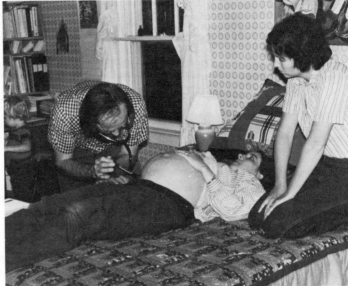

Sam Aronson

FOR THE EXPECTANT FATHER
by the Maternity Center Association
6-panel brochure, Illus.

from
Maternity Center Association
48 East 92nd Street
New York, NY 10028
single copy 25 cents
15 cents each for 10-99
10 cents each for 100 or more
request list of publications

This brochure points out the many ways fathers can become involved in pregnancy and birth, helping to lay the foundations for a strong family life. These include talking about worries and problems, learning about the events of pregnancy and birth, going to meet the doctor, being sensitive to the mother's emotional changes and needs, attending childbirth classes together, preparing for natural childbirth and participation in labor and delivery, and helping with housework and

baby care. A list of additional reading and resources is included.

"Naturally, the physical and emotional changes resulting from pregnancy affect expectant mothers most directly, but fathers-to-be have anxieties and stresses of their own. Some of these center on shared practical questions . . . Other concerns, more personal and emotional, may be unexpected: Are you ready for additional responsibilities? How will your wife react in the months ahead? Will the coming of the baby change your relationship? As in other major turning points in life, certain old, unresolved problems may begin to surface, creating additional sources of emotional discomfort.

"Learning about the events of pregnancy and the part you can play will help reduce some of your apprehensions. At the same time, it will draw you and your wife even closer as a couple."

GETTING INVOLVED

Becoming involved with your partner's prenatal care can help give a real physical dimension to the pregnancy for you. Ask your midwife or doctor to show you how to palpate (feel) and auscultate (listen) to the fetus during prenatal visits. You can also do this at home. Pressing firmly but gently on a pregnant woman's abdomen won't harm her or the baby and you will be able to feel the baby kick and move under your hands in the later months of pregnancy. Listening to the baby's heartbeat with a simple stethoscope or a fetoscope will also help let you know that there is "really someone in there."

Pregnancy after 30

Susan Ritchie, editor

Perhaps because I was born when my parents were 41 I have never viewed pregnancy after 30 as an exceptional phenomenon. But delaying parenthood until the 30's or 40's certainly was the exception years ago whereas today it is a growing trend. The women's movement, women's career plans, improved general health, and more reliable birth control methods have all contributed to delayed childbearing.

What are the risks involved in pregnancy after 30? Since delayed first pregnancy is a relatively new phenomenon, the statistics about risk factors for over-30 women may not accurately describe today's generation of women. It may be the case that women who delay childbearing by choice represent a different population than women of previous generations whose lateness in having their first baby may have been due to reproductive problems or ill health. On the other hand, the older a woman is, the more likely it becomes that her ova (eggs) have aged or been exposed to environmental contaminants or that her body is not as strong and healthy as before. Women should not ignore the statistics which indicate higher maternal and infant complications for over-30 women, but it is also important to assess the "risk" status of each woman as an individual.

The books reviewed in this section can provide needed information on both the medical and personal factors involved in pregnancy after 30. And the existence of these books attests to the growing acceptance and support for this trend. But over-30 parents will still find it necessary to dig a little deeper for the special information they need, as we await new research results and analysis from this generation. (SR)

(Editor's Note: In reviewing the material for this section, I am struck by the tendency to emphasize the "risk" factors in pregnancy after 30. Many pregnant women over 30 are in excellent health and can be considered good candidates for non-interventive, normal childbirth, including home birth and other alternatives. Many childbirth educators and other professionals feel it's important to evaluate your own risk status *as an individual* and not be pressured into a high-technology approach to pregnancy and birth simply because your age alone puts you into a "high-risk" *category*. JIA)

PARENTHOOD AFTER THIRTY
451 Vermont
Berkeley, CA 94707
415/524-6635 or 525-1586

This project is sponsored by the Office of Family Planning of the state of California and the Foundation for Comprehensive Health Services. It's designed to help professionals better serve their clients who are women and couples over 30 by providing professional training, consumer education materials, educational presentations, consultation and technical assistance, and resource materials. The following materials are available. (JIA)

Parenthood After Thirty: There is a Choice, 11 page booklet
$3.00

Annotated Bibliography, 21 pages (included in Resource Manual)
$3.00

Resource Manual, 130 pages
$15.00

Parenthood After Thirty? brochures
*Yes: I Do Want to Become
a Parent* $.50
No: The Childfree Option .50
There is a Choice .75

"WHAT YOU CAN DO TO MINIMIZE YOUR RISKS

Get a Medical Check-up Before You Try to Conceive.
Wait Three Months After Stopping The Pill Before You Try to Get Pregnant.
Develop a Healthy Body.
Find Out Where to Get Quality Medical Care.
Consider Amniocentesis If You Are Over 35."

—from *Parenthood After Thirty? There is a Choice*

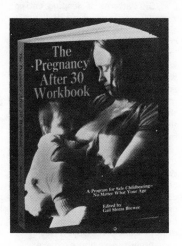

THE PREGNANCY AFTER 30 WORKBOOK: A Program for Safe Childbearing—No Matter What Your Age
Gail Sforza Brewer, editor
1978, 233 pages, Illus.

from
Rodale Press
33 E. Minor Street
Emmaus, PA 18049
$10.95 pap.

In a way, the book is mis-named since so much of the excellent information it contains will be useful for every pregnant woman regardless of age. There is so much to learn from each one of the chapters that you ought to consider reading this book before you become pregnant or early in your pregnancy. The first chapter is specifically aimed at the over 30 group, discussing risks and medical technologies. The following chapters cover the "no-risk" pregnancy diet (by Tom Brewer, M.D.), exercise for pregnancy and beyond, cooperative childbearing, breastfeeding and "pregnancy means parenting," which discusses emotional preparation for parenting during pregnancy. Each chapter is written by an expert in the field and most include recommended readings or references to other books on the subject. In the margins throughout the book, there are anecdotes and comments from several couples about their pregnancies, births and parenting experiences, which enhance the text. Also included are: a nutrition quiz, labor readiness scale, listing of preferences in childbirth, a questionnaire on hospital policy, and checklists for emotionally surviving pregnancy and parenting. These tools contribute to a very "take-charge" attitude and will be of interest to childbirth educators as well as parents. (SR)

". . . statistics tell us that older women are two-and-a-half times more likely to have an abruption of the placenta (a condition in which the placenta separates from the wall of the uterus before the baby is born). But they do not tell us that all mothers over the age of 30—sick and well, rich and poor, well-nourished and malnourished—have been used to set this figure. They don't say that abruptions are the result of poor nutrition during pregnancy, and that many of the older women who experience abruption do so because they have many mouths to feed and, so, eat poorly themselves during later pregnancies.

"The point is that an individual woman will *only* become a high risk for an abruption if she is malnourished, but the statistics do not distinguish between the risks of this condition for the well fed and the risks for those whose diets are inadequate. Instead, the statistics present the problem strictly on the basis of age. We prefer to base our expectations for an individual woman's pregnancy on her own medical history and current health status. Statistics alone have little validity as guidelines for the management of individual pregnancies.

"As far as actual labor goes, the only important contraction is the one you're having. Deal with each one as it presents itself, then let it go. Never predict the future of your labor. This contraction may be the last. Never think back to contractions you have already dealt with. They will never return. Stay in the present time and focus your attention on what you can do to release tension *now.* One of the absolute tip-offs that you are completely relaxed is when you find yourself drooling on the pillow.

"Another way of turning away from parenting is by focusing on the future. While pregnant, we dream of sweet little babies; when the kids are infants, we cannot wait until they learn to walk; when toddlers, the goal is nursery school; when 6 to 10, we hope they will soon be able to do their share of the housework and take care of themselves; when preteens and teens, we anticipate the day they move out; and then, we anxiously await grandchildren. Each stage of parenthood has its problems, to be sure, but coping by looking to the future for solutions is escape. The irony of it is that we can escape the positive features of parenthood: intimacy, play, touching and holding, the beauty of young bodies, sharing, and growth, but we cannot escape most of the annoyances: the noise, chaos, slow pace, bills, unpredictability, responsibility of thinking for others, disruptions of home and lifestyle, interference with career, and so forth. Using escape to improve the parenting experience accents the negative and mutes the positive."

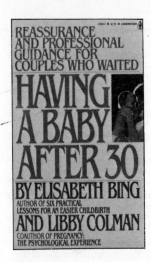

HAVING A BABY AFTER 30
by Elisabeth Bing and Libby Colman
1980, 174 pages

from
Bantam Books
666 Fifth Avenue
New York, NY 10019
$2.95 pap.

Written by a childbirth educator and a psychologist who is known for her writings on the emotional aspects of pregnancy and childbirth, this book covers the main concerns about pregnancy and childrearing after age 30. The authors use comments and insights from pregnant couples and new parents in this age category to illustrate the more factual parts of the text. They give attention to the medical considerations pertinent to those over 30, the special emotional concerns of "older" parents, questions of parenting and working or not working, and the impact of a baby on the life and marriage of couples in their 30's. They are quick to point out the many variations which couples have found or chosen in dealing with the changes that the choice of having a child brings. A bibliography is included which lists books on pregnancy and birth, childbirth preparation, childcare and other related topics. (SR)

"The birth of the first child certainly brings a radical change in lifestyle, especially to a woman who has been working. This change can be feared or it can be eagerly anticipated. Many women have told us that the whole adventure seemed like 'starting a whole new lifestyle.' During pregnancy, this was exciting, even wonderous. One mother-to-be said, 'Maybe I'll be a totally different person. I don't really know what to expect.'

"We have been struck by the number of people who choose to have a baby when they are ready for a change in their own life, when they feel ready to move into a new phase of their own development. . . .

"Life at home with a baby is radically different from the life of most thirty-year old, childless people. Old patterns of sleeping, eating, working, and playing are all disrupted. Over and over again new parents remark in amazement that taking care of an infant is the hardest job they have ever done. It consumes more time and energy than anyone can possibly anticipate. This may be as true for a woman in her thirties as for one in her twenties. A thirty-seven-year-old woman remarked:

'I now have a respect for mothers that I never had before. I was always a little contemptuous of them and didn't understand why you couldn't easily combine work and a career with being a parent. I felt I knew what hard work was. After all, didn't I work seven days a week and sometimes twelve hours a day at that? What a shock to find it was *nothing* compared to the work of mothering. I tried to describe it to someone who had no children, and said it was a little like what the "Burma March" must have been like. The erosive quality of the tiredness is unlike anything I've ever known. Knowing that I *must* answer to another person's needs is totally exhausting.'

> "Life at home with a baby is radically different from the life of most thirty-year old, childless people."

"While the role of father is often defined by externals, by earning the money and giving the family its last name, these are not the only involvements that men can feel. When a man is intimately involved with his wife's pregnancy, the entire process can take on physical overtones for him as well as for his wife.

'When I heard she was pregnant, I became afraid I was too old to be a good father. I'm nowhere near as healthy and active as I was when I was 18. How am I ever going to be a good father? Will I be able to keep up with my kids? Will I have the strength to meet the demands of fatherhood? I made up my mind to become healthier.

'The first day, I went out to the Central Park Reservoir and jogged around. I jogged over a mile. I was relieved I was able to run that whole way. I knew then that I could be healthy enough to be a good father. I've continued to jog. I've given up smoking, I watch my diet, and I try to be as informed about health as I can. I want to live and be healthy. I feel I have an obligation to a child and to his brothers or sisters to be a healthy parent. I also want to have life and energy left for my own life.' "

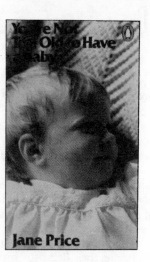

Jane Price

YOU'RE NOT TOO OLD TO HAVE A BABY
by Jane Price
1978, 147 pages

from
Penguin Books
625 Madison Ave.
New York, New York 10022
$2.95 pap.

Jane Price and her husband became parents in their 30's. Before making this decision, they gathered information about medical risks and some other pros and cons of becoming parents at that age. This information, as well as further research and interviews with couples, became the basis for their book. Price examines the trend of later child-bearing in American society—how it came to be, factors which contributed to it and the noticeable shift toward continuing this trend. She points out how advances in medical technology and further understanding of genetic inheritance can aid couples in making the parenthood decision. She also points out that being healthy to begin with, getting good prenatal nutrition, avoiding smoking and drugs, along with being well-informed about pregnancy and childbirth, are the basic and significant pluses which will lead to a healthy baby and mother. While much of the information in this book does not differ significantly from that in other books on the same subject, there was one chapter which stood out for me—"After the Baby's Born: How Does the Late-Blooming Family Fare?" In this chapter, Price examines the thoughts which I am also considering at this time—how much energy does it take? have an only child or more? are children of older parents different? what about illness and death, the generation gap, and older grandparents? Price is very open and nonjudgmental in presenting this material, encouraging couples to think about these issues and describing the thoughts and feelings of couples she

interviewed. Clearly she has been there and is trying to light the way for others. Also included is a list of books on pregnancy, childbirth and childrearing which she especially recommends to older couples. (SR)

"While older couples may have a somewhat harder transition to parenthood, they can draw on resources that may make coping with children easier in the long run. One way they compensate is by summoning their patience and maturity, bolstered by the realization that their child was wanted and planned for. According to Virginia Barber and Merrill Maguire Skaggs, who studied women's reactions to motherhood, 'We learned that women who became mothers in their late twenties and thirties, rather than younger, often found the frustrations of living with an infant more tolerable, perhaps because the child was more intensely desired, or because they had a more mature view of time or of their life and goals.'. . .

> "While older couples may have a somewhat harder transition to parenthood, they can draw on resources that may make coping with children easier in the long run."

"Delaying parenthood gives women an edge as jugglers, but much more is needed to change what is fundamentally at stake, the persistence of outdated definitions of male and female roles. If women are to achieve equality with men, we need a society where men have as much responsibility for the children and the home as women, where combining career and family is an issue for *both* parents. . . . Delaying parenthood has worked to better the position of women, but true equality between the sexes will require further transformation of our institutions and values.

"Each woman puts her own value on her career. If she has other consuming interests besides her work, she should be free to pursue them. The main point is that her potentialities not be limited by a constricting motherhood role. Arthur Campbell, deputy director of the Center for Population Research at the National Institute of Child Health and Development, has said, 'A girl pregnant at age sixteen has 90 percent of her life script written for her.' By delaying parenthood, women have more of a chance to develop a set of options in the way they lead their lives. We could say, 'A woman pregnant at age thirty-six writes 90 percent of her life script herself.'"

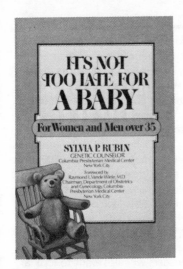

IT'S NOT TOO LATE FOR A BABY:
For Women and Men Over 35.
by Sylvia P. Rubin
1980, 274 pages, Illus.

from
Prentice-Hall
Englewood Cliffs, NJ 07632
$14.95 hd.

Sylvia Rubin writes about pregnancy after 30 from her perspective as a genetic counselor and instructor in Clinical Obstetrics and Gynecology at Columbia-Presbyterian Medical Center. She advises genetic counseling for prenatal diagnosis for any woman 35 years or older as well as for couples with any question about hereditary defects, a family member with genetic disease, or complications during the pregnancy (exposure to rubella, medications or X-rays in early pregnancy). She advises genetic couseling because she feels it can reduce fears and anxieties by helping the couple understand what risks *do* exist and what *can* be done prenatally. She discusses the techniques of ultra-sound and recommends that pregnant women 35 and older have an amniocentesis performed, while deemphasizing questions about the safety of these procedures. In her chapter on genetics, Rubin notes several defects which can occur (including Down's syndrome), their genetic basis, and detection. In the appendix she lists the many hereditary diseases that can be diagnosed prenatally. Other technical chapters review drugs and pregnancy, complications during pregnancy which can result in fetal complications, fetal monitoring procedures, and nutrition, all with a strong emphasis on reliance on medical technology. She also includes chapters on the psychology of pregnancy, the over-35 reaction to it, a quick review of some methods of childbirth, thoughts on after the baby comes, and some observations gleaned from obstetricians about patients who are over 35. Throughout the book she shares couples' personal experiences to illustrate her points. While readable for the lay person with some previous understanding of genetics, this book could also be a valuable reference book for childbirth educators and other professionals involved in counseling pregnant couples. (SR)

"Margaret was apprehensive as she put on the sac-like hospital gown in preparation for the ultrasonography. The physician then placed a jelly-like substance on her abdomen which helped to conduct the sound waves. The doctor then proceeded to use a stethoscope-like instrument which was attached to the ultrasonography equipment itself, running it back and forth, slowly moving it slightly each time, until the whole width of the abdomen was covered. This same method was repeated up and down the abdomen as well. She did watch the transmission on the television-like screen, but she could not make out anything that remotely resembled what she envisioned the fetus would look like. The obstetrician and the nurse became very excited, however, and she watched them point to two round areas on the screen. The only word she understood was 'twins.' The doctor then explained to her what they suspected and went on to confirm this fact with additional scanning. Every minute or so Polaroid photographs were taken of the screen projection for a permanent record. The obstetrician called in her husband, John, to show him the first pictures of their babies. . . .

"There is a basic agreement among most of the obstetricians this author has consulted regarding pregnant women who are over the age of 35. From their own point of view they find them, as a group, more cooperative, more motivated, and, in general, more apt to take better care of themselves. They are, from a medical standpoint, a very satisfying group to follow. Their maturity reveals a healthy concern for themselves and their babies.

"There is disagreement among the obstetricians regarding the incidence of complications. This, however, is more a reflection of their own patient populations. Every physician agreed that complications were more a function of the age as a group *per se* rather than a function of the pregnancy itself. And with good obstetrical prenatal care, complications can be carefully monitored, controlled, and sometimes even avoided."

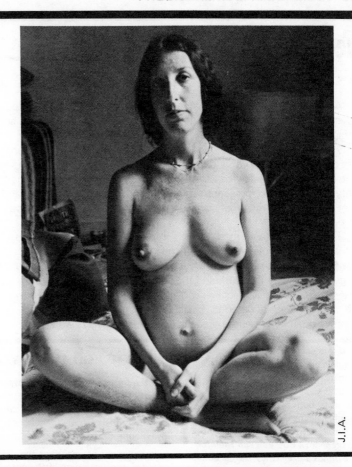

J.I.A.

SOONER OR LATER: The Timing of Parenthood in Adult Lives
by Pamela Daniels and Kathy Weingarten
1982, 366 pages

from
W.W. Norton
500 Fifth Avenue
New York, NY 10036
$14.95 hd.

Daniels and Weingarten are a developmental psychologist and a clinical psychologist respectively, who conducted a study of how the timing of parenthood (first baby at 20, 30, 40) affects the couples, their marriage, their careers, and their experiences as parents. Though medical issues are briefly covered, this book is mainly about the personal impact of parenthood on people's lives. (JIA)

"Today, as parents of young children, the mid-life couples we met are basically pleased, even thrilled, with their situation. They feel 'deeply blessed' to be parents at their age. But their age has a dark side too, and they were aware of this. As we have seen, the mid-life, family-timing pattern may reflect involuntary delay and circumstantial infertility as often as programmatic postponement; uncertainties and anxieties related to the experience of amniocentesis can create harrowing moments during pregnancy. Once their infants were safely born and these issues had faded into memory, the mid-life parents cited only one age-related draw-back, for the present—their energy level. 'I think I'm more tired than I might be if I were younger. Maybe it's just the demands of life with a preschooler. But I think that ten years ago I would not have felt the same fatigue at the end of the day that I do now. . . .'

"The early-timing parents in our study differed in their assessment of missing out on the freedoms of the early adult years. Some felt that they had forfeited valuable moratorium time for self-absorption, experimentation, and testing their readiness to make permanent commitments. Others believed that the middle adult years are the time to be without children—as seasoned people in the prime of life. By contrast, the late-timing and mid-life parents were virtually unanimous in their conviction that the 20s are the years to be free and unencumbered by the cares of parenthood. Most parents whose first child was born in their late 20s or early 30s would time the moment just that way again. However, for parents who did not have their first child until their late 30s or early 40s, the preparental freedom that had felt wonderful and right in their 20s was tinged with restlessness or regret as they approached 40. And, perhaps because they had not one but two decades of nonparental time before having a child, mid-life parents did not yearn to return to it as some of the late-timing parents did."

Teenage Pregnancy

Susan Ritchie, editor

A teenage pregnancy is like any other pregnancy in that it started when an egg and a sperm got together and it can possibly result in an infant's birth about nine months later. Pregnancy in anyone's life may not come quite at the right time. But pregnancy in a teenager's life can have special problems. The statistics show that more than one million American teenagers will become pregnant this year, that only one out of five pregnant teens *planned* to become pregnant, and that pregnancy is the most common reason for teenage girls to drop out of school.

There are increased medical risks for the pregnant teenager (possibly anemia, toxemia, etc.) and for the infant (possible low birth weight, prematurity, etc.). Because her body is still growing, there is greater risk to her health and the baby's than in an adult pregnancy. Economic and social problems add to the risk for this new life and the teenage parents. This is not to say that there are not positive aspects to teenage pregnancy. Some teenagers want to be pregnant and to become parents. Some feel it is a turning point in their lives, when they begin to accept responsibility for their action. For this group the aim of pregnancy care is to minimize the physical risks through attention to good nutrition and prenatal care and education. But for the others, those who did not want to become parents, this physical care must be given along with information on prevention of pregnancy, and on how to cope with it physically, emotionally, and socially.

The books and pamphlets in this section describe the overall problem of teenage pregnancy and offer some ideas and solutions. There is quite a lot of information available for parents and for those who work with pregnant teenagers but a noticeable lack of material suitable for teenagers themselves, especially those with limited reading skills. There is even less written for teenage fathers and their special problems and interests. We have included some of what is available and hope that it will be useful. Teenagers will also want to look at the other sections of this *Catalog,* for more detailed information on pregnancy, labor and birth, and family planning.   (SR)

If you suspect you're pregnant, getting a pregnancy test done as soon as possible will give you more time to consider your options. A missed menstrual period, breast tenderness, morning sickness and fatigue can all be signals from your body that you are pregnant. But *you can't tell for sure unless a pregnancy test is done.* For a description of these tests, see the index. If you don't know where you can have a test done, look in the yellow pages of the phone book (under "Birth Control") or ask a friend. The following places usually perform pregnancy tests. If they don't, ask them who does in your community.

*Birth Control Information Centers (like Planned Parenthood, Birthright, and birth control and abortion clinics)
*local health department clinics
*private physicians
*home pregnancy test kits available at drugstores

When you call, ask for the following information:

1. When can I bring in a urine sample? (It should be about a half a cup of your first urine of that morning. Put it in a clean, dry jar and keep it in the refrigerator or in a cool place if you can't take it for testing right away.)
2. If you are going to have a blood test, when can it be done?
3. How much will the test cost?
4. When can I call back/stop by for the results?
5. Is parental notification or consent required?
6. How many days past a missed menstrual period should I be able to get accurate results from the test (know the day when your last menstrual period started)?

IF YOU THINK YOU'RE PREGNANT

7. If the first test is negative (shows I'm not pregnant) should I have a repeat test at a later date to make sure? (Pregnancy tests can read falsely negative if done too early.)

If you're not pregnant, see the index for information on birth control to make sure you stay unpregnant until you want to have a baby.

If you are pregnant and you want to be, that's great. See the section about prenatal care (listed in the index).

If you are pregnant and you're not sure you want to be, you have several alternatives.

1. Continue the pregnancy and keep the baby
2. Continue the pregnancy and place the baby with adoptive parents
3. Have an abortion

It's important for you to seek medical care as soon as possible after you know you're pregnant. If you decide to continue with the pregnancy, you can avoid many potential problems by obtaining prenatal care, finding out about what foods to eat, what drugs and medications to avoid, and what's happening in your body during pregnancy, labor and birth. See other sections of this *Catalog* for information on all these subjects.

You may also need some financial help. You will need medical care, food, clothing and supplies throughout your pregnancy, at the time of the birth and for you and your child afterwards. If you don't have much money available, call the Department of Social Services in your area as soon as possible to get an appointment to see if you're eligible for 1) medicaid,

2) public assistance, 3) food stamps, and 4) Aid to Families with Dependent Children. Explain your situation and ask for the earliest possible appointment. Check with social services or the local health department about the WIC program (Women, Infants, Children program which provides additional foods to pregnant and nursing mothers and their children) and see if there is a local program for pregnant teenagers (it may be sponsored by the "Y" or Cooperative Extension, etc.). If you're in school and want to stay there, some communities have special classes you can join to learn about baby care along with your other subjects. Be persistent in finding people and places where you can be helped—they exist and you need them now.

If you decide to have an abortion, you'll want to plan for it as soon as possible. Ask about abortion services at the place where you had your pregnancy test done. If they can't help you, check the yellow pages of the phone book under "abortion information" or "birth control information centers." See the section on family planning for more information.

If you don't know what you want to do, the most important thing to remember is that you should make a decision and *do something.* Think about what your options are, what feels right for you. It may help to talk with someone about it—a friend, your boyfriend, your mother, a teacher at school. If you can't find someone you know to talk with about your pregnancy or if you want to discuss it further, there are several possibilities:

*pregnancy counselors at clinics such as Planned Parenthood, the health department, etc.
* a school counselor
* a counselor at a local family service

If you continue the pregnancy but aren't sure you want to put the child up for adoption, consider foster care arrangements until you make your decision. Or if you have the baby and realize you can't take care of the child right then, but plan to in the near future, consider foster care. Foster care can be arranged through many many agencies, such as United Community Services, department of child welfare, and religious organizations. They can tell you what arrangements can be made, what legal rights you have, and how to go about it.

If you want to continue with the pregnancy and have someone adopt the baby after birth, realize that there are people in the world who can't have children for some medical reason and would be willing and glad to adopt the baby. Children are adopted legally through government-authorized adoption agencies or private adoption agencies and through lawyers and state judges. Agencies which deal with adoption and can help you are:

* your state's department of child welfare
* local adoption agencies
* religious organizations (like Catholic Charities, Federation of Protestant Welfare Agencies, United Federation of Jewish Philanthropies)

Organizations which deal with infertility may be able to put you in touch with couples who want to adopt a baby. See the section on infertility in the *Catalog.*

CHILDBIRTH: A TEENAGER'S GUIDE
by Margot Edwards
1979, 4 pages, Illus.

from
the pennypress
1100 23rd Avenue East
Seattle, WA 98112
$.50
$20. per 100

This is only a 4-page pamphlet but it's packed with information on labor and birth—what it's like, what to do, and how to do it. There are only a couple of illustrations but the written descriptions are very clear and in a style which should be readable for most teens. (SR)

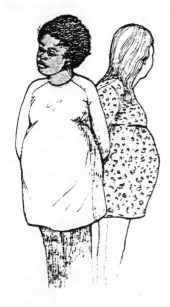

"... First, the uterus has a neck like a coke bottle which is called a cervix. The cervix has to get wider for the baby to get out. You see, the cervix opens with the contractions; that's the only reason the muscle gets hard—to pull open the cervix. In the cervix is a plug made out of mucus like the mucus in your nose. This plug stops up the cervix when you're pregnant to keep germs from getting into the house where the baby lies. The plug can be pink or whitish with bloody streaks. It is called the 'show.' It doesn't hurt at all when it comes out."

"Open the gate to let the baby out. If you tighten your body and close the gate, you will feel pain. If you feel the baby's head passing and you think you will split, that is normal. Do not be afraid. It may feel like burning for a few seconds; that will pass soon. Remember when we pulled the corners of our mouths, stretching our lips? It burned; that's how this feels. You will be so glad when the baby is born, and you'll know you worked very hard for this."

TEENAGE PREGNANCY: A Resource Kit
by Janis Wood Catano
1979, 100+ pages, Illus.

from
Prepared Childbirth Association of Nova Scotia
P.O. Box 5052 Armdale
Halifax, Nova Scotia
B3L 4M6 Canada
$3.50 (Canadian funds)

"*The Resource Kit* is a series of illustrated informational hand-outs designed for adolescents. These handouts can be used in a variety of teaching formats, and each is accompanied by a brief introduction for teachers and a short bibliography including reference to relevant audio-visual aids. The topics covered are:

1. Prenatal Care—Health Care During Pregnancy
2. Pregnancy and Fetal Development
3. Nutrition
4. Pre- and Post-natal Exercise, Posture and Comfort Measures
5. Labour and Delivery
   I What Happens During Childbirth?

SOME THINGS REALLY CAN HURT YOUR BABY — THESE ARE

DRUGS   SMOKING

X-RAYS   ALCOHOL

SICK PEOPLE   V.D.

YOUR BABY'S HEALTH AND FUTURE DEPEND ON HOW WELL YOU TAKE CARE OF YOURSELF—AND HIM WHILE YOU ARE PREGNANT. BE GOOD TO YOURSELF AND YOUR BABY!

   II What Can I do to Make Childbirth more Comfortable?
6. Post-partum
   I "Hey! I'm not Pregnant Any more!"
   II The Newborn Baby

LABOR AND BIRTH: A Guide for You
by Linda Todd
1981, 50 pages, Illus.

ICEA Bookcenter
P.O. Box 20048
Minneapolis, MN 55420
$2.50 plus $1.00 postage
bulk rates available

Linda Todd is the Chairperson of ICEA's Community Outreach Committee. Through this easily read new booklet, she does an impressive job of "reaching out" to discuss labor and birth. Lovely and clearly drawn illustrations by Vivien Cohen highlight important points and make the anatomy of the body during pregnancy easily understood. Wherever possible Todd includes short accounts from mothers and fathers describing their labors and births. She covers everything—from how to get ready for birth and what labor is like to bonding, recovery after birth, hints for new parents and information on adoption. Guidelines are given on how to be informed during the time of pregnancy and labor. This is an excellent booklet for teenagers as well as for adults. (SR)

"I was in labor for 23 hours. During hard labor, I got panicky and started to cry. That sure didn't do any good. So, from then on, I tried to relax and remember my breathing. That helped a lot!"

"... No woman should have to suffer in labor to prove she is womanly or will be a good mother. No woman should have to suffer in childbirth to prove she is worth being cared for or to make up for anything done in the past. Childbirth is when

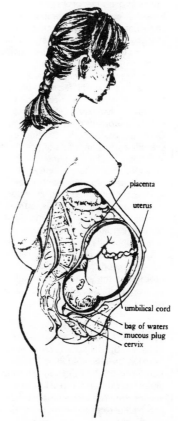

placenta

uterus

umbilical cord

bag of waters
mucous plug
cervix

7. Choices, Chance, Changes: Thinking About Tomorrow

A curriculum guide to prenatal education for teachers is also included.
"In the course of writing my thesis in Health Education, I had the readability of the *Resource Kit* evaluated using the READS Program ... developed at the Atlantic Institute of Education. The average grade level score was 6.17, which means that readers with a grade 6 reading ability would be able to read and understand the material in the *Resource Kit* to the extent that they could respond correctly to 75% of questions asked about it." —author Janis Catano

This book is printed in a large format (8½ x 11) and the pages are perforated and intended to be reproduced for distribution as class "hand-outs." Topics are covered thoroughly but without an overwhelming amount of detail. Line drawings with captioned question and answer sessions between a pregnant teenager and her older sister (who is a nurse) illustrate much of the material. (SR)

a mother and baby meet for the first time. The more joy there can be, the better for both. . . .

"Classes were so helpful. We felt ready when the time finally came. My boyfriend and I had done a lot of hiking in the mountains so the picture that compared the work of labor to climbing the mountain was perfect. In many ways, our experience in childbirth was like climbing a 13,000 foot peak. Lots of preparation, more hard work, and even more excitement when it's done. However, our baby was a better outcome than my usual sore feet!

"If you are faced with a choice about raising your baby or placing your baby with adoptive parents, you may want some help. This can be such a hard decision. Sometimes it is easier if you can talk to other mothers who have faced similar choices. Two agencies in the United States which may be able to offer one-to-one or group counseling are: Lutheran Social Services and Children's Home Society. In Canada, the Children's Aid Society has similar programs. . . .

"If you have made a choice to place your baby with adoptive parents, you may wonder what will be best for you and your baby after birth. Should you see your baby? Hold your baby? Care for your baby during your hospital stay? There are no easy answers. It is important that you know you can do these things. It is best to *follow your feelings* rather than to do what others tell you would be best. Talk your choices over with others you trust. That can be a big help."

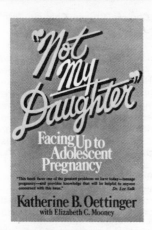

NOT *MY* DAUGHTER: Facing Up to Adolescent Pregnancy
by Katherine B. Oettinger
1979, 184 pages

from
Prentice-Hall
Englewood Cliffs, NJ 07632
$9.95 hd

If parents wait too long for their preteens and teens to start asking questions about sex, pregnancy, and other related issues, the first question may be "I'm pregnant, what should I do?" Katherine Oettinger asks parents to think seriously about where their teenagers get their sex education. "Off the bathroom walls or from the guys at school," replied one young man. Oettinger advocates early communication about sexuality between parents and children, as well as discussions in school and through peer counseling groups. Oettinger bases her recommendations on her experiences as former Chief of the Children's Bureau of the Department of HEW and as the first Deputy Assistant Secretary for Population and Family Planning. Her book is full of concrete examples and ideas on parent-child communication and she also discusses dealing with adolescents' feelings, birth control when needed, and what options are available if a pregnancy does occur. Both positive and negative aspects of each option are considered. A resource guide lists books, pamphlets, and films which parents and people who work with teens will find extremely useful. (SR)

"By the time our children are ready for kindergarten, they should know that pregnancy, not the stork, precedes childbirth. This quite naturally leads to the information that a baby grows inside the mother. The story of the miracle of birth can unfold before the child is 8, and from there it is possible to build a foundation for knowledge of human sexual relations."

TEENAGE SEXUALITY, PREGNANCY AND CHILDBEARING
Edited by Frank F. Furstenberg, Jr., Richard Lincoln and Jane Menken
1981, 423 pages, Illus.

from
University of Pennsylvania Press
3933 Walnut Street
Philadelphia, PA 19104
$22.95 hd

This book is an anthology of 28 articles which appeared in *Family Planning Perspectives*, a bimonthly publication of the Alan Guttmacher Institute. They give an overall view of research in the areas of teenage pregnancy and childbearing in the 1970's. The book is divided into four sections: 1) trends and their interpretation, 2) the consequences of early parenthood, 3) locating the problem/defining the solution, and 4) sources of resistance and change. Topics covered include patterns of sexual experience, pregnancy and contraceptive use; health effects of early pregnancy; psychological factors in unwanted pregnancy; pregnancy prevention services; and teenage pregnancy and the law. (SR)

"The educational and informational materials available to adolescents who are pregnant or the parents of a newborn infant are few and, for the most part, inappropriate. It is time that commercial companies, government agencies and public and charitable organizations that publish 'new mother' materials review them with an eye toward the needs of the one million teenagers who become pregnant each year. Do their booklets deal with choice of abortion in an evenhanded way? Do they explain how birth control methods work and where to obtain them? Do they discuss the early symptoms of pregnancy, and how to get a pregnancy test? Do they talk about the possibility of miscarriage? Do they identify resources for job, child care and educational counseling, as well as sources of medical care and economic help? Do they explain reproductive physiology, especially its relationship to the risk of pregnancy, and the various gynecological and obstetrical procedures the young woman is likely to undergo in the course of her pregnancy? . . .

"The cost of adding the capacity to clinic programs to serve one-half million additional adolescents each year has been estimated at $35 million for 1979, $74 million for 1980 and $118 million for 1981. Given the well-documented long-term adverse consequences of an unintended birth for the teenage mother and her baby, the cost to individuals, and to society, of *not* adding this capacity is enormous."

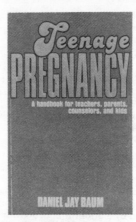

TEENAGE PREGNANCY: A Handbook for Teachers, Parents, Counselors, and Kids
by Daniel Jay Baum
1980, 157 pages

from
Beaufort Books, Inc.
9 East 40th Street
New York, NY 10016
$6.95 pap.

Lawyer and educator Daniel Baum presents the alarming facts and figures on teenage pregnancy, then briefly examines important aspects of the problem, including why teenagers get pregnant, the special problems of teenage mothers and fathers, and providing sex education and birth control. Baum looks at what the law has to say about teenage pregnancy, abortion, birth control and marriage, considers the options of abortion and relinquishing the baby for adoption, and describes what kinds of help are available for young mothers who keep their babies. Baum concludes with some thoughts on how parents can help their teenage children to become responsible adults. A reference list after each section provides guidance for further reading. (SR)

"Dr. Cowell would like to change the ways we try to help the younger teenager. She was quoted in *The Medical Post*:

" 'What we have is a marketing problem in failing to sell contraception to this population. We are coping with the pleasures of recreational sexual activity and with therapeutic abortion. It's a sad comment on the state of affairs that teenagers think it's easier to get a therapeutic abortion than practice contraception.'

"Perhaps the energies —and funds ——of those concerned about teenage pregnancy should be devoted to persuading society to accept the widest possible distribution and availability of condoms to young boys. Many are too shy to carry a package to the—probably female—cashier in a drugstore. Dispensing machines in schools, sports facility locker rooms, theatres, wherever teenagers congregate, might prevent tragedies."

MANAGING TEENAGE PREGNANCY: Access to Abortion, Contraception, and Sex Education
by James E. Allen with Deborah Bender
1980, 332 pages, Illus.

from
Praeger Publishers
521 Fifth Avenue
New York, NY 10017
$29.95

This book describes a research project evaluating the differences between two North Carolina communities' efforts to deal with the issue of teenage pregnancy. The authors' conclusions will be very useful to any community or agency planning to provide services in sex education, pregnancy, and abortion to teenagers. One study community, "Farmville," had an above-average rate of teenage pregnancies and births while the other, "Southern City," had a very low rate. The authors show that this difference was in very large part due to the differences in availability of contraception, sex education, and information in each community. Southern City focused on what the need was, made services available with little fuss, provided those services at little or no cost, did not require parental consent, funded the services on a county level, and had a number of community agencies involved in the issues and in providing services. In contrast, the Farmville system often prevented teens from seeking care. A startling example was that of obtaining a pregnancy test. In Southern City, it was done by taking an early morning urine sample to the Health Department lab any weekday, fee $3.00, results available in three hours, age not a factor (this was one of four alternatives in that community). In Farmville a call to the Health Department led to a wait if two periods had not yet been missed, the need for parental consent if under 18, referral to the patient's family physician, if any, if not an appointment with Social Services to determine Medicaid or Title 20 eligibility, then a clinic appointment and exam to check for pregnancy. The pregnancy test was free in this case, but the rigmarole beforehand kept many teenagers from getting the services they needed. (SR)

"Teens said they need the following:
Knowledge about how to prevent pregnancy,
Someone to talk to,
Access to free or low-cost contraceptives,
Pills that do not cause cancer,
Partner's early awareness of whether the other is using birth control,
Better prenatal care,
Information on how to care for children, and
Help in dealing with anger about pregnancy."

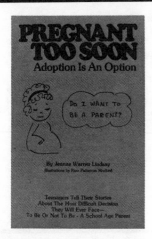

PREGNANT TOO SOON: Adoption
is an Option
by Jeanne Warren Lindsay
1980, 204 pages, Illus.

from
EMC Publishing
180 East 6th Street
Saint Paul, MN 55101
$5.95 pap.

Jeanne Warren Lindsay is the
school teacher/coordinator for a teen
mothers program at a high school in
California. She has gathered much of
the material for this book from students in her own and other programs.
Lindsay explores the how's, why's,
when's, and feelings of teenage mothers on being pregnant and deciding
to relinquish a baby for adoption.
Along with these topics she also discusses adoptions via agencies or independently, the possibility of relatives adopting the baby, fathers'
rights, relinquishing a toddler for
adoption, and provides a few stories
from adoptees and adoptive parents.
Throughout the book she makes a
very conscious effort to relate what
the feelings of all concerned might be
in the area of adoption. She uses the
young women's and men's own stories to illustrate her points. It's a
thoughtful book and well worth reading by anyone concerned about the
adoption option for unplanned pregnancies.   (SR)

"If you are releasing a child, you
need to know what the grieving process is. You will have to go through
it. You should realize what the
stages of grief are . . . to realize it's
OK to deny your grief, to be angry,
to be depressed, to feel rejected.
And finally, if you go through these
stages and you don't try to bury your
grief, you will feel acceptance. It's
OK to have these feelings. That's
been so important to me, to work
through these feelings no matter how
long it takes."

PLANNED PARENTHOOD FEDER-ATION OF AMERICA
810 Seventh Avenue
New York, NY 10019

Planned Parenthood offers several
pamphlets and posters on teenage
sexuality and pregnancy. Titles in-
clude:
Pregnancy Resource Books
    Considering What To Do
    Caring for Two
    Deciding on Abortion
Teensex? It's OK To Say No Way
What Teens Want to Know But
    Don't Know How to Ask
Basics of Birth Control
About Childbirth
Don't Make Your Growing Pains
    Labor Pains (poster)
Prices range from 25 cents to
$1.00 for single copies and bulk
rates are available. Write for a com-
plete publications catalog.   (JIA)

TEENAGE PREGNANCY: What
Can Be Done?
by Irving R. Dickman
1981, 28 pages, Illus.

from
Public Affairs Pamphlets
381 Park Avenue South
New York, NY 10016
50 cents
bulk rates available

This pamphlet discusses the consequences of teenage pregnancy,
gives a brief summary of what
schools can do to provide sex education, and describes the varied programs available for teens in birth control and during pregnancy. The auth-
or reminds us that federal funds for
abortion, sex education and family-
planning are currently being cut back
and he challenges educators and parents to work to find answers to help
young people in these areas.   (SR)

". . . there are still many girls
who seek enhanced self-esteem
through a closeness and a sharing
that they have been led to believe
'sex' will provide. At best, they are
getting mixed messages and confusing signals from the world around
them. They do hear the voices warning of the evils or the harm of premature sexual activity. Much more
often, however, they are confronted
by TV programs, including prime-
time soap operas, based largely on
sex and violence. Commercials add
the subliminal message of an almost-
universal advertising approach that,
to take one product as an example,
all but says 'better blue jeans mean
better sex.'"

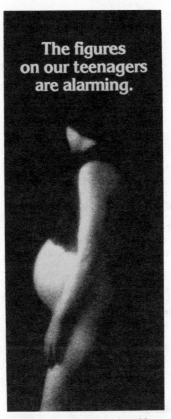

Cover of a pamphlet produced by
the New York State Department of
Health.

TEENAGE PARENTS
by Margot Edwards
90 pages

from
the pennypress
1100 23rd Avenue East
Seattle, WA 98112
$3.75
bulk rates available

"Primarily for those working
with pregnant teens or young mothers, this book contains discussions
of the unique social and health problems of teen parents; descriptions
of several programs for pregnant mi-
nors; ways to motivate and teach
childbirth education and parenting;
and a description of childbirth written as a teenager might describe it
to another teenager. There are numerous quotations from teenage discussions throughout the book which
enhance one's understanding of their
unique situation."

TEENAGE PREGNANCY: EVERY-BODY'S PROBLEM
1979, brochure
DHEW Pub. No (HSA) 79-5619

from
Public Health Service
Bureau of Community Health Ser-
vices
Rockville, MD 20857
single copy free

This brochure provides educators
and parents with statistics on teen
pregnancy, consequences of early
childbearing, and an outline of preventive services aimed at both education and contraception. Included is
an annotated list of organizations
which can provide further information and services.   (SR)

THE HASSLES OF BECOMING A
TEENAGE PARENT
1978, brochure
DHEW Pub. No. (HSA) 78-5624

from
Public Health Service
Bureau of Community Health Ser-
vices
Rockville, MD 20857
single copy free

Written for the teenager, this
brochure presents the facts on conception, on staying *un*pregnant—
what methods work and which don't
(with a quick sentence or two on
why)—as well as a short review on
venereal disease. It's a start for teenagers who need some basics.   (SR)

HELPING TEENAGE PARENTS
PREPARE FOR CHILDBIRTH
by Linda Todd
9 pages
free with SASE

SUPPORT FOR TEENS
by Christine Scanlan
2 pages
free with SASE

TEENAGE PREGNANCY
special issue of *ICEA Sharing*
20 pages
$1.00 single issue

These resources and other materials on teenage and outreach teaching
are available from:
Community Outreach Committee
Int'l Childbirth Education Assoc.
c/o Linda Todd, Chair
3139 Irving Avenue South
Minneapolis, MN 55408
                                 (JIA)
"You don't have to try to reach
all of the million teens who will get
pregnant this year. One or two
would make a difference . . ."
                          —Linda Todd
                          ICEA Sharing

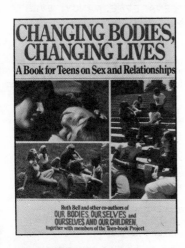

CHANGING BODIES, CHANGING LIVES: A Book for Teens on Sex and Relationships
by Ruth Bell
1980, 242 pages, Illus.

from
Random House
201 East 50th Street
New York, NY 10022
$7.95 pap.

Finally, a super-comprehensive book for teenagers on sex and relationships. This new book, from the co-authors of *Our Bodies, Ourselves,* gives an impressive amount of information on these two subjects, with the feelings, thoughts and questions of teenagers woven throughout. As an adult, it is sometimes difficult not to sermonize to teenagers about sex, pregnancy and related issues—this book doesn't. If you are a teenager, this book will be a wonderful source of information and help. If you're an adult, and you can get a copy away from a teenager long enough to read it, you'll be reminded of the many thoughts, feelings, difficult times, body changes, and different reality you experienced as a teenager. The important philosophy which is continuously expressed by this book includes 1) acceptance of teenagers and all their thoughts and feelings, 2) an emphasis on not hurting or exploiting yourself or other people, and 3) the importance of learning to be responsible for yourself and your actions. To give an idea of the scope of this book the table of contents is listed below. Especially relevant to this section of the *Catalog* is the chapter on teenage pregnancy.

"A NOTE TO PARENTS: Many parents have an underlying feeling that sex information will shock or disturb their children, or even worse, that it will interest them too much. Some fear that if we give young people information about sex, it will make them rush out and 'do it.'

"It's natural to think that way, but it isn't what happens. Good sex education, which means to us sex education that is about real people going through real-life situations, doesn't encourage anybody to go out and get wild. In fact, studies show that teenagers who are taught about sex, birth control, VD and body functions are *less* likely to get pregnant before they want to, *less* likely to catch VD and *less* likely to engage in thoughtless sexual activity than teens who haven't had that education. It's when we don't teach teens and preteens about sex and their bodies that they get into trouble. . . .

"The teenage years can be pretty hard on the way parents and children get along together. Although your feelings about your parents and their feelings about you will probably remain strong throughout, they are usually not *only* positive feelings. In fact, there may be times when you feel very definitely unloving toward each other, times when you each feel completely misunderstood or unappreciated, times when you can't even believe how much anger there is between you.

"The reason for all these intense feelings is not so hard to understand. It comes from what your relationship is all about in the first place. Parents try to raise children who'll be able to leave them and live independently when they get old enough. But they feel it's their responsibility to take care of and protect their children until they *are* able to live on their own. Children need their parents but they also want to grow up, have more independence, live on their own. The problem for both sides is: when to hold on to each other and how much and when to let go . . . .

"If you as a boy helped to create a pregnancy, then you may have strong feelings at this time too. It's natural to want to be part of the decision; it's natural, also, to feel very confused. You may in fact be feeling very left out because all the attention is on the girl. She's the one who gets pregnant, she's the one who has to go for the test, and she's the one who has to have the abortion or go through the childbirth. You may feel that there's no role for you in this process, but that's not true. If you care, if you want to be a part of it, you can participate. You also have a responsibility to the girl to help her in any way you can. Sixteen-year-old Stanley told us:

'I know some guys skip town or drop out of sight for a while if they get a girl pregnant, but, man, I figure if you were there for the fun you ought to be there for the hard part too. My girl needs me now. I can't let her down.' "

MODEL PROGRAMS

ADOLESCENT PROGRAM
Booth Maternity Center
6051 Overbrook Avenue
Philadelphia, PA 19131
215/878-7800

The Salvation Army's Booth Maternity Center began as a place for unwed mothers to find shelter and medical care. Though social needs have changed and Booth now offers family-centered maternity care to all women, the Center has developed a special new program for teenagers to provide prenatal care and classes, social services, labor and delivery care in the hospital, postpartum visits, baby care classes, and discussion groups. Care is provided primarily by nurse-midwives and involves personalized education and support. Contact Booth for literature and more information on their adolescent program.   (JIA)

"A study has been recently completed of the first 52 participants of Booth's Adolescent Program. The participants were compared with those of a matched sample who received care at Booth Maternity Center before the special Teen Program was developed. Significant differences were found in the participants of the new program. The study showed lower numbers of neonatal and intrapartal complications among participants in the new program. There were higher numbers of prenatal and postpartum visits. Over half of the mothers (54%) in the present program were breastfeeding their babies at the time of the postpartum check up, as compared to 28% of the control group. Eighty-three percent of the clinic group had decided on a birth control method, contrasted to 50% of the control group."

ADOLESCENT FAMILY CENTER
Rush Presbyterian St. Luke's Medical Center
1753 W. Congress Parkway
Chicago, IL 60612
312/942-8775

The adolescent family center offers prenatal care and classes and complete birth care provided by a certified nurse-midwife. Family planning and social services are also available. Health care providers who are interested in providing a similar service may wish to contact Laurie Stortz-Driscoll, CNM at the center.
                                (JIA)

". . . The Adolescent Family Center is a private non-sectarian facility. It has been in operation since February, 1974, and is funded through the Chicago Foundlings Home.

"Health care is provided through a team approach. A physician, social worker and nurse-midwife work together with each patient. A personal touch prevails: each girl is seen by the same nurse midwife and social worker each time she comes

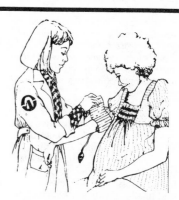

to the Adolescent Family Center.

"These professionals provide a supportive environment in which each girl can work through the specific problems of her prenatal and postpartum periods. In addition, they assist each girl with her maturation process; help the girl and her family prepare for the future; and respond to her individual needs, keeping in mind the importance of the ethnic, economic, and social aspects of her life."

Outreach

Susan Ritchie, editor

Information on various aspects of pregnancy and childbirth isn't always easy to obtain. Some of the barriers may be cultural, socio-economic or educational. Outreach teaching and education can help increase access to vital information that everyone should be able to have when they need it, or before. There *are* pamphlets on pregnancy in Spanish, there *are* parenting booklets for people who read at a second grade level, there *are* expectant mother's classes in some prisons, and there *are* classes for pregnant teenagers who may be faced with decisions about motherhood, adoption and foster care. Knowledge gives us more power in our decision-making and in what will happen with ourselves, our children and our families. Everyone has a right to that knowledge and these resources discuss ways it can be made more accessible to everyone. (SR)

NEW READERS PRESS
1320 Jamesville Avenue
Box 131
Syracuse, NY 13210
free catalog

The New Readers Press, a division of Laubach Literacy International, produces pamphlets and books for adults with low-level reading skills. Their catalog includes pamphlets on *Having a Baby* and *So-easy-to-read Parenting*. Topics include conception and pregnancy, prenatal care, giving birth, the first six weeks, the baby and the family, unwed mothers, and family planning. (SR)

COMMUNITY OUTREACH COMMITTEE
Int'l Childbirth Education Association
c/o Linda Todd, Chair
3139 Irving Avenue South
Minneapolis, MN 55408

This committee provides additional materials on outreach teaching which can be obtained by sending a self-addressed, stamped (two stamps) envelope to Linda Todd at the address above. (Include one SASE for each paper requested.) Current titles include the following.

REACHING OUT TO WOMEN IN PRISON
by Elaine Anthony
3 pages

Briefly discusses setting up childbirth preparation classes in prisons and lists major points to discuss with prison staff (nutritional needs in pregnancy, labor support, bonding).

CHILDBIRTH EDUCATION IN RURAL AREAS
by Terry Steinmetz
8 pages

Discusses needs and problems in rural areas, strategies for meeting needs, teaching methods, and further resources.

SETTING UP AN OUTREACH CLASS
by Linda Todd
10 pages

The nitty-gritty details of setting up an outreach class, including funding sources, publicity, and content areas.

SOURCES OF SPANISH LANGUAGE RESOURCES FOR CHILDBIRTH AND PARENT EDUCATION
ICEA Community Outreach Committee
5 pages

Lists books and pamphlets available from organizations in the U.S. and distributors with films in Spanish on childbirth and parent education.

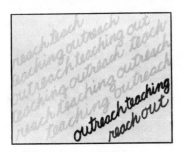

OUTREACH TEACHING
Edited by Barbara McCormick
1979, 110 pages

from
ICEA Bookcenter
P.O. Box 20048
Minneapolis, MN 55420
$6.00 plus $1.25 postage

Differing cultural, socioeconomic and educational backgrounds may be factors which influence a person's approach to pregnancy and childbirth and thus to prepared childbirth classes. CEA of Greater Minneapolis-St. Paul, under the auspices of the International Childbirth Education Association, has put together a valuable guide for teaching childbirth classes in outreach situations. The authors have themselves taught such classes and relate their own experiences—mistakes and triumphs—which makes for very enjoyable reading as well as providing a background for anyone planning to do similar work. The fundamental factors are outlined: working within the setting and with hospital/clinic personnel, the teaching staff (responsibilities, preparation, salaries, etc.), communicating with students, class content, types of classes, and giving support to the laboring woman. Two chapters— "The Pregnant Adolescent" and "The Relinquishing Mother"—will be of special interest to those working with teenagers. The resource section of the book includes a suggested bibliography for childbirth educators involved in outreach, commu-

nity services which can be valuable to clients and classes, a brief outline of various teaching methods, the body signs, feelings and needs of preg-pregnant women in the three trimesters, and two possible course outlines. (SR)

"... the problem here is not dealing with those who approach us for education; it is making ourselves available to those who do not seek out preparation. It means seeking them out, going to them, reaching out."

"... In a broad sense, outreach is designed to better meet the particular needs of any learner who may not be comfortable or learn well in a couple-oriented, middle-class environment. The learner's discomfort may have to do with socioeconomic status. It sometimes coincides with marital status. It sometimes coincides with age. Perhaps the learning disadvantage is general, pertaining to all kinds of learning; perhaps it is specific, involving an inability to assimilate information about a traumatic pregnancy and any related subjects. Sometimes it is not a matter of discomfort but the positive advantage of working through a major change in life with the support of others making similar changes."

"When discussing nutrition in pregnancy, focus on getting your money's worth in food buying, eligibility for food stamps or participation in the WIC program, location of local food coops and thrift stores and the existence of any local food commodity programs. Obviously,

finding ways to get nutritious foods is as much a need as knowing what good foods you should eat . . . ."

"The problem here is not dealing with those who approach us for education; it is making ourselves available to those who do not seek out preparation. It means seeking them out, going to them, reaching out.

"Reaching out is not reaching down. If we think hard enough about differences between ourselves and any potential class member, we can easily feel threatened by learners with less education or money, and by those with more. We have something any woman looking forward to labor can use. Focused on that reality, differences become hazy and are matters of circumstance more than anything else.

"If one of the values of using aids is to make the information real, a real body to demonstrate obstetrical landmarks or describe musculature or function must be the most valuable aid of all. The childbirth educator is always her own best aid. Her comfort in using her body and her attitude toward a woman's body and how it functions contribute to the comfort of the entire class. She can convey trust and encourage participants to feel good about themselves, their bodies, and how their bodies function. She will find an additional important advantage to using her body as a teaching aid: it is something she can always count on to be available."

"Where direct contact with inmates is not possible, you may be able to set up a 'pen-pal' correspondence between childbirth educators and inmates."

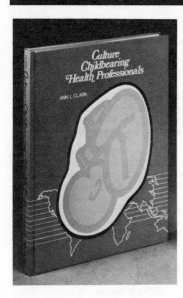

CULTURE, CHILDBEARING, HEALTH PROFESSIONALS
Edited by Ann L. Clark
1978, 190 pages, Illus.

from
F.A. Davis Company
1915 Arch Street
Philadelphia, PA 19103
$22.00 hd.

Health care in our country is delivered, for the most part, by white middle-class people with European backgrounds. What this group regards as "normal" and acceptable influences the type of care patients receive, even those from other cultures. But other cultures have different ideas about pregnancy, birth, baby care, and family life which must be taken into account for at least two reasons: 1) it's harder to provide good care when unspoken assumptions about health and disease differ between patient and provider, and 2) just because ideas are "different" doesn't mean they are "wrong"—we all have much to learn from each other.

Culture, Childbearing, Health Professionals provides an introduction to the effects of cultural beliefs on childbearing and presents a series of essays on the distinctive childbearing practices and attitudes of nine American ethnic groups: the American Indian, the Afro-American, the Chinese-American, the Japanese-American, the Mexican-American, the Puerto Rican, the Filipino-American, the American-Samoan, and the Vietnamese. (JIA)

"Although menstruation is a time when a black woman thinks she is 'sick,' pregnancy is thought to be a state of wellness. This is one of the reasons for the delay, on the part of many black women, in obtaining prenatal care. Therefore, in the South, a woman is expected to work in the fields until she is ready to deliver, while in the North, women wish to continue working, but are more restricted by employer policies. Because pregnancy is seen as a physiological process, many women are not convinced that prenatal care is that important. Since prenatal care is regarded by these women as a "passive" type of medical care, their interest and cooperation are often half-hearted. Some young women have said to me, 'When I come to the clinic, "they" never do anything but feel my stomach and then that's it. . .'

"One experience that may be very frightening to the pregnant woman is the pelvic examination. Most traditional cultures reject the idea of a man's viewing the genitals of someone other than his mate. Male physicians in Mexico have learned to do a physical examination through cloth by means of a gown that extends from the patient's neck to her ankles. Pelvic examination is not acceptable to many Mexican-American women or their mates, so it is not done without strong indication. Women physicians, of whom there are many in Mexico, and midwives may examin the pelvis internally without fear of censure. . . .

"The four Sansei [third generation Japanese-Americans] also stated that they believed that pregnancy was a normal process. Two of the Sansei selected care from a contemporary health delivery system. Both obtained prenatal care from the Kaiser Health Plan, either under the care of a physician or a nurse-practitioner. A private physician was not consulted, owing to their particular insurance coverage with Kaiser and the fact that additional expenses would be incurred. The other two Sansei sought the services of a family physician for initial physical examination and laboratory work. They requested his opinion of their chances for a normal birth at home, and hearing that the overall chances were very good, they elected the care of lay midwives. The major motivations for seeking a home birth were spiritual and economic ones. They wished the intimacy and closeness of the home environment and control to prevent separation from the baby. They believed that pregnancy was a natural process, and wanted to maintain the sense of naturalness found in the home. The women added that the standard hospital fees were prohibitive.

"All four of these Sansei complied well with the dietary and activity suggestions made by their health counselors. The two women who elected home birth modified some of the suggestions related to diet, because both were vegetarians and one of them suffered from a milk allergy. Many Asians have similar milk lactose intolerances and may need guidance in securing adequate amounts of calcium."

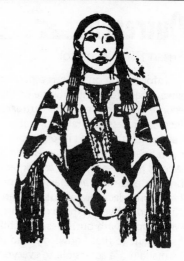

WOMEN'S DANCE HEALTH PROJECT
c/o Marcie Rendon
2713 Delaware SE
Minneapolis, MN 55414
612/623-1845

"Women's Dance Health Project began as a group of women who came together to work with other Indian women in self-help health care, prenatal counselling, health advocacy and family-centered birthing alternatives. As a community-based organization, through direct experience and necessity, we have gained a working knowledge of incest counselling, battering, alcoholism, healthy sexuality and other important and often misunderstood areas. We now offer in-service workshops, lectures, and classes on the following topics:
Direction of Native American Women Today
Pre-Natal Care
Incest
Battering
Sexuality
Political Awareness for Women
Cycles—Women's Relation to Mother Earth

Family Involvement in Birth
Self-Help Health Care
Alcoholism/Chemical Dependency
Natural Birth Control
Preventive Family Health Care
Sterilization

These topics are offered in a culturally and spiritually relevant atmosphere."

NATIVE WOMAN POSTER: This full color poster is 17" x 22". Copies are available for $3.00 each from Akwesasne Notes, Mohawk Nation, Rooseveltown, NY 13683.

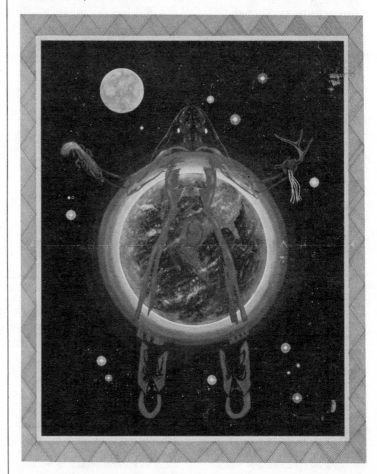

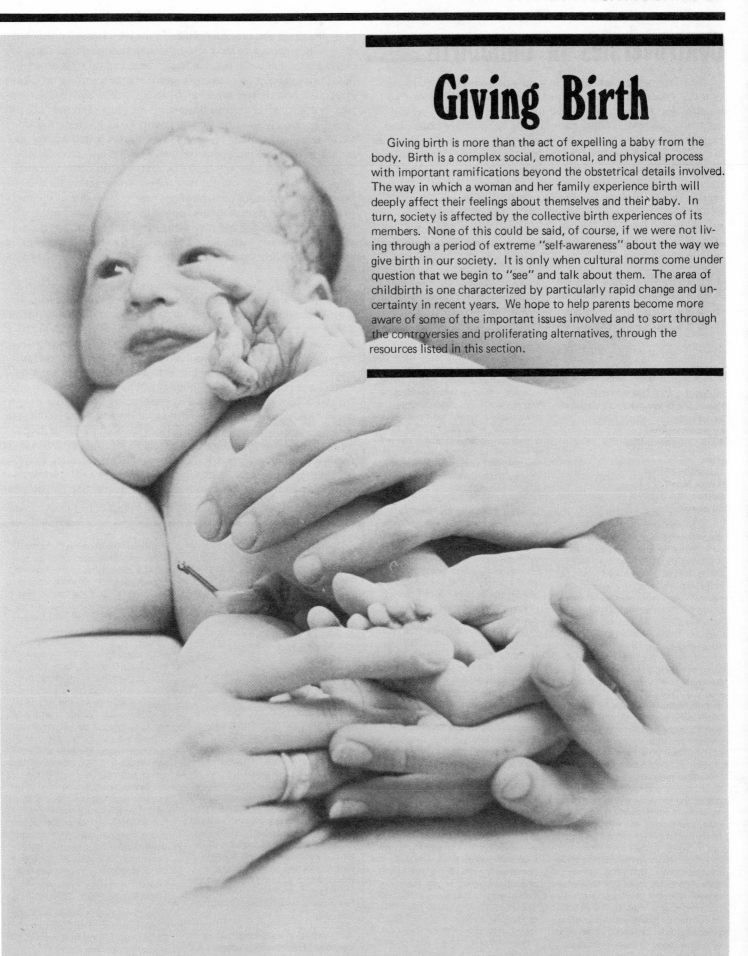

Giving Birth

Giving birth is more than the act of expelling a baby from the body. Birth is a complex social, emotional, and physical process with important ramifications beyond the obstetrical details involved. The way in which a woman and her family experience birth will deeply affect their feelings about themselves and their baby. In turn, society is affected by the collective birth experiences of its members. None of this could be said, of course, if we were not living through a period of extreme "self-awareness" about the way we give birth in our society. It is only when cultural norms come under question that we begin to "see" and talk about them. The area of childbirth is one characterized by particularly rapid change and uncertainty in recent years. We hope to help parents become more aware of some of the important issues involved and to sort through the controversies and proliferating alternatives, through the resources listed in this section.

Controversies in Childbirth___

American birth practices are in a state of tremendous controversy today. An increasing number of consumers and childbirth "advocates" feel that virtually everything which is done in American maternity hospitals is either harmful or unnecessary or both. The basic thing wrong with the hospital approach, according to its critics, is that it interferes or "practices routine interventions" in a process which is inherently normal and requires no intervention (except in the small minority of abnormal cases). Of course, if routine intervention in normal birth produced better birth outcomes, it would be justified. But many studies and our own birth statistics have shown that intervention does not "improve" birth. The net effect of all the drugs and procedures used in obstetrics today, many critics feel, is to *introduce risks* into otherwise normal births, cause psychological and physical harm in many cases, and do so at an enormous financial cost to consumers, insurance carriers, and tax-payers. Physicians who defend American birth practices argue that our infant mortality rates have declined in recent years. But the U.S. still ranks very poorly in world statistics, with 12 to 16 Western countries having lower infant mortality rates. Our high-technology approach to birth has not compared well with the low-intervention, midwife-oriented approach used in countries with better statistics. Many critics have pointed out that the routine practices used in American hospitals for birth have not been proven safe or necessary. Most procedures have developed either through hospital and staff needs for convenience and easy management of patients or through medical "tradition," without being subjected to the kind of rigorous scientific investigation which could show whether they are of any benefit.

Parents today find themselves facing a confusion of arguments and counter-arguments concerning the safety of hospital birth. It is often tempting to simply put our faith in our doctors and institutions rather than take on the major responsibility for birth ourselves. Many parents feel uncertain about questioning or challenging the advice of the medical professionals who care for them. We need to realize, however, that medical practices and opinions are not always correct and parents and their children will pay a high price for any "mistakes" which are made. Being "responsible" in childbirth doesn't mean that you have to abandon the medical system altogether or face the prospect of a painful labor without relief. It does mean that parents should make an effort to inform themselves about the risk of common obstetrical practices and drugs and try to choose the safest alternatives available in their community. The books, pamphlets and government studies listed in this section can help parents in becoming informed consumers of maternity care.

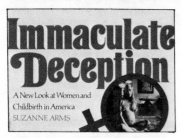

IMMACULATE DECEPTION: A New Look at Women and Childbirth in America
by Suzanne Arms
1975, 318 pages, Illus.

from
Houghton Mifflin
2 Park Street
Boston, MA 02107
$6.95 pap.

This is an angry book, born of the author's shock and sense of loss over the badly-managed and all-too-typical hospital birth of her first child. It is also an inspired work, lucidly exposing the "immaculate deception" American women have believed for so long—that birth is an inherently dangerous process which must be "improved" on by medical science. Arms outlines the history of childbirth, describes the development of "Birth's Machine Age" in America, and shows us very clearly that the claims made for the safety and necessity of hospital birth just don't stand up to scrutiny. She argues strongly for the return of childbirth to the skill and control of women, both as mothers and as midwives.

Some childbirth educators are reluctant to recommend this book to their students, for fear it will be too disturbing for those planning a hospital birth. I think parents *should* read it, and do so early in pregnancy, so that what they learn can be put to use in planning their own birth.

"The unspoken assumption of obstetrics today is that what is predictable is certainly more safe than what is not. And the process of birth is not predictable enough. In an effort to control birth and make it predictable, obstetrical science has devised a routine series of interferences designed to "improve" upon the normal birth. The obstetrician thus patterns his practice in normal birth after his practice in abnormal birth, forcing the majority of women to undergo procedures that are unnecessary for all but a few women. This makes the birth process a more predictable operation for the doctor, even though any interference can create a greater risk to the woman than the original problem it was intended to solve. Whether interferences are worth the risk is a question only the physician—certainly not the mother—can answer, since any interference is a medical procedure. But in her reliance upon her doctor's authority, the pregnant woman is seldom aware that such decisions are being made over her prone body.

"What she does hear, if she is lucky, is that such 'improvements' are made for her safety or her child's, and that preventive interferences are the doctor's way of turning sloppy old nature into a clean, safe science. He may explain that obstetrical science is simply a 'just-in-case' game of playing the odds in her favor: just in case you hemorrhage, we'll give you simulated hormones before you expel the placenta; just in case your perineum tears, we'll make a nice clean incision before delivery; just in case labor tires you out, we'll give you an early sedative; just in case you need general anesthesia (for an emergency Caesarean), we'll keep a vein open and stop you from eating and drinking throughout labor, even if it takes twenty-four hours; and just in case you totally lose control, we'll knock you out right now. Hearing this, the pregnant woman cannot help but believe that normal birth is loaded with unpredictable horrors that only her doctor can prevent.

"The result is that birthing mothers have given up their responsibility in *normal* birth to obstetricians, who have then turned the normal into the abnormal for the sake of preventive procedures, which in turn have caused greater (but more predictable) risks, and this in turn has required even more preventive technology to interfere further with what was once a natural and uncomplicated process requiring no interference at all."

CHILDBIRTH: Alternatives to Medical Control
Edited by Shelly Romalis
1982, 262 pages

from
University of Texas Press
Box 7812
Austin, TX 78712
$22.50 hd
$ 8.95 pap

This is an exceptionally fine collection of essays on birth in North America as it is affected by social, cultural, and political forces. Carefully edited and referenced, the book is more than a catalog of the ills of modern medical maternity care, but provides a framework for understanding the social context of birth and the history of the philosophies which are now so aggressively opposed. The conflict between physicians and women over who should control birth has now become so heated and so visible that it is of interest to the dissectors of society—sociologists and anthropologists—who attempt to bring their skills and insights to bear on the childbirth controversy as a cultural phenomenon.

"In spite of the widespread acceptance of childbirth preparation, in spite of the growing numbers of nurse-midwives, in spite of all the interior decorating of labor rooms, obstetrical intervention is increasing, not decreasing. Fetal monitoring has become routine in the few years since its introduction; the Caesarean section rate has gone up astronomically; epidural anesthesia is often considered a routine adjunct to Lamaze breathing techniques. One of the ways in which reform has been coopted stems from the focus on ambiance for the individual laboring woman rather than the principles of medical decision-making. Nowhere is this more clear than in the current management of Caesarean sections. The Caesarean section rate is at an all-time high in the United States, approaching 30 percent in some teaching hospitals. Concurrently, hospitals are starting to offer 'father-attended' Caesarean sections and spinal anesthesia, in the name of 'family-oriented' maternity care. Certainly this is progress for the individual woman having a Caesarean section. But is a warmer, cozier Caesarean section the real issue?"

from "Awake and Aware, or False Consciousness: The Cooption of Childbirth Reform in America" by Barbara Katz Rothman

BIRTH CONTROL AND CONTROLLING BIRTH: Women-Centered Perspectives
Edited by Helen B. Holmes, Betty B. Hoskins, and Michael Gross
1980, 338 pages, Illus.

from
The Humana Press
P.O. Box 2148
Clifton, NJ 07015
$14.95 hd
$ 7.95 pap

This book is based on talks presented at a conference on "Ethical Issues in Human Reproduction Technology" held in June, 1979, at Hampshire College in Amherst, Massachusetts. The participants are mainly feminist, consumer-oriented women who are active in the women's health movement. The first half of the book is devoted to issues in contraception. The second half includes presentations on childbirth technology and on the social control of childbirth, given by Norma Swenson, Dorothy Wertz, Yvonne Brackbill, David Banta, Ina May Gaskin, and others. The information on childbirth procedures and drugs will be useful for parents and childbirth teachers.

"The ethical issues in birth technology today center on two basic questions: 1) who should have the ultimate authority to make decisions and 2) should resources be used to provide high technology, such as fetal monitors, to everybody, or should there be a reallocation of resources toward providing basic care? The answer to these questions depends in part upon one's belief about nature. At the present there is a complete polarity between most of the obstetrical profession, which seeks greater safety through more crisis technology, and a radical group of families who wish to avoid the conventional medical system altogether and have their births at home.

"If this polarity is ever to be resolved, women and doctors are going to have to agree about whether birth is a natural process or a potential disease, and about what percentage of births is normal . . . . The problem is that medicine lost the sense of nature so long ago that it is going to be very difficult to regain it. There is very little research on normal birth outside the hospital environment. It is possible that we do not even know what normal birth is, aside from the elaborate structures that our technological culture has erected around it."

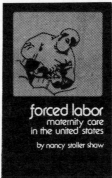

FORCED LABOR: Maternity Care in the United States
by Nancy Stoller Shaw
1974, 166 pages, Illus.

from
Pergamon Press
Maxwell House, Fairview Park
Elmsford, NY 10523
$9.75 pap.

As I write, Nancy Shaw is struggling to gain tenure in the sociology department at the University of California at Santa Cruz. At issue is whether her work, including this study of maternity care, is "theoretical" enough to be considered seriously by the sociology community. Women's studies and concerns are often put down in this way, but *Forced Labor* remains a very important and influential study of the way women receive care in the hospital. Shaw conducted her fieldwork for this study in 1967 at hospitals in the Northeast. She followed maternity patients through their prenatal care, labor, delivery and postpartum care, observing interactions between patients and care givers. Her conclusion is that hospital maternity care is systematically dehumanizing and relies

on medical monopoly, the specialization and fragmentation of care, the hospital setting itself, technology, and the staff's use of power and status to rob women of control in childbirth.

"The needs of the staff are for docile, willing patients, who allow them to keep the floor working smoothly, and the different components of the medical, nursing, administrative, and nursing staffs to all get their jobs accomplished with a minimum of conflict.

"The classifications of the patients have already been pointed out. Those who approximate the most desirable combination of social characteristics are treated most like humans; those who are similar to the least liked patient type are treated most like animals or non-persons. What is desirable or valuable to a doctor may not be so to a student nurse, although the basic positive orientation toward marriage, whiteness, education, Protestantism, and youth is shared by all. Part of the evaluation of patients is how much work they require; the easiest are the best liked. Physical effort is more tolerable than emotional output and interruptions in routine.

"The patient's contribution—passivity, aggression, or cooperation with her labor and the staff—also affects the extent of dehumanization in her new identity and treatment. As we shall see, the basic approach of the hospital to the laboring woman is to treat her as a child who neither understands herself nor can help herself. Occasionally, she may be handled and discussed as a pre-rational, dangerous animal. To recognize and treat her as an adult—with individual power over her self—is the hardest job of all."

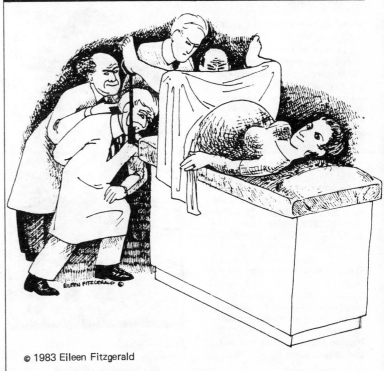

© 1983 Eileen Fitzgerald

MATERNITY CARE IN FERMENT:
Conflicting Issues
by The Maternity Center Association
Martin Kelly, editor
1980, 150 pages

from
Maternity Center Association
48 East 92nd Street
New York, NY 10028
$5.00 pap.

"Fifty distinguished professionals in medicine, public health, nurse-midwifery, nursing, and other fields, as well as . . . consumer representatives" met in a seminar to celebrate the 60th anniversary of the Maternity Center Association, and this book is based on a transcript of the proceedings. Included are talks, group reports, and discussions on technology and alternatives in maternity care, patient/provider relations, and health care delivery. The book will be mainly of interest and use for health care providers and planners.

"While the remarkable decline in mortality has been ascribed to the intervention of physicians, there's considerable question as to whether medicine can take any of the credit. True, the arrogant behavior of a Meigs, in deliberately walking with unwashed hands from the autopsy room to the delivery room, has disappeared. But that only means that doctor-borne diseases of that kind have been ended. There's only a statistical relationship, an association, between hospital deliveries, physician-assisted deliveries and the lowering of infant and maternal mortality. European experiences bear out the fact that higher standards of living and careful exclusion of high-risk cases can result in a remarkable lowering of infant and maternal mortality, even with home deliveries and midwifery.

"There's also some evidence that physicians in many instances do harm: the induction of labor, the uses of anesthesia, forceps, fetal monitoring—all carry added risk to the mother and child. Perhaps they have a place in obstetrics, but their use is too extravagant, too widespread, too uncontrolled. The rising caesarean rate is inexcusable. Concentration on technology diverts attention, money, and appropriate organized assistance from the generality of obstetrical care, continuing the scandalously differential rates of mortality among the poor and minorities."

from "Providing Choice in Childbirth" by George A. Silver, M.D.

Obstetrical Practices

SOME CONSEQUENCES OF OBSTETRICAL INTERFERENCE (1977)

THE INFLUENCE OF MATERNAL POSITION ON TIME OF SPONTANEOUS RUPTURE OF THE MEMBRANES, PROGRESS OF LABOR, AND FETAL HEAD COMPRESSION (1979)

THE INFLUENCE OF MATERNAL BEARING DOWN EFFORTS DURING SECOND STAGE ON FETAL WELL-BEING (1977)
by Roberto Caldeyro-Barcia
24 pages, Illus.

from
BIRTH Reprints
110 El Camino Real
Berkeley, CA 94705
$2.00

Roberto Caldeyro-Barcia is a past president of the International Federation of Gynecologists and Obstetricians and works with the World Health Organization in Uruguay. For many years he has studied the effects of obstetrical interference in the birth process, particularly the use of artificial rupture of the membranes, the lithotomy position, and too-vigorous maternal bearing-down efforts. Three of his papers on these subjects were published in BIRTH and are reprinted together along with letters to the editor from childbirth educators, physicians, and others. Readers will need to be familiar with some medical terms (vena cava, late deceleration, parietal and occipital bones, etc.) but in general these papers are an excellent introduction to the problem of *iatrogenic* or "doctor-caused" problems in birth.

"It is a fact that in the last forty years more artificial practices have been introduced which have changed labor from a physiological event into a very complicated medical procedure, in which all kinds of drugs and manoeuvers are done, sometimes unnecessarily. Many of them are potentially damaging for the baby and even for the mother."
(from *Some Consequences...*)

"As many people are aware, until late in the 18th Century most women in the world adopted an upright position during the first, second and third stages of labor. This might have been standing, sitting, kneeling or squatting, but always with the trunk more vertical than horizontal.
"In 1738, the French obstetrician, Francois Mauriceau, proposed the recumbant position in bed to replace the sitting position on the birth stool. Since Mauriceau was the obstetrician to the Queen of France, he was able to impose this position, which then became popular throughout Europe and spread across the Atlantic. According to the book of Mauriceau, the recumbent position was introduced to facilitate the management of labor by the accoucheur and NOT because it might be beneficial for the mother or the fetus. . . ."
(from *The Influence of Maternal Position. . .*)

"We have learned that we should recommend that parturient women be instructed to bear down as they feel the need, without trying to produce very strong or prolonged (longer than six seconds) efforts, and without complete closure of the glottis. The second stage of labor proceeds

"...artificial practices... have changed labor from a physiological event into a very complicated medical procedure..."

more slowly when the woman bears down in this way, but the fetus is in excellent condition. I do not see any reason for speeding up second stage when the fetus is handling it well. Another advantage to a longer second stage is that it gives the perineum more time to stretch slowly and the need for episiotomy is very markedly reduced."
(from *The Influence of Maternal Bearing-down Efforts . . .*)

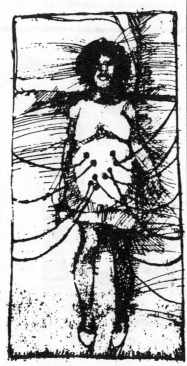

PEG AVERILL

THE CULTURAL WARPING OF CHILDBIRTH: A Special Report on U.S. Obstetrics
by Doris B. Haire
1972, 36 pages, Illus.

from
Int'l Childbirth Education Association
P.O. Box 20048
Minneapolis, MN 55420
$1.50 plus 1.00 postage

Doris Haire is a medical sociologist and well-known "fetal advocate" who has traveled throughout the world observing childbirth practices and has extensively studied the medical literature on common obstetrical practices. Her conclusion in this report is that most of the procedures being used in American maternity hospitals have not been scientifically proven safe or necessary in the management of normal labor and that most are, in fact, harmful. Her list of harmful or unnecessary procedures includes the following:

1. Withholding information on the disadvantages of obstetrical medication.
2. Ambivalent prenatal counseling on breast-feeding.
3. Permitting the mother to face childbirth uninformed of ways in which she can help herself to cope with the discomfort of labor and birth.
4. Requiring all normal women to give birth in the hospital.
5. Elective induction of labor.
6. Separating the mother from familial support during the labor and birth.
7. Confining the normal laboring woman to bed.
8. Shaving the birth area.
9. Withholding food and drink from the normal unmedicated woman in labor.
10. Professional dependence on technology and pharmacological methods of pain relief.
11. Chemical stimulation of labor.
12. Moving the normal mother to a delivery room for birth.
13. Delaying birth until the physician arrives.
14. Requiring the mother to assume the lithotomy position for birth.
15. The routine use of regional or general anesthesia for delivery.
16. Fundal pressure to facilitate delivery.
17. The routine use of forceps for delivery.
18. Routine episiotomy.
19. Early clamping or "milking" of the umbilical cord.
20. Routine suctioning with a nasogastric tube.
21. Apgar scoring by the accoucheur.
22. Obstetrical intervention in placental expulsion.
23. Separating the mother from her newborn infant.
24. Delaying the first breast-feeding.
25. Offering water and formula to the breast-fed newborn infant.
26. Restricting newborn infants to a four hour feeding schedule and withholding night time feedings.
27. Preventing early father-child contact.
28. Assigning nursing personnel to mothers or to babies (rather than to mother-baby couples).
29. Restricting intermittent rooming-in to specific room requirements.
30. Restricting sibling visitation.

For each of the practices listed above, Haire provides a brief discussion of the harmful effects and concludes with a listing of 102 medical references to support her opinion. This report was published by ICEA as a booklet in 1972 and I obtained a copy in 1976 while planning the birth of my first child. The report became the conclusive factor in my decision to give birth at home.

"According to the National Association for Retarded Children there are now 6,000,000 retarded children in the United States with a predicted annual increase of over 100,000 a year. The number of children and adults with behavioral difficulties or perceptual dysfunction resulting from minimal brain damage is an ever growing challenge to society and to the economy. While it may be easier on the conscience to blame such numbing facts solely on socioeconomic factors and birth defects recent research makes it evident that obstetrical medication can play a role in our staggering incidence of neurological impairment. It may be convenient to blame our relatively poor infant outcome on a lack of facilities or inadequate government funding, but it is obvious from the research being carried out that we could effect an immediate improvement in infant outcome by changing the pattern of obstetrical care in the United States. It is time that we take a good look at the overall experience of childbirth in this country and begin to recognize how our culture has warped this experience for the majority of American mothers and their new-born infants."

COSTS AND BENEFITS OF ELECTRONIC FETAL MONITORING: A REVIEW OF THE LITERATURE

by David Banta and Stephen Thacker
April, 1979, 31 pages,
(DHHS Pub. No. (PHS) 79-3245)

from
National Center for Health Services Research, Publications and Information Branch
3700 East-West Highway, Rm. 7-44
Hyattsville, MD 20782
single copy free

This report was prepared for the National Center for Health Services Research (NCHSR) by David Banta, M.D., of the Office of Technology Assessment and Stephen Thacker, M.D., of the Center for Disease Control. In brief, the authors conclude that there is no evidence to show that electronic fetal monitoring (EFM) is of any benefit in low-risk labors, but that the risks of EFM are substantial, including an association with increased rates of cesarean section. The report covers the history of fetal monitoring, the accuracy (or inaccuracy) of current EFM methods, the impact of EFM on infant and maternal outcome, the risks to mother and fetus, costs of EFM, and projections for the future. A list of 296 references is included. This landmark report has caused professional and consumer organizations alike to issue revised policy statements on the use of EFM.

"Replacing nursing care with electronic devices could be expected to produce negative reactions. Haverkamp *et. al.*, noted: 'Very close physical contact with the patient was necessary for the nurse to auscultate fetal heart tones adequately. This was not true to the same degree with the monitored group. Nursing attention to the gravida with respect to maternal comfort, emotional support, and "laying on of hands" could have a significant impact on the fetus. . . . The authors have the impression that the reassuring psychological atmosphere created by personal nurse interaction and the absence of the recording machine in auscultated patients contributed to the excellent infant outcome in auscultated patients.' Indeed, a growing minority of women are demanding delivery without interference and are turning to midwives and home delvery to find such human support...

"Careful review of the literature indicates little increased benefit from EFM compared to auscultation. This is not surprising, given the lack of precision of EFM for the diagnosis of fetal distress, and the general difficulty in separating normal fetal stress during labor from fetal distress. If EFM has benefit, it appears to be for low birth weight infants, but no RCT (randomized, controlled, clinical trial) of its use in this group has been carried out.

ELECTRONIC FETAL MONITORING

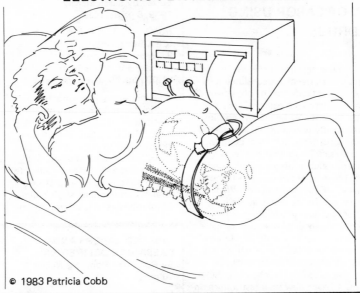

© 1983 Patricia Cobb

LISTENING AS A FETUS BECOMES A BABY

by Earl B. Abrams
1979, 4 pages, Illus.
(HHS Pub. No. (FDA) 80-4019)

from
Food and Drug Administration
Office of Public Affairs
5600 Fishers Lane
Rockville, MD 20857
single copy free

This reprint from the September 1979 issue of *FDA Consumer* discusses the controversy over the use of electronic fetal monitoring for low-risk mothers. One of the important reasons why EFM is used routinely in hospitals, despite its problems, is that hospitals don't have enough staff to provide careful, continuous personal monitoring of laboring women using a stethoscope or fetoscope. The article also points out that EFM is an ultrsound device and that the FDA has doubts about the safety of ultrasound use.

"On the negative side, the mother may feel highly restricted by all the attachments, and the relative immobility imposed by the monitoring devices can itself lead to complications. Also, the mechanical, depersonalized aspect of the internal devices may cause the mother to become depressed or afraid. In addition, there is a risk of infection. And artificially rupturing the amniotic sac can require additional medical or surgical measures, creating otherwise avoidable complications."

"The risk from EFM is substantial, especially but not wholly through the increased CSR (cesarean section rate) that its use apparently engenders. We estimate the addition to the annual cost of childbirth to be $411 million if 50 per cent of deliveries are monitored electronically."

ICEA POSITION STATEMENT ON ELECTRONIC FETAL MONITORING

(*ICEA News*, Vol. 20:4, November 1981, 3 pages)

from
Int'l Childbirth Education Association
P.O. Box 20048
Minneapolis, MN 55420
$1.00 plus 60 cents postage for back issues of *ICEA News*

ICEA has studied the use of electronic fetal monitoring (EFM) and developed the position that "EFM should not be a routine procedure and should be avoided unless indicated by a specific medical condition." Their position paper includes a discussion of the technique of EFM, cost-benefit factors, use in high-risk cases, accuracy, effect on cesarean rate, psychological responses to EFM, complications, and alternatives. A list of 24 references is included.

"The proper clinical management of women who are not monitored electronically in labor should always include periodic auscultation (use of stethoscope or fetoscope) by the nurse, midwife, or physician. The Task Force on Predictors of Fetal Distress confirms that this is an 'acceptable' method of determining the condition of the fetus for low-risk women and emphasizes that in no way should EFM use 'be a substitute for clinical judgement.' If a woman chooses not to use EFM, which is her legal right, she should discuss the matter with her birth practitioner well in advance of the expected birth.

"It has been suggested that if staff limitation preclude periodic auscultations as stated here, parents may consider hiring a highly trained special duty nurse or monitrice to perform the job."

THE NURSES' ROLE IN ELECTRONIC FETAL MONITORING

NAACOG Technical Bulletin No. 7
July 1980, 6 pages

from
Nurses Association of the American College of Obstetricians and Gynecologists (NAACOG)
600 Maryland Ave., SW, Suite 200
Washington, DC 20024
$2.00 plus 50 cents postage
request complete publications list

This technical bulletin outlines the nurses' role in interpreting fetal heart rate patterns, and in providing care to the monitored woman. The bulletin acknowledges the controversy over routine use of EFM and stresses the importance of nurses' education and skill in making EFM more accurate.

"The nursing care of a monitored patient is essentially the same care given any patient during labor, with a few additional considerations for those factors relating directly to the monitor. How you integrate a machine (the EFM) into the intimate, emotional, and stress-producing aspects of labor and delivery is important. The nurse needs to be sure that the monitor does not receive more care than the patient."

THE CURRENT ROLE OF CONTINUOUS ELECTRONIC FETAL HEART RATE MONITORING IN LABOR

(ACOG Committee Statement)
March 1979, 4 pages

from
Resource Center
The American College of Obstetricians and Gynecologists
600 Maryland Ave., SW No. 300
Washington, DC 20024
free

In response to "numerous controversial reports on the efficacy of electronic fetal monitoring (EFM) the ACOG Committee on Obstetrics: Maternal and Fetal Medicine considered the question and issued this "state-of-the-art opinion." The Committee concluded that the available literature showed some benefit of EFM for "high-risk" patients and no benefit for "low-risk" patients. The committee felt that possible benefit in low-risk cases would be difficult to assess, however, "since fetal demise during labor is such a rare event (1-5/1000 term infants), it would require many thousands of patients in experimental and control groups to demonstrate a benefit of continuous EFM if mortality alone is used as an endpoint." The Committee recommends that "the physician and/or patient may choose to use continuous EFM even in low risk situations." The risks of EFM are defined as "minimal" and are not discussed.

ELECTIVE INDUCTION OF LABOR USING OXYTOCIC DRUGS

On June 21, 1978, the FDA's advisory committee on Fertility and Maternal Health Drugs held hearings to consider the use of oxytocic drugs for the elective induction of labor. Doris Haire, representing both ICEA and the National Women's Health Network, was among those who testified about the dangers of induced labors, including the risk of prematurity, greater incidence of prolapsed cord, and increased risk of fetal hypoxia (lack of oxygen). She said,

"It is unfortunate that few Americans outside of, and many within the obstetric specialty, realize the relationship between the use of oxytocic drugs (which are uterine stimulants) and the oxygenation of the fetal brain. During a normal contraction the contracting uterus constricts, or 'pinches off,' the blood vessels which pass through the uterine muscle wall as they carry the mother's oxygenated blood to the placenta. Despite this constriction of the blood vessels, the oxygen supply from the mother's circulation to the fetus usually remains at a relatively constant, normal level and the fetal heartrate remains essentially unchanged. This occurs because nature has provided a protective biologic mechanism whereby an extra supply of the mother's oxygenated blood is 'stored up' in the intervillous space of the placenta during the intervals *between* contractions. This storing-up process can only take place when the maternal blood is flowing freely to the placenta. During the next contraction the oxygen from the stored reserve of maternal blood is transferred to the fetal bloodstream as needed.

"Normal uterine contractions vary in their frequency and intensity during labor. There appears to be a biochemical interaction between the maternal and fetal physiology which regulates the frequency and intensity of the uterine contractions to meet the oxygen needs of the fetus. The administration of synthetic oxytocin can interfere with this protective mechanism."

Dr. Lewis Sullivan, representing the American Society for Psychoprophylaxis in Obstetrics, also testified, saying:

"The term 'elective induction' refers to artificially starting labor, in the absence of any medical condition requiring such an action, with resultant vaginal delivery of the fetus. While there are many justifications given for elective inductions, there is general agreement that as currently practiced, the major considerations are convenience for the physician and sociopsychologic pressures from the patient. While there is nothing inherently wrong with these reasons, the procedure itself must be shown to be safe for mother and fetus to justify such arbitrary action. One of the most ancient axioms in medicine is 'First, do no harm.' We feel that experience with elective inductions using oxytocic drugs as reflected in the medical literature reveal the procedure to be dangerous and fraught with hazards which far outweigh any potential benefits."

As a result of this hearing, the FDA issued new label restrictions on the use of injectable oxytocin (oxytocin given by mouth is no longer acceptable), which were published in the October/November 1978 issue of *FDA Drug Bulletin*. The revised product labeling alerts doctors that oxytocic drugs should no longer be used for elective induction of labor.

Using an oxytocic drug, like Pitocin, is now an "unapproved use" of an approved drug. A physician who does this may be more vulnerable to a charge of medical malpractice if mother or baby are harmed. Unfortunately, in spite of the new labeling, elective induction using oxytocic drugs is still common. An acquaintance of mine recently gave birth to her first child on a Christmas eve and wondered why she was the only occupant of the maternity floor. "Oh, all the other girls had themselves induced," said a nurse, "so they and their doctors could be home for Christmas."

MORE RESOURCES ON INDUCTION

BENEFITS AND HAZARDS OF THE NEW OBSTETRICS
T. Chard and M. Richards, eds.
1978, Lippincott Co.

INDUCTION OF LABOR WITH OXYTOCIN: Effects on the Fetus
ICEA Review
c/o ICEA Bookcenter
P.O. Box 20048
Minneapolis, MN 55420
$1.00 plus 60 cents postage

THE DIGNITY OF LABOUR?: A Study of Childbearing and Induction
by Ann Cartwright
1979, Tavistock Publications
(distributed in the U.S. by Methuen)

AMNIOTOMY
Edited by Susan McKay
1979, 8 pages, Illus.

from
ICEA Bookcenter
P.O. Box 20048
Minneapolis, MN 55420
$1.00 plus 60 cents postage

Amniotomy is the practice of artificially rupturing the amniotic membranes (bag of waters) during labor. The procedure is done to induce labor to start, to "speed along" an established labor, and more commonly today, to allow for attachment of an internal electronic fetal monitor to the baby's scalp. Amniotomy is virtually routine in American hospitals, yet the studies abstracted in this issue of *ICEA Review* (Summer, 1979) show that amniotomy can cause many adverse effects, including abnormal dips in fetal heart rate during labor, abnormal molding of the baby's head, reduction in fetal oxygen and blood supply, and an increased risk of postpartum infection. In his concluding commentary, Dr. Ricardo Schwarcz, of the World Health Organization, argues that artificial rupture of the membranes should not be done in normal labors, or at least not until the first stage of labor is complete and the birth of the baby is imminent.

INDUCED LABORS AND CAESARIAN DELIVERIES
By Rosemary Romberg Wiener
10 pages

from
Rosemary Romberg Wiener
6294 Mission Road
Everson, WA 98247
45 cents plus business size self-addressed stamped envelope
bulk rates available

This two part information "handout" discusses the use of induced labor and cesarean section when labor does not progress normally. In simple lay terms, Weiner describes the commonly used techniques for inducing labor, including "stripping the membranes," rupturing the membranes (amniotomy), the use of an oxytocic drug, and "home remedies" for inducing labor including castor oil, enema, and herbs. She discusses the reasons for inducing labor and the special management of artificially induced or augmented labors, including the use of electronic fetal monitoring,

INDUCTION OF LABOR
(NAACOG Technical Bulletin No. 4)
1979, 4 pages

from
Nurses Association of the American College of Obstetricians and Gynecologists (NAACOG)
600 Maryland Ave., SW, Suite 200
Washington, DC 20024
$2.00 plus 50 cents postage
request complete publications list

This bulletin is intended to provide labor and delivery nurses with guidelines for assisting with the induction of labor, either by amniotomy or use of intravenous oxytocin drip. The bulletin describes how the procedures are to be carried out and how to handle complications of induction, which are listed as 1) prolapsed umbilical cord, 2) fetal hypoxia, 3) precipitate labor, and 4) rupture of the uterus.

Stimulating a Slow Labor —alternatives to pitocin

Cooperate with your body
- *identify and overcome inhibitions to giving birth*

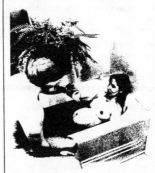

Take a warm bath or shower

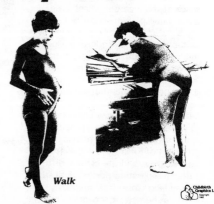

Walk

Create a non-stressful atmosphere with guaranteed privacy for ½ hour or more
- *kissing and cuddling, nipple stimulation*
- *massage and relaxation techniques*

MATERNAL POSITION

MATERNAL POSITION DURING LABOR AND BIRTH
Edited by Susan McKay
1978, 8 pages

from
ICEA Bookcenter
P.O. Box 20048
Minneapolis, MN 55420
$1.00 plus 60 cents postage
bulk rates available

Sitting, squatting, standing, and kneeling are the common "natural" positions for childbirth in our species. Only under physician care and only in recent decades have women been required to lie down on their backs for delivery. The supine position is more convenient and power-enhancing for the doctor, but has serious adverse effects on the mother and baby, including supine hypotension (lowered blood pressure) and reduced blood and oxygen supply to the fetus. This issue of *ICEA Review* (Summer, 1978) examines the question of maternal position and includes abstracts of eight papers from the medical literature, in general showing the advantages of the upright position for labor and delivery.

"Disadvantages of the dorsal position during labor and birth have been recognized for some time. However, the following event is still commonly observed when a woman in active labor is admitted to the labor room, routinely placed on an external fetal monitor, and immobilized flat on her back to obtain an optimal tracing:
"The nurse may, after noticing an abnormality in the tracing, ask her to turn to her side. The monitor then returns to recording normal tracings and is credited with preventing an abnormality that would probably not have existed if the woman had been allowed the freedom of assuming whatever position she felt was comfortable."

THE RISKS AND BENEFITS OF EPISIOTOMY: A REVIEW
by David Banta and Stephen B. Thacker
(*BIRTH*, Vol. 9:1, Spring 1982)
6 pages, Illus.

from
BIRTH
110 El Camino Real
Berkeley, CA 94705
$4.00, single issue copy

Banta and Thacker's first study in the area of obstetrics concerned electronic fetal monitoring (see index). They now turn their attention to episiotomy, as an example of a "low-capital" procedure which is done "at great expense for uncertain benefit." Episiotomy involves cutting through the perineal tissue to enlarge the vaginal opening during birth. It is "the second most common surgical procedure done in the United States after cutting the umbilical cord." Banta and Thacker review the history of the procedure and the current medical literature and find that there is no data to support the claims made for benefits from routine episiotomy (these include ease of repair, fewer third-degree lacerations, prevention of fetal brain damage, and prevention of pelvic relaxation). A list of 44 references is included.

". . . episiotomies are done frequently in the United States despite the absence of data to support such routine use. Moreover, there are significant risks associated with episiotomy that have not been adequately studied. What, then, is an optimal episiotomy rate for the United States? In birthing centers where nurse-midwives have primary responsibility, the episiotomy rate runs between 15-25 percent, with rates of third-degree lacerations of 3-4 percent and rates for first-or-second-degree lacerations requiring repair of 25-30 percent. In the absence of better data, our judgment is that the U.S. episiotomy rate could be reduced by more than half without causing harm to either mothers or babies . . . ."

BRAIN DAMAGE BY ASPHYXIA AT BIRTH
by William F. Windle
1969, 10 pages, Illus.

from
Scientific American Offprints
W.H. Freeman and Co.
660 Market Street
San Francisco, CA 94104
$. 60 each
request complete catalog

William Windle, a researcher at New York University Medical Center, subjected newborn rhesus monkeys to artificial asphyxia by reducing thei their supply of oxygen during birth. He then observed the results on their behavior and later autopsied the monkeys to examine their brains. Windle found that even in monkeys who had been asphyxiated for very short periods, required no resuscitation, and appeared to be normal, there was "minimal" structural brain damage. He concludes that human infants may be similarly damaged by asphyxia at birth and notes that certain obstetrical practices contribute to asphyxia, especially the practice of giving birth in the supine position (lying on the back), and the practice of rapidly clamping the umbilical cord before the placenta has delivered.
"The monkey experiments described in this article have taught us that birth asphyxia lasting long enough to make resuscitation necessary always damages the brain. This could be proved, however, only by histological examination. A great many human infants have to be resuscitated at birth. We assume that their brains too have been damaged. There is reason to believe that the number of human beings in the U.S. with minimal brain damage due to asphyxia at birth is much larger than has been thought. Need this continue to be so? Perhaps it is time to reexamine current practices of childbirth with a view to avoiding conditions that give rise to asphyxia and brain damage."

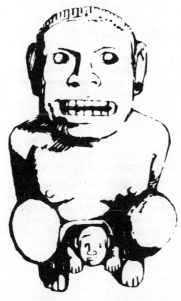

Ixcuina, the Aztec goddess of childbirth, in the physiological squatting position for birth.

EPISIOTOMY

EPISIOTOMY: Physical and Emotional Aspects
Edited by Sheila Kitzinger
1981, 55 pages

from
National Childbirth Trust (publisher)
Birth & Life Bookstore (order source)
P.O. Box 70625
Seattle, WA 98107
$5.00 plus 1.00 postage

This booklet presents eight papers by English midwives and physicians and American psychologists, edited by Sheila Kitzinger for the National Childbirth Trust (9 Queensborough Terrace, London W2 3TB, England). The authors question the routine use of episiotomy for childbirth and discuss how to manage delivery to minimize perineal tears, how to perform an episiotomy so that it heals better and with less discomfort, and how to educate birthing women about their pelvic floor muscles and about post-episiotomy sexual adjustment. Written in research paper format, the booklet includes illustrations of the repair of a midline episiotomy incision, tables of research results, and references.
"The second stage of labour should be conducted with the objective of retaining an intact perineum—or at most only minimal lacerations.
"The most important factors in making this likely are a peaceful atmosphere, education of the mother, self-control and skilful (sic) verbal encouragement on the part of whoever is delivering the baby." (Chloe Fisher)

SOME WOMEN'S EXPERIENCES OF EPISIOTOMY
by Sheila Kitzinger with Rhiannon Walters
1981, 20 pages

from
National Childbirth Trust (publisher)
Birth & Life Bookstore (order source)
P.O. Box 70625
Seattle, WA 98107
$2.00 plus 1.00 postage

Sheila Kitzinger and her research assistant, Rhiannon Walters, have conducted a preparatory study of 1,795 English women to find out how women experience episiotomy and its subsequent discomfort and how episiotomy women compare with those who had tears or no injury to the perineum. Results are presented through personal comments from mothers, tables, and discussion. References are included.
" 'I found the after-effects of the stitches the most draining part of childbirth. I felt full of energy and completely well just after the birth, a bit tired when the milk came in, but when my stitches began to hurt I started to feel very tired and limp.' "
"Episiotomy causes women often unnecessary pain at and following delivery. It does not, despite claims to the contrary, avoid tears, does not improve the condition of the perineum in the weeks following childbirth, may interfere with the mother's initial relationship with her baby and the start of breastfeeding and can adversely affect the couple's sexual relationship for a long time after."

Drugs in Labor

by Susan Ritchie

The following tables describe the effects of some of the most commonly used drugs in labor and delivery. It is important to note that most drugs given to pregnant women cross the placenta and may be present in the baby at birth. The ability to excrete these drugs varies from mother to mother and from infant to infant. These tables describe only drugs used in labor and delivery and not during the nine months of pregnancy. See index for information on medications and their effects during pregnancy. If you are taking any medications during pregnancy and/or have any physical conditions such as asthma, diabetes, etc., different effects than those described below may occur. Explore this further with your doctor, midwife, or birth attendant. Remember that all medications must be selected and used properly and judiciously, if they are used at all.

Definitions:

CNS depression = central nervous system depression, i.e., lessening of brain activity

Vasomotor depression = decrease in circulation, decrease of blood pressure caused by dilated blood vessels.

All medications are listed by their generic names (general chemical or common name). Trade names are given in parenthesis.

SEDATIVES

Medications which exert a soothing or tranquilizing effect: e.g. alcohol, meprobromate, barbiturates.

Examples of Barbiturates

Pentobarbitol sodium (Nembutal)
Secobarbital (Seconal)
Amobarbital (Amytal)
Phenobarbital (Luminal Sodium)

Use

To relieve anxiety and promote sleep in early or false labor. (Note: these should *not* be used within one to two hours of delivery. Also, barbiturates do not lessen the strength or frequency of contractions appreciably.)

Possible Adverse Effects

To Mother—Do not cause amnesia but may confuse or distort recollection; possible respiratory and vasomotor depression; may have hangover feeling.

To Baby—Possible respiratory and vasomotor depression; may have transient effect on baby's ability to regulate temperature and suck; if used late in first stage or early in second stage, may cause severe CNS depression; Brackbill and Broman have found that use of Seconal is associated with behavioral effects such as hypoactivity and low emotional reactivity in four and seven year olds.

NARCOTIC ANALGESICS
Medications which relieve pain

Examples

Morphine—most potent in general use

Meperidine (Demerol)—intermediate potency

Codeine—least potent

Use

For pain relief, sedation and rest. No amnesic effects. Within 15 minutes after an intramuscular injection the maximal effect of most narcotic analgesics is felt: effect lasts about two hours. (Note: Sizable doses should not be given within one to two hours of delivery. Also, none should be given after full dilation in a first time mother or after 7-8 centimeters dilation in a multipara.)

Possible Adverse Effects

To Mother—may cause nausea, vomiting, lightheadedness and dizziness. The drug manufacturers advise that women given these medications should lie down to minimize the above problems. Also, respiratory depression, constipation, urinary retention, decreased blood pressure, shock.

To Baby—depression of respiration, may require resuscitation. Brackbill and Broman have found that Demerol is related to increased failures on relatively difficult test items on the Stanford Binet IQ test and on some fine motor tests at four years of age, and to lower scores on spelling and reading achievement tests at seven years. (Note: there are narcotic antagonist drugs available which can reverse the narcotic effects of the above medications. If labor is more rapid than expected one of these drugs will help reduce respiratory depression in the baby. Examples: Nalorphine [Nalline], Levallorphan [Lorfan], Naloxane [Narcan].)

ANALGESIC POTENTIATING DRUGS (ATARACTICS)

Examples

Promazine (Sparine)
Hydroxyzine pamoate (Vistaril)
Promethazine (Phenergan)

Use

To add to desirable effects of analgesics, decrease undesirable effects. Prevent and/or control nausea and vomiting.

Possible Adverse Effects

To Mother—Impair alertness, increase drowsiness, increase dryness of mouth, increase or decrease blood pressure, create sensitivity to light.

To Baby—Brackbill and Broman have found that Phenergan is associated with lower verbal IQ scores and achievement test scores in seven-year-olds.

AMNESICS
Medications which cause loss of memory.

Example
Scopolamine

Use

To inhibit secretions. reduce excitement and produce amnesia in preparation for general anesthesia. Scopolamine has no analgesic effect, so an analgesic is usually given along with it.

Possible Adverse Effects

To Mother—may *cause* excitement, hallucinations, possibly delirium. Almost no recall of recent events. Dryness of mouth and throat. Urinary retention. Increased heart rate.

To Baby—decreased oxygen to baby, making fetal monitoring essential. Brackbill and Broman found same effects as for Demerol; also associated with lower IQ scores on the WISC (Wexler Intelligence Scale for Children), lower scale scores on information comprehension, vocabulary, and block structures.

REGIONAL ANESTHESIA
Medications which cause loss of sensation in certain parts of the body.

Use

For local pain relief in labor and delivery, for repair of episiotomy. (Note: resuscitative equipment and drugs should be readily available when any local anesthetic is used.)

Examples

Procaine (Novocain)
Tetracaine (Pontocaine)
Mepivacine (Carbocaine)
Lidocaine (Xylocaine)
Bupivacaine (Marcaine)

Possible Adverse Effects

To Mother—nervousness, dizziness, blurred vision, tremors, drowsiness, convulsions, unconsciousness, respiratory arrest, decreased blood pressure, cardiac arrest.

To Baby—respiratory depression, decreased heart rate, fetal distress. Brackbill and Broman have found that inhalant plus conduction (regional) anesthesia is related to lower reading scores in seven-year-olds.

Types of Regional Anesthesia

● *Paracervical Block:* Used after the cervix is greater than 5 but less than 8 centimeters dilated. Used for pain relief in lower uterus, cervix and upper vagina. Little or no effect on labor. Adverse effects as above. Procaine (Novocain) is often used for this block. Bupivacaine should not be used for this block as it can lead to fetal distress.

● *Pudendal Block:* Done during second stage as presenting part descends through cervix. Eliminates vaginal and perineal sensation. (Note: the bearing-down reflex is lessened or lost with this block.)

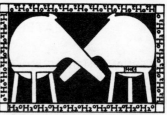

● *Spinal Anesthesia* (Saddle Block): Used to alleviate pain during late first stage and all of second stage. Mother remains conscious, however she cannot feel contractions, so must be told when to bear down, etc. Episiotomy and low forceps will be used for delivery. Increases tendency for bladder and uterine atony, also headache. Novocain or Pontocaine often used.

● *Epidural (including Caudal) Anesthesia:* Used during well-established first stage and second stage to alleviate pain. Mother remains conscious, muscle relaxation achieved, headaches rarely occur. However, mother will need coaching regarding when to push as she cannot feel the contractions. Episiotomy and low forceps used at delivery. Occasionally depression of contractions may result. (Note: special training and experience are required to administer epidural anesthesia.) Bupivacaine often used.

GENERAL ANESTHESIA
Medication which affects entire body; person is unconscious

Intravenous Anesthetic Drugs
Not used in delivery because they cross the placenta very rapidly.

Inhalation Anesthetic Drugs
Halothane (Fluothane)—most potent inhalation anesthetic. Must be administered by an anesthesiologist. Increases risk of postpartum hemorrhage because it relaxes uterus so much; also can be toxic to liver and heart of mother.

Cyclopropane—very explosive; must be administered by an anesthesiologist; may cause nausea, vomiting, heart rhythm irregularities.

Ethyl ether—hazardous, should not be used.

Combination Anesthesia for C-Sections

A combination of thiopental, nitrous oxide-oxygen, succinylcholine. An anesthesiologist must administer it; good tolerance and rapid resuscitation of mother and baby reported.

No drugs are *necessary* for the conduct of normal labor. The drugs listed above are used to alleviate pain and anxiety, but do not improve the medical outcome of the pregnancy. Women who are prepared for labor through education about its processes and the use of relaxation techniques, can learn to cope with the normal pain of labor without using drugs.

HOW THE FDA DETERMINES THE "SAFETY" OF DRUGS—JUST HOW SAFE IS "SAFE"?
by Doris Haire
1980, 8 pages

from
American Foundation for Maternal and Child Health
30 Beekman Place
New York, NY 10022
$1.00

This report is so important that I am listing it twice in this *Catalog* (for review in the section on Drugs and Other Hazards, see index). Following is a press release issued by the American Foundation for Maternal and Child Health (AFMCH) concerning this report:

"A new report, *How the FDA Determines the 'Safety' of Drugs— Just How Safe is 'Safe'?*, was the focus of a Congressional hearing on July 30th (1981). The investigation arm of the House Committee on the Science and Technology held the hearing to question various experts as to the adequacy of the testing methods used to evaluate the effects on the child's subsequent neurological development of drugs used in obstetrics. All agreed that none of the drugs used in obstetric care today have been subjected to a well controlled, scientific evaluation and found to be safe in regard to the neurological development of the child exposed to the drugs in utero.

The report went unchallenged in its contentions that:

● FDA ignores its own guidelines for evaluating the neurotoxicity of obstetric drugs
● Most health professionals do not know how to tell from the package insert whether or not a drug has been approved by the FDA as safe for use in obstetrics
● FDA fails to make it clear that a 'Usage in Pregnancy (or Obstetrics)' section in the package insert does not indicate FDA approval for that use
● Less than a dozen drugs have been approved by the FDA as safe for use in obstetrics
● FDA permits manufacturers to use evasive wording in the package insert—wording which implies safety for the child when no such evidence exists
● The most dangerous adverse effects of obstetric drugs are frequently omitted from the package insert or are buried in inappropriate sections
● FDA's new Pregnancy Categories A, B, C, D and X for obstetric-related drugs are vague and misleading

"The report, written for consumers, places particular emphasis on teaching expectant parents how to identify those drugs which have or have not been approved by the FDA for obstetric use. As a result of the Congressional hearing and the broad distribution of the new report, an increasing number of women will undoubtedly question the safety of drugs offered to them during labor and delivery."

MEDICATIONS USED DURING LABOR AND BIRTH: A Resource for Childbirth Educators
by Avis J. Ericson
1978, 36 pages

from
Int'l Childbirth Education Association
P.O. Box 20048
Minneapolis, MN 55420
$3.00 plus $1.00 postage
bulk rates available

This very useful booklet begins with a discussion of the use of medication in labor and the mechanism of effects on the fetus (placental transfer, absorption, metabolism, etc.). It goes on to describe in detail the dose, use, maternal side effects, labor side effects, placental transfer, and fetal or newborn side effects of over 50 commonly used drugs (both generic and brand names are given). Included are: sedatives, tranquilizers, analgesics, narcotic antagonists, local anesthetics, anticholinergics, induction agents, inhalation agents, oxytocics, and lactation suppressants. There is also a section on administration techniques and on methods for discussing labor medication with prospective parents.

"Much of the public has been lulled into a false sense of security regarding drugs. Merely because a drug is available for use does not mean it is safe and carries no hazard to mother or child. Indeed, the American Academy of Pediatrics' Committee on Drugs has warned that there is *no* drug which has been proven safe for the unborn child. The Food and Drug Administration (FDA), responsible for drug approval in the United States, presently has no regulations regarding drugs and the childbearing woman.

"Prior to the FDA's 1962 amendments to the Food, Drug, and Cosmetic Act, approval for marketing new drugs was relatively easy. Testing for fetal and neonatal effects was not required. Since that time, there have not been any systematic attempts by the FDA or drug manufacturers to gather the information necessary to establish or refute short-term and long-term safety. The majority of medications used during labor and birth were marketed prior to the 1962 amendments."

"To generate discussion on medications, some instructors request that during the coming week, couples ask physicians their views on medication, what ones they are likely to use, if any, etc., and report back at the next class. Discussion is then drawn from their comments, and the responsibility of discussing the topic with the physician prior to the onset of labor is underscored."

MEDICATION CHART
Compiled by Betsy K. Adrian and Nada Logan Stotland, M.D.
20" x 18"

from
American Society for Psychoprophylaxis in Obstetrics (ASPO)
1411 K Street, NW, Suite 200
Washington, DC 20005
$2.00 each, $80.00 for 50

This over-sized chart is designed for use by childbirth educators. It describes briefly the effects of commonly used drugs in labor and delivery, including general and regional anesthesia, sedatives, tranquilizers, amnesics, and analgesics. Parameters listed include therapeutic effect, effect on labor, side effects on mother and fetus or newborn, placental transfer, and methods of administration.

EPIDURAL ANALGESIA
Edited by Rosemary Cogan
1981, 8 pages, Illus.

from
Int'l Childbirth Education Association
P.O Box 20048
Minneapolis, MN 55420
$1.00 plus .60 postage

Epidural block is one of the newer forms of anesthesia for childbirth. It is done by injecting a local anesthetic drug between the vertebrae of the lower back, into the epidural space of the spinal column. In some cases it can provide complete relief from labor pain, but critics are concerned about harmful side effects to mother and baby. This issue of *ICEA Review* (August, 1981) examines the controversy by abstracting 13 papers on the subject.

BRACKBILL-BROMAN REPORT

"Because of . . . inherent difficulties no completely safe and satisfactory method of pain relief in obstetrics has yet been developed." So states the current edition of *Williams' Obstetrics,* a widely used medical textbook. And yet, because the burden of proof has historically rested with consumers to prove that drugs are unsafe, rather than with pharmaceutical companies and doctors to prove that they are safe, many drugs being used for pain relief in labor have never been tested or proven safe for use with women in labor and their effects on children are not known. The Food and Drug Administration (FDA) is charged with the responsibility of regulating drugs, including those used in childbirth. However, as recent controversies over the use of birth control pills, estrogens, caffeine, etc., have shown, the FDA may not always regulate in the best interest of the public.

On March 20, 1979, the Anesthetic and Life Support Drug Advisory Committee of the FDA met for the first time to discuss the as yet unpublished study by Drs. Yvonne Brackbill and Sarah H. Broman on obstetrical medication and its effect on child development in the first year of life. The task of the committee, composed entirely of surgeons and anesthesiologists, was to decide whether labelling and physician package inserts for obstetrical drugs should be revised to reflect the finding of the Brackbill-Broman study that such medications have negative short-term and long-term effects on children.

Speaking before the committee, Dr. Brackbill (of the Department of Psychology, University of Florida) emphasized four points from the study: 1) obstetric drugs have negative effects on child behavior, 2) these effects are related to the drug dosage, 3) drug effects are most noticeable when children attempt difficult tasks, and 4) drug effects do not tend to disappear with age. Dr. Brackbill noted that, contrary to popular perception, the use of obstetrical medication in this country is *increasing*, and urged the committee to revise the labeling for obstetric drugs to reflect the findings of the literature.

This presentation touched off a controversy which is continuing. Members of the committee and others in the medical profession were extremely critical of Brackbill for making her results available to the public before the study had been accepted for publication in a medical journal. Critics feared that women might refuse to accept medication or "necessary" cesareans if they had access to revised information of the risks of drug use in labor. One physician characterized Brackbill's public comments as "shrill and strident." On the other side, Brackbill's work has been strongly supported by consumer and women's health organizations, many of which sent representatives to the FDA hearing. These people spoke out against the use of obstetric drugs which have never been proven safe.

Copies of the final Brackbill-Broman report were supposed to be available after the hearing in 1979, but the study has yet to be released. To place your name on the mailing list to receive a copy of the final study, contact:
Sylvia W. Shaffer, Chief
Office of Scientific and Health Reports
National Institute of Neurological and Communicative Disorders and Stroke
National Institutes of Health
Bethesda, MD 20205

This controversy points up serious questions about the ability of the FDA to regulate obstetric drugs (see Doris Haire's report on this page).

THE FEDERAL GOVERNMENT INVESTIGATES
OBSTETRICAL PRACTICES

OBSTETRICAL PRACTICES IN THE UNITED STATES, 1978
Hearing transcript
1978, 226 pages

from
U.S. Government Printing Office
Washington, DC 20402
single copy free

On April 17, 1978, the Subcommittee of Health and Scientific Research of the Committee on Human Resources of the U.S. Senate met to examine obstetrical practices in the U.S., especially the use of fetal monitors, the rising cesarean rate, elective induction of labor, and the use of drugs in pregnancy and labor. The Subcommittee hearing was chaired by Senator Edward M. Kennedy, who expressed concern about the poor infant mortality rate in the U.S. and the effects of obstetrical practices on the health of the newborn. Pointing out that the use of ultrasound, for example, has become widespread in obstetrics *before* being proven safe, he said. "As in many areas of medicine, the development of obstetrical technology far outstrips our capacity to assess its appropriate value. As a result, common practice is established before appropriate practice can be defined." Senator Kennedy proposed the creation of a National Institute of Health Care Research to evaluate the appropriateness of health care technologies.

Witnesses at this hearing included Donald Kennedy, FDA Commissioner and others representing the FDA; Dr. Roberto Caldeyro-Barcia of the World Health Organization, accompanied by Doris Haire and others concerned about the hazards of obstetrical practices; Ervin Nichols and others representing the American College of Obstetricians and Gynecologists; Yvonne Brackbill, speaking on the long-term effects of labor drugs; and others. The transcript includes the complete text of Doris Haire's *The Cultural Warping of Childbirth* and other important materials.

"Monitoring, for the mother, increases not only the cost of her delivery, but decreases the naturalness of that delivery; decreases her mobility while in labor; requires that she receive care in a rather large hospital complex thereby limiting her choice of a place in which to have her baby; and significantly increases the probability that she will have major surgery (Cesarean section) during delivery.

"I feel that fetal monitoring gives the doctor and nurse information. More information doesn't necessarily give a better outcome. It seems that in the OB patient, the more information you receive the more anxious you become about its significance and the more aggressive to ameliorate the problem so every piece of information that looks irregular problematically is like a red flag to a conscientious physician to get in there and do something. C-sections are done by conscientious people who are nervous, not knife-happy.

"Finally, I fear that obstetricians may create a credibility gap and a crisis of confidence by overselling the public on high technology and aggressive obstetrics, especially when a number of people are dropping out of the system altogether and having what appear to be reasonably healthy outcomes. This would be a grave disservice to the public and medicine. . . ."
Testimony of Dr. Albert D. Haverkamp

"Like a snowball rolling downhill, American obstetric care has gradually accumulated an ever-increasing amount of obstetric interventive practices which, however well intentioned, have never been shown by properly controlled evaluation to be in the best interests of mothers and their offspring. The

"... we have reached a point in obstetric care in this country which is considered barbaric by many European and American health professionals."

process has been so gradual that we have reached a point in obstetric care in the country which is considered barbaric by many European and American health professionals. . .

"Having observed obstetric care in 37 countries, I can say without hesitation that it is no accident that an infant born in the United States is more than twice as likely to die during the first day of life than is an infant born in the Netherlands or Japan—countries where many children are born at home or in maternity homes and where the midwives make a maximum effort to avoid interference in the intricate process of checks and balances of human parturition, even in hospital obstetric units."
Testimony of Doris Haire

A REVIEW OF RESEARCH LITERATURE AND FEDERAL INVOLVEMENT RELATING TO SELECTED OBSTETRIC PRACTICES
by the Staff of the U.S. General Accounting Office
September 1979, 92 pages, Illus.

from
U.S. General Accounting Office
Distribution Section, R. 1518
441 G. Street, NW
Washington, DC 20548
single copy free

In response to the April, 1978, Senate hearing on obstetrical practices, General Accounting Office (GAO) conducted a survey of research literature and federal and private involvement in evaluating the risks and benefits of five selected obstetrical practices: elective induction of labor, medication to relieve labor pain, preventive use of forceps, routine electronic fetal monitoring, and increasing use of cesarean section. For each practice, the GAO staff presents a description, indications for use, extent of use, research results (in each case these are described as "inconclusive"), and the extent of involvement by federal agencies and professional organizations. The overall picture presented is that very little is known about the safety of commonly used obstetrical practices.

"FDA has no mandatory system for getting drug warnings to patients. Current drug labeling is for physicians, and FDA requires that it contain warnings, contraindications and possible adverse reactions from drugs. However, FDA has no control over a physician's actual use of a drug or of the drug's use with patients."

EVALUATING BENEFITS AND RISKS OF OBSTETRIC PRACTICES: More Coordinated Federal and Private Efforts Needed
by the Comptroller General of the United States
September, 1979, 68 pages, Illus.

from
U.S. General Accounting Office
Distribution Section, Rm. 1518
441 G Street, NW
Washington, DC 20548
single copy free

In this companion volume to the General Accounting Office (GAO) Staff report (above), the Comptroller General calls for better evaluation of obstetrical practices. The report concludes that the federal government lacks "a coordinated strategy or overall research plan for evaluating obstetric practices or educating the public on their benefits and risks. Long-term research necessary to prove the safety of various obstetric procedures for infant development is generally not being funded by the Government. The Comptroller General calls on Congress and the Department of Health, Education and Welfare (now Health and Human Services) to make efforts to provide better evaluation and control of obstetrical practices.

"Methods used in childbirth to facilitate labor and delivery have become a controversial issue in the United States. Many have questioned the necessity, benefits, or safety of some of the procedures. Critics cite hazards which are associated with some of these obstetric practices or point to differences in use of particular practices within

"Methods used in childbirth to facilitate labor and delivery have become a controversial issue in the United States. Many have questioned the necessity, benefits, or safety of some of the procedures."

the United States or between the United States and other countries. Some of these countries have lower infant mortality rates than the United States, which some say indicates a need to re-examine the childbirth methods used here. Representatives from the medical community, on the other hand, say that U.S. obstetrical practices have contributed to the declining U.S. perinatal (fetal and infant) mortality rate. They claim that the benefits derived from using those practices exceed any risks associated with them.

"How babies are delivered is an important national concern. Each year more than 3 million deliveries occur in the United States. Obstetric practices used during these births may improve the chances for mother and baby to come through the birth process healthy. But on the other hand, these same practices may contribute to perinatal mortality, birth injury, or permanent injury to the child, and may contribute to injury to the mother."

OVERSIGHT ON EFFORTS TO REDUCE INFANT MORTALITY AND TO IMPROVE PREGNANCY OUTCOME
Hearing Transcript
1980, 700 pages

from
U.S. Government Printing Office
Washington, DC 20402
single copy free

On June 30, 1980, the Subcommittee on Child and Human Development of the Committee on Labor and Human Resources of the U.S. Senate met to "examine the overall efforts by the federal government and certain medical services to reduce infant mortality, birth defects, and improve pregnancy outcome." In his opening statement, Chairperson Senator Alan Cranston outlined seven goals which the government hoped to achieve: 1) improve health care and living standards for disadvantaged mothers, 2) work to prevent low birth-weight, 3) improve prevention, detection, and treatment of birth defects, 4) "develop better methods of assuring the safety and efficacy of various obstetric drugs and practices," 5) assure access to family planning services, 6) assure access to early and continuing prenatal care, and 7) improve public health education about health habits that effect pregnancy.

Speaking specifically to the fourth point, Doris Haire, representing the National Women's Health Network and Sally Tom of the American College of Nurse-Midwives, testified at the hearing. Doris Haire expressed concern about the harmful effects of obstetrical drugs and other practices which can cause brain damage by reducing oxygen flow to the fetus during labor (see excerpt from Ms. Haire's testimony below). Sally Tom spoke of the value of utilizing nurse-midwives to provide low-cost, high-quality care during pregnancy and birth. She described several studies showing that the use of nurse-midwives increases patient use of prenatal care services and decreases the incidence of prematurity, low birth weight, and neonatal death.

"Senator Cranston: Did you say there is a higher rate of maternal and infant deaths in the hospital affiliated with a medical school?"

"Ms. Haire: Yes."

"Senator Cranston: What is your explanation?"

"Ms. Haire: I feel it is intervention.. If you go into any teaching hospital, you find there is a tremendous amount of obstetric intervention. Sometimes it is done for staff convenience. Many times it is done merely because someone needs the teaching experience. We advise women to sign their name on the consent form—adding, 'neither I nor my baby shall be used as teaching or research subject without my informed consent.' Just teaching mothers to write those few words would do a tremendous amount to reduce the poor outcome that we see in teaching or in large obstetric services."

"The primary goal of care during a healthy labor should be the support of the normal physiology and psychology of labor and birth. This includes provision of adequate nutrition and fluid intake during labor and assumption by the mother of positions which facilitate her comfort and the process of labor. Receiving care during labor from competent, trusted care providers and having one or more supportive family members present greatly increases a woman's comfort and control.

"Another important component of supporting the natural process of labor is careful monitoring of maternal and fetal condition and the progress of labor. This does not mean only the use of electronic fetal monitoring; it may mean the use of the fetoscope, the doptone."
—from the testimony of Sally Austen Tom, Certified Nurse-Midwife

---

"Few American children are born today as Nature intended them to be. With rare exception, newborn infants in the U.S. have been subjected to the direct or indirect effects of an awesome armamentarium of central-nervous-system depressants, uterine stimulants, and interventive procedures such as amniotomy (artificial rupture of the membranes), forceps extraction, etc. Most of these drugs and procedures can deprive the fetal brain of oxygen, or disrupt the integrity of the fetal brain.

"Intervention has become so much a part of American obstetric care that in one highly regarded New York hospital the neonatologist reports that 50% of the newborn infants admitted to the intensive care newborn nursery came from mothers who were diagnosed as normal when they entered the hospital in labor.

"I have observed obstetric care in 44 countries. I can say without hesitation that it is no accident that an infant born in the U.S. is more than twice as likely to die during the first day of life than is an infant born in The Netherlands or Japan. In those countries obstetric drugs are seldom used. The sensitive, skillful support of the midwife greatly reduces or eliminates the mother's need for obstetric drugs. Therefore, the mother remains relatively ambulatory—intermittently resting, walking or sitting—facilitating the normal progress of labor.

"Nature has provided the parturient and her fetus a sequence of intricate biochemical checks and balances to help assure the normal progress of labor and birth, and the newborn infant's adjustment to extrauterine life. In the U.S. iatrogenic (physician caused) disruptions of these protective mechanisms frequently adversely affect the newborn infant's ability to initiate and sustain normal breathing, to self-regulate its body temperature, to eliminate bilirubin from its blood and brain, etc. These disruptions in the basic life-sustaining mechanisms can seriously impair the infant's subsequent neurologic development.

"It is difficult to read the scientific literature without coming to the conclusion that obstetric drugs and procedures, however well intended, contribute to the enormous number of neurologically impaired children in the U.S.—children who are retarded, autistic, learning disabled, hyperkinetic, severely, emotionally disturbed, or who exhibit consistent erratic or psychopathologic behavior."

from the testimony of Doris Haire, representing the National Women's Health Network in *Oversight on Efforts to Reduce Infant Mortality and to Improve Pregnancy Outcome,* a hearing before the subcommittee on Child and Human Development, Committee on Labor and Human Resources, United States Senate, June 30, 1980.

EFFECTS OF PRESCRIPTION DRUGS DURING PREGNANCY
Hearing Transcript
1981, 244 pages

from
U.S. Government Printing Office
Washington, DC 20402
single copy free

This hearing was misnamed—it should have been titled "Effects of Drugs during Pregnancy *and Labor*." Over half of the transcript (almost 150 pages) consists of testimony presented by Doris Haire, representing the National Women's Health Network. She presents invaluable information on the hazards of using drugs for pain relief during labor and on the inadequacy of FDA regulation of such drugs. The hearing was held by the Subcommittee on Investigation and Oversight of the Committee on Science and Technology of the U.S. House of Representatives, chaired by Congressmember Albert Gore of Tennessee.

"Mr. Gore:... Mrs. Haire I see on your list of drugs commonly used in obstetrics on page three Scopalamine. Is that still used?

"Ms. Haire: Obstetricians will usually tell you that the drug is no longer used, but nurses tell me, definitely, that it is being used. It is something I think most hospitals are ashamed of, but, nevertheless, Scopalamine is being used.

"Mr. Gore: When my wife and I attended to the birth of our first child we went through the American Society of Psychoprophylaxis and Obstetrics, or LaMaze classes, and the effects of that medication were described as being the woman continues to experience the pain but her memory of it is obliterated afterwards. She is so completely disoriented and so forth she cannot recall the pain. Is that a fair description of the bizarre effect of that drug?

"Ms. Haire: That is the 'desirable' effect.

"Mr. Gore: That is what they want to happen?

"Ms. Haire: I think it is tragic that many women miss the most ego-building experience a woman could possibly have. The sad thing is that many women must be treated by a psychotherapist after being administered Scopalamine during childbirth—because the drug tends to cause nightmarish effects when the mother reflects on her obstetric experience. For some women there is just enough recall to produce psychological problems. There are now psychotherapists in New York who deal only with women who have been traumatized by their childbirth experience."

"Mr. Shamansky: Doris, you made a statement on page 23 to the effect that 1 out of 10 children has some kind of impairment. Are you convinced that a high proportion or a low proportion is the result of administering drugs during pregnancy or during the delivery?

"Ms. Haire: I cannot give you specific quantity. I feel a significant proportion of these children are the result of obstetric medication given, with the best of intentions to women during labor. Whether the drug, in itself, does the harm or whether it works synergistically with other obstetric stresses would have to be evaluated, but there is no doubt in my mind that a large proportion of the learning disabled and brain-injured children in the United States are the result of obstetric drugs."

Cesarean Section

Cesarean section is the ultimate intervention in childbirth. Instead of pushing her baby out through her vagina, the woman's abdomen and uterus are opened surgically and the baby is removed through the incision. In the truest sense, the doctor "delivers" the baby.

Before this century, cesarean sections were rarely performed because of the great dangers of infection and death for the mother. For the small percentage of women with serious difficulties in childbearing, the improvements in surgical technique which have made cesarean section a safer procedure have been truly life-saving, both for mother and baby. But unfortunately, as with so many innovations in medicine, a procedure which was developed to help high-risk mothers and babies is now being used, at alarming rates, with women who are not at significant risk. In the 1950's the cesarean section rate in our country was about 4 percent. However, in the 1970's, the cesarean rate began to climb sharply, going from 5% in 1968 to 12.8% in 1977. In 1980 the national rate was estimated to be about 18% with large hospitals having rates of 20 to 40%. Critics of the rising cesarean rate feel that many of the cesareans being done now are unnecessary. Many factors have been implicated in the rising rate, including increasing diagnosis of "failure to progress" in labor, repeat cesareans, cesarean for breech position, increasing diagnosis of "fetal distress" (associated with increased use of electronic fetal monitoring), the increasing use of obstetrical intervention in normal birth, insurance reimbursement for surgical birth, doctor's fear of malpractice suits, economic incentives of doctors and hospitals, increasing use of obstetricians (a surgical specialty) rather than general practitioners or midwives for normal births, and needs for "teaching material" in medical school affiliated hospitals.

An unexpected cesarean delivery can be emotionally devastating for the woman who hoped for a normal birth, and the recovery from major surgery can make the postpartum adjustment and new baby care more difficult. Many cesarean support groups have arisen to help women deal with the aftermath of a cesarean birth. These groups and others have worked toward the goal of "family-centered cesarean" care in which the mother is awake under regional anesthesia for the procedure and the father is with her in the operating room. But as the cesarean section rate continues to climb, many parents and childbirth educators are realizing that "cesarean prevention" information must now become an integral part of preparation for childbirth.

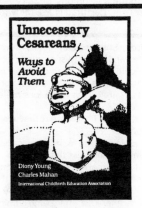

UNNECESSARY CESAREANS:
Ways to Avoid Them
by Diony Young and Charles Mahan
1980, 27 pages, Illus.

from
ICEA Bookcenter
P.O. Box 20048
Minneapolis, MN 55420
$1.50 plus $1.00 postage
bulk rates available

This booklet should be considered required reading for all childbirth preparation classes. The cesarean rate is approaching 25% in many parts of the country. This means your chances are 1 in 4 of having a cesarean just by walking in the hospital door! It's no longer enough for parents to think, "It won't be me." It's also time to stop accepting the cesarean delivery as a normal or even desireable way of having a baby. *Unnecessary Cesareans* addresses both issues, stressing the importance of "cesarean prevention" as a necessary part of childbirth education, and providing specific information on why many cesareans are unnecessary and can be avoided. The authors discuss the reasons behind the recent rise in cesarean births ("high-tech" approach to birth, "defensive medicine," more diagnoses of "failure to progress"), and analyze how current hospital practices directly contribute to high cesarean rates. Induced labor, the supine position for labor, electronic fetal monitoring, and use of labor drugs all begin the interventionist "scenario" which, increasingly, leads to a cesarean. Specific guidelines are provided for preventing cesareans through consumer-oriented preparation in pregnancy and a "physiologic" approach to labor. Recommendations are offered for the management of breech presentation, cephalopelvic disproportion (CPD), vaginal birth after cesarean, elective repeat cesarean, emergency cesarean, and the options for family-centered cesarean, baby care, and recovery. A summary check-list makes it easy for parents to see the important issues at a glance and a glossary of terms and list of references and additional reading are included.

"If your labor slows down and contractions weaken, try nonmedical alternatives such as position changes; walking; warm shower; nipple stimulation (which can activate beneficial, natural oxytocin production); change in environment; and removal of any person whose presence is stressful. Resist pressures to use obstetrical drugs and intervention unless medically warranted. Avoid the use of medically administered oxytocin to speed up labor because this can precipitate maternal and fetal complications. Rest is recommended for prolonged first stage of labor.

"Your partner can help the progress of labor by expressing love and encouragement, kissing and cuddling, massaging thigh and abdominal muscles deeply during and between contractions, giving reassurance that your body is adequate to the task, giving accurate feedback about how you are responding to your contractions, and reminding you of the goal of this work; privacy with your partner is an added helpful measure.

"Do not allow yourself to feel 'rushed' or 'pressured' by hospital or attending personnel. If medical procedures or intervention are suggested because 'labor isn't progressing,' insist on more time and try nonmedical alternatives. In this situation a third person as an advocate can provide needed support."

THE CAESAREAN EPIDEMIC:
Who's Having This Baby, Anyway—
You Or The Doctor?
by Gena Corea
June 1980, 8 pages

from
Mother Jones Reprint Service
625 Third Street
San Francisco, CA 94107
$1.00 plus .35 postage for two copies (minimum order), additional copies, .25 each.

Gena Corea does not mince words in this angry, hard-hitting article on the rising incidence of caesarean deliveries. She lays the blame squarely on obstetrical intervention, doctor's greed, and sexist attitudes about women. Corea points out that some women have been accused of "child abuse" for attempting to refuse a "necessary" caesarean and sees a strong relationship between current right-to-life sentiment and attitudes which place the welfare of the fetus above that of the mother. Special features are included on "Engineering a Caesarean," "A Feeling of Being Raped," and "Stopping That Knife."

"From the figures alone it seems clear that the C-section delivery is no longer being used as an emergency birth method to save the life of mother or child. Rather, the demands of birth technology and the medical technocracy are now taking precedence over the best interests of mother and infant . . . .

"Indeed, so enthusiastic are some doctors about doing Caesareans that they talk as if there were something wrong with women who want to have their babies the old-fashioned way. 'It may well be that during the next 40 years the allowing of a vaginal delivery or attempted vaginal delivery may need to be justified in each particular instance,' write Drs. John Sutherst and Barbara Case in the April, 1975 issue of the British Journal *Clinics in Obstetrics and Gynaecology.* And in an American journal last year, in an article entitled 'The Fetal Right to Live,' four Israeli obstetricians suggest that an 'occult reason' may lie behind a woman's refusal of a Caesarean section. 'It is probably that the patient hopes to be freed in this way of an undesired pregnancy,' they write. Other possible reasons for this strange reluctance to undergo a C-section, the doctors speculate, may be 'fear of surgery, prejudice, ignorance, difficulty with the language or inadequate rapport between doctor and patient.'

"Physicians refer to C-section deliveries as 'from above' and vaginal deliveries as 'from below.' Dr. Helen Marieskind, author of a report prepared for the Department of Health, Education and Welfare (HEW), relates that while she was conducting interviews for her study on the rising Caesarean rate, obstetricians repeatedly asked her: 'What's so great about delivering from below, anyway?'"

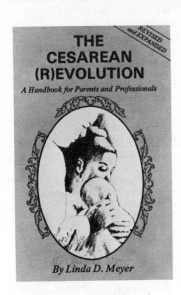

THE CAESAREAN (R)EVOLUTION: A Handbook for Parents and Professionals
by Linda D. Meyer
1981, 170 pages

from
The Chas. Franklin Press
18409 90th Avenue West
Edmonds, WA 98020
$5.95 plus .75 postage, pap.

Linda Meyer begins her book by describing a "typical" caesarean delivery (for breech) and contrasts it with her model for a more sensitive and flexible approach. She goes on to discuss the relation between Caesarean delivery and a great many other factors, including medication, patients' rights, fathers' participation, the role of friends and relatives, nutrition, grief, postpartum depression,

mothering disorders, sterilization, the obstetrician, the pediatrician, the anesthesiologist, respiratory distress, breastfeeding, bottlefeeding, and vaginal delivery after caesarean. An extensive set of appendices provides information on terminology, caesarean education, support groups, guidelines for counseling caesarean parents, class outline, a hospital questionnaire, and more.

"Friends and relatives can be a terrific boon to the caesarean mother or an albatross around her neck. She needs their support and help so much, and yet frequently such is not forthcoming. She is recovering from major surgery, and she may be very sensitive about having had a caesarean. These are the two most important things one should remember when dealing with the post-surgical mother . . . .

"What specifically can you do?
1. Let her know that you care about her.
2. Let her know she can depend on you.
3. Offer to come in for an hour or two daily to straighten the house, cook dinner, shop for groceries.
4. Take her older child(ren) for the afternoon or overnight.
5. Bake her a casserole.
6. Take her to the doctor.
7. Be sure she is eating well, even if you have to fix it.
8. Organize her friends or neighbors so that each one helps out one day apiece.
9. Take all the children including the infant, if she wishes, for an afternoon so she can get some much-needed sleep.
10. Do her laundry.
11. Be available to listen."

CESAREAN CHILDBIRTH: A Handbook for Parents
by Christine Coleman Wilson and Wendy Roe Hovey
1981, 272 pages, Illus.

from
Signet Books
New American Library
1301 Avenue of the Americas
New York, NY 10021
$3.50 pap.

This book began in 1977 as a self-published booklet, distributed by the authors, both of whom had experienced cesarean births. Wilson and Hovey place their emphasis on information which will help the couple cope with and understand their cesarean delivery. They provide an introduction to issues in childbirth today, including the role of the consumer. They discuss the reasons for cesarean delivery and provide information on choice of anesthesia, father's participation, recovery, new baby care, emotional responses, and repeat cesarean. Advice is offered on starting a cesarean support group and on guidelines for family-centered cesar-

ean programs for hospitals.

"Acceptance sometimes disappears after it has arrived. You may feel as though you have completely resolved all your feelings about the birth, only to have them reappear when an unmedicated vaginal birth is shown on TV, or your friend shows you the pictures of her easy, prepared birth in the local hospital's birthing room. Being reminded of what you missed can bring some of the old feelings back, but they will drift away again.

"Often Cesarean parents are told, 'Having a healthy baby is all that matters.' This trite phrase has a hollow ring to the woman whose disappointment about having surgery is very fresh, or to the father who feels cheated because he could not greet his child at birth. But for some parents, the stage of acceptance begins when they can say, 'Having a healthy baby really is all that matters.' For others, the regrets that accompany the birth continue to coexist with the enjoyment that the baby brings."

THE CESAREAN BIRTH EXPERIENCE
by Bonnie Donovan
1978, 241 pages, Illus.

from
Beacon Press
25 Beacon Street
Boston, MA 02108
$5.95 pap.

Whether cesarean education should focus on "accepting" and coping with high cesarean rates is a subject of much debate and caused Bonnie Donovan to provide an update for her book, emphasizing her opposition to the "skyrocketing incidence" of cesareans and providing information on vaginal birth after cesarean. She goes on, in the main part of the book, to describe and explain the cesarean delivery itself, covering indications, the role of emotional stress in unanticipated cesareans, hospital tests and procedures, fathers in the operating room, making a good beginning in the recovery room, bonding and breastfeeding, and the postpartum period. She also provides a class outline for cesarean preparation classes.

"RECIPE

Take: two parents-to-be who may experience a temporary panic as they contemplate the responsibilities of parenthood and their unpreparedness for taking care of a newborn
Add: a dash of fear that the baby may be born less than perfect
Fold in: the parents' guilt that they are having negative thoughts in the first place
Combine: the ordinary trepidations of anyone about to have surgery
Take away: books, films, and slides concerning this alternative birthing method (because there haven't been any)
Remove: classes in prepared childbirth designed to meet the special needs of these parents (because no one thought they were needed)
Beat in: two lumps of confusion on behalf of maternity personnel who are not quite certain about their roles in caring for a patient who is both postpartum and postsurgical
Throw in: anxiety, tension, myths and misinformation—and the often harrowing experiences of others
Separate: parents just when they need each other's love and support most
Optional: one or more previous cesarean deliveries
Wheel: your mixture into an operating room and keep there for about one hour, or until done
Yield: one cesarean section, one hopefully healthy baby, and two traumatized parents."

IMPACT OF CESAREAN CHILDBIRTH
Edited by Dyanne D. Affonso
1981, 296 pages, Illus.

from
F.A. Davis Company
1915 Arch Street
Philadelphia, PA 19103
$15.95 hd.

This book is a collection of essays, directed mainly to professionals, on the impact of cesarean childbirth on the family, health professionals, and society. The contributors discuss the physical and psychological effects of cesarean birth on the mother, the father and the baby, the impact on obstetrics, nursing and anesthesia services, and the implications for society.

". . . cesarean childbirths can create degrees of confusion regarding the social role of the woman and her family in the birth event. In the past, cultural norms defined what the woman's role would be in effecting vaginal birth, and how the social environment assisted in facilitating vaginal birth. However, a cesarean childbirth appears to place the control of the birth into the domain of society's experts—obstetricians, anesthesiologists, and nurses. The woman may perceive that her active participation has been relinquished. For example, whereas with a vaginal delivery a woman can expect to 'labor and push her baby out,' with a cesarean she may feel 'the obstetrician delivers the baby. . . .'

"Our lifestyles involve a continuous confrontation with change. We are constantly expending energies to achieve different levels of adaptation. Amidst an environment in which change is the expectation, we yearn for experiences that will bring some degree of stability, predictability, and order. Nature and the natural order of initiating and terminating life are perceived to have a degree of order and stability. The current movement of 'return to nature' as manifested in health foods, herbal medicines, and conservation of wildlife resources may be viewed as attempts to regain stability and order. There once was a time when the two experiences perceived to unite every individual's contact with order and predictability were birth and death. Every human was considered to be brought into the world by some natural course of activity (viewed as a vaginal birth process) and then leave through death. As cesarean childbirths rapidly increased, the sense of stability and order associated with the natural process of birth became altered and perceived by many as being lost."

from "Impact on Society: Sociological Significance of Cesarean Childbirth" by Dyanne Affonso

CESAREAN SUPPORT AND PREVENTION GROUPS

Listed below are national organizations which provide referrals, support, and information on cesarean birth. These groups can let you know about local support groups for cesarean mothers; provide information on avoiding unnecessary cesareans and on vaginal birth after cesarean (VBAC); and provide newsletters, pamphlets, books and other resources.

In searching for a local support group, it may be a good idea to contact more than one of these national organizations since some may refer only to their own affiliate groups. The following guidelines will also help you get the best service.

1. In addition to your full address and zip code, give specific information on where you are located (county, nearest big cities, etc.).

2. Specify exactly what kind of information you need (cesarean prevention?, family-centered cesarean, VBAC?) since different support groups vary in their emphasis.

3. Enclose a self-addressed, stamped envelope with every request for information. These are non-profit organizations with shoe-string budgets, usually run by mothers who volunteer their time to provide a free referral service.

4. Consider becoming a member, making a contribution, or buying publications from groups which have been helpful to you. Your contribution will make it possible for more women to receive information.

CESAREAN BIRTH ALLIANCE
39 Denton Avenue
East Rockaway, NY 11518
Hotline:
Barbara Brown-Hill, 516/593-7556
Forwarding phone number, 516/627-1636

The Cesarean Birth Alliance provides an excellent packet of information on cesarean section and vaginal birth after cesarean for $15. and provides individual telephone counseling ($10. per hour) and referrals to home VBAC attendants. Classes and workshops are also available.

CESEREAN PREVENTION MOVEMENT
P.O. Box 152
University Station
Syracuse, NY 13210
315/424-1942

"Our primary goal is to reduce the skyrocketing cesarean rate in the United States by educating and supporting couples who are having children. When a cesarean is necessary it is a lifesaving technique, but it has become far too common a practice. By reducing the primary cesarean rate and increasing the vaginal birth after cesarean (VBAC) rate we can accomplish our goal."

The Cesarean Prevention Movement is currently working with a professional librarian to develop an annotated bibliography of resources on cesarean birth, with information on how these resources may be obtained through the inter-library loan systems of local libraries.

CESAREAN PREVENTION CLARION
$15./year for individuals. Includes membership in CPM.

THE CESAREAN CONNECTION
P.O. Box 11
Westmont, IL 60559
312/968-8877

"The Cesarean Connection (is) an organization dedicated to cesarean childbirth education. Cesarean parents, cesarean childbirth educators, cesarean support groups and interested professionals in allied fields from across the country and Canada are utilizing the Connection as a means of communicating and keeping abreast of new developments affecting the cesarean childbirth experience."

The Cesarean Connection offers a "Cesarean Childbirth Education Aids Guide" for $.50 plus SASE, a monthly *Bulletin* newsletter for $12. a year, and a listing of cesarean support groups serving the United States and Canada, for $5. postpaid.

CESAREAN BIRTH COUNCIL INTERNATIONAL, INC.
P.O. Box 6081
San Jose, CA 95150
415/343-4044

"The Cesarean Birth Council International, Inc., is a support group specifically designed to meet the needs of parents experiencing Cesarean childbirth, and to provide educational assistance pre and postnatally for Cesarean parents."

Less geared toward prevention than some of the other groups, the CBCI helps mothers with planned and unplanned cesareans better cope with the experience. Services include prenatal classes, telephone counseling, rap groups, a quarterly newsletter, audio visual aids, lectures, local chapters, and literature.

CESAREAN/SUPPORT, EDUCATION AND CONCERN
22 Forest Road
Framingham, MA 01701
617/877-8266

"Cesarean/Support, Education, and Concern (C/SEC), Inc., is a non-profit organization committed to improving the cesarean childbirth experience. The goals of our organization are: 1) to provide emotional support for cesarean delivery families, 2) to share information and promote education on cesarean childbirth, cesarean prevention, and VBAC, and 3) to change attitudes and policies which affect the cesarean childbirth experience."

COUNCIL FOR CESAREAN AWARENESS
5520 S.W. 92nd Avenue
Miami, FL 33165
205/596-2699

"We seek to educate the birthing public and the health care professionals who serve them about cesarean birth. Our purposes are: 1) to try to prepare every birthing couple for the possibility of a cesarean birth so they know what their options are and can prepare ahead of time for a positive birth experience if they wind up with a cesarean, 2) to educate the birthing couple as to their birthing alternatives and the possibilities of winding up with a cesarean in an (a) conventional hospital setting, (b) alternative in-hospital setting, (c) out-of-hospital setting, with an eye toward cesarean prevention, and 3) to provide support, information, and help to couples who seek vaginal births after cesareans (which should be the majority of those who've had previous cesareans). It goes without saying that the people who serve the birthing couple should be so educated."

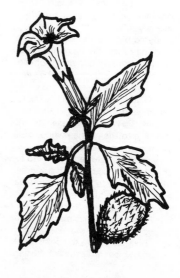

1981 CESAREAN UPDATE
36 pages

from
BIRTH
110 El Camino Real
Berkeley, CA 94705
$2.50

This group of four articles first appeared in *BIRTH* (formerly *Birth and the Family Journal*) and is now offered as a reprint. Articles include:

Enkin: "Having a Section is Having a Baby"
Conner Shearer: "Teaching about Cesarean Birth in Traditional Childbirth Classes"
Cohen: "Minimizing the Emotional Sequelae of Cesarean Childbirth" plus reference charts of complications of cesarean to mother and baby.
Conner Shearer: "NIH Consensus Development Task Force on Cesarean Childbirth: The Process and the Result"

CESAREAN BIRTH—A SPECIAL DELIVERY
by Kathy Keolker
1979, 4 pages

from
the pennypress
1100 23rd Avenue East
Seattle, WA 98112
50 cents single copy
$20. per 100

This flyer explains the common reasons for a cesarean and describes the surgical procedure. Advice is offered on the recovery period, breast-feeding, the first weeks at home, the father's role, and vaginal birth after cesarean. Included is a summary list of options for "family centered" cesarean.

"Cesarean birth is becoming more common. While recognizing that it is major surgery with all its inherent risks and concerns, having a cesarean baby can be a fulfilling birthing experience when done with sensitivity and concern for the needs of the family."

YOUR CESAREAN DELIVERY:
A Cesarean Mother's Guide to Recovery During Her Hospital Stay
by Kris A. Berger
1981, 20 pages

from
PEACE & HOME Association of Wichita, Inc.
P.O. Box 18363
Wichita, KS 67218
$1.50

This useful booklet provides advice on moving, walking, pain, medication, emotions, breastfeeding and other aspects of the immediate post-cesarean period. Childbirth educators would do well to have a few copies on hand for their students who have an unexpected cesarean delivery.

HOW MOTHERS FEEL

"I didn't have any trouble at all with my cesarean. I was up and walking around five hours after surgery. I didn't have any anesthesia related complications. Therefore I wasn't depressed, though some women are. After 24 hours of Lamaze-trained labor. I was satisfied with the outcome. I saw the baby right after his first bath and was, able to nurse him the next day. I have a tendency to take a bad experience and make it something good. After all, I got a baby and that was what I wanted. I thought I wouldn't really care if I had another cesarean, but after my vaginal birth for my second child I realized that there was no comparison. With my second child the bonding was so terrific because I really saw the baby come out of my body! There was a strong, spontaneous attachment. It took me weeks before I had that feeling with my first baby. Having a VBAC was like a bonus, having a baby and also *seeing* it some out! Now I feel like I have had a good experience and a fantastic experience."

—Rochelle Maucher

"I had a long and very supported VBAC labor at home. I loved it. But after transition I couldn't get the baby's head down. I went from full dilation to half dilation and stayed there. Then we noticed my cervix was swollen and protruding, so we decided to go to the hospital. The doctor on call was a VBAC mother herself and would have supported continuing the labor. But the chief of obstetrics insisted that I have pitocin, an IV, an internal pressure monitor, a fetal monitor, etc. I felt those things might cause fetal distress so I decided to go ahead with another cesarean. I asked for an epidural and the anesthesiologists spent a long time trying to argue me into a spinal, which I refused. My husband was not allowed into the operating room. When the baby was born, they took him away too quickly. I was not able to bond. It was as terrible as it could be. I spasmed in the neck and shoulders and asked for a very small dose of Demerol. Instead they gave me a massive dose of Demerol and Valium and I became unconscious. My whole family was dispersed—the baby to the nursery, me to my room, my husband home, and my older son to his grandmother's. Everyone was alone that night. That was the most terrible thing. I checked out after only two days to try to reassemble my family."

—Rachel Neulander

"I have a tendency to take a bad experience and make it something good. . . I thought I wouldn't really care if I had another cesarean, but after my vaginal birth for my second child I realized there was no comparison."

"The surgery was bad enough but going home to take care of two babies even before I was fully or even slightly recuperated set me up for five months of personal agony. In retrospect it may have been because I was told to keep off my feet for the two months prior to the twins' birth because I was having mild contractions. I went into surgery a vegetable and came out the same. The boys weighed 7½ pounds each and were 21 inches long. I did a great job for them but not so great for me.

"Many C-section patients complain that people care very little how they feel and only come to the hospital to see the baby and it's true. Relatives were ANNOYED that I had to ask them to leave because I was in pain or that I was in too much pain to answer the phone for two days following surgery."

—Sharon Poidomani

ENGINEERING
A Play in Two Acts

Address inquiries to:
Marcia Slatkin
P.O. Box 60
Shoreham, NY 11786

Marcia Slatkin was outraged by reading "The Caesarean Epidemic," (see index) and wrote this black comedy about the way unnecessary cesareans are "engineered," Contact her for information on performance rights.

"Doctor: Mrs. Ramos, I'm afraid we're going to have to do a cesarean.
Mrs. Ramos: But I'm fine, I don't want a cesarean.
Doctor: My dear, I'm the physician. And your baby's heart rate is slightly affected.
Mrs. Ramos: (loudly) But I've had the urge to push already. I've been panting and breathing and holding back but I've had the urge to push.
Doctor: Nonsense, Mrs. Ramos, you weren't more than 5 centimeters dilated less than a half hour ago. Your baby's heart is at stake, Mrs. Ramos.
Mrs. Ramos: My baby's heart rate is fine. It's loud as sin on that machine! And I'm fine. And I'm starting to push. I'm pushing (screams). I'm having this baby now!!!!
Doctor: Nurse, IV sedative, please. (Nurse injects woman, who continues to scream.)
Mrs. Ramos: (screaming) No Cesarean. I want to push. Leave me alone.

I'm having this baby now. (Nurse pulls up her gown, starts to shave her stomach) Leave me alone. What are you doing (screaming at the top of her lungs) I'm pushing. The baby is coming!
Nurse: We're just shaving your stomach dear. (wheels her into the hall, around set to the lit up delivery room sign. As she wheels her, the anesthesiologist comes with a mask. He puts it over her face, and we see the woman struggle, then suddenly relax and go limp. She is wheeled around the platform so that we no longer see her)

* * *

"(A loud wail of a newborn infant is heard from the delivery room. The crying of the infant continues, the nurse comes running in to the special treatment room, breathless.)
Nurse: I'm so sorry, Doctor. John and I were talking, and we thought she was under. But she's stronger than we suspected. Suddenly, she turned over on the table, squatted down and started to push, grunt and push. That baby was born on the table, without any assistance. Incredible. She's holding him now, nursing. She won't let me take it away.
Doctor: Damnation. I might have known she would try something like that. Nothing is going right today. All right, I'll be right there. Keep everyone calm. After all, it could be worse. . ."

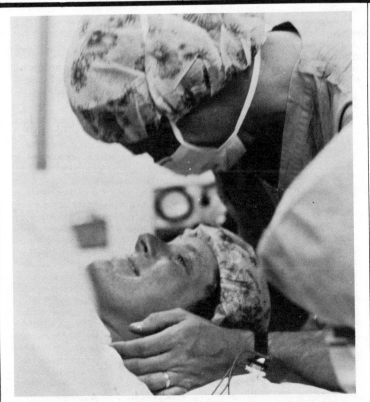

Illustration from *Cesarean: A Special Birth*, a slide series with audio cassette, available from BABES, c/o Deanna Sollid, 59 Berens Drive, Kentfield, CA 94904. Reproduced with permission.

CESAREAN POEMS
by Marion Cohen
1980, 4 pages, Illus.

from
Mothering Reprints
P.O. Box 2208
Albuquerque, NM 87103-2208
75 cents
bulk rates available

Marion Cohen is poetry editor for *Mothering Magazine* and has written many poems based on her childbirth experiences.

"When they said We're gonna hafta take the baby she started screaming hysterically She thought they meant actually take the baby away from her (Ya know, put it up for adoption) So they explained to her Oh no We don't mean take the baby permanently We mean take it temporarily Take it out of your body But she wouldn't calm down She just went on Screaming"

"Aw come on whatchu cryin' for? You didn't get a hysterectomy Just a Cesarean You haven't been spayed Just sectioned They didn't fix it so you can't pull in more children Just so you can't push them out Why all the weeping?"

AN EVALUATION OF CAESAREAN SECTION IN THE UNITED STATES
by Helen I. Marieskind
June 1979, 283 pages

from
Clara G. Schiffer
Room 447F8
HHS-HHH Bldg.
Washington, DC 20201
single copy free

Helen Marieskind is a health administrator and until recently was editor of *Women and Health* journal (see index). This report was prepared for the Department of Health, Education and Welfare (now Health, and Human Services) and is based on a review of the medical literature, interviews with physicians, and additional data analysis. Marieskind identifies and discusses the major factors which have contributed to the increasing rate of cesarean-section. These, in order of significance, are:

1. Threat of Malpractice Suits
2. Obstetrical Policy in the U.S. of Repeat Cesarean Section
3. Obstetrical Training
4. Belief in Superior Outcome from Cesarean Section
5. Changing Indications for Cesarean Section
6. Age, Parity and Fertility Characteristics
7. Economics
8. Obstetric Technology
9. Birth Weight
10. Women with Severe Medical Conditions
11. Herpes II
12. Miscellaneous Factors

Marieskind offers a series of thirteen recommendations for reducing the incidence of cesarean section, including improved data collection on cesarean deliveries and related obstetrical practices, changes in obstetrical training and review, the encouragement of family-centered birthing programs in all hospitals, uniform federal reimbursement for physicians regardless of type of delivery, and greater use of midwives.

"Many articles report that women who have given birth by means of a Caesarean section feel profound guilt, hostility toward the infant, regret, a sense of failure and of helplessness, especially as many of them do not even know the reason for their Caesarean. While it is unlikely that all women experience all of these feelings, such feelings have been reported to be even stronger among women who have had to have a Caesarean after a trial of labor, and most particularly among women who have gone through prepared childbirth classes. Such conflicts, when they do exist, are not surprising, considering the influence of the promotion of natural childbirth. This is not to say that unmedicated childbirth should not be encouraged in the interests of a healthy infant and mother; it is to say that the hidden message which leaves women who do not deliver vaginally feeling guilty is not constructive to maternal and, ultimately, infant well-being. Several researchers have noted that some women interviewed have blamed themselves for the Caesareans, feeling that, 'if only I had tried a little harder' they could have delivered vaginally. One researcher noted that women seemed to be in a grieving process because they had had no active part in the delivery. . . '

"The increase in Caesarean sections has fostered other efforts at easing psychological costs: the development of Caesarean classes in prepared childbirth courses, community-based support groups for Caesarean mothers and numerous articles, films and books on the 'Caesarean birth experience.' . . . Interestingly, these classes, groups and literature seem markedly uncritical of the rising Ceasarean section rate. Obviously it is to some extent dysfunctional to ask a recent surgical patient to consider whether her surgery was, indeed, necessary. However, the consistent lack of questioning also becomes dysfunctional for equipping women to be responsible health care consumers, informed and aware of their rights as patients and cautious of the potential for abuse inherent in any surgical procedure. . . .

"During the course of interviews a frequent reason given by physicians for the Caesarean section rate increase was that residents were not trained in normal obstetrics and were ill-prepared to manage labor. . . ."although many of the physicians interviewed recommended that prospective controlled trials were needed to assess the risks and benefits of increased Caesarean section use, most stressed that even if they were done and current practice demonstrated as unwarranted, few physicians would change. Habits and beliefs are already formed and the specter of suits for past unnecessary interference too great. . . . As the literature and physician opinion continue uncriticized and unevaluated, use of Caesarean section becomes more routine and entrenched; physician practice, resident training and patient acceptance of increased rates become more firmly established. The prevailing standards of practice in the community are set and it is then considered malpractice and possibly unethical to deviate."

THE FEDERAL GOVERNMENT INVESTIGATES CESAREAN-SECTION

FINAL REPORT OF THE TASK FORCE ON CESAREAN CHILDBIRTH
1980, 550 pages

from
Pamela Driscoll
Office of Research Reporting
National Institute of Child Health and Human Development (NICHD)
Bldg. 31, Room 2A-32
Bethesda, MD 20205
single copy free

A draft of this report was prepared by the Task Force on Cesarean Childbirth, to serve as a working document at the Consensus Development Conference on Cesarean Childbirth sponsored by the National Institutes of Health in September, 1980. It was later published in final form along with the consensus conference recommendations. The report includes an introduction to the history and current incidence of cesarean delivery, a discussion of important medical factors in cesarean delivery (mortality, anesthesia, dystocia, fetal distress, repeat cesarean, breech presentation), information on the psychological effects of cesarean birth on mothers, infants, and the family, and a discussion of the ethical, medicolegal, and economic concerns relating to cesarean birth.

The following recommendations are taken from the summary statement on cesarean childbirth published along with the Task Force report.

"In the absence of fetal distress, management of dysfunctional labor may include such measures as patient rest, hydration, ambulation, sedation, and use of oxytocin, prior to considering cesarean birth.

"There is a compelling reason to examine the diagnostic category of dystocia because of its prominent association with the increase in primary cesarean birth rate and the absence of a survival advantage for the cesarean births over 2500 grams. . . .

"In hospitals with appropriate facilities, services, and staff for prompt emergency cesarean birth, a proper selection of cases should permit a safe trial of labor and vaginal delivery for women who have had a previous low segment transverse cesarean birth. Informed consent should be obtained before a trial labor is attempted. . . .

"Vaginal delivery of the term breech should remain an acceptable obstetrical choice for delivery when the following conditions are present:
(a) anticipated fetal weight of less than 8 pounds;
(b) normal pelvic dimensions and architecture
(c) frank breech presentation without a hyperextended head; and
(d) delivery to be conducted by a physician experienced in vaginal breech delivery. . . .

"Although overall maternal mortality is extremely uncommon (9.9 deaths/100,000 births in 1978), cesarean birth carries two to four times the risk for mortality when compared with vaginal delivery. Some maternal mortality following cesarean birth is related to maternal illness rather than to the surgery. Maternal mortality rates are still underreported. Cesarean birth is a major surgical procedure with morbidity greater than vaginal delivery. Infections constitute the greatest portion of this morbidity. . . .

"Choices for the kind of anesthesia should be available and discussed among patient, obstetrician, and anesthesiologist. In particular, where not medically contraindicated the patient should have the option of receiving regional anesthesia. . . .

"There is limited research concerning the psychological impact on parents following cesarean birth. Nevertheless, surgery is clearly an increased psychological and physical burden when compared with a normal vaginal delivery. In addition, negative responses from mother and father have been reported in the available retrospective studies. In some hospitals, family centered maternity care has been extended to the cesarean birth family, and in these cases there is no evidence of harm to the mother, neonate, or father. The presence of fathers in the operating room and closer contact between mother and neonate appear to improve the post-cesarean behavioral responses of the families. One consistent finding from small scale studies of post-cesarean birth families is the greater involvement of fathers with their infants. Improved educational programs for all families so that they may understand the cesarean birth, and specific educational programs for previous cesarean birth families, are methods to improve the birth experience. . . .

"The courts should recognize that if a vaginal delivery resulted in a 'less than perfect' baby, this does not necessarily mean that the physician was negligent for not performing a cesarean birth."

VAGINAL BIRTH AFTER CESAREAN

In Europe vaginal birth after cesarean (VBAC) is common, but in the U.S. the dictum has been, "Once a cesarean, always a cesarean." This is changing, as more women question the necessity of a repeat elective cesarean. Some researchers feel that the risk of a trial of labor is in fact lower than the risks of repeat surgery. And, the rate of uterine rupture is only about .5%, much lower than most people realize. More doctors are offering VBAC services to their patients, but many regard the previous cesarean patient as a high-risk case and conduct VBACs with the kind of "aggressive management" of labor which may result in another cesarean. For this reason some cesarean parents are now having their vaginal births after cesarean at home.

The Cesarean Birth Alliance, the Cesarean Prevention Movement, the Council for Cesarean Awareness and C/SEC (all listed under "Cesarean Support and Prevention Groups") provide information on vaginal birth after cesarean (VBAC).

NANCY WAINER COHEN
10 Great Plain Terrace
Needham, MA 02192
617/449-2490

Nancy Cohen is a one-woman "organization." She was a co-founder of C/SEC (see index) and left that group some years ago to devote her energies to the promotion of vaginal birth after cesarean (VBAC). Cohen's first child was born by cesarean, her second vaginally in a hospital, and her third vaginally at home. She believes strongly in the safety of VBAC and her approach to education includes correcting misinformation that leads couples to fear VBAC (especially the "myth" of catastrophic uterine rupture), and developing psychological attitudes and tools to cope confidently with labor.

Nancy Cohen offers the following services. When writing to her for information, please include a self-addressed, stamped envelope.
VBAC and Cesarean Prevention Classes, 8 week course, held in Needham
Concentrated Saturday Workshops, for couples living out-of-state
Traveling Lecture and All-Day Workshop available for booking
Telephone Counseling for VBAC and cesarean prevention
Class Packet of information on VBAC
There is a fee involved for each of these services. Write for more information.

> ". . . in most cases, attempting a vaginal birth is less risky than automatically performing another cesarean."

"There is much research to substantiate the theory that a VBAC can be accomplished in a very high percentage of cases, and that in most cases, attempting a vaginal birth is less risky than automatically performing another cesarean. We are reminded that the United States is one of the only countries where repeat cesarean is practiced, and that many cesareans in our country could be prevented. To accomplish a VBAC requires that we be informed, educated, and determined. The decision about a vaginal birth ultimately rests with the informed woman (or couple) who considers her past birth history, the present pregnancy and other factors. Although a vaginal birth is not available to all women who have had cesareans, it is important to realize that the dictum 'Once a cesarean, always a cesarean' is a worn-out cliche. It is unfortunate that many women find out after they have had three or four cesareans that a vaginal delivery would have been possible. More and more, couples are questioning the practice of repeat cesareans, in an effort to avoid giving birth surgically. They are challenging the old dictum with extremely encouraging results."

from "Vaginal Birth Following A Cesarean?" a fact sheet by Nancy Cohen, 1980.

SILENT KNIFE: Cesarean Prevention and Vaginal Birth After Cesarean (VBAC)
by Nancy Wainer Cohen and Lois J. Estner
1983, 480 pages, Illus.

from
J.F. Bergin Publishers
670 Amherst Road
South Hadley, MA 01075
$29.75 hd.
$14.95 pap.
plus 1.00 shipping

As I write, this book is not yet available for review, but I hear from those in the cesarean prevention movement that Silent Knife is excellent. Write for a brochure.

VAGINAL BIRTH AFTER CESAREAN
by Kathy Keolker
1981, 4 pages

from
the pennypress
1100 23rd Avenue East
Seattle, WA 98112
$.50 single copy
bulk rates available

Kathy Keolker discusses the risks and benefits of VBAC and outlines who may be a candidate. She discusses the role of fear in anticipating a vaginal delivery and stresses that at least 50 to 70% of women can have a VBAC, according to current studies. Advice is offered on choosing a supportive doctor, making a birth plan, dealing with the stresses of labor, and accepting the possibility of another cesarean.

HOME BIRTH AFTER CESAREAN
by Kathy Neetz
1981, 2 pages, Illus.
(Summer 1981 issue of Childbirth Alternatives Quarterly)

from
Childbirth Alternatives Quarterly
c/o Ashford
Bin 62, SLAC
Stanford, CA 94305

Kathy and Phil Neetz had their first child by cesarean and ultimately came to feel that the surgery had been unnecessary. In preparation for their second birth, they attended a Saturday workshop with Nancy Cohen in Massachusetts (traveling from Brooklyn to attend) and made plans for a home delivery attended by a midwife. Phil is a minister and their Christian faith was an important factor in giving them the confidence to give birth naturally at home.

"I had been quiet with Joshua's labor, but this time I was really vocal and it felt great. Also, I had done Lamaze breathing before. This time I did whatever felt right with each contraction—sometimes slow and sometimes more rapid, using no set pattern.

"It was when I saw Caleb's head in the mirror as he was slowly descending and lightly touched it that I knew we were going to do it. A few more good pushes and Caleb was born. Praise God!"

GUIDELINES FOR VAGINAL DELIVERY AFTER A CESAREAN CHILDBIRTH
(ACOG Committee Statement)
January 1982, 4 pages

from
Resource Center
The American College of Obstetricians and Gynecologists
600 Maryland Ave., SW, No. 300
Washington, DC 20024
free

Vaginal birth after cesarean (VBAC) is common in Europe but very uncommon in the U.S., where the American College of Obstetricians and Gynecologists (ACOG) estimates that 99% of all cesarean mothers have repeat cesareans for their subsequent births. In response to consumer demands for VBAC, the ACOG Committee on Obstetrics: Maternal and Fetal Medicine studied the literature and concluded that VBAC is "an option appropriate for consideration." The Committee states, "Specific data on the risk of vaginal birth after a prior low transverse uterine incision are limited but suggest that the risk of maternal mortality from uterine rupture is almost nonexistent and the risk of perinatal death is relatively small."

"First, why might a woman consider a vaginal birth? The reasons are varied. Her previous cesarean may have been emotionally or physically difficult, she may have had a bad experience with medication, she may wonder if it was truly necessary, her partner may have been excluded, she may have been separated from her baby. She may simply be looking for a better experience this time. All these reasons are good ones, as there are many documented benefits of vaginal birth after cesarean. A review of the literature indicates that the current maternal mortality rate with elective repeat cesarean is 18/100,000, which is 1.2 times greater than with vaginal birth after cesarean. Infection rates in mothers after cesarean birth range from 10 to 65%, and are much lower after vaginal birth."

The following guidelines are given for physicians and hospitals which wish to provide VBAC services:
"The woman and her physician should fully discuss the options of a trial of labor early in the prenatal course to allow for appropriate planning.

The indication for the prior cesarean birth should be a nonrepeating condition, e.g., patients with previous cesarean birth for fetal distress or for failure to progress without documented feto pelvic disproportion.

The type of previous uterine incision should have been documented to be a low segment transverse type.

The pregnancy should be a singleton with a vertex presentation and a fetal weight estimated to be less than 4,000 grams.

There should be no other obstetric, medical or surgical history or physical findings that contraindicates labor and vaginal delivery.

There should be capabilities for continuous fetal heart rate and uterine activity monitoring throughout labor.

The patient should understand that it may be necessary to terminate the trial of labor and proceed with cesarean section."

Patient's Rights

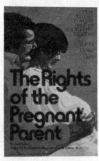

THE RIGHTS OF THE PREGNANT PARENT (Revised Edition)
by Valmai Howe Elkins
1980, 304 pages

from
Schocken Books
200 Madison Avenue
New York, NY 10016
$6.95 pap.

No woman should give birth in a hospital without first reading this book. Valmai Elkins is a childbirth educator who became angry when so many of her students did not have the kind of birth they'd hoped for. She describes the history of childbirth practices, the methods of prepared childbirth, the common procedures and drugs used in hospitals, and carefully details the basic "human rights" to which she believes all pregnant couples are entitled. These include:

1. The right to a supportive doctor.
2. The right to a healthy baby.
3. The right to childbirth education.
4. The right to a shared birth experience.
5. The right to childbirth with dignity.
6. The right to family-centered maternity care.

Most valuable is the chapter, "How to Get the Childbirth You Want," which provides step by step guidelines for choosing medical care and working with hospital staff. Many anecdotes are included to show how couples used what they learned to affect hospital policy. It all adds up to what Elkins calls "ultra-prepared childbirth."

"Valerie and Serge Poulard didn't see the need for routine fetal monitoring or an IV, because Valerie was not a high-risk pregnancy. When Valerie signed the [hospital consent] form, she added, 'all procedures to be carried out only with my complete understanding of the need for such.' The Poulards were at a hospital where IV's and monitors are used almost routinely, and Valerie bypassed them because of this clause: instead, the fetal heart rate was monitored by a nurse.

"The 'subject to my complete understanding of procedures involved' clause is useful if you want to avoid

any of the hospital 'routines.' But be careful to make your decisions after careful thought, to avoid 'faddiness' and be aware that in sidestepping routine you take on yourselves responsibility for anything which goes wrong. (I have never heard of a case where bypassing a routine led to anything undesirable.) In the event of a complication, medical staff should explain procedures so that you give your 'informed consent' with full understanding of the need.

" 'In my case the clause was a safeguard because as it turned out I did not have to resort to it,' says Valerie. 'The nurses were surprised when I told them that I had the doctor's permission to bypass routines. They respected our decisions and were supportive—except for one nurse who really wanted to shave me, something I had requested not be done. When it's all boiled down, nobody can force you into these procedures.' "

OBSTETRIC TESTS AND TECHNOLOGY: A Consumer's Guide
by Margot Edwards and Penny Simkin
1980, 8 pages, Illus.

from
the pennypress
1100 23rd Ave., East
Seattle, WA 98112
$1.00 single copy
$40.00 per 100

This leaflet provides an excellent introduction to the risks and benefits of the many obstetrical tests which parents will confront during pregnancy and labor. Covered are the estriol determination series, oxytocin challenge test, non-stress test, amniocentesis, tests for fetal lung maturity, roll-over test, ultrasound, and electronic fetal monitoring. The authors stress the importance of informed consent and decision making. An additional list of references to accompany this leaflet is available by sending a self-addressed, stamped envelope to the publisher, the pennypress.

"Before consenting to a test, parents should know something about it, and whether its benefits exceed its risks. Tests are ordered to rule out and diagnose problems. Results of the tests may imply a decided action if problems exist. One means of deciding whether to have a test is to ask if the results will alter the physician's plan for care and/or treatment, or if his/her decision on how to proceed depends on the results of a particular test. If so, how? If not, then perhaps the test is not necessary. Parents are often asked to sign a consent or release form for certain tests, and signing should be based upon an informed consent."

INFORMED CONSENT FOR OBSTETRIC DRUGS

In 1978, New York became the first state to have a law requiring informed consent for obstetric drugs. The law (Section 2503 of the Public Health Law) reads:

"The physician or nurse-midwife to be in attendance at the birth of a child shall inform the expectant mother, in advance of the birth, of the drugs that such physician or nurse-midwife expects to employ during pregnancy and of the obstetrical and other drugs that such physician or nurse-midwife expects to employ at birth and of the possible effects of such drugs on the child and mother."

The law was passed largely through the efforts of Doris Haire, of the American Foundation for Maternal and Child Health; and Estelle Cohen, a woman whose second child suffered permanent brain damage probably as a result of a labor which was electively induced with an oxytocic drug. Haire and Cohen hope that the New York law will serve as a model for other states. Under the law, the physician or nurse-midwife is responsible for *initiating* a discussion of drug risks and benefits with every obstetrical patient, whether or not the patient herself requests such information. Unfortunately, the experience of childbirth groups on Long Island and in the New York metropolitan area has been that doctors are not initiating such discussions, and are in violation of the law either willfully or through ignorance.

A similar bill has been introduced on the federal level to help provide women across the country with more access to information on obstetrical drugs. The bill, HR6341, was introduced by Congressperson Jonathan

Bingham of New York on January 30, 1980, at the urging of his constituent, Estelle Cohen. The introduction to the bill states:

"To amend Title V of the Social Security Act to require States to provide women access to their obstetric medical records and current information on obstetrical procedures, to amend the Federal Food, Drug, and Cosmetic Act to require the dissemination of information on the effects and risks of drugs and devices on the health of pregnant and parturient women and of prospective and developing children, and to provide for a study on the delayed long-term effect on child development of obstetrical drugs and procedures administered to or used by pregnant and parturient women."

Unfortunately, it has been difficult to persuade other members of Congress that the bill is important and should be considered in committee hearings, a first step toward approval. In addition, Mr. Bingham left office at the end of 1982 and it is not clear who will now sponsor the legislation. Readers may consider writing to their own representatives in Congress to urge that hearings be held.

For more information on Estelle Cohen and the New York law on obstetric drugs, see "Estelle Cohen: A Woman Who Fought Back," by Janet Isaacs Ashford, in the Fall 1980 issue of Childbirth Alternatives Quarterly (see index).

For a copy of Congressperson Bingham's proposed bill on obstetric care, request HR6341 from:
House Documents Office
Washington, DC 20505

**THE PREGNANT PATIENT'S BILL OF RIGHTS
THE PREGNANT PATIENT'S RESPONSIBILITIES**
by Doris Haire
4 pages

from
ICEA Bookcenter
P.O. Box 20048
Minneapolis, MN 55420
$.20 plus .60 postage
bulk rates available

This bill of rights and responsibilities is an essential tool for women who want to ensure a safe, satisfying pregnancy and birth experience. Doris Haire has provided an excellent discussion of the elements of informed consent and a 16-point bill of rights and 12-point list of responsibilities.

"American parents are becoming increasingly aware that well-intentioned health professionals do not always have scientific data to support common American obstetrical

practices and that many of these practices are carried out primarily because they are part of medical and hospital tradition. In the last forty years many artificial practices have been introduced which have changed childbirth from a physiological event to a very complicated medical procedure in which all kinds of drugs are used and procedures carried out, sometimes unnecessarily, and many of them potentially damaging for the baby and even for the mother. A growing body of research makes it alarmingly clear that every aspect of traditional American hospital care during labor and delivery must now be questioned as to its possible effect on the future well-being of both the obstetric patient and her unborn child."

PLANNING YOUR BABY'S BIRTH
by Penny Simkin and Carla Reinke
1980, 4 pages

from
the pennypress
1100 23rd Avenue East
Seattle, WA 98112
$.50 single copy
$20.00 for 100

Planning Your Baby's Birth features a 3-page discussion of the important issues in birth planning and preparation and a 1-page chart of "Choices in Childbirth" which lists birth practices and procedures side by side under the headings "Medical Pathway" and "Physiologic Pathway."

"Under 'Medical Pathway' are listed hospital routines and procedures that are widely used with women in childbirth. These are not always used for medical reasons. Sometimes these routines are used not because something has gone wrong, but just in case something should go wrong, or for medico-legal reasons. Sometimes they are used simply as a matter of staff convenience. Sometimes these routines are habits from the past when birth involved surgical technique, sterile surroundings, and general anesthesia. Of course, every hospital does not routinely use each procedure, but they are mentioned here because they are in wide use in North America. Find out which routines prevail in your hospital. Birth centers and home birth services have fewer routines, mainly because of their physiologic orientation toward birth. If you do not have a birth plan, you may expect that your birth will be managed by the routines of your doctor and hospital."

CONSIDERATIONS FOR HOSPITAL BIRTH
8 pages
$.35 plus SASE

BIRTH CHOICES
1981, 4 pages
$.25 plus SASE

from
Rosemary Romberg Wiener
6294 Mission Road
Everson, WA 98247
bulk rates available

These two pamphlets are part of Wiener's series of class "hand-outs" for childbirth educators (see index). *Considerations for Hospital Birth* describes 14 common hospital birth practices, explaining the medical rationale and consumer alternatives. *Birth Choices* considers hospital birth, birthing centers, and home birth, providing a list of advantages and disadvantages of each method.

"It is . . . very important to discuss what you want in your birth experience, and make arrangements for

MAKING A BIRTH PLAN

these things in advance of your actual admission. It is not a good idea to start asking for a number of things after you are in the hospital and in labor. Labor requires your complete attention and concentration and should be as peaceful and undisturbed of an experience as possible. Besides, the nurses in the hospital don't make the rules and probably will not feel that they are free to do things differently for you. Fighting a nurse who is trying to give you an enema or pubic shave will probably get you nowhere and will make everyone miserable. Trying to ask for special things while you are in labor, and perhaps encountering disappointment over not getting what you want can be very disturbing and upsetting to the course of labor."

PREPARED CHILDBIRTH PREFERENCES
by the Long Island ASPO Professional Coalition
1981, 2 pages

from
Prepared Childbirth Preferences
P.O. Box 424 North
1614 Grand Avenue
North Baldwin, NY 11510
$.50 each
bulk rates available

Fifty-two specific procedures and requests are listed, with two spaces beside each for the woman to initial her preference and the physician to initial his/her approval. Items include the role of the labor coach, comfort measures in labor, hospital routines, fetal monitoring, bonding, and rooming-in. The list is especially geared to Lamaze-trained couples planning a hospital birth.

"Today's childbearing woman is often an enlightened medical consumer seeking a teamwork relationship with her obstetrician. This *Prepared Childbirth Preferences* form has been developed as a prenatal dialogue guide, establishing clearly those options which the pregnant couple specifically desires; and which of those options the professional staff is able and willing to provide . . . .

"Before resorting to oxytocics, let me try stimulation of a sluggish labor by non-invasive means: position changes, ambulation, removal of stressful staff member, privacy with coach and his loving touch, progressive relaxation."

PREGNANCY/CHILDBIRTH CHECKLIST
by Dana Shilling
1980, 8 pages

from
Plaintext
41 Mercer Street
Jersey City, NJ 07302
$2.00 for single copy
$4.00 for complete Family Health Package which includes *Pregnancy/ Childbirth Checklist, Choosing a Doctor, Doctor-Patient Check-list,* and *Hospital Patient's Check-list.*
bulk rates available

Plaintext's check-list is a well-prepared form for recording informa-

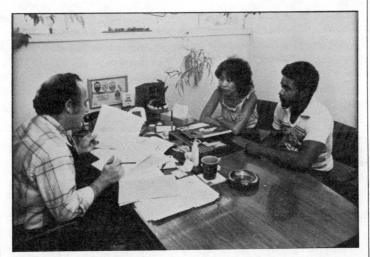

© 1983 Rodger F. Ewy/EGA Inc.

tion and preferences for childbirth. Part I, "Choices in Childbirth," lists 17 specific options with room to fill in a definition, advantages and disadvantages, and your choice for each one. The format encourages consumers to do their own reading and research in order to "fill in the blanks." Options include place and attendant for birth, different labor medications, and different methods for unmedicated childbirth. "Problems of Pregnancy and Childbirth" lists 12 common medical problems with room to note a definition plus "How to Recognize It," and "How to Cope." Prenatal Care Notes are provided for 10 visits with room for dates, exam and lab results, and discussion. Part 4 is for recording "Facts About the Hospital or Maternity Center" and Part 5 is a "Labor Record."

Plaintext editor, Dana Shilling, is a Harvard trained lawyer and in a letter says, "The techniques for making up a plain English checklist about *anything* are pretty much the same: read all you can, to identify the issues (after all, since it's a check-list, I don't take sides; I just try to let people know the areas of controversy), figure out the information needed to make an intelligent choice, and arrange the information for maximum accessibility."

COOPERATIVE CHILDBIRTH PREFERENCES
by Gail Sforza Brewer
1978, 2 pages

from
Cooperative Childbirth Network
16 Sunset Drive
Bedford Hills, NY 10507
$.15 plus SASE

Excerpted from the *Pregnancy-After-30 Workbook* by Gail Brewer, this check-list lists 14 "preferences" for labor and 14 for birth side by side with a "rationale" which explains the advantages of each.
"Preference 4. Refrain from routine use of IV fluids.
"Rationale 4. Well-nourished mothers have expanded plasma volume and stored fluid as prophylaxes against dehydration and shock. A mother who gives birth spontaneously, without analgesia or anesthesia, and breastfeeds her baby at birth rarely hemorrhages. IV interferes with relaxation.
"Preference 11. Allow membranes to rupture spontaneously.
"Rationale 11. Forewaters provide a cushioning effect, equalizing pressure on the baby's head during contractions. Excessive molding of the head is caused by unequal pressure after amniotomy. Artificial rupture commits staff to delivery by schedule and increases the risk of infection to mother and baby."

HOSPITAL BIRTH CHECK-LIST

Prepared with assistance from Ruth Longacre and materials supplied by
HOMEBIRTH, INC., Boston University Station, P.O. Box 355, Boston, MA 02215.

MORE AND MORE COUPLES are preparing for "natural child-birth" and attending childbirth classes, in hopes of a joyous, normal birth. *But,* more and more routine procedures and drugs are being used in hospital births today and the cesarean section rate is very high (20 to 40 percent, depending on the hospital). So couples who plan to give birth in a hospital will need to make careful preparations during pregnancy to make sure that the hospital birth experience is safe and satisfying for them. If you want to avoid routine obstetrical interventions which may be harmful or unnecessary in normal birth, your plans must be worked out and discussed with your care givers *before* labor begins. Labor is not a good time to begin making changes in hospital routine. Start working now to make sure that your doctor and the hospital staff understand and will cooperate with your plans for your birth. It may be difficult or frustrating to change established policies, but remember that your efforts will also benefit the women who come after you.

A GOOD FIRST STEP is to make a list of your needs and concerns (include special treatment you *want* as well as routine treatment you *don't* want) to help clarify these issues in your own mind. Take a look at some of the books and "birth plans" listed in the section on Patients' Rights in this *Catalog* for guidance in learning about the risks and benefits of obstetrical practices. It is wise to read and investigate standards of maternity care as early in pregnancy as possible, or even before. With your list of requests firmly in mind or on paper, you will be in a better position to choose a supportive doctor for your prenatal care.

THE NEXT STEP is to choose your doctor/midwife and hospital carefully. Find out which hospitals in your area have the most flexible maternity programs (family-centered care, birthing rooms, rooming-in, etc.) and interview the professionals affiliated with the best hospitals. In a non-emergency situation, you may want to travel some distance to get the best birth experience. At your first prenatal visit, ask the doctor or midwife how s/he feels about the things which are most important to you (natural childbirth, fathers in the delivery room, breastfeeding, etc.). If you find you must change doctors, do so as early as possible. It is also important to choose the best, most supportive childbirth preparation class available. Look for an instructor with a strong, consumer-oriented approach. She may be able to offer you invaluable information on how other couples have been treated at local hospitals. It may be a good idea to choose a course sponsored by an independent childbirth organization rather than one sponsored by the hospital. (See section on choosing a childbirth educator in the section on childbirth preparation.)

AS YOUR DUE DATE APPROACHES, it is important to work out specific details in advance with both your doctor and the hospital. Don't take anything for granted. Discuss with your doctor exactly how you expect the birth to be handled. Present your list of requests to your doctor. It may be a good idea to set up a separate appointment to be able to take the time to sit in the doctor's office, with your husband or labor coach, to go over the details of the birth. You don't want to be sitting half-dressed on an examining table and you don't want to be made to feel rushed. Discuss your requests with your doctor carefully, resolve any differences of opinion, and have the list attached to your medical records. Also bring a copy of your list with you when you are admitted to the hospital. This is important, since the hospital staff may be reluctant to honor special requests if your doctor is not available during labor to confirm them. Find out in advance exactly what the routine policies of your hospital are. It may be that many of your requests are already accepted practice, or it may be that none of them are. If the hospital staff is not cooperative, your doctor's orders can help override any routine procedures.

WHAT IF THERE ARE NO DOCTORS OR HOSPITALS in your area which will honor your requests? Many couples faced with this problem choose to give birth at home or in a free-standing birth center, if such services are available. If you decide to continue with your plans to deliver in a hospital, however, it is important to know what your rights are. According to the ACLU's handbook on patients' rights (see index under *The Rights of Hospital Patients*), all hospital patients have the right to refuse any medical treatment. Under these circumstances, the hospital is still obliged to continue care within the limits of the patient's refusals. If you are forced to simply refuse certain treatments, expect to be badgered by the staff, but remember that refusal is your legal right. Hospital "rules" are simply the hospital's own policies and do not have the force of law. It is your right to refuse any drug or other medication and to refuse most routine procedures such as aftificial breaking of the membranes or the use of an electronic fetal heart monitor. Patients may not dictate treatment, however, so if the hospital resists, you cannot demand a Leboyer birth or rooming-in, for instance. If your hospital's policies are very bad, your best course may be to check in as late in labor as possible and leave as soon as possible after birth.

EVEN IF YOU HAVE WORKED OUT YOUR PLANS carefully in advance with both doctor and hospital, you may still encounter problems while you are actually in labor. Make sure that you and your husband or other labor coach are in agreement about how to handle difficulties. For instance, you might say to your labor coach in advance, "If I am in pain and the staff is encouraging me to accept drugs, please remind me that labor will be over soon, that we can get through the next contraction, and that I really don't want to take a chance on harming the baby. Help me to be firm when I'm under stress and act as my advocate with the staff." If you are asked to sign a consent form, make sure you write in an extra clause to protect your right to informed consent. You might write in, "No drugs or procedures to be used without my informed consent." If your own doctor is unavailable when you check in, make sure to explain your plans to whoever is caring for you. Remember to act firmly, insist on your rights, and be prepared to say NO if unacceptable procedures are offered or pressed.

HOSPITAL SURVEYS

The Mother's Center of Hicksville, New York, conducted a hospital survey of ten local hospitals with maternity units, asking fifty specific questions about facilities, staff and services. Results were published in table form and made available to the public. For more information on conducting a hospital survey in your area, contact the Mothers' Center, Old Country Road and Nelson Ave., Hicksville, New York 11801.

The following is a list of specific requests which many parents have found useful. Refer to the resources listed in this *Catalog* for more specific information on the advantages and disadvantages of the procedures listed here.

1. Omit shaving the pubic hair or routine use of an enema.
2. Allow use of juice and light food during labor and other comfort measures, such as ice chips, a face cloth, heating pad, extra pillows, ice pack, etc. Omit routine intravenous fluids.
3. Don't offer sedatives, tranquilizers, analgesics, or anesthetics unless medically necessary.
4. If labor is slow or long, allow alternative treatment (walking, change of position, rest, etc.) before considering speeding the labor with drugs.
5. Allow the fetal membranes to rupture spontaneously.
6. Use frequent auscultation with a fetoscope to monitor the baby's heartbeat, rather than routine electronic fetal monitoring.
7. Allow the mother to walk and be upright during labor and assume any comfortable position.
8. Allow mother to assume most comfortable position for delivery (side lying, on all fours, squatting, sitting up, etc.) without use of stirrups or hand cuffs.
9. Allow use of the same room for labor, delivery and recovery.
10. Provide dimmed lights and warm temperature in birthing room, if desired by parents.
11. Permit use of personal clothing for labor and birth and for the baby.
12. Permit husband and/or other coach-companions in labor, delivery, and recovery.
13. Allow siblings to participate in the birth, stay over in the hospital if necessary, and have visiting privileges.
14. Allow use of a camera in labor and delivery and admittance of a person other than coach to operate it.
15. Permit the father or other companion to receive the baby as it is being born and to cut the umbilical cord.
16. Use massage, hot compresses, and non-lithotomy position (flat on the back) to avoid tearing of the perineum. Avoid routine epsiotomy.
17. Delay cutting the cord until it has stopped pulsing and emptied of blood.
18. Allow adequate time for spontaneous delivery of the placenta. Do not use routine drugs or pulling, or manual extraction.
19. Give the baby immediately to the mother on the delivery table, so that she may nurse and warm the baby with her body.
20. Delay eye treatment for several hours to permit parent-infant bonding and use less harmful alternatives to silver nitrate, such as erythromycin or tetracycline ointments.
21. Use a local anesthetic for post-episiotomy stitches, if necessary.
22. Reduce or eliminate time spent in recovery room. Permit immediate and continued rooming-in for whole family.
23. Facilitate an early newborn examination by pediatrician, to permit early discharge from the hospital, 2 to 6 hours after delivery, barring complications.
24. If baby is discharged early from hospital, schedule routine PKU testing for 7-14 days after birth, since testing in first 1-3 days of life will not be accurate.
25. Omit routine shot of Vitamin K for newborn. If circumcision is desired, delay it until baby is at least one week old, when blood clotting ability is normal.
26. If cesarean-section is necessary allow use of regional anesthesia, husband and/or companion in operating room, no parent/infant separation if baby is healthy, immediate breastfeeding, and rooming-in.
27. If the baby requires intensive care: keep parents constantly informed of baby's condition, allow parents to stay over in the hospital, transfer mother and baby together to a high-risk center, allow parents to assume as much of the baby's care as possible, feed baby with breast milk (provide breast pump when necessary) and allow breastfeeding as soon as possible, discharge baby from intensive care unit at earliest possible time.

A Personal Experience
by Ruth Longacre

When I became pregnant with my third child I knew more about birth and what choices I had. I also had more confidence in myself as a woman. At first, we planned for a home birth and a midwife friend of mine agreed to attend. But we finally decided to use the birthing room at a small, private hospital because of the complications of the pregnancy of the last child (he was premature) and because I had experienced a miscarriage about a year before. It was a painful decision because I knew that the atmosphere of an uncomplicated home birth could not be duplicated in the hospital. The decision was difficult also because we already belonged to a community health plan which covered maternity expenses only at an affiliated hospital, which I would not use because of its rigid, unbending birthing practices. The payments for the private hospital had to come out of our own pockets.

The most important thing to me, though, was that the baby never leave my arms. The early separation from my first two babies was the most distressing part of my hospital care. We also wanted Rio and Jesse Jesse, who were then six and four, to be with Ron and me at the birth. Because I was seeing a very unusual and sensitive doctor, we were pleased to have his okay for the childrens' presence in the birthing room. There was also a great deal of support from the nursing supervisor. However, we still needed permission from the State Department of Public Health which, after many letters and phone calls, was finally granted.

We wrote a letter to our doctor, outlining our requests for labor, birth, and the postpartum period as we had discussed them with him. Because of our preparation and the cooperation of our doctor and the hospital staff, we were able to achieve the birth we wanted. Afterwards, I wrote this letter of thanks to the hospital director:

'Dear Sir,

'I would like to take this opportunity on behalf of my family and myself to express our appreciation for receiving the kind of birthing experience that we had anticipated and had worked so hard to achieve.

'Our child was welcomed into a calm, quiet, unhurried atmosphere, with as little as possible intervention by the nursing staff. The two older children viewed the birth with awe and immediately surrounded the new child, forming a bond and making the transition of accepting a new sibling very easy and untraumatic.

'Dr. _____ had cared for me during my prenatal period with both compassion and obstetrical competence. This kind of individualized care made the prenatal months easy to flow through, knowing I had both an advocate and a skilled physician on my team.

'I hope that my family's experience will open the door for other families to have the same choices, so that they can feel they have some control over their birthing experience and can experience childbirth with dignity.

Ruth Longacre, 1978'

(Editor's Note: Ruth gave birth to her fourth child [and first daughter] at home. Pictures of her labor and birth appear in the section on home birth.)

THE RIGHTS OF HOSPITAL PATIENTS
The Basic ACLU Guide to a Hospital Patient's Rights
by George J. Annas
1975, 246 pages

from
Avon Books
959 Eighth Avenue
New York, NY 10019
$2.50 pap.

A major component of the rights of hospital patients is the right to refuse treatment. This is especially important in maternity care, where so many hospital "routines" are potentially harmful. Many patients are intimidated into accepting unwanted procedures and drugs by staff members who say, "It's hospital policy!" But as Annas points out, "Patients may refuse to permit any medical or surgical procedure from being performed on them regardless of the opinions of their doctors as to the advisability of the treatment." This book uses a question and answer format to explain the legal rights of hospital patients and includes a chapter on the special concerns of women.

"Inside the hospital, the woman in labor has all the rights of any other hospital patient. As such she cannot be given any specific types of treatment without her consent and has the right to refuse specifically recommended procedures. She has, for example, the right to refuse any and all drugs before and during delivery or to fully participate in deciding which drugs will be used on her, at what time, and in what doses."

A PATIENT'S BILL OF RIGHTS

from
American Hospital Association
840 N. Lake Shore Drive
Chicago, IL 60611
free flyer

This 12-point bill of rights was developed and approved by the American Hospital Association and hospitals which are members of the Association are expected to honor and support these rights for their patients.

"The patient has the right to receive from his physician information necessary to give informed consent prior to the start of any procedure and/or treatment. Except in emergencies, such information for informed consent should include but not necessarily be limited to the specific procedure and/or treatment, the medically significant risks involved, and the probable duration of incapacitation. Where medically significant alternatives for care or treatment exist, or when the patient requests information concerning medical alternatives, the patient has the right to such information. The patient also has the right to know the name of the person responsible for the procedures and/or treatment."

MEDICAL RECORDS: GETTING YOURS
A Consumer's Guide to Obtaining Your Medical Records
by Maria Sarath, Melissa Auerbach and Ted Bogue
1980, 63 pages

from
Public Citizen/Health Research Group
2000 P Street, NW, Suite 708
Washington, DC 20036
$2.50 pap.
bulk rates available

If you've had a bad hospital birth experience, you may want to take a look at your hospital medical records to find out what went wrong and how it can be prevented next time. Many women are surprised to learn from their records that they received drugs without being informed at the time. Because hospitals and doctors are often reluctant to provide access to medical records, Public Citizen (a Ralph Nader organization) has published this guide to help patients know their rights. The guide explains why access to records is important and provides a step by step guide to getting your records, with a survey of the relevant state laws (access is governed by state law and each state is different), plus a guide to federal access and advice on obtaining employee records.

"Call the health care provider (in a hospital, the medical records department) whose records you wish to see and ask what procedures you should follow to obtain access. Some hospitals may have established procedures which are not specified in any state law. For example, you may be told to go in person to the hospital's medical records department or to put your request in writing first (which also may be required by state law).

"If anything the doctor or hospital tells you is not consistent with the law in your state, you should immediately point it out, citing the statute. For this purpose, it would be advisable to have a copy of this book's description of your statute (if there is one) in front of you when you call.

"For all telephone conversations, you should write down the date and time of the phone call, the name of the person you talked to, and what you were told. Such documentation may be valuable later."

CONSUMER GUIDES FOR CHILDBIRTH

NAPSAC CONSUMER GUIDE: To Alternative Birth Services
by Penny Simkin, with revisions by Jamy Braun and Lee Stewart
1982, 38 pages

from
NAPSAC International
P.O. Box 267
Marble Hill, MO 63764
$2.00
bulk rates available

This *Consumer Guide* is included with the complete Directory of Alternative Birth Services, published by NAPSAC (see Index), but it is also available as a separate publication. The guide provides an introduction to current issues in childbirth and the role of the consumer, and provides guidelines for choosing a birth attendant and childbirth educator and for deciding where and how to give birth.

"Standing orders from each physician in the hospital deal with such things as: when, what, and how much medication or anesthesia to give; prepping procedures—enema, shave, etc.; the use of intravenous fluids; the fetal monitor; and other procedures the nurse does. If you do not wish to be treated according to standing orders, this will have to to stated on your chart, and you should be prepared to remind the staff of this. It is an excellent idea to write out a Birth Plan, describing how you would like your childbirth experience to be. . . . A good Birth Plan takes time and study; let your doctor know you are preparing it. Write it in a style that reflects a cooperative and reasonable attitude. Then, approximately three to four weeks before you expect to give birth, or sooner if you know what you want, go over it with the doctor. Be willing to consider alternatives presented by your doctor. It should then become part of your medical record which will be with you when you are in labor."

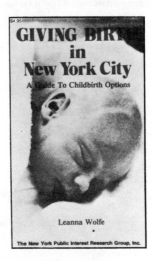

GIVING BIRTH IN NEW YORK CITY: A Guide to Childbirth Options
by Leanna Wolfe
1981, 93 pages, Illus.

from
NYPIRG Publications
9 Murray St., 3rd floor
New York, NY 10007
212/349-6460
$4.95 plus $1.05 postage
bulk rates available

This guide was published as a project of the New York Public Interest Research Group (NYPIRG), a non-profit research and advocacy organization directed by New York state college students. It contains descriptive listings of alternative birth services in the New York City area, including hospital-based midwifery services, home birth services, and birth centers. This part of the guide will be directly useful to people who live in the metropolitan area. But the sections on financial resources for birth (insurance, medicaid, etc.), and the listings of useful books and national organizations will be helpful to people anywhere. The Appendix includes a glossary of terms, a sample "Birth Plan," the "Pregnant Patient's Bill of Rights," and information on New York state's model law on informed consent in childbirth. Activists around the country will find this guide an extremely useful model for the production of similar local guidebooks.

"In the United States, partly as a result of the women's and consumers' movements, there is a growing emphasis on more natural, personalized childbirth. Central to the movement are midwives, health care professionals who provide family planning services, childbirth education, prenatal and postpartum care, as well as attending normal labors and deliveries. Midwifery is based on an understanding of pregnancy and childbirth as part of the life cycle rather than as an illness. The psychological, social, and cultural needs of women and families are viewed with respect. Nutritional and health maintenance information is considered a vital part of prenatal care. By carefully attending a woman through pregnancy and labor, midwives can minimize the need for drugs. Midwives are taught to screen for potential problems, to recognize problems if they arise, and to use available technology when necessary. Physicians are consulted if needed."

Alternatives in Childbirth

Alternatives to routine hospital birth practices have come about during the past twenty or so years due to intense consumer pressure and due to competition among physicians and hospitals caused by falling birth rates. Alternatives range from the modest changes made by family-centered maternity programs in hospitals to the radical challenge to hospital birth presented by home births without medical assistance. This section will explore and provide resources on some of the many alternatives currently available in settings and attendants for birth.

Family-centered Care

Family-centered maternity care generally means a program in which the emotional needs of the family are considered to be as important as the medical management of the birth. Programs may range from the simple permission for fathers to be present in the labor and delivery rooms to well-defined, non-interventive programs for hospital "birthing-rooms."

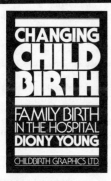

CHANGING CHILDBIRTH: Family Birth in the Hospital
by Diony Young
1982, 480 pages

from
Childbirth Graphics, Ltd.
P.O. Box 17025, Irondequoit Div.
Rochester, NY 14617-0325
$18.95 pap.

Diony Young is a well-respected childbirth advocate whose previous works include *Bonding: How Parents Become Attached to Their Baby* and *Unnecessary Cesareans: Ways to Avoid Them* (see index for reviews). In *Changing Childbirth* she gathers together and discusses the voluminous material now available on the benefits of the family-centered approach to birth, with the sole intention of helping consumers and providers who are working to change hospital policies. Young provides the extensive documentation and background childbirth advocates need to overcome resistance from institutions. Young describes the basic principles and background of the family-centered program and devotes a chapter to each important component. She covers the following topics: sharing birth with a partner; childbirth education; the labor lounge and maternal position in labor; gentle birth; the effects of selected obstetrical practices; hospital

birthing rooms; in-hospital "alternative birth centers"; siblings at birth; rooming-in and bonding; postpartum education; visitation by siblings and grandparents; family-centered care for the family with a premature, handicapped, or dead baby; models for single room care; early discharge; and effects of regionalization of maternity care. Ms. Young concludes with excellent and specific information and guidelines for providers and consumers on how to implement change along with an extensive set of appendices with position statements, sample programs, protocols, etc., from varied institutions and professional and consumer organizations. This book will be an invaluable resource for those who are working to humanize birth care in the hospital. (Also see excerpt on last page of this *Catalog*.)

"Individualized care for each childbearing woman and her family is the crucial element of a family-centered program of maternal and newborn care. To achieve this goal, every member of the childbirth team must undertake a commitment to identify the particular emotional and social needs of each pregnant woman and her family. This priority must be equated with considerations for safety. As Post observes, 'Every child has the right to be well and safely born, but this does not contravene the right to be born in a nurturing and emotionally supportive environment.'"

"It has been demonstrated that not only do family-centered maternal/newborn policies promote and maintain family wellness and relationships, but they also appear to provide significant preventive elements in terms of later parenting. Considerable evidence now exists that separation of mother and infant early in the life of the infant is a major factor in child abuse."

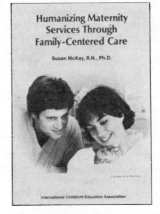

HUMANIZING MATERNITY SERVICES THROUGH FAMILY-CENTERED CARE
by Susan McKay
1982, 28 pages, Illus.

from
ICEA Bookcenter
P.O. Box 20048
Minneapolis, MN 55420
$3.50 plus $1.25 postage
bulk rates available

This excellent new booklet from ICEA will be very helpful for consumer advocates, health planners, and others who are working to implement family-centered maternity care programs in their communities. Susan McKay provides descriptions, rationales, and supporting references for the major components of the family-centered approach, including prenatal care and education, the alternatives in birth care and setting (in-hospital birthing rooms, the Single Unit Delivery System, the traditional labor and delivery

suite, out-of-hospital birth centers, home birth, and the use of midwives), family-centered care for high-risk families and for cesarean birth, siblings at birth, and postpartum care. Lovely photographs by Alison Wachstein illustrate important aspects of family-centered care.

"The development of birthing rooms and alternative birth centers [within the hospital] has had widespread influence on maternity services because of their emphasis on humanized family-centered care. Birthing rooms and ABC's may be located within the labor and delivery suite, in the postpartum area, or entirely separate from the obstetrical facility—in which case the unit may be separately staffed.

"Because of the immediate availability of hospital backup, birthing rooms and ABCs can provide safety in childbirth in conjunction with a full range of family-centered options. The decor, while appreciated, is less important than is the emotional climate (Malone, 1980, pg. 31). Cohen (1980) found in a series of 67 interviews with parents who had their babies in alternative birth centers that the homelike atmosphere wasn't of major importance; instead the availability of support person, other children in the family, and immediate and uninterrupted contact with the newborn were the important care components. Also cited by interviewees was the increase in self-confidence which occurred when the woman was able to participate actively in the decisions surrounding birth and self-care."

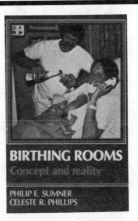

BIRTHING ROOMS: Concept and Reality
by Philip E. Sumner and Celeste R. Phillips
1981, 213 pages, Illus.

from
C.V. Mosby Company
11830 Westline Industrial Drive
St. Louis, MO 63141
$12.95 pap.

Because of increasing consumer dissatisfaction with hospital birth and the trend toward out-of-hospital

birth, hospitals competing for maternity patients have been more or less forced to offer alternatives, including the in-hospital "birthing-room." Directed mainly to health professionals, this book offers a background to the concern for "birth environment" and describes how hospital birthing room programs work in practice: the physical set-up (many different "birthing beds" are described); the staff; and how drugs, anesthesia and electronic fetal monitoring can be incorporated into the birthing room setting. Also included are interviews with families, thoughts on instituting changes in hospital care and nursing practices, questions and answers about birthing room practice, and descriptions (including protocols and risk criteria) of several functioning birthing room programs. In this book, hospital birthing rooms are promoted as "a happy compromise to home birth." However, consumers should make sure, in evaluating local birthing room services, that they are not being offered the usual hospital treatment camouflaged by wallpaper, drapes, and potted plants.

THE CYBELE SOCIETY
Suite 414, Peyton Building
Spokane, WA 99201
509/838-2332

The Cybele Society is a national organization for maternity care professionals and institutions which are supportive of family-centered maternity care. This organization works to promote and help implement family-centered programs through consultation and site visits (working with architects, administrators, physicians, and nurses), self-study Continuing Medical Education programs, conferences and workshops, resource center services, and publications. Professional membership fees range from $50 to $250.

"Family-oriented maternity care is becoming accepted as standard medical practice, as health care providers see that family-centered care is also better medical care. A new population of mothers experiencing childbirth with little or no anesthe-

sia, with labor ambulation, and with physiologic labor and delivery positions presents an exciting research opportunity. Information gathered so far strongly suggests that a physiologic approach may be a good deal safer for mother and baby."
—from Loel Fenwick, M.D., Executive Director, *The Cybele Report*, Winter, 1982.

THE CYBELE CLUSTER SYSTEM:
Single Room Maternity Care for High and Low Risk Families
by Loel Fenwick and Ruthie Dearing
1981
$4.75 plus $1.00 postage

FAMILY-CENTERED MATERNITY CARE: How To Achieve It
by Jan Bishop
1980
$3.25 plus $1.00 postage

THE CYBELE REPORT
quarterly newsletter
$10.00 a year

All Cybele Society publications above are included in cost of membership, but are also available to non-members at the prices listed.

GUIDELINES FOR ESTABLISHING A HOSPITAL BIRTH ROOM
9 pages
from
American College of Nurse-Midwives
1522 K Street, NW, Suite 1120
Washington, DC 20005
$2.75

These guidelines, presented in outline form, were developed by the American College of Nurse-Midwives Clinical Practice Committee to assist Certified Nurse Midwives and others in establishing nurse-midwifery services in the hospital birth room setting.

THE DEVELOPMENT OF FAMILY-CENTERED MATERNITY/NEWBORN CARE IN HOSPITALS
by the Interprofessional Task Force on Health Care of Women and Children
June 1978, 10 pages
from
Interprofessional Task Force Secretariat
ACOG
600 Maryland Ave., SW, Suite 300
Washington, DC 20024
single copies free

This is a Joint Position Statement prepared by representatives of the American Academy of Pediatrics, the American College of Nurse-Midwives, the American College of Obstetricians and Gynecologists (ACOG), the American Nurses' Association, the Nurses Association of ACOG, and endorsed by the American Hospital Association. It defines family-centered maternity care (FCMC) from the point of view of professional health care providers. The Statement describes the potential components of an in-hospital FCMC program, which include preparation for families and hospital staff and a "family-centered program within the Maternity/Newborn Unit." Definitions are offered for the following components: family waiting room, diagnostic-admitting room, birthing room, labor room, delivery room, recovery room, and postpartum "New Family Unit."

"Family-centered maternity/newborn care can be defined as the delivery of safe, quality health care while recognizing, focusing on, and adapting to both the physical and psychosocial needs of the client-patient, the family, and the newly born. The emphasis is on the provision of maternity/newborn health care which fosters family unity while maintaining physical safety."

PACKAGING AND MARKETING MATERNITY CARE: Some Characteristics of the System
by Pauline Donnelly Harnden
1982, 3 pages, Illus.
(from the Winter 81-82 issue of *Childbirth Alternatives Quarterly*)

from
c/o Ashford
Bin 62, SLAC
Stanford, CA 94305
$2.00 per back issue copy

Pauline Harnden is a member of ICEA's Health Planning and Legislation Committee and works with Advocates for Childbearing Rights in Connecticut to improve consumer's options for maternity care. In this article she looks at the response of the maternity care system to consumer demand for more family-centered approaches, and discusses the negative impact of some inherent characteristics of the medical system in meeting that demand, including *competition* among hospitals and practitioners, *co-optation* of concepts from the alternative birth movement, *commodification* of childbirth (turning birth care into a commodity which can be bought and sold), and *coercion* used by medical professionals against parents and alternative practitioners.

"To change the image of routinized, high technology childbirth, part of the acute care hospital OB unit has been repackaged, borrowing concepts from the alternative birth movement. Such principles from the health model of birth as childbirth education, family participation, natural birth, and mother/infant bonding have been incorporated in the new Family Centered Maternity Care policies. Major physical changes in design and decoration of hospital units have produced hospital birthing rooms and even units called birth centers. Overt displays of technology have become covert, hiding in 'homelike' closets, or behind pleasing drapes and plants. In some cases, nurse midwives have been hired to attract consumers and to help build bridges between staffs and administrations trying to coordinate two distinctly opposite models of birth care. Hospitals have achieved differing degrees of commitment and success at incorporating these new concepts into their birth service. Generally speaking, however, as a marketing strategy, Family Centered Maternity Care has been successful and patients have responded very positively to the new mode. Some birth reformers find that the original humanistic concepts which emphasize attitudinal and interpersonal dynamics, as well as family participation, have become distorted in the transition to the hospital setting. This is due to the difficulties acute care hospitals face in superimposing such a model on a bureaucratic, technological and commercial base."

BOOTH MATERNITY CENTER
6051 Overbrook Avenue
Philadelphia, PA 19131
215/878-7800
Sally Branca, Public Relations

A pioneer in family-centered maternity care, Booth Maternity Center is owned and operated by the Salvation Army. It began as Booth Memorial Hospital, a facility in which unwed mothers could live and give birth. As the need for this kind of service declined, Booth opened its doors to all women and in 1971 began an innovative nurse-midwifery birth and training program. Ruth Wilf, of the Childbirth Education Association of Greater Philadelphia, Ruth Watson Lubic, and Kitty Ernst of the Maternity Center Association assisted. Booth became one of the first hospitals to encourage women to give birth naturally, with midwife support, and fathers actively involved. Now, work has been completed on Booth's new birthing rooms, involving an extensive renovation of the second floor of the hospital into a "birthing floor." The new area includes two birthing "suites" which each include a sitting room for family and friends, a birth room and a kitchenette. The usual stay for birthing room families is 24 hours, as opposed to the customary 2 to 3 days. The new floor also includes labor, delivery, and recovery rooms and is fully equipped for cesarean section. (In 1981 Booth's cesarean rate was 8 percent, well below the national average.) Booth also provides a model parenting program (see index).

Interested professionals and others who would like to know more about Booth's programs may contact Sally Branca at the address and phone above.

POSITION PAPER ON PLANNING COMPREHENSIVE MATERNAL AND NEWBORN SERVICES FOR THE CHILDBEARING YEAR
by the International Childbirth Education Association
December 1978, 16 pages
from
ICEA Bookcenter
P.O.Box 20048
Minneapolis, MN 55420
35 cents plus 60 cents postage

ICEA prepared this paper to clarify its position on family-centered care, partly in reply to the American College of Obstetricians and Gynecologists statement (see right) and in response to plans for the "regionalization" of maternity care services which would reduce access to small, local maternity units.

"ICEA believes that a comprehensive approach to low-risk childbirth (1) must provide safe, low-cost alternative models of maternity and newborn care both in and out of the hospital that meet a variety of family needs and life-styles, and (2) must provide expectant parents with an informed choice and control of where and how they give birth. . .

"Planning for maternal and newborn services and facilities must include a careful examination of recent findings concerning quality, management, safety, outcome, and economic aspects of maternal and newborn care. . . Controlled studies have not demonstrated that the acute care setting of the hospital necessarily provides the safest, most psychologically beneficial, and most economical environment for low-risk, normal childbirth."

A MODEL PROGRAM FOR FAMILY-CENTERED HOSPITAL CARE
by Jane Dwinell

Gifford Memorial Hospital, in Vermont, offers what many believe to be a model program of family-centered, low intervention care. The following article, describing Gifford's program, was written by Jane Dwinell, Head Nurse. Readers may contact her directly for more information.

Gifford Memorial Hospital
44 S. Main Street
Randolph, Vermont 05060
802/728-3366

"Birth at Gifford Memorial Hospital is a special event. Since opening the first Birthing Room in Vermont, the birth rate at Gifford has more than doubled. Couples are coming from all over the state of Vermont—from as far away as Bennington (100 miles) Burlington (65 miles) and St. Johnsbury (65 miles)—as well as from New Hampshire and New York State. We provide the atmosphere and care for birth as no one else does in Vermont, possibly even New England and the whole United States.

"There were 143 births at GMH in 1977. That year the Birthing Room opened on December 29th and in 1978 the birth rate jumped to 205 with 50% of those births in the Birthing Room. In 1979 a second Birthing Room was opened. In 1981 there were 369 births, with 80% Birthing Room usage. Because of the overwhelming response to this method of childbirth, we have undergone renovations to have five Birthing Rooms.

"Our renovated unit provides us with a unique obstetrical suite which portrays our attitude about birth. When a woman comes to us in labor, she is given a room—*and there she stays until she goes home*. Our Birthing Rooms are not just used for labor and birth with a transfer to another area after birth or in case of complications. The family remains together for their entire stay without the annoyance of being moved (approximately 24-36 hours after birth). Even if a woman gives birth in the delivery room or operating room by necessity or choice, she still returns to the room she previously occupied. Our rooms are not filled with special or expensive equipment but are furnished simply and comfortably. Instrument trays for the birth as well as other necessary items are located in a bureau drawer. Emergency equipment is placed outside the door when birth is imminent. The baby stays with the family in their room unless it needs to be in the nursery for observation or procedures, or at the parents' request. Our nursery is fully equipped to handle many problems but if a baby is very sick, it would be transferred to a Neonatal Intensive Care Unit.

"Our unit is small enough that we can handle birth this way. The nursing staff, physicians and nurse-midwife feel that our personal care provides the best for the new family. By feeling comfortable in their surroundings, by staying in the same place and having the same nurses care for them throughout their stay, the family develops a strong trust and bond with the staff which allows labor to go better, less complications to happen at birth, and bonding, feeding and baby care to be established more easily.

"Although people choose to birth at Gifford because of our Birthing Rooms, the lack of *routine* interventions (i.e. enemas, preps, IVs, episiotomies, circumcisions) and the inexpensive cost, most people say they come for the excellent personal care given by the nurses. Each laboring couple is monitored personally by a nurse, not a machine. The nurse is there to provide psychological and physical comfort as well as to keep her eye on the condition of mother and baby. Couples know that it is *their* birth, that nothing will be done "to" them, that all interventionist procedures deemed necessary (i.e. pitocin augmentation, artificial rupture of membranes, forceps, IVs, episiotomies, Caesarean Section) will be discussed and explained first. Even in the case of an emergency, there is still time to remain human and explain what is happening and why. Because people remain in control of their own labor, we have less need for these interventions and the associated complications and in turn have healthy moms and babes. Our primary Caesarean Section rate is 6% and the total rate (including repeats) is only 10%. Fathers are allowed to be present in the operating room and the hospital sponsors a special class to prepare them for their experience. Because the family stays together for this birth and postpartum recovery, in combination with our low rate of Caesarean births, the women who need them do not have as much of the associated guilt attached with "was it really necessary" because if a Caesarean was done at Gifford they know that everything else was tried first and that the surgery was *absolutely necessary*.

"Two family practice physicians and a certified nurse-midwife provide the bulk of the obstetrical care. Most of the homebirth midwives use them for back-up. Excellent prenatal care is provided, paying close attention to exercise, diet, good habits, and relationships. Family, children and friends are encouraged to participate actively during this time. Women and their support people attend childbirth preparation classes. They explore their feelings and beliefs about childbirth and come prepared to take responsibility for their own labor and birth.

"When the woman and her family arrive at the hospital in labor, they are encouraged to be up and around, take walks, eat as desired, drink plenty of fluids, and take long hot showers. A nurse monitors the labor, keeping track of the well being of mother and baby in sensitive and professional ways. She listens to the baby's heartbeat frequently, takes the mother's vital signs as necessary, encourages the woman in various ways—to walk or to rest, to shower or to drink more, to change breathing techniques. The nurse does whatever need be to help the labor go smoothly and as quickly as possible. When birth is imminent she notifies the birth attendant who arrives to assist in the final stages. Few stitches are necessary after the baby has been gently eased out with perineal massage and hot compresses (60% of women in 1981 had intact perineums). The baby is held warmly by the mother and the cord is cut by the father after it has stopped pulsating. The family is left alone to enjoy their new addition with the nurse discreetly nearby to answer questions and make sure mom and babe are stable. Babies can stay with their mothers as much as they want and all procedures needed are discussed first. The nurse continues to care for the whole family for the rest of their stay (which can be as short or as long as they want) and teaches them all they need to know about baby care, feeding and postpartum adjustment.

"The obstetrical unit of Gifford Memorial Hospital provides an important service to the local community as well as to all Vermonters who care about the birth of their children. Many women cannot or do not want to birth at home and Gifford has proven that a hospital can provide a safe humane alternative. We are proud of the care that we provide and would be pleased to share our knowledge with other health professionals who also care."

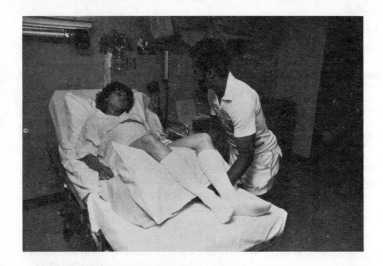

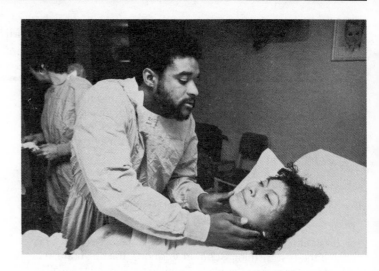

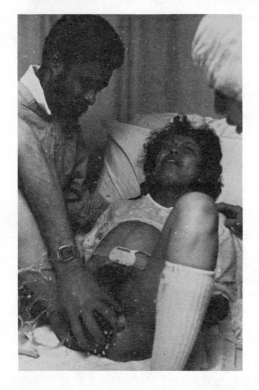

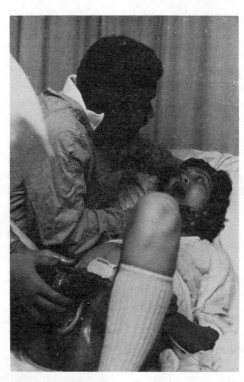

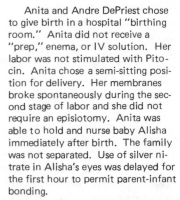

Anita and Andre DePriest chose to give birth in a hospital "birthing room." Anita did not receive a "prep," enema, or IV solution. Her labor was not stimulated with Pitocin. Anita chose a semi-sitting position for delivery. Her membranes broke spontaneously during the second stage of labor and she did not require an episiotomy. Anita was able to hold and nurse baby Alisha immediately after birth. The family was not separated. Use of silver nitrate in Alisha's eyes was delayed for the first hour to permit parent-infant bonding.

Photographs ©1983 Rodger F. Ewy/ EGA Inc.

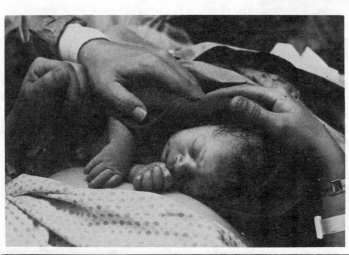

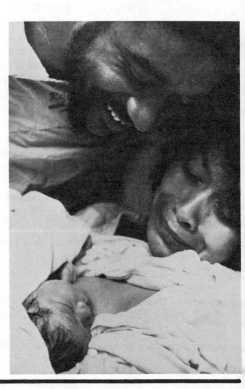

BIRTH STORY

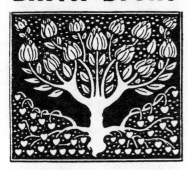

LAMAZE AND LEBOYER IN A HOSPITAL BIRTHING ROOM

The Birth of Dorothy Ida Gambrell
Thursday, June 22, 1978, 2:30 p.m.

Carole Gambrell

When I wanted to learn how to ski, I took out every book in the library on skiing. When I was going to redo my kitchen, I read everything I could on the subject. So, naturally, when we decided to have children I began reading everything on pregnancy and childbirth.

"By the time I became pregnant at age thirty-two, I had formed very definite ideas about what I did and did not want. Ideally, I would have chosen a home birth. I had read studies of animals that showed that if a mother were moved during labor it lengthened the duration of labor and increased the number of complications. Noise, bright lights and activity all seemed to have the same effect. Unfortunately, all these things are part of an average hospital birth. In two of the hospitals I later visited, the mother was first taken to a labor room—a stark, well-lit room containing only a bed. When birth was imminent, she was transferred from the bed to a "stretcher" table, wheeled to the delivery room and transferred to the delivery table. The delivery room looked like an operating room. A long table with stirrups stood in the middle of the room under bright lights. All around tiles gleamed and chrome glistened. Once the baby was born, the mother was transferred again to the stretcher and wheeled to the recovery room—which in one case was a hall. None of this seemed very conducive to a short, pleasant labor. It also did not go along with my belief in childbirth as a normal, healthy process, not an illness.

"The problem with having a home birth on Long Island was that there was only one doctor I had heard of that would attend a home birth and there were only two qualified midwives, both of whom worked in Manhattan and sometimes had trouble making it out to Suffolk County in

time for the birth. A home birth was out for me. I knew I didn't have the strong personality necessary to blaze new trails and convert a doctor to my way of thinking. Also, partly because of my age, I was nervous about being too far from a hospital's emergency resources.

Realizing my first option was out, I tried to find a doctor who would go along with my requests. Basically I wanted to be left alone. Every procedure I had read about had its bad side effects. It was a matter of weighing the risks against the benefits. It seemed that too many procedures that were very valid and essential in special situations were being used routinely. There were cases of doctors inducing labor for their own or the mother's convenience only to find themselves with a premature baby because the due date was incorrect. Some drugs that are given to reduce pain only decrease your ability to concentrate and to help in the pushing stage, which, in turn, increases the need for medical help, such as forceps, during the delivery. The forceps, in turn, can harm the baby. Almost any drug you take can be absorbed by the fetus. This can be very harmful to a baby with other problems and, even in a healthy child, can have subtle but long-term effects. Many episiotomies are much worse than the small tear you may receive during birth. Shaving the pubic hair can cause irritation and infection. Both the I.V. and the fetal monitor leave you fairly immobile on a bed. The list goes on and on. I had decided I wanted no prep, no episiotomy, no I.V., no drugs, no fetal monitor—unless necessary for a specific medical reason.

"I was lucky in finding a female obstetrician who not only agreed with, but even encouraged, my feelings. Her emphasis was on preventative care. Throughout my pregnancy, she had me exercising, eating well and, above all, reading as much as I could about childbirth. To her, pregnancy was a miracle to be enjoyed.

"In 1977 she had helped set up one of the few birthing rooms on Long Island, at Smithtown General Hospital. The idea appealed to me, although I did visit the two other hospitals she was affiliated with before making my final decision. The visits reinforced my first inclination. The differences in philosophy between the three were amazing. In one you were treated like an invalid and given an unbreakable rule for everything—you couldn't get out of bed once you were admitted, you had to have an I.V., etc. The second hospital was a little less rigid, but only Smithtown left most decisions up to the mother and her doctor. My choice was an easy one.

"Of course, I realized that if I wanted to have a noninterventionist

birth, I had to do everything I could during my pregnancy to mitigate any problems. I ate well-balanced meals. At the end of nine months I never wanted to see lettuce again. I exercised—walked, rode my bike, and did daily exercises to prepare the muscles used during pregnancy and childbirth. I took prenatal classes at the Mother's Center where I could share my questions with other expectant mothers and experts. I took Lamaze classes, which were some of the most helpful things. We were taught exercises, breathing and methods of concentration to help with the birth and the accompanying pain. We were given information about the physical and medical sides of pregnancy and birth. But most of all, we were taught what to expect so that we would not be afraid. We were given self-confidence.

"My labor began when my water broke at 1 a.m. on Thursday, three weeks before my due date. We had just attended our last Lamaze class and been given a baby shower the day before. After thumbing through my birth books to make sure I wasn't supposed to call the doctor, I got a banana and yogurt to eat and returned to bed. By 6:30 A.M. the contractions were getting stronger so I decided it was time to wake my husband and let him know what was happening. We gave the doctor a quick call and I ate another banana. (For some reason I had a strange image of myself developing "debilitating" hunger pains half way through labor.)

"During this stage of labor I walked or changed position between each contraction. I tried every conceivable position—on my knees, leaning against the bed, lying on the floor, etc. This is something I wouldn't have felt comfortable doing in a hospital, even in a birthing room. I had severe back labor from about 9:00 to 11:00. Luckily, we had just covered this in our Lamaze class the night before. Rich pressed on the small of my back, as hard as he could, sometimes using his hands, sometimes his feet.

"At 10:30 Rich called the doctor again. The contractions were very intense and were, we thought, about two minutes apart. (We weren't completely sure we were timing them correctly.) The doctor, assuming "first baby panic," didn't believe it was time to go to the hospital yet. I hadn't warned her of my English habit of understatement. She told us that if we still felt we wanted to go in an hour, to come to her office.

"In an hour we were at her office. I was over five centimeters dilated. We were sent directly to the hospital.

"At the hospital I was taken straight from admissions to the birthing room. I was even given my choice of two birthing rooms—a choice I didn't appreciate at the time.

The one I chose contained a hospital bed, a large stuffed chair and a couch with matching curtains in a colonial print. There was a very homey feel to the place. After I had changed into the hospital gown, the nurse reappeared with Rich, who was now wearing his hospital clothes. Together they helped me into bed.

"The doctor arrived next. She tried to encourage me to sit in the chair, but by then I wasn't going to move an inch. She asked if I was tired. When I said no, she agreed to forgo the I.V., since I was so close to delivery. This is the one thing she would not agree to before.

"From then on Rich and I were left alone, except for an occasional nurse's head popping in to see if we were okay. I lay on my back doing my panting breathing and concentrating on a tile in the ceiling. The pushing stage began about 12:30 P.M. It did not seem like a great improvement over the previous stage. I was getting tired and thinking about changing my mind about having a baby. At this point I probably would have taken drugs, if it hadn't been for my Lamaze instructor. She had warned us that at this stage the drugs would not alleviate the pain, they would only decrease my ability to concentrate and push. I knew I was in the last stage and would be done soon. Toward the end our nurse suggested attaching the fetal monitor for a few minutes to help me time my pushing. She helped for those few minutes and then left.

"When our daughter's head began to crown, Rich and I were alone. Rich ran into the hall and got our nurse. Our doctor was not available, so the two nurses who had been with us since we arrived were the only ones present with Rich and me when Dorothy was born. At 2:30 P.M., two and a half hours after we entered the hospital, our six pound, eleven ounce daughter emerged.

"We had asked for a Leboyer birth, so Dorothy was placed on my stomach as soon as she was born. Rich and I were encouraged to stroke her. After a few minutes the umbilical cord was cut. Rich and one nurse took Dorothy to the side of the room to give her her bath. By then the doctor had arrived. She cleaned me up and gave me the two stitches I needed.

"After that, Rich and Dorothy and I were left alone in the birthing room for two hours. There was a phone by the bed, so we called our parents to tell them they had a granddaughter who was half an hour old. The rest of the time was spent staring at our daughter's tiny fingers or stroking her long black hair. From time to time I would try to breast feed her, but she wasn't interested.

"At 5:00 P.M. we were taken from the birthing room for the first time—Dorothy to the nursery, Rich

(continued on p. 94, bottom left)

Birth Centers

In 1975, the Maternity Center Association (MCA) opened the nation's first freestanding birthing center, the Childbearing Center, in their townhouse in Manhattan. Since then, more than 1000 births have taken place at the center, providing parents with what director Ruth Watson Lubic calls a "safe, satisfying and economical alternative to hospital care."

The Childbearing Center began as a "demonstration project," the latest in a long line of important projects initiated during the Maternity Center's illustrious 60-year history. (For more information on the MCA, see index.)

Many see the birth center concept as a "compromise" offered by professionals who recognize and appreciate parents' disenchantment with hospital birth, but who fear the practice of "do-it-yourself" home birth which many parents have turned to as their only alternative. The birth center attempts to offer the "best of both worlds," providing the warmth of flexible, family-centered, midwifery care in a home-like setting combined with the security of professional assistance and emergency back-up.

Consumer response to this model of care has been good and interest in birth centers has grown rapidly. MCA reports that in mid-1981 there were seventy-four birth centers operating in twenty-six states, and at least twenty more in the planning stage. MCA has received a major grant to coordinate birth center activities and networking (see opposite page). Unfortunately, there has been resistance from the medical establishment, particularly from obstetricians, who view nurse-midwifery and birth centers as a direct threat to their professional and economic control over maternity care. MCA's Childbearing Center was vigorously opposed by many professional groups and individuals and was not granted permanent establishment by the public Health Council until almost three years after it was proposed. In addition to physician resistance, birth centers have had to overcome the problems of obtaining third party reimbursement (by insurance carriers, Blue Cross/Blue Shield, Medicaid, etc.) for their services. Other problems include obtaining state licensure (many states do not have statutes specific to birth centers), favorable review by local Health Systems Agencies, arranging hospital back-up, and generating start-up and operating funds.

At this point, the birth center concept can be considered very "new" and struggling to become established. Only a small percentage of parents will find a birth center in their community, though many will travel hundreds of miles, perhaps arranging to live-in with friends or relatives, in order to use the nearest birth center. In order to find the birth center nearest you, consult the NAPSAC Directory of Alternative Birth Services (see index) or contact the International Childbirth Education Association (see index).

BIRTH STORY (cont'd)

and I to my hospital room, dinner, and visitors. I felt terrific—as if I could dance down the hall. It wasn't until the next day that the muscle soreness set in.

"I stayed in the hospital for two days. During most of that I had Dorothy and Rich with me. We even got a little extra attention. The nurse who had delivered Dorothy brought her daughter in on her day off to visit "her baby."

"Although there was pain, I remember Dorothy's birth as a totally posi-

tive experience. I had gotten everything I wanted. I feel it was as close to a home birth as possible, without actually being one."

(Editor's Note: Carole Gambrell is the mother of two girls and works as a librarian at the State University of New York. She planned another "birthing room" birth for her second child, but baby Yvonne came so fast that Carole had to deliver by herself at home, before either her husband or the ambulance could reach her. It was a little scary but everything turned out okay.)

COMPETITION AMONG HEALTH CARE PRACTITIONERS: The Influence of the Medical Profession on the Health Manpower Market, Volumes I and II
by Levin and Associates, Inc.
1982

from
Federal Trade Commission
Public Reference Branch, Room 130
Washington, DC 20580
free

This report was commissioned by the Federal Trade Commission to examine the problems of the restraint of free trade in medical care which may be caused by the existence of a firmly-entrenched professional medical establishment. Volume II of the report looks specifically at the Childbearing Center of the Maternity Center Association in New York City, describing the Center's difficulties in starting up and overcoming opposition from the medical profession. The following quote is taken from a preliminary version of the report, published in the *CBCN News* (see next page). For more information on restraint of trade against nurse-midwives see index.

"... in almost five years of operation, the Childbearing Center has overcome numerous obstacles and has demonstrated that safe, efficient care can be provided to low-risk mothers in a context utilizing teams of physician and non-physician professionals. In so doing, it has increased consumer access to alternative delivery systems."

BIRTHING CENTERS: Alternative in Obstetric Services for Indiana
by Pragmatics, Inc.
December 1978, 59 pages

from
Blue Cross and Blue Shield of Indiana
Health Services Information Dept.
Health Economics Division, 9K
120 W. Market Street
Indianapolis, IN 46204
single copies free

This report was prepared for Blue Cross/Blue Shield of Indiana and provides an introduction to the birth center concept and discusses current consumer reactions to conventional obstetrical practices. Medical safety issues of hospital versus home birth are discussed with birth centers, both in-hospital and free-standing, seen as a possible compromise. The authors describe factors which influence the establishment of birth centers (consumer demand, competition, attitudes of providers, third-party payment, licensure) and develop scenarios for the possible growth of birth centers in Indiana. The effects of birth centers on health care costs are also discussed. A bibliography and sample screening criteria are included.

GUIDELINES FOR ESTABLISHING AN ALTERNATIVE BIRTH CENTER
ACNM Clinical Practice Committee
10 pages

from
American College of Nurse-Midwives
1522 K Street, NW, Suite 1120
Washington, DC 20005
$2.75 plus .55 postage

Guidelines to consider in establishing a birth center are presented in outline form, including determining need/demand, establishing a planning group, developing a manual for philosophy, staffing and protocols, developing physical plans, budgeting, and implementing plans. Suggested equipment and supplies are listed and sample birth center budget categories are included.

IDEAS AND MODELS

The birth center idea is so new that there are no books yet available solely devoted to this subject. But listed below are several "chapters" on birth centers, included in books on childbirth. These provide varying visions of the "model" birth center concept and reality. (See the index under book title for *Whole Birth Catalog* reviews of these books.)

IMPLEMENTING A MEDICALLY SOUND CHILDBEARING CENTER
Problems and Solutions
by Myrtle E. Hosford

in *21st Century Obstetrics Now!*
David and Lee Stewart, eds.
NAPSAC, 1977

THE CONTINUUM CONCEPT:
Home, Hospital and Birth Center Care, All Within a Single Service
by Eunice K.M. Ernst, J. Robert McTammany, Thomas M. Ebersole, Myra M. Farr, Ester T. Mack, and Sandra Perkins

STARTING A CHILDBEARING CENTER IN YOUR COMMUNITY
by Mary Helen Carroll

in *Compulsory Hospitalization or Freedom of Choice in Childbirth*
David and Lee Stewart, eds.
NAPSAC, 1979

ANATOMY OF A BIRTH CENTER
by Irene Nielsen

in *Kaleidoscope of Childbearing*
Penny Simkin and Carla Reinke, eds.
the penny press, 1978

YOUR SISTER HAS TWINS!
by Suzanne Arms

in *Immaculate Deception*
by Suzanne Arms
Houghton Mifflin, 1975

A HOLISTIC BIRTH CENTER
by Leni Schwartz

in *The Life of the Unborn*
by Leni Schwartz
Richard Marek Pub., 1980

COOPERATIVE BIRTH CENTER NETWORK
Box 1, Route 1
Perkiomenville, PA 18074
215/234-8068
Eunice K. M. Ernst, Director

The Cooperative Birth Center Network (CBCN) was launched in 1981 with a 2-year grant awarded to the Maternity Center Association, which provides leadership for the project. The Network is directed by Kitty Ernst, a certified nurse-midwife who has long worked with the Maternity Center. In the Network's first newsletter (November, 1981), Ms. Ernst describes how the Network came about:

"The need for a birth center network just became apparent in the Summer of 1979. During a tour of fourteen birth centers across the United States, the need for a central resource and support system to draw on for assistance, information and problem sharing was expressed at all centers. The work of each center represented total commitment by the pioneers who struggled to serve the childbearing parents making the decision not to give birth in the acute care setting of the hospital. One had the sense that the first waves of a movement toward change in the system for delivery of maternity care services was underway. Most centers were alone in their struggle. Few enjoyed any support from the powerful institutions and organized professional societies. Such is the path chosen

by those who dare to change the status quo.

"Data, we need data!' was the most frequent cry...."

The goals of the Network are to:
* promote a wider public understanding of the birth center concept
* create a cooperative resource and information network for dissemination of the model at the operational level
* develop standards or recommendations for regulations for the guidance of public health officials, policy planners and insurance carriers.

The Network provides much needed assistance to those who are working to establish or maintain birth centers in their communities. Services include:
* On site and telephone consultation
* A Repository Inventory (samples of materials used by birth centers, like bylaws, risk criteria, standing orders, budgets, client handouts, sample newsletters, funding efforts, etc.)
* Assistance in community education and outreach
* Initiation and response to media contacts
* Exploration of accreditation by relevant professional associations
* Standardized forms for collecting and processing data
* Resource to insurance carriers
* Procurement of liability coverage
* Developing recommendations for regulations for licensure
* Regional workshops which will address financing, management, oper-

ation and marketing of alternative birth services
* Assistance to consumer organizations seeking birth center information
*Coordination of birth centers as educational sites for nurse-midwifery students and graduates

The Network's newsletter, *CBCN News,* is available to birth centers and others interested in the birth center concept who would like to be placed on the mailing list. However, parents should please take note that the Network does not supply a list of the names of birth centers around the country and cannot yet handle consumer requests for information on how to find a birth center. To find a birth center in your area, refer to the *NAPSAC Directory of Alternative Birth Services* (see index) or contact the International Childbirth Education Association (see index).

INFORMATION FOR ESTABLISHING STANDARDS OR REGULATIONS FOR FREE STANDING BIRTH CENTERS
1982, 12 pages
(in CBCN News, Vol. 1, No. 2 & 3)

from
Cooperative Birth Center Network
(see address above)
$2.00

This paper was written to provide information on the characteristics of birth centers for people who are trying to start a center, for professionals

who need guidelines for practice in birth centers, and for governmental bodies which are responsible for regulation and licensing of birth centers. The information is based on six years of experience with operating birth centers and is presented as the current "state-of-the-art." Contents include a recommendation, rationale, and sample regulation for each of the following topics: authority, definitions, licensure process, organization, facility, administration, services, and evaluation.

"It is recommended that the definition differentiate the free-standing birth center from birth rooms, birthing suites, and other short-stay, in-hospital, high technology or acute care birth facilities; and emphasize professional, personalized, preventive care for healthy expectant mothers and their babies as opposed to a concept of 'fast and cheap processing' of maternity care."

THE FREE-STANDING BIRTH CENTRE
by Anita B. Bennetts
1982, 3 pages
$1.00

In 1980 a national collaborative study was conducted of more than 4000 births in eleven birth centers. It was published in *The Lancet* and reprints may be obtained from Cooperative Birth Center Network (CBCN).

A PLAN FOR ESTABLISHING A BIRTH CENTER

GUIDELINES FOR BIRTH CENTERS

Kitty Ernst, of the Cooperative Birth Center Network, is concerned that Birth Centers maintain high levels of quality with regard to the training and expertise of the staff, the physical set-up of the center, and back-up and support services. In states where lay midwives are unlicensed or poorly regulated, people with little or no training may call themselves "midwives" and open "birth centers." Likewise, physicians can operate a "birth center" out of their offices, without providing midwifery services and without having to conform to the safety and quality regulations which govern hospitals. Ernst urges that consumers take responsibility for evaluating the quality and safety of birth centers in their area. The following recommendations were developed by the Birth Center Task Force of the Health Planning Council of Greater Boston, in 1978. They may serve as useful guidelines for the evaluation of birth centers by consumers.

1. The birth center shall be freestanding (i.e., separate from a hospital) and non-profit.
2. The birth center shall be family-centered and shall provide prenatal, intrapartum, and postpartum care and education.
3. The birth center shall be community-based and community-controlled (governed by a board of consumers and providers).
4. Primary caretakers at the birth center shall be nurse-midwives. Physicians shall be available for consultation and back-up as necessary. (Editor's note: in some states non-nurse midwives are licensed and regulated by the state government to provide professional midwifery services.)
5. The birth center shall have essential life support equipment and emergency transfer capability.
6. The birth center shall have arrangements for back-up with one or more hospitals.
7. Ideally, the birth center site shall be chosen so as to serve childbearing women from mixed socio-economic backgrounds.
8. Provisions will be made to serve women and families with special needs (physical, linguistic, cultural, spiritual, etc.).

For a complete copy of the *Report of the Birth Center Task Force of HSA IV*, write to:
Health Planning Council of Greater Boston
294 Washington St.
Boston, MA 02108

BIRTH CENTERS: A Sampling of Philosophies and Services

THE BIRTH CENTER
Women's Health Center
3418 Staunton Avenue, SE
Charleston, WV 25304
304/344-9834

"It is our desire to bring the focus in childbearing back to where it belongs—to the mother, the father, the baby and the family that the birth is creating . . . .

"We encourage your active participation and your right to a dignified birth experience.

"We believe this can best be accomplished through a family-centered maternity program that allows the family to have informed choices . . . .

"Labor is allowed to progress naturally with medical intervention kept to a minimum."

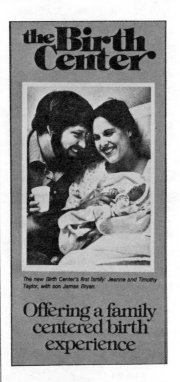

The new Birth Center's first family: Jeanne and Timothy Taylor, with son James Bryan.

Offering a family centered birth experience

THE BIRTHPLACE
4708 Aurora Avenue North
Seattle, WA 98103
(206) 633-0884

"The Birthplace is an alternative birth center dedicated to providing high quality, individualized care to childbearing families . . . The Birthplace provides complete prenatal care. Clients are encouraged to participate actively in their own care, and are considered partners in the health team . . . After the birth the parents and their newborn infant are not separated. Physical contact during this special time has been recognized as being very important to the attachment process between parents and their infant . . . "

FAMILYBORN: A Center for Birth and Women's Health
2688 State Highway 27
North Brunswick, NJ 08902
201/821-6200

"Familyborn believes that childbearing is a healthy process and that it belongs within the sphere of the family. Active participation in prenatal care and delivery enables a woman to manage her birth with confidence and control.

"Familyborn provides the safety of modern science and the security of traditional wisdom. The thorough medical training, practical experience and personal concern of the certified nurse-midwife give her a clear perception of the needs of each family . . . .

"We are a non-profit organization, founded by consumers, and staffed by sensitive, supportive Certified Nurse-Midwives. Based on a philosophy of assuming responsibility for oneself, good nutrition, and extensive education, we believe childbearing to be a natural physiological process of a healthy body. Birth is one of the single most important moments in the life of a family, and should be treated with sensitivity and respect. We at Familyborn provide the setting, emotional support, education, and medical expertise to help make this event as special as possible. All prenatal care is given by Certified Nurse-Midwives, back up care and consultation by supportive OB-GYN's. Labor and birth are at the center, families are never separated, and go home six to twelve hours postpartum."

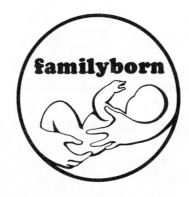

THE BIRTH PLACE
1220 University Drive
Menlo Park, CA 94025
415/326-7603 and 326-7609

"The Birth Place meets all state safety standards for normal childbirth in an out-of-hospital setting. Since any medication given to a mother in labor is known to be a potential hazard to mother and baby, pain medications for labor aren't used at The Birth Place. Instead we give mothers the emotional support they need to go through labor without drugs.

"Childbirth education is the foundation for natural, unmedicated childbirth. In a natural, unmedicated birth there is seldom any need for the use of resuscitation equipment. However, The Birth Place has this equipment on hand if it's needed. Should the need arise for transfer to hospital, ambulance service is available to Stanford Medical Center, just two miles away. The practitioners at The Birth Place will transfer mother and baby before a problem is left to develop into an emergency."

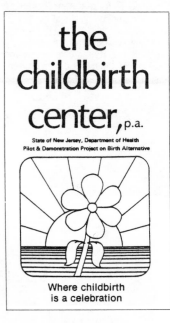

the childbirth center, p.a.

State of New Jersey, Department of Health
Pilot & Demonstration Project on Birth Alternative

Where childbirth is a celebration

THE CHILDBIRTH CENTER, P.A.
291 S. Van Brunt Street
Englewood, NJ 07631
201/567-0810

"The Childbirth Center is founded on the concept of family-centered maternity care where childbirth is a celebration. . . It is an alternative to hospital delivery, offering prenatal care as well as delivery in a home-like atmosphere to families expecting a normal birth. All members of the family are encouraged to participate in the birth experience."

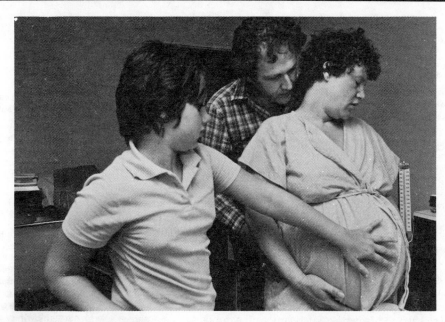

Certified Nurse-Midwife Lonnie Holtzman
Morris gave birth to her second child in her own
birth center, The Childbirth Center in Englewood,
New Jersey (see previous page). Lonnie's husband
and ten-year-old daughter were with her for the
birth and she was attended by her nurse-midwife
partner at the Center and a back-up physician.
These photographs show one of the important reasons why midwives who are also mothers are
uniquely qualified to attend women in childbirth.

Photographs © 1983 Carol Halebian

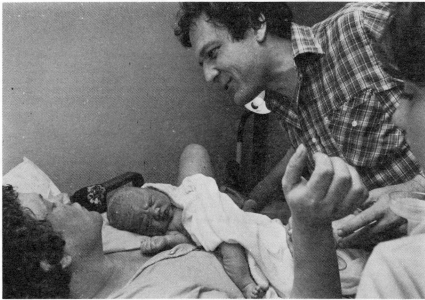

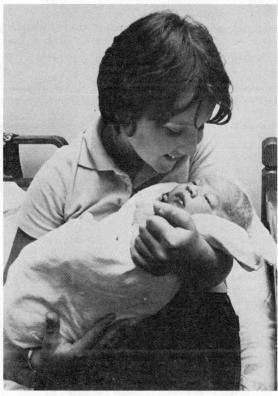

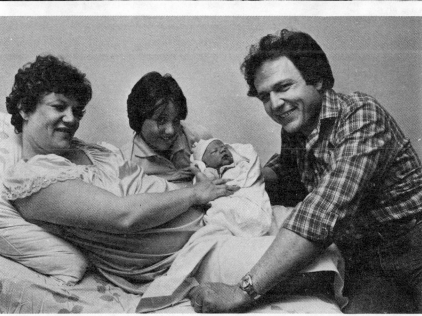

Nurse-midwives

A nurse-midwife is a registered nurse who has received additional training in midwifery. She becomes a certified nurse-midwife (CNM) by becoming certified according to the requirements of the American College of Nurse-Midwives. CNM's are licensed in 48 states and can provide independent management and care for "essentially normal" women and babies, both during pregnancy, labor, birth and the postpartum period and through family-planning and "well-woman" gynecology services.

Most CNM's attend births in hospitals, though some also practice in birth centers or attend home births. Though parents are usually very happy with nurse-midwife services, opposition to nurse-midwifery practice by the medical profession has restricted their practice, making it difficult for CNM's to obtain hospital delivery privileges or to work comfortably in alternative settings.

Because nurse-midwives are trained in "normal childbearing" they tend to be more protective of the normal processes of childbirth and less likely to intervene than are obstetricians. This is because of their differing philosophy and also because CNM's are not permitted to use certain interventions (i.e. forceps or cesarean-section). However, because of their medically oriented training and perhaps also because of the pressure of constant scrutiny, from the medical profession, CNM's are often more likely to intervene or refer a patient to a physician than are lay-midwives, many of whom are now becoming licensed in states with new lay-midwifery legislation. Important questions of how and where midwifery should be practiced will be vigorously debated in the coming years.

SAFETY

"In the early 1960's a CNM practice was established as a pilot project in Madera County, California. Special legislation made nurse-midwifery legal for the duration of the project. Certified nurse-midwives were introduced as the only new variable in the medically understaffed county's health care system. The mothers served by the project were primarily agricultural workers.

"During the first 18 months of the project, the Madera County prematurity rate dropped from its previous level of 11 percent to 6.6 percent and the neonatal mortality rate

"During the first 18 months of the nurse-midwifery project, . . . the neonatal mortality rate dropped from 23.9 per 1,000 live births to 10.3 deaths per 1,000 live births."

dropped from 23.9 deaths per 1,000 live births to 10.3 deaths per 1,000 live births. There was a significant increase in attendance at prenatal clinics during the pilot project. Mothers who had had no prenatal care and who were cared for during labor and delivery by nurse-midwives experienced a neonatal death rate of 26.8 per 1,000 live births. The neonatal death rate for mothers who had no prenatal care was 50.6 per 1,000 live births after the project ended and nursemidwifery care during labor was no longer available.

"Despite these good results, the California Medical Society opposed legalization of nurse-midwifery, and the nurse-midwives had to leave at the end of the project. After they left, the prematurity rate increased by almost 50 percent and the neonatal death rate tripled. . . ."

from the testimony of Sally Tom, of the American College of Nurse Midwives, in *Nurse Midwifery: Consumers' Freedom of Choice* (see index).

WHAT NURSE-MIDWIVES DO

NURSE-MIDWIFERY IN CONTEXT
by Ruth Watson Lubic
12 pages

50 cents single copy
bulk rates available

The Maternity Center Association (MCA) established the first U.S. school of nurse-midwifery in 1931. In this pamphlet, MCA director Ruth Lubic describes the growth of nurse-midwifery since then, the barriers to nurse-midwifery practice (including 12 "myths" about midwives), and current trends in maternity care which influence the practice of nurse-midwives.

"Myth No. 4. Nurse-midwives can be utilized only in the care of low-income patients; the more affluent will never accept such care.

"During the years of slow growth, nurse-midwifery practice was restricted to high-caseload settings such as municipal hospitals, where assistance in providing care was readily welcomed, or to rural areas where physicians were in short

"... mothers seem to appreciate the value nurse-midwives place on education during and for the childbearing cycle."

supply. Today, with a crisis in the delivery of health care not only implicitly recognized but explicitly acknowledged, professionals are seeking a variety of solutions. Where nurse-midwifery services are offered in a team framework, the acceptance by mothers of all socio-economic backgrounds is enthusiastic. . . .

"In particular, mothers seem to

appreciate the value nurse-midwives place on education during and for the childbearing cycle. And may I suggest that if physicians introduce a nurse-midwife colleague and educate patients concerning her role, she will be welcomed and appreciated in any setting. . . ."

Both publications are available from:

MATERNITY CENTER ASSOCIATION
48 East 92nd Street
New York, NY 10028

DEVELOPING MATERNITY SERVICES WOMEN WILL TRUST
by Ruth Watson Lubic
1975, 4 pages, Illus.

single copy free

This article originally appeared in the *American Journal of Nursing*. It describes the dissatisfaction of women with conventional maternity care and explains how nurse-midwifery can help by providing safe options for alternative care.

"Nurse-midwifery management of the entire childbearing experience offers an unusual opportunity for establishment of trust between care receivers and care givers. In this manner the validity and acceptance of teaching, which at times can be only theoretical and not applied until a future time, are ensured. Nurse-midwives then, are *with* a family through one of its most exciting and gratifying life cycle events, sharing in the joy at the climax of the reproductive miracle as well as being supportive through the days of expectation and the trials of settling a newborn into the family."

FILMS

MIDWIFE
Produced by Michael Anderson
16mm color film, 26 minutes

Distributed by
Michael Anderson
402 San Francisco Blvd.
San Anselmo, CA 94960
415/454-8099

This film documents the work of two nurse-midwives who share a home and hospital birth practice. The special nurturing care of midwives is emphasized.

DAUGHTERS OF TIME
Produced by Durrin Films, Inc.
16mm color film, 29 minutes, 1981

Distributed by
New Day Films
P.O. Box 315
Franklin Lakes, NJ 07417
201/891-8240

This excellent new film describes the practice of three modern nurse-midwives, who provide birth care in three different settings—the home, a hospital "birthing room," and a birth center. The film includes excerpts from the Congressional hearing on nurse-midwifery held on December 18, 1980 (see index).

AMERICAN COLLEGE OF NURSE-MIDWIVES

AMERICAN COLLEGE OF NURSE-MIDWIVES
1522 K Street, NW, Suite 1120·
Washington, DC 20005
202/347-5445

The American College of Nurse-Midwives (ACNM) is the professional organization for nurse-midwives in the United States. The college conducts an annual convention, administers national certification examinations, accredits nurse-midwifery educational programs, provides membership services, and produces publications for its members and the public.

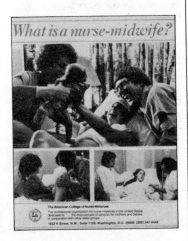

WHAT IS A NURSE-MIDWIFE?
brochure
single copy free

This 6-panel brochure is beautifully illustrated with photographs of nurse-midwives at work: providing prenatal care, attending births, and counseling and teaching families. The brochure describes the training of nurse-midwives and what services they provide. It lists the schools where ACNM accredited programs of nurse-midwifery are taught and lists 23 ACNM publications available on competencies and standards for practice.

"The nurse-midwife stays with the woman during labor in order to provide comfort measures and emotional support as well as to supervise and evaluate the progress of the labor The nurse-midwife will encourage the father or other support person to assume as active a role as possible in the labor and birth process. The CNM makes every effort to facilitate the natural forces of labor in a non-interfering manner and to ensure that the couple's birth plans are implemented as long as progress continues within the range of normal. However, the CNM is prepared to intervene or to consult with a physician should the course of labor deviate from what is considered safe

for mother or baby. The nurse-midwife may provide pain-relieving medications as appropriate for the needs of the client."

JOURNAL OF NURSE-MIDWIFERY
Bimonthly Magazine

Suscription Department
Elsevier North Holland, Inc.

52 Vanderbilt Avenue
New York, NY 10017
$21.00 for individuals
$42.00 for institutions
(make checks payable to the
Journal of Nurse-Midwifery)

The *Journal of Nurse-Midwifery* is the "official voice" of the ACNM. It includes articles on nurse-midwifery, parent-child health, obstetrics, well-woman gynecology, family planning and neonatology, including good coverage of alternative birth issues and practice. The *Journal* also includes letters and editorials, a legislative exchange and news updates, journal abstracts, and media reviews. Sample copies are available upon request from Elsevier North Holland.

WHERE IS NURSE-MIDWIFERY TAUGHT?

(information supplied by the American College of Nurse-Midwives)

Booth Maternity Center
6051 Overbrook Avenue
Philadelphia, PA 19131
215/878-7800, ext. 71

College of Medicine and Dentistry of New Jersey
School of Allied Health Professions
Nurse-Midwifery Program
100 Bergen Street
Newark, NJ 07103
201/456-4249, 4298

Columbia University Graduate Program in Maternity, Nursing and Nurse-Midwifery
Department of Nursing, Faculty of Medicine
Columbia-Presbyterian Medical Center
622 West 168th Street
New York, NY 10032
212/694-3529

Cleveland Metropolitan General Hospital
Nurse-Midwifery Service
c/o Department of Ob-Gyn
3395 Scranton Road
Cleveland, OH 44109
216/459-5342

Emory University
School of Nursing
Atlanta, GA 30322
404/329-6917

Frontier School of Midwifery and Family Nursing
Frontier Nursing Service
Hyden, KY 41749
606/672-2901

Georgetown University School of Nursing
Graduate Program, Growing Family Nurse-Midwifery
3700 Reservoir Road, NW
Washington, DC 20007
202/625-3559

Medical University of South Carolina
Nurse-Midwifery Program, College of Nursing
171 Ashley Avenue
Charleston, SC 29403
803/792-2200, 3093

Meharry Medical College
Nurse-Midwifery Program
Department of Nursing Education
1005-18th Avenue, N
Nashville, TN 37208
615/327-6497, 6494

St. Louis University
Department of Nursing
Graduate Program in Nurse-Midwifery
3525 Caroline Street
St. Louis, MO 63104
314/664-9800

State University of New York
Downstate Medical Center
College of Health Related Professions
Nurse-Midwifery Program
Box 93
450 Clarkson Avenue
Brooklyn, NY 11203
212/270-1359, 1360

United States Air Force (USAF Nurses only)
Nurse-Midwifery Program
Malcolm Grow USAF Medical Center
Andrews Air Force Base, MD 20331
301/981-6104

University of Arizona
College of Nursing
Tucson, AZ 85721
602/626-7481

University of California at San Diego
Primary Care Nurse Practitioner Program
Nurse-Midwifery Component
University Hospital, H-813
225 Dickinson Street
San Diego, CA 92103
714/294-6113

University of California at San Francisco
San Francisco General Hospital
Room 6B30
1001 Potrero Avenue
San Francisco, CA 94110
415/821-5106 or 647-7828

University of Colorado Health Sciences Center
School of Nursing Graduate Program
Nurse-Midwifery Tract
Box C 288
4200 East 9th Street
Denver, CO 80262
303/394-7880, 8654

The University of Illinois at the Medical Center
College of Nursing
Department of Maternal-Child Nursing, Nurse-Midwifery Program
P.O. Box 6998
Chicago, IL 60680
312/996-7937

University of Kentucky
College of Nursing
760 Rose Street
Lexington, KY 40536
606/233-5406, 6620

University of Miami
School of Nursing
1540 Corniche
Coral Gables, FL 33124
305/284-2830

University of Minnesota
3313 Powell Hall
500 Essex Street, SE
Minneapolis, MN 55455
612/376-8472

University of Mississippi
Nurse-Midwifery Education Program
265 Woodland Hills Bldg.
Jackson, MS 39216
601/987-4823

University of Pennsylvania
School of Nursing
Nursing Education Building
420 Service Dr., SW
Philadelphia, PA 19104
215/243-4335

University of Southern California
LA County-USC Medical Center
Women's Hospital Room 8K5
1240 N. Mission Road
Los Angeles, CA 90033
213/226-3386, 3387

University of Utah
College of Nursing
Graduate Major in Maternal and Newborn Nursing and Nurse-Midwifery
25 South Medical Drive
Salt Lake City, UT 84112
801/581-8274

Yale University
Maternal-Newborn (Nurse-Midwifery) Program
855 Howard Avenue, Box 3333
New Haven, CT 06510
203/436-3782

NURSE-MIDWIFERY
by Helen Varney
1980, 654 pages, Illus.

from
Blackwell Scientific Publications
C.V. Mosby, Distributor
11830 Westline Industrial Drive
St. Louis, MO 63141
$37.50

This is the first textbook written specifically for the education of American nurse-midwives. Until now, nurse-midwifery instructors and students have had to piece together information from obstetrics texts and English midwifery texts, neither of which speak to the way nurse-midwifery is practiced in the U.S. This book fills the gap and will be of interest not only to midwifery students but to those who want to understand how nurse-midwives are different from doctors and from their sister lay-midwives.

Helen Varney, head of the nurse-midwifery program at Yale, begins with a history and description of the profession of nurse-midwifery. Midwifery has always been practiced, but at the turn of the century in America (not in Europe), traditional midwives were outlawed in most states, due to pressure from the young and growing male medical profession. The first domestic program to train nurse-midwives began in the 1930's and today there are about 25 programs in universities and hospitals which teach nurse-midwifery.

Varney goes on to describe the "management" by nurse-midwives of prenatal care, the intrapartal period, the newborn, the postpartum period, and the "interconceptional" period (family-planning). The text is well-illustrated and organized and describes the anatomy and physiology of birth as well as providing specific guidelines for the practice of nurse-midwifery. A final section describes 26 specific "skills" which are used by nurse-midwives.

"As the nurse-midwife specializes in management of the essentially normal childbearing woman, the nurse-midwife has perfected skills which promote and facilitate the normal processes of childbearing, as well as those which may be obstetrically indicated. For example, the nurse-midwife has the knowledge, judgement, and skills required for either performing pudendal blocks, delivery in lithotomy position, and cutting and repairing episiotomies or providing the alternative of delivering over an intact perineum in dorsal position with no or minimal analgesia and/or anesthesia while coaching the patient in her breathing or any combination of these choices. Such decisions are made in conjunction with the patient and within the obstetrical limits of safe-

NURSE-MIDWIVES IN PRACTICE—PHILOSOPHIES AND SERVICES

"The nurse-midwife provides care for the normal mother during pregnancy and stays with her during labor, providing continuous physical and emotional support. She evaluates progress and manages the labor and delivery. She evaluates and provides immediate care for the normal newborn. She helps the mother to care for herself and for her infant; to adjust the home situation to the new child, and to lay a healthful foundation for future pregnancies through family planning and gynecologic services. The nurse-midwife is prepared to teach, interpret, and provide support as an integral part of her service."

Nurse-Midwifery Service
UCSD Medical Center
San Diego, California

* * *

"To me, the special difference you made during pregnancy and childbirth was the extra time you spent, time to talk during our prenatal visits, to be there through the entire labor and delivery, to spend time during your postpartum checks and even a moment for a phone call or two after I returned home. It was truly personalized care and much appreciated."

from *Nurse-Midwives: Comments from Moms and Dads*, produced by the nurse-midwifery program at Family Hospital, Milwaukee, Wisconsin.

"I am a certified nurse-midwife in private practice providing care to families desiring homebirth. I also do well-women gynecology exams... Although I work in collaboration with several area obstetricians, my practice is my own, and is based on the philosophy that childbirth is most often a healthy process that should occur within the family unit. I also feel strongly that my role is to offer support, information, and guidance while the birthing couple maintains control of their experience."

Certified Nurse-Midwife
Pittsburgh, Pennsylvania

* * *

"Midwives have been delivering babies for centuries. Today's certified nurse-midwife is still actively involved in providing family centered maternity care, but she has added another dimension to her practice: well-woman gynecology.

"For the woman who needs routine gynecological or family planning services, the nurse-midwife offers an alternative to traditional medical care."

Nurse-Midwifery Practice
Hospital of the University of Pennsylvania, Philadelphia, Pennsylvania

* * *

"The nurse-midwives accept as maternity clients only healthy women experiencing normal pregnancy.

The nurse-midwife provides complete prenatal care, manages the labor and birth in the client's home or hospital, and offers postpartum follow-care, plus family planning. All clients are expected to take an active role in preparing for their baby's birth... Parents also make major decisions about birth procedures: who will be present, the delivery techniques to be used and how the baby will be welcomed into the family. The nurse-midwife provides constant monitoring of the labor and advises the parents of any needed medical procedures. Complications of pregnancy or labor are immediately referred to the care of a physician."

Maternity Center Associates
Bethesda, Maryland

* * *

"The Nurse-Midwives believe that responsiveness to the individual needs and desires of the childbearing family is an essential ingredient in good maternity care.

"The Nurse-Midwives will make all of their knowledge and skills available to participants in the practice to bring about a fulfilling birth experience, recognizing that the goal of all childbearing families is a healthy mother and baby."

Nurse-Midwifery Care of Orange County
Santa Ana, California

---

ty as dictated by the patient's condition.

"Currently, nurse-midwives are again listening to consumer concerns and desires and are in the forefront of developing alternatives to the all too frequently typical sterile, pathologically-oriented obstetrical units in hospitals. Alternatives are being sought which will provide all the safety features and emergency equipment for both mother and baby if needed and which will utilize the advantages, while modifying or avoiding the disadvantages, of the present in-hospital health care system. Such alternatives include promoting obstetrical team (physician/nurse-midwife) efforts geared towards deliveries in the labor room, or specifically designed family-oriented birthing rooms, and early discharge from the hospital, family-oriented maternity homes with emergency equipment and arrangements with nearby hospitals, and carefully selected home deliveries with arrangements for transportation and a back-up hospital....

"One of the hallmarks of a nurse-midwife is the constant care she/he

"One of the hallmarks of a nurse-midwife is the constant care she/he gives to the woman throughout labor."

gives the woman throughout labor. This does not mean remote control management of the woman but, rather, an active and participating presence in the room both to manage the care of the woman obstetrically and to provide or facilitate the provision of indicated supportive care. Women's horror stories of being left alone in fear and in pain without knowing what was going on, with only an hourly check of the blood pressure and fetal heart tone and a 'mashing' of her abdomen for comfort and company, are anathema to the nurse-midwife. This sort of trauma experienced by a woman in labor may have a negative psychological effect upon her for the rest of her life and upon her relationship with the child whom she may see as the causative factor for her trauma.

"It has been said that effective supportive care is worth 100 to 200 milligrams of Demerol, two to three hours of labor duration, and uncountable psychological benefits.

"Lesser and Keane identified five needs of a woman in labor as follows:

1. bodily or physical care
2. sustaining human presence
3. relief from pain
4. acceptance of attitudes and behavior
5. information and reassurance of a safe outcome for herself and her baby."

RESTRAINT OF TRADE AGAINST NURSE-MIDWIVES

Restraint of the practice of nurse-midwives by physicians was the focus of a hearing held December 18, 1980, by the Subcommittee on Oversight and Investigations of the U.S. House Committee on Interstate and Foreign Commerce. The hearing, conducted by Congressmembers Albert Gore, Jr., and Barbara Mikulski, centered around a case in Gore's home state of Tennessee in which two nurse-midwives who attempted to set up an independent midwifery service for in-hospital birth were denied admitting privileges at local hospitals and their back-up physician suffered cancellation of his malpractice insurance. Nurse-midwives Lonnie Holtzman Morris of the Childbirth Center in Englewood, New Jersey, Ruth Watson Lubic of the Maternity Center Association in New York, and Marion McCartney of Maternity Center Associates in Bethesda, Maryland all testified on the problems certified nurse-midwives (CNM) have had in their states. Other witnesses included Judy Norsigian of the National Women's Health Network, Sally Tom of the American College of Nurse Midwives, and Warren Pearse of the American College of Obstetricians and Gynecologists, who was asked to explain why ACOG had supported efforts in New Jersey to restrict the practice of nurse-midwives.

Susan Sizemore and Victoria Henderson, the two Tennessee nurse-midwives involved, have joined with the Consumer Coalition for Health, a Nashville based, non-profit consumer organization, to work on filing a lawsuit in Federal Court alleging restraint of trade. In October, 1981, a fundraising event was held to raise money for legal fees. Over 1000 people attended and $15,000 was raised in one evening, demonstrating tremendous community support for the midwives.

For more information or to make donations contact:
Consumer Coalition for Health
Nurse-Midwifery Project
P.O. Box 120582, Acklen Station
Nashville, TN 37212

NURSE MIDWIFERY: CONSUMERS FREEDOM OF CHOICE
Hearing before the Subcommittee on Oversight and Investigations of the Committee on Interstate and Foreign Commerce, House of Representatives December 18, 1980, 180 pages

from
U.S. House of Representatives
Subcommittee on Oversight and Investigations
Committee on Interstate and Foreign Commerce
Washington, DC 20515
202/225-4441
single copy free

This is the complete text of the hearing on nurse-midwifery chaired by Albert Gore and Barbara Mikulski.

(from Susan Sizemore's testimony) "We still provide midwifery services to the disadvantaged poor at Metropolitan Nashville General Hospital and we will continue to do so. Apparently it is quite acceptable to the medical community of Nashville for poor women to receive our services. In fact, they are the only ones who indeed have a choice. Self-paying or non-medicaid third-party paying clients do not have this choice, they must be delivered by an obstetrician if choosing any one of a number of hospitals for delivery . . .

Mr. Gore: ". . . What we have here is a case where a lot of consumers have asked for the service that you are attempting to provide?"

Ms. Sizemore: "Yes."

Mr. Gore: "They want the service. It is cheaper, arguably safer, at least as safe, and yet the established medical community or some members of that established medical community have forced you to go out of business by denying you the opportunity to practice, and they have made professional life so miserable for the doctor with whom you were associated that he felt it necessary to move to another State?

I believe that is an outrage."

Ms. Sizemore: "It is real hard to understand it and to gain some perspective on it, other than to come to the conclusion that many people in medicine in Nashville choose not to work collegially with nurse-midwives . . ."

* * *

Mr. Gore: "Let the record be clear on this point. The medical community appears to have no objection whatsoever, based on quality or any other matter, where poor women are concerned. Where there is not a substantial economic stake involved, it is perfectly all right, apparently, for certified nurse-midwives to assume complete direction, control, whatever words of art you want to use. The controversy only arises where middle-income women or upper-income women hear about the alternatives provided by and associated with certified nurse-midwives, when they would otherwise be going to and paying fees to obstetricians, is that right?"

Ms. Sizemore: "That seems to be the problem . . . ."

MIDWIVES ALLIANCE OF NORTH AMERICA-M.A.N.A.

"In an effort to improve the quality of maternal/infant health care in the United States, midwives from all over the country have joined together in an unprecedented organization, The Midwives Alliance of North America (M.A.N.A.). Certified nurse-midwives and lay midwives from all parts of the U.S. formed the group in Lexingon, Kentucky, during the week of April 25-30, 1982.

The idea for such an organization developed from an October, 1981, meeting in Washington, DC, between nurse-midwives and lay midwives. The meeting was called by Sister Angela Murdaugh, president of the American College of Nurse-Midwives, who felt that dialogue between the two groups needed to be established. The core group of midwives present at the 1981 gathering (from Washington, California, Texas, Tennessee, Georgia, and Massachusetts) agreed on the need for a professional organization which would create a strong alliance among all midwives. They decided on an open meeting in April, coinciding with an annual convention of the American College of Nurse-Midwives.

Several hundred midwives were present at these open meetings in Lexington. After considerable discussion, the following purposes were developed:

1. To expand communication and support among North American (including Canadian) midwives.
2. To form an identifiable and cohesive organization representing the professional midwife on a regional, national and international basis.
3. To promote guidelines for the education and training of midwives, and to assist in development of midwifery educational programs.
4. To promote guidelines for basic competency in practicing midwives.
5. To promote midwifery as a quality health care option for women and their families.
6. To promote research in the field of midwifery care.
7. To establish channels for communication and cooperation between midwives and other professional and non-professional groups concerned with the health of women and their families.

Membership in M.A.N.A. is open to all midwives, students, and supporters of midwifery. In the future, membership may be categorized. Eventually a certification process may be made available for practicing midwives. The communication vehicle for M.A.N.A. will be *The Practicing Midwife*. New pages will be added for M.A.N.A. news and input.

M.A.N.A. would like to hear from local, state or regional midwifery groups, as well as individual midwives, who want to offer input. The ideal is a national organization which will represent the grassroots groups that have been forming around the country."

(Information taken from press releases circulated during the Summer of 1982.) For additional information or to join M.A.N.A. contact:
Midwives Alliance of North America
c/o Concord Midwifery Service
30 South Main Street
Concord, NH 03301

To contribute articles and ideas to *The Practicing Midwife* contact:
The Practicing Midwife
c/o Ina May Gaskin
156 Drakes Lane
Summertown, TN 38483

Lay Midwives

A midwife is a person who assists women in childbirth. There have probably always been midwives, for as long as people have lived together in social groups. In times past (and still today) a midwife arises spontaneously from the people, to take on her role of helping in childbirth. Sometimes she learns her skills from her mother or by apprenticing to an older midwife. Sometimes she is simply a woman who has witnessed many births and borne children herself and becomes known to the other mothers in her community as a sympathetic helper. Often a midwife has other healing functions in the community—she may cultivate and prescribe herbs and be sought for advice on infertility or an unwanted pregnancy. It is thought that during the witch-hunts of the Middle Ages, many midwives and women healers were among the victims. Until this century, childbirth was considered the province of midwives alone, and men were not allowed to assist at births. However, with the rise of the medical profession, midwives were outlawed for the first time in history and only in North America, an unusual situation which is now beginning to reverse itself.

After the suppression of midwives in the United States, midwives in Europe continued to be professionally trained in the science and skills of obstetrics. Midwives in the few U.S. states which did not outlaw them continued to practice as "granny" midwives, most often in poor, rural areas unserved by doctors. In the 1930's the profession of nurse-midwifery was created in the U.S. to reintroduce the midwife, but as a person with medical nursing training. In the 1960's, in response to the growing demand for home birth attendants, self-trained midwives arose from the counter-culture communities of northern California and Boston and throughout the United States. Called "lay" midwives, these women are often young mothers who have given birth at home themselves and who learn their skills through a combination of practical experience (attending births, apprenticing to another midwife) and studying the anatomy and physiology of pregnancy, labor, and birth. In most states the practice of lay midwifery is illegal and lay midwives are always subject to fear of harassment and prosecution and forced to practice without adequate medical back-up. However, during the 1970's some states began to reevaluate their old midwifery laws, based on consumer demand and new studies showing that infant and maternal death rates are lower when midwives handle the majority of normal births. States such as Washington, New Hampshire, and Rhode Island have issued new laws which license and regulate lay midwives. Now these new "Licensed Midwives," lay midwives, and nurse-midwives are joining together to work toward the reestablishment of midwifery as the model of care for birth in America. This section describes many of the books, organizations, schools, and skills developed by lay midwives.

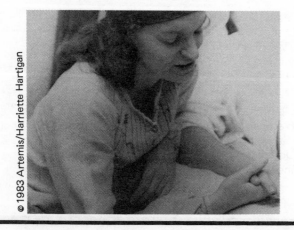

© 1983 Artemis/Harriette Hartigan

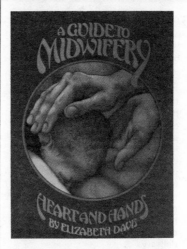

A GUIDE TO MIDWIFERY: HEART AND HANDS
by Elizabeth Davis
1981, 216 pages, Illus

from
John Muir Publications
P.O. Box 613
Santa Fe, NM 87501
$9.00 pap., discounts available

This is the first book devoted solely to the practice of lay midwifery, written by a San Francisco lay midwife who practices in an open, supportive community. The book will be extremely useful in a practical sense but will also be of tremendous historical interest in years to come as a document of the resurgence in America of the ancient art of women helping women at birth. Davis describes the ways in which women become lay midwives (self-study, labor coaching, schools and study groups, apprenticeship) and provides guidelines for setting up a practice. She then describes prenatal care, attending at birth, and postpartum care, as commonly practiced by the modern American lay midwife. Her emphasis is on the emotional factors in birth (heart) and on the midwife's practical, manual skills (hands). Many excellent illustrations and photographs complement the text, and there is a complete set of birth record forms in the Appendix. This book will be invaluable for midwives, both lay and nurse, and should be required reading for obstetricians who are not familiar with how normal birth can be managed in the absence of hospital "technology." Parents, especially those planning a home birth, will also be enlightened by Davis's advice on helping mothers and fathers cope with pregnancy, labor and birth. I am disturbed by the aggressiveness of some of Davis's techniques (for instance, I wouldn't want anyone to be massaging deeply inside my vagina during second stage!) but on the whole this is an excellent guide to the *art* of midwifery.

"Now, while you are going through your procedure of 'massage, squeeze out the compress, pour the oil and massage again,' how's the baby doing? This is, after all, the factor that determines the amount of time you have to spend on keeping the perineum intact. Your fetoscope should be conveniently hanging around your neck, and if you have the type that has the forehead brace you can listen to the baby during a contraction and keep your hands free to support the perineum as it starts distending. But this is almost too much to coordinate, this feeling and massaging without quite being able to see what you are doing, while also attempting to count out the rate of the fetal heartbeat. Most midwives work in pairs so these tasks can be divided, allowing each partner a chance to rest more frequently, squeeze out another hot compress, or to center down and breathe deeply before going on to the next task. . . .

"It's important that the midwife acknowledges the incredible demands that her work places on her mate, as well as the stresses placed on her family. Running off at inopportune moments can be hard on small children, and really rough on the nursing baby-mother unit. Not to mention the obvious; more than once I've been interrupted by the phone call in the middle of lovemaking that was super great or much needed. In fact, the phone rings constantly, bearing messages of varying and sometimes questionable urgency. Occasionally I find myself saying as I reach for the receiver, 'Don't let this be a heavy one' or even half seriously, 'I hope no one's in labor.' Usually this is because my own family needs energy; I have shopping or cleaning to do or want simply to relate without interruptions. Being prepared for 'the phone call' means keeping one's self, home, and family in a constant state of readiness. All midwives should consider (and reconsider) limiting their practice to a level that is workable overall. For me, this is currently around four births a month, which gives me time to integrate new learning from each birthing, catch up on sleep, get the family back in kilter, and generally bliss-out and rejuvenate myself before going on."

LAY MIDWIFERY SCHOOLS

The following schools offer "in-residence" training for lay midwifery. Write for more information on the program, fees, and for applications for admission.

INSTITUTE FOR MIDWIFERY STUDIES
P.O. Box 1694
Tacoma, WA 98401
206/272-7038

Sponsored by the Association for Childbirth at Home, International, this new school is applying for approval for Washington State licensure.

NEW MEXICO MIDWIFERY TRAINING INSTITUTE
P.O. Box 26174
Albuquerque, NM 87102

A formal 2-year education and apprenticeship program.

NORTH TEXAS SCHOOL OF MIDWIFERY
814 Dalworth
Grand Prairie, TX 75050
214/263-0299

THE MATERNITY CENTER
1119 E. San Antonio
El Paso, TX 79901
915/533-8142

Lay midwifery is legal in Texas, which enables lay midwife Shari

Daniels to operate this unique center serving a largely Mexican-American population in El Paso. The midwifery training program lasts for one year and involves class work as well as a high case load of births, which take place at the Center's clinic and in homes. Students must be able to speak Spanish.

SEATTLE MIDWIFERY SCHOOL
2611 NE 125th Street, Suite 207
Seattle, WA 98125
206/365-4092

The Seattle Midwifery School offers midwifery training for non-nurse-midwives. Graduates are approved to take the Washington State Licensing Exam to become licensed midwives. Training is from two to three years in duration. At least one year of didactic training is given, through courses taught by health care professionals, and at least one year of clinical training, through apprenticeship to a "preceptor" is required. Prospective students should contact the School in Spring to find out when the next class will begin.

SONOMA COUNTY SELF-STUDY MIDWIFERY TRAINING PROGRAM
13140 Frati Lane
Sebastopol, CA 95472
707/874-2857 and 707/829-1131

Nan Ullrike Koehler has developed this three-year midwifery training program, which involves one year of reading and home study, one year of directed research and courses from outside sources, and one year of apprenticeship.

TRAVELING WORKSHOPS

The following workshops are offered throughout the country. Write for information on fees, current calendar schedule, or to arrange a workshop for your community.

SHARI DANIELS MIDWIFERY INTENSIVE SEMINARS
c/o The Maternity Center
1119 E. San Antonio
El Paso, TX 79901
915/533-8142

Shari Daniels gives 5-day seminars in midwifery skills which cover history taking, prenatal care, normal labor, complications, and being a midwife. Materials include sample client hand-outs and films of births at the Maternity Center are shown.

INFORMED HOMEBIRTH MIDWIFERY SKILLS WORKSHOPS
P.O. Box 788
Boulder, CO 80306
303/449-4181

5-day intensive workshops are taught by a pair of lay midwives.

Skills covered include: prenatal care, evaluating risk, monitoring labor, psychological support, complications, suturing, record-keeping, newborn exam, etc. Materials and hand-outs are included in fee.

ASSOCIATION FOR CHILDBIRTH AT HOME, INTERNATIONAL INTENSIVE SEMINARS IN MIDWIFERY SCIENCE AND SKILLS
P.O. Box 39498
Los Angeles, CA 90039
213/667-0839 and 213/660-2539

5-day seminars are taught by a team of three lay midwives and by local guest professionals and offered for beginning and intermediate level midwives and for advanced and very experienced midwives. Classes include extensive use of audio-visual aids and cover normal pregnancy, labor, postpartum and the newborn, complications, case review, and emergency management.

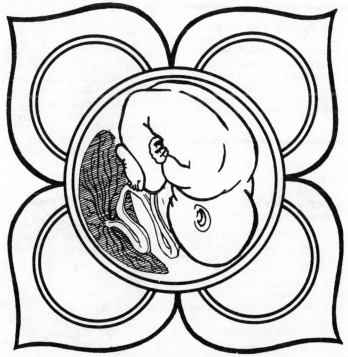

Drawing courtesy of Jennifer Stapleton-Houston

INTERNATIONAL DEFINITION OF A MIDWIFE

(Accepted by the Council of the International Confederation of Midwives in 1972 and by the General Assembly of the International Federation of Gynaecology and Obstetrics in 1973)

"A midwife is a person who, having been regularly admitted to a midwifery educational programme, duly recognised in the country in which it is located, has successfully completed the prescribed course of studies in midwifery and has acquired the requisite qualifications to be registered and/or legally licensed to practise midwifery. She must be able to give the necessary supervision, care and advice to women during pregnancy, labour and the postpartum period, to conduct deliveries on her own responsibility and to care for the new born and the infant. This care includes preventive measures, the detection of abnormal conditions in mother and child, the procurement of medical assistance and the execution of emergency measures in the absence of medical help. She has an important task in health couseling and education, not only for patients but also within the family and the community. The work should involve ante-natal education and preparation for parenthood and extend to certain areas of gynaecology, family planning and child care. She may practise in hospitals, clinics, health units, domiciliary conditions or in any other service."

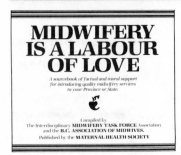

MIDWIFERY IS A LABOUR OF LOVE

A sourcebook of factual and moral support for introducing quality midwifery services to your Province or State

Compiled by
The Interdisciplinary **MIDWIFERY TASK FORCE** Association
and the **B.C. ASSOCIATION OF MIDWIVES.**
Published by the **MATERNAL HEALTH SOCIETY**

MIDWIFERY IS A LABOUR OF LOVE: A Sourcebook of Factual and Moral Support for Introducing Quality Midwifery Services in Your Province or State
Compiled by the Interdisciplinary Midwifery Task Force Association and the B.C. Association of Midwives

from
Midwifery Task Force Treasurer
1244 Shorepine Walk
Vancouver, British Columbia
V6H 3T8, Canada
$8.50 plus $1.00 postage
(make checks payable to Midwifery is a Labour of Love)

The practice of midwifery, even by certified nurse-midwives, is not legal in Canada. In Spring, 1980, a conference was held in Vancouver, B.C. to help build support for Canadian midwifery education and services. This book is a transcript of the proceedings and includes talks on the practice and scope of midwifery given by Gerrit Jan Kloosterman (an obstetrician from the Netherlands), Jean Donnison (author of *Midwives and Medical Men*), Ruth Watson Lubic (director of the Maternity Center Association of New York), and Canadian parents and midwives. Also included is a set of international, Canadian, and U.S. position papers and advisories on midwifery, and extensive references and tables.

"It is incredibly difficult to stay and offer one's self silently as a companion in those awesome hours and months of waiting. A high degree of emotional and spiritual maturity is required. A Zen Buddhist monk might be better qualified than a doctor or a nurse to stand waiting in the face of such elemental forces as a labouring woman, an expectant father, a birthing baby. It is a supreme skill to do nothing when that is required. It is even more difficult to integrate in one person the social, emotional and psychic skills required with the specialised body of knowledge essential to a birth attendant.

"I believe midwives *are* the people who embody these skills most comletely. They are here working among us already. It is time we recognized the value of their practice and supported their growth. . ."
—from "Why Parents Need Midwives," by Eleanor Quirk, New Denver, British Columbia, Mother and Registered Nurse.

For more information on midwifery in British Columbia contact:

INTERDISCIPLINARY MIDWIFERY TASK FORCE ASSOCIATION
926 School Green
Vancouver, BC
V6H 3N7, Canada

BRITISH COLUMBIA ASSOCIATION OF MIDWIVES
1053 Douglas Cres.
Vancouver, BC
V6H 1V4, Canada

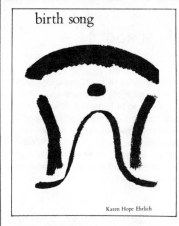

birth song

Karen Hope Ehrlich

BIRTH SONG
by Karen Hope Ehrlich
1979, 50 pages, Illus.

from
Karen Hope Ehrlich
P.O. Box 956
Ben Lomond, CA 95005
$5.00 plus 75 cents postage
10 or more for $4. each

This is a collection of poems about birth and midwifery written by lay midwife, Karen Ehrlich. The poems are all beautiful and insightful and deal with both the joyous and painful aspects of being a midwife. These poems will provide inspiration and strength to practicing midwives, who are sometimes overwhelmed by the heavy emotional demands and responsibilities of attending births.

"My Soft Hands

i have felt life
try to pass out of my hands
i have coaxed it back with my hands
to take up its long residence
as long as a lifetime

i have urged the breath from my own
     lungs
into life hanging tipsily
on the razor edge of life's crossing

my head aches
with the smashing hopes and long
     beginning
of a virus

i have felt woman's blood of all life
pour out of bodies
in a warm bath
a sensual jangling bath over my hands
thick as carpet

i harbor unshed tears
from the deepest part of my sex
that has been wounded
at the tortured shapes of women
in the throes of battle
with life's purest crossing

my soft hands with haloed fingers
eager to stroke away pain
eager to give thanks for a joyous
     entry"

SILK'N'THREADS
8200 Oak Avenue
Ben Lomond, CA 95005

Janice Aylsworth, of Silk'N' Threads, is a mother and former midwife, who now does silk-screening, producing a series of T-shirts with artwork and slogans, including "Support Your Local Midwife" and "I was Born at Home." These T-shirts are sold by the California Association of Midwives to raise money for efforts to legalize lay midwifery in California and can also be ordered directly from Silk'N'Threads. Other interested groups can request information on bulk rates. Write for a brochure with current prices. T-shirts are available in infant's, children's, women's, men's, and maternity sizes, in cotton and cotton blends.

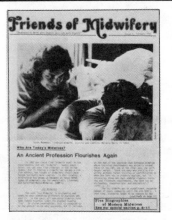

FRIENDS OF MIDWIFERY
P.O. Box 18643
Seattle, WA 98118
$10.00 per year

This excellent new quarterly newsletter is published by the Seattle Midwifery School. Issue No. 2, February, 1982, contained a description of Washington state's new midwifery law, consumer guidelines for evaluating a midwife, and five biographies of "modern midwives," practicing in Washington, including nurse-midwives, foreign-trained, and domestic lay and licensed midwives.

"Parents should feel secure that their attendants are: 1) capable technicians; 2) knowledgeable about the normal; 3) able to recognize problems and able to rectify them or know when medical help must be sought; 4) understanding of the individual needs and desires of each woman/couple; 5) flexible enough to respond to these individual needs and desires; 6) respectful of the rights and responsibilities of parents to be the ultimate decision makers; 7) empathetic toward the great changes taking place in the woman's/couple's lives. Your midwife can and should fulfill all these expectations. It used to be—and still is in many parts of the country—a matter of choosing which physician and which hospital to give birth in, and anyone lucky enough to locate a midwife would often engage her services regardless of her attributes. Here and now, however, we have a *range* of choices when selecting a midwife, for today's midwives function in a variety of settings and offer a variety of services. . ."
—from "What to Ask Your Midwife" in *Friends of Midwifery*, Issue 2.

NATIONAL MIDWIVES ASSOCIATION
1119 E. San Antonio
El Paso, TX 79901

The National Midwives Association is an offshoot of activities at the Maternity Center in El Paso. The Association works to provide information and support for its members, holds conferences, publishes a monthly newsletter, and makes referrals for parents wanting a lay midwife. Write for more information.

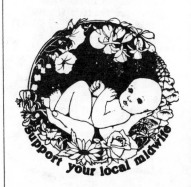

MIDWIFERY SKILLS BOOKS

from
Informed Homebirth
P.O. Box 788
Boulder, CO 80306

Informed Homebirth has recently published a series of four books on midwifery skills, written by Anne Frye and Valerie Hobbs, lay midwives who teach the Informed Homebirth Midwifery Skills workshops. The books are available separately at the prices listed below plus $1.00 each for postage or $3.16 postage for four books sent together. These books are designed to provide useful, technical information to practicing lay midwives.

PRENATAL LAB WORK FOR LAY MIDWIVES (Second Edition)
by Anne Frye
1982, 72 pages, Illus.
$7.00

Covers tests a midwife can do herself, working with a laboratory and lab test results (blood tests, rubella, venereal disease, pap test, etc.), working with a doctor and obstetric diagnostic tests (x-ray, ultrasound, amniocentesis, etc.), and tests for infant well-being. Included are charts showing normal ranges and an annotated bibliography.

COMPLICATIONS OF LABOR AND DELIVERY
by Valerie Hobbs
1982, 58 pages, Illus.
$7.00

Covers the management of malpresentations, bleeding, obstetrical emergencies (prolapsed cord, fetal distress etc.), labor dystocias, and neonatal abnormalities including respiratory distress. Includes contributions by Ina May Gaskin on management of breech deliveries and by Mau Blossom on "manual removal of a partially detached placenta."

SUTURING FOR MIDWIVES
by Anne Frye
1981, 29 pages, Illus.
$5.00 pap.

Covers equipment and techniques for repair of lacerations and episiotomies.

HERBS FOR WOMEN: A Guide for Lay Midwives
by Valerie Hobbs
1981, 30 pages
$5.00 pap.

Provides an introduction to the use of herbs and how to gather and prepare them. Lists herbal remedies for "female balance," pregnancy, labor, postpartum, and breastfeeding. Includes a list of books and herb supply companies.

STANDARDS OF PRACTICE FOR LAY MIDWIVES

1. Know basic anatomy and physiology, in particular the female reproductive system and the neonate.
2. Know how to recognize and manage normal pregnancy, labor and birth.
3. Be familiar with possible complications, know your limitations and be willing to call a more knowledgeable and experienced person for back-up.
4. Be able to assess the needs of the neonate. Be able to provide the necessary care or refer to a more competent practitioner.
5. Use risk factor assessments to determine candidacy for home births. Inform and encourage women with high risks to obtain appropiate care. It is the midwife's prerogative to refuse service to a mother who may present a risk. Be objective in your decision to protect the mother, fetus and yourself.
6. Attend peer review meetings in your region.
7. Attend a minimum of 50 hours of workshops or class time in continuing education per year.
8. Maintain records including history, lab, pregnancy, birth and the post-partum.
9. Provide high quality prenatal, intrapartum and postpartum care (at least through one month).
10. Provide information on individual practice so that an informed choice can be made. This should include:
    A. Education
    B. Experience
    C. Back-up
    D. Financial needs
    E. Responsibilities of pregnant woman/couple
    F. Roles and responsibilities of midwife
11. Have adequate transportation, communication and be available at all times and/or have reliable back-up
12. Make sure that your pregnant women/couples are educated on:
    A. Choices in health care, including PKU test and eye prophylaxis
    B. Changes in pregnancy
    C. Good nutrition and health practice
    D. Natural childbirth
    E. Breastfeeding and newborn care
    F. Parenting
    G. Family Planning

Reproduced with permission from *Birthing*, the newsletter of the Oregon Midwifery Council (Vol. 4, No. 16).

FACING THE WORST
by Elizabeth Depperman Gilmore
1980, 3 pages

from
Mothering Reprints
P.O. Box 2208
Albuquerque, NM 87103-2208
75 cents
10% discount for 10 or more

Facing the possibility of death is one of the most difficult tasks of expectant parents and those who help them. Midwife Elizabeth Gilmore uses her personal experience to illustrate some of the important issues.

"When my thoughtful friend, Helen, told me she had worries about her birth, I defined midwifery to her and described my style. My primary task is to assist her birth and do everything in my power to avoid emergencies and to cope with any emergencies that do arise. Second, I am willing to keep her company, if she feels comfortable with my brand of honesty. I am a listener. I listen with all my senses to what she says both verbally and physically. I then repeat to her what I hear so that she can make the best use of the information. I tell her what I see and what my experience and knowledge have taught me about the choices of each given situation. I also tell her when I'm seeing something I don't understand or do not know how to handle.

" 'There is always time to tell the parents what's up,' I point out. Courses of action can be suggested and parents and midwives together choose the best one. It is the parents who will live with the outcome. 'Above all,' I reminded Helen, 'we must both understand that there are no guarantees. We must be absolutely sure that you want to give birth at home. I must be absolutely sure I want to keep you company.' "

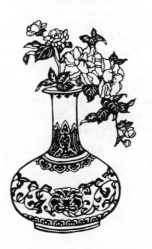

APPRENTICE ACADEMICS
24310 Pine Canyon
Spring, TX 77380

Apprentice Academics is a midwifery correspondence course, developed by lay midwife Carla Hartley. It is intended to help provide training for lay midwives, in turn to help meet the demand for knowledgeable attendents for home birth. The course is self-paced and includes a study guide and course evaluation. Requirements include the definition of vocabulary words, book reports, quizzes, research assignments, and technical questions. The course takes about a year to complete. Write for application and information on fee.

"The Apprentice Academics program offers more than technical preparation for midwifery—practical aspects of handling a midwifery practice are included. The curriculum is varied and thorough—HOWEVER— no amount of academic preparation can substitute for the supervised 'hands on' experience that is absolutely essential to midwifery training. Completion of the Apprentice Academics program is intended as preparation for, or as a compliment to, experiential training with a practicing midwife."

LAY MIDWIFE ORGANIZATIONS

In many states lay midwives are coming together to promote midwifery and support each other and also to provide parents with referrals to competent birth attendants. Listed below are the associations which responded to my request for information. I sent letters to many other state associations but some of my letters were returned marked "moved, left no forwarding address," so this is obviously an area of great flux. I would like to hear from state midwives' associations for future editions of the *Catalog.*

ARIZONA ASSOCIATION OF MIDWIVES
1248 E. Broadmor
Tempe, AZ 85282
602/966-8275

"We are an Association of Arizona Midwives dedicated to promoting safe home birth in the state through:
1. Encouraging communication between midwives
2. Developing educational programs for midwives
3. Educating the public and other professionals regarding midwifery and home birth
4. Supporting legislation in favor of midwifery, childbirth alternatives, and the rights of childbearing families.

We would also be glad to serve as a midwives' referral center to those those looking for a good midwife in Arizona."

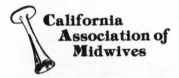

CALIFORNIA ASSOCIATION OF MIDWIVES
P.O. Box 3306
San Jose, CA 95156

The California Association of Midwives (CAM) has been working hard to promote legislation to legalize and regulate lay midwives in California, and also provides support for the many California midwives who have been arrested (see "Legal Cases Involving Lay Midwives" on next page). CAM publishes an excellent newsletter with national midwifery news and updates, articles, book reviews, and letters. CAM also refers parents to birth attendants.

The following information is taken from the CAM brochure:

"We believe that compulsory hospitalization infringes on one of the basic rights of parenthood: the right to choose the birthing environment and care best suited to individual needs. Present data indicates that planned homebirth is a safe and responsible alternative. Midwifery has arisen in response to public demand for competent homebirth attendants.

"We put forth our code of ethics as the highest form to strive for in our art. It is the goal, not an exclusion. We agree among ourselves that this is a distillation of those qualities that are valuable in midwifery.

* To be competent.
* To recognize our limits.
* To be open to the criticism of others and to examine ourselves.
* To listen.
* To respect privacy and protect intimacy
* To be invisible and protect the birth process, and to guard, cherish, and respect the people involved."

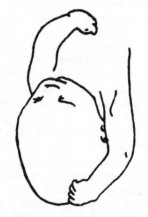

OREGON MIDWIFERY COUNCIL
3839 Pacific Avenue, No. 189
Forest Grove, OR 97116

The Oregon Midwifery Council works to support lay midwives in Oregon and publishes an excellent newsletter called *Birthing* which includes much useful information on midwifery standards, risk criteria, home birth midwife/client agreements, etc. Subscriptions are available for $15. a year, $12. for nonmembers.

THE ASSOCIATION OF TEXAS MIDWIVES
P.O. Box 702
Palestine, TX 75801
214/825-3509

"The Association of Texas Midwives is an organization of persons currently practicing, learning, or sup-

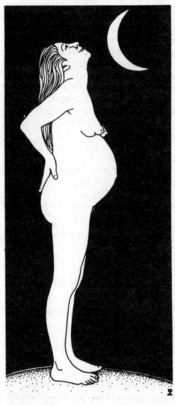

porting midwifery in Texas. The enclosed brochure states our objectives, as well as some areas of ATM activity, including a quarterly newsletter, lay midwifery certification program, and state-wide referrals. ATM membership is based on the concept of 'Informed choice'; each Associate member is required to file an Informed Choice Agreement, which is open for public review and inquiry. ATM will gladly provide information for consumers concerning home birth, midwifery, and birth alternatives in Texas."

ONTARIO ASSOCIATION OF MIDWIVES
20 London Road West
Guelph, Ontario
N1H 2B5, Canada
519/837-2796

The Ontario Association of Midwives publishes an excellent newsletter called *Issue* which contains much useful information for practicing midwives. The following code of ethics is taken from the Summer/Fall 1981 number of *Issue*.

The Ontario Association of Midwives also produces a *Whole Birth Catalogue* which is a mail-order supply source for books, birth supplies, midwifery equipment, clothing, herbs, vitamins, etc. Send $1.50 to OAM for a copy.

"MIDWIVES CODE OF PROFESSIONAL ETHICS

"Aspiring to serve birthing women and their families, I vow to:

"1. Diligently study all areas concerning birthing women—pregnancy, nutrition, labour, birth, breastfeeding and any related areas of study—so that my knowledge may be of service to my clients.
2. Respect the right of the birthing woman to be in control of her choices concerning birth. I will educate; I will not impose my own values on her against her will when she is at her most helpless.
3. Respect equally the life of mother and baby and do nothing to harm either life.
4. Comply with all legal requirements and work within the law to provide for the free exercise of my midwifery skills, in as far as I can do this without violating another section of this code.
5. Serve as the guardian of the normal in birth, alert to possible complications but always on guard against arbitrary interference in the birthing process for the sake of convenience, custom or the desire to use human beings in scientific studies and training.
6. Respect the ongoing interaction between birthing women and their babies and their families and strive in every way not to interpose myself between these relating family members.
7. Seek to work efficiently and with good will with doctors, nurses, nurse-midwives and others in the medical health field to ensure the best over-all care for birthing women and their families.
8. Share my knowledge and skills with others who wish to become midwives, and be honest and accurate with them in evaluating their competence.
9. Honor the confidence of any of those who come into contact with me in the course of my work and regard what I see and hear as inviolable, remembering always however that my highest loyalty is owed to my client and not to my own reputation or to my professional health colleagues.
10. Refuse to allow a woman's ability to pay, social prestige, marital status, or personal habits to become the primary reason for granting or refusing my services. I vow that the primary determinant will remain her need, and my capacity to provide appropriate care."

LEGAL CASES INVOLVING LAY MIDWIVES

Since the beginning of the home birth movement in the late 1960's, concerned women in communities across the country have taken on the responsibility of learning about birth, in order to meet the needs of parents for skilled home birth attendants. But since the practice of non-nurse midwifery is illegal in many states, lay midwives are vulnerable legally; several have been arrested and charged with practicing medicine without a license and, in cases where a baby died, some have been charged with murder. Many within the home birth movement view these arrests as a form of harrassment. Arrests have often been made as a result of complaints made by physicians and hospitals, not by parents. In general, however, the courts have been in sympathy with parents' right to choose home birth and midwifery services and most midwives have been exonerated. Listed below are highlights of some recent cases, which point up some of the important issues involved.

MARIANNE DOSHI—CALIFORNIA

Marianne Doshi, a lay midwife from San Luis Obispo, was charged with murder and practicing medicine without a license, in 1978. The charges resulted when a baby Doshi helped deliver died in a hospital five days after being born at home. Many supporters attended Doshi's hearing and on October 20, 1978, all charges against her were dropped. Judge Richard C. Kirkpatrick made the following remarks for the record:

"I really feel that we have a segment of our society that wants to choose an alternative to what the California Medical Association, or the American Medical Association, or the medical profession, wants to provide, as far as the birth of children goes. And I think these people probably have that right under our Constitution. . . .

"I am convinced, . . that had that child died in the hospital, or at home under a doctor's care, that we would have had a thousand doctors lined up between here and Los Angeles willing to testify that the doctor provided medical treatment according to the standard of care. I think this was a circumstance that happened, and it is very unfortunate; but I think, from reading the medical testimony, it is something that just could not have been prevented."

CAROLLE BAYA—FLORIDA

Carolle Baya, a Florida Lamaze instructor and home birth attendant, was charged with practicing midwifery without a license, in 1979. She pleaded not guilty, and Judge Richard O. Watson ruled in her favor by declaring that the Florida statutes on midwifery enacted in 1931 were unconstitutional because they were too vague.

During the August, 1979, hearing, dozens of women and children crowded the courtroom to show their support for Baya. In his six-page opinion, Judge Watson described Baya as "an intelligent, serious, 32-year-old unlicensed midwife. . . who maintains a sizable birth-related library, has read extensively, taught Lamaze or prepared childbirth, observed numerous births, assisted a registered nurse for one year, and attended a number of women in home births. . . It is difficult to imagine a more suitable candidate for midwifery licensing." Under the 1931 statute, the practice of lay midwifery in Florida is legal so long as the midwife is licensed. At the time of her arrest, Carolle Baya had been attempting, unsuccessfully, to obtain licensing as a lay midwife for two years.

With regard to the midwifery statutes, Watson wrote: "No reasonable person can determine from the face of the statute exactly what must be done in order to become licensed. Essentially the statute and rules require an applicant to satisfy HRS as to the applicant's qualifications. Yet there are no standards against which qualifications can be measured nor any way for the applicant or a Court to determine when HRS should be satisfied with the qualification in question. Due process protects citizens against statutes so vague that citizens of ordinary intelligence must necessarily guess at its meaning."

At present, Watson's ruling applies only to his own judicial circuit, although judges in other circuits can cite the Baya case as a precedent if similar cases arise in their jurisdiction. The State and the HRS did not appeal the ruling, and Carolle Baya went on to found a maternity center to provide home birth services. She and other midwives in the state are working to achieve new midwifery legislation in Florida.

For more information contact:
Carolle Baya
c/o The St. Augustine Maternity Center
P.O. Box 2085
St. Augustine, FL 32084

JOANN RUIZ—CALIFORNIA

Joann Ruiz, a nurse and lay midwife, was indicted on a felony charge of practicing medicine without a license in June, 1980. The charge resulted when a woman whom Ruiz had counseled during pregnancy developed metabolic toxemia of late pregnancy and experienced a seizure.

A preliminary hearing was set for Ruiz; however there was a great public outcry against bringing Joann Ruiz to trial. The Sacramento "Bee" carried an editorial in its July 8, 1980 edition, arguing for proper licensing of lay midwives:

"With thousands of California parents objecting to the overmedicalization, the too-frequent surgery, and the impersonal and uncaring atmosphere in hospital obstetrics wards, there is an obvious demand for midwives.

"However, despite the well-documented evidence that competent midwives are at least as capable as doctors of dealing with the vast majority of pregnancies and births . . . only a handful of nurse-midwives have been trained in California and only 165, mostly trained elsewhere, have been licensed. It should thus be no surprise that as many as 500 midwives are practicing here illegally. . . .

"The situation cries out for recognition and quality controls, not repression and harassment. For the public's protection, midwives must be trained and licensed, not kept underground. . . .

"Despite all its talk about childbirth safety, the medical community is not meeting the public's safety needs by insisting that the number of licensed midwives be strictly limited and that those who do practice be kept under the control of doctors. Joann Ruiz may or may not be a competent midwife, but as long as she and other midwives are subject to prosecution rather than licensing review, her patients will never know."

On August 12, 1980, Ruiz and her attorney met with the State's District Attorney to arrange a settlement and all felony charges were dropped. Under the terms of the settlement, Ms. Ruiz may practice midwifery if she obtains a signed set of "standardized procedures" from a California physician. As a registered nurse, this will enable her to practice midwifery under a provision of the California Nurse Practice Act which allows for "independent and overlapping functions for nursing."

DELEA BURNS—CALIFORNIA

Delea Burns, a lay midwife from Reseda, was convicted on three counts of practicing medicine without a license in 1981 and was sentenced to serve 30 days in jail and three years probation. She is the first lay midwife ever to be sentenced to a jail term. The charges came about when a woman whom Burns had attended at home, died of an air embolism at a hospital after the birth. Burns was not prosecuted or considered responsible in that death. She appealed her sentence and is being supported by the California Association of Midwives.

CAROL WARNOCK—VERMONT

A Vermont lay midwife, Carol Warnock, was acquitted of a charge of practicing medicine without a license in July, 1981. Charges were brought by the state attorney in response to a complaint by obstetrician Alan Ayer, who was the physician on duty when Warnock brought a home birth mother with postpartum bleeding to the hospital for treatment. Until this case, Vermont midwives "had maintained an uneasy truce with the medical establishment." But as a result of the charges brought against Warnock, midwives are reluctant to talk openly about their work. Lay midwives are not licensed in Vermont and their legal status is not clear.

ROSALIE TARPENING—CALIFORNIA

In August, 1981, lay midwife Rosalie Tarpening was convicted of practicing medicine without a license. She had originally been charged with murder in connection with the death of a baby born in her home in November, 1979. However, during the course of testimony it appeared that the baby was not stillborn, as Tarpening had thought, but had died in the hospital after administration of oxygen at too high a concentration. The murder charge and another charge of grand theft for accepting a fee were dropped. But after 14 hours of deliberation, the jury in Madera County returned a verdict of guilty in the remaining felony charge of practicing medicine without a license. Judge Clifford Plumley ordered that Tarpening not attend any births for a period of two years. Detailed accounts of Tarpening's case appear in the Winter 1981 issue of *NAPSAC News* (P.O. Box 267, Marble Hill, MO 63764) and in the Winter, '82 issue of *Mothering* magazine (P.O. Box 2208, Albuquerque, NM 87103).

NEW MIDWIFERY LEGISLATION IN THE STATES

Many states are reevaluating their older laws and statutes which outlawed the practice of lay midwives (sometimes called "granny midwives"). Several states have ordered "sunset reviews" of outmoded laws and consumer groups are working hard to achieve favorable new legislation. Some of these efforts, along with related organizations and resources, are listed below.

CALIFORNIA

In 1981, a bill to license lay midwives (SB670) was introduced into the State Legislature of California. The Midwifery Practice Act of 1981 was designed to provide licensing for midwives with non-nurse training. In a letter from the State's Department of Consumer Affairs, which supports the proposed legislation, the background of the bill is given: "While the State of California presently licenses nurse-midwives to practice, the practice of midwifery as it has been historically defined is currently illegal in this state. Our legislative initiative is designed to enhance maternity-care consumers' freedom to choose from among a set of alternative birthing services. . . . The bill is premised on the assumption that normal childbirth is a function of wellness not of disease, and therefore can be handled by health professionals trained to practice within the scope of normal childbirth." Unfortunately, the bill was defeated in the California Senate Health and Welfare Committee on April 28, 1981, and supporters are now working on another attempt at passage of the legislation.

The bill was authored by State Senator Barry Keene, Democrat of Mendicino County, who estimates that 40% of babies born in his county are delivered by midwives. (The Califonia Association of Midwives estimates that there are about 600 lay midwives practicing covertly in the state.) The bill was supported by the California State Department of Consumer Affairs, the California Association of Midwives, and by women's health groups around the state. It was opposed by the California Medical Association, which has long opposed the practice of midwifery.

For more information and for a copy of the proposed legislation contact:
Patricia Ternahan
Department of Consumer Affairs
1020 N Street
Sacramento, CA 95814
and
Califonia Association of Midwives
P.O. Box 3306
San Jose, CA 95156

CONNECTICUT

In 1979, the Legislative Program Review and Investigation Committee of the Connecticut General Assembly conducted a "sunset review" of regulations governing a variety of health-related professions, including midwifery. The old law, written at the turn of the century, was seen to be outmoded and the Committee, after hearing public testimony and reviewing other information made the following recommendations:
1. Repeal current midwifery statutes, Chapter 377.
2. Direct the Public Health Committee to:
    * Study the issues of home birth and lay midwifery practice; and
    * Report legislation during the 1980 legislative session to establish an appropriate regulatory mechanism for lay midwifery, consistent with Model Legislation, which would allow consumers the choice of safe home birth and lay midwifery services.

A copy of the "sunset" committee's report on midwifery, *Regulation of Midwives, Vol. 1-2*, may be requested from:
Connecticut General Assembly
Legislative Program Review and Investigations Committee
Legislative Office Building
18 Trinity Street
Hartford, CT 06115
203/566-8480

KENTUCKY

The Kentucky Committee on Midwifery Reform, a consumer group, is working to achieve legislation to regulate the practice of lay midwifery in the state. A proposed act has been written by the Kentucky Legislation Research Commission, and must now go through the process of sponsorship, hearings, and ratification. In their grant proposal to gain funding for promotion of the legislation, the Committee says:

"Awareness of one's personal health and health of family has increased dramatically in the past 20 years. It has resulted in the realization that alternatives in health services are not only desired but warranted. Childbearing is one area in which most all would agree health providers are not 'cure oriented' but rather monitors of a natural phenomenon aided by knowledge of and counseling in nutrition, hygiene, and physical and mental conditioning. Normal pregnancy and childbirth are not medical problems and as such do not by definition require medical solutions. Midwives have been the primary health providers for women for more than 2000 years. Low income women are seeking midwives

as a proper, healthy alternative to escalating costs, overcrowded facilities and budget altered health agencies. Midwifery legislative reform in Kentucky will provide for safe standards of practice by competent, trained midwives and insure the maintenance of professionalism by requiring continuing education."

For more information contact:
Kentucky Committee on Midwifery Reform (Nancy Singler, director)
Route 1, Box 249B
New Haven, KY 40051
502/549-3400

WASHINGTON STATE

A bill which licenses lay midwives in Washington was passed by the state legislature in the Spring of 1981. The new law adds "midwife" to the list of persons who can be licensed as "health care providers" and sets up a midwifery advisory committee consisting of one obstetrician, one other physician, one certified nurse-midwife, three midwives licensed under the new law, and one public member. According to the new law, "Any person shall be regarded as practicing midwifery within the meaning of this chapter who shall render medical aid for a fee or compensation to a woman during prenatal, intrapartum, and postpartum stages or who shall advertise as a midwife by signs, printed cards, or otherwise. Nothing shall be construed in this chapter to prohibit gratuitous services. It shall be the duty of a midwife to consult with a legally qualified physician whenever there are significant deviations from the normal in either the mother or the infant." Candidates for midwife licensing must be graduated from an accredited midwifery program, have a minimum of three years of midwifery training, and meet certain minimum educational requirements. A student midwife can obtain a permit to practice under supervision after having cared for 50 women, and must care for another 50 before being fully licensed. Licensed midwives may obtain and use prophylactic ophthalmic medication, postpartum oxytocic drugs, and local anesthetics. Nurse-midwives in the state are also licensed and practice under a different law.

For a copy of Washington's new midwifery law, regarded by many as a model for legislation contact:
State of Washington
Joint Legislative Bill Room
Olympia, WA 98504
(request Substitute House Bill No. 316)

WASHINGTON STATE MIDWIFERY COUNCIL
1512 Langridge Avenue
Olympia, WA 98502
206/943-8607

Florida, New Hampshire and Rhode Island have also recently passed legislation to license and regulate lay midwives.

MIDWIFERY AND THE LAW
by Pacia Sallomi, Angie Pallow and Peggy O'Mara McMahon
1982, 34 pages, Illus.

from
Mothering Publications
P.O. Box 2208
Albuquerque, NM 87103
$3.50

The staff of *Mothering Magazine* has compiled this report on the legal status of nurse and lay midwives in the U.S. Included is a state-by-state summary of the law, a description of any pending legislation or court cases, and a listing of contact people/ organizations, including groups which advocate lay midwifery and home birth. Also included is a large map which shows the legal status of lay midwifery at a glance, and listings of lay midwifery schools, helpful organizations, resources, and research sources. The first edition of this report appeared in the Fall, 1981 issue of *Mothering Magazine* and has been updated. The report is intended to help midwives organize and work for legislation in their states and also to help consumers locate a competent birth attendant.

"As midwifery grows and matures in a state, the midwives tend more to see themselves as professionals in the positive sense of the word and to want to practice to the full extent of their craft with good medical backup, peer communication and the use of emergency measures necessary for good outcome. As midwives evolve, they tend to want some system of accreditation, either by their peers or through their state legal system. This helps their public definition as they become more visible and the demand for their services grows. . . .

It is not hard to see that, indeed, midwifery is 'winning.' There are many state organizations, many successful legal precedents being established, as well as an increasing number of consumers expressing interest in alternative births. The goal here is not one of conversion to home birth, but one of consumer choice. It is a stronger society, just as it's a stronger family, which allows for differences of opinion and respects a variety of ways to experience the same phenomena. 'Nature fulfills herself in a variety of ways, lest one good custom corrupt the world.' "

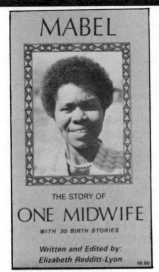

MABEL: The Story of One Midwife
by Elizabeth Redditt-Lyon
1982, 159 pages, Illus.

from
Red Lyon Publications
6940 NW Oak Creek Drive
Corvallis, OR 97330
503/753-5019
$5.00 pap. plus $1.00 shipping
$9.00 hd. plus $1.00 shipping
15% discount to childbirth educators
40% discount to booksellers

Mabel Dzata was educated and professionally trained as a midwife in her native Ghana (where she attended 3000 births) and came to live in northwestern Oregon, where she has attended many home births, beginning in 1978. Elizabeth Redditt-Lyon, one of Mabel's "clients," has lovingly written and published this book describing Mabel's background and the important features of her practice in America (30 birth stories are included). Mabel's definition of what is normal in childbirth is broad and through this book we are able to contrast her cultural attitudes toward birth with those of the U.S., as well as get a picture of what home birth is like on the West Coast and how Mabel was embraced by and has adapted to it.

"... a man bicycled into the clinic one morning. He told Mabel that his wife had entered labor and had been pushing for three days without birthing the baby.

"Mabel left immediately in the clinic ambulance for their home in a village off the main road between Yeji and Kumasi. ...When she arrived at their home, Mabel briefly examined the woman. She saw that the woman was very swollen from pushing for so long. Mabel decided it would be best to bring the couple back to the clinic.

"At the clinic, Mabel examined the woman more thoroughly, 'The shape of the woman's abdomen didn't look right. I was really scared, Mabel recalls. 'I thought she might have a ruptured uterus.' To test this possibility, Mabel touched her abdomen in different places and asked the woman if she felt pain. Fortunately, the woman answered that she did not.

"Following a hunch, Mabel asked her, 'How long has it been since you urinated?'

" 'Not since I began to push, three days ago,' the woman had answered. Mabel immediately cleaned the woman and catheterized her. 'She had gallons of urine,' Mabel comments.

"Following this procedure, Mabel did an internal exam. The woman had not been fully dilated when she began pushing. As a result, her cervix had swelled, preventing the baby from working its way into the birth canal. By now, the woman's contractions were mild. She was weak, so Mabel offered her food. In addition, Mabel set up an IV and asked the woman to lie quietly on her side.

"As the contractions came in greater strength, Mabel instructed her to pant and to breathe, but not to push. Two hours later, the woman told Mabel that she now felt like pushing. Finally, her cervix was fully dilated. But, Mabel still asked her to push slowly. Soon after, to everyone's relief, a beautiful, healthy baby was born."

"Wendy and Chuck Rak realized they would have a breech delivery only three weeks before the baby's due date. . . .

" 'The news of the breech shattered my confidence,' Wendy confides. 'Three things you need for a successful home birth are confidence, support, and good health. I was scared to death.'

"Chuck arranged a meeting time with Mabel. Two days later, he and Wendy drove to Corvalis to talk with her. Wendy remembers that meeting. 'After reviewing my x-rays and examining me, she was convinced we could have another successful home birth.' Chuck was also impressed with Mabel's qualifications. 'We decided to ask Mabel to help deliver,' Wendy says.

"Throughout her labor and delivery, Wendy felt confident and secure. She credits much of this feeling to having a loving and supportive birth team. 'The most noteworthy part of the experience,' Wendy adds, 'was Mabel's attitude that a frank breech is a normal presentation and any healthy woman with a large enough pelvis can have a successful vaginal delivery. Her confidence became my confidence.'

. . ."One family member who was present at the birth of Angela Natalie was Wendy's mother, Mrs. Teresa Walter. 'This was a unique experience for me,' she says, 'as I had all five of my children in hospitals, never dreaming of a home birth. One never is too old to learn!' Teresa participated by helping Wendy with her breathing during labor and by making sure the receiving blankets were warm. 'Mabel with her quiet, but knowing attitude . . . brought about a wonderful birth process. I just felt everything was going right and would succeed,' Teresa says.

"Succeed it did and amazingly well because Angela Natalie was no small baby for either a breech or head-down delivery. She weighed nine pounds (4.0 kg) and measured twenty inches (53 cm) in length."

". . . midwifery is much more than developing particular techniques or routines for birth even when these are more humane and health-oriented than conventional hospital procedures. There are many more qualities that are essential in a good midwife, qualities like empathy, affection, and love of family. These can only be cultivated; they cannot be taught. After Ferne Godshall gave birth to her second baby, Elizabeth, she composed a list of qualities she appreciates about Mabel. She could have been detailing some of the most important qualities that every birth attendant should possess.

1. Her quiet observation
2. Her love of family
3. Her ability to provide positive reinforcement
4. Her compassion and empathy for another
5. Her loving and heartfelt manner of being
6. Her quiet, humble professionalism."

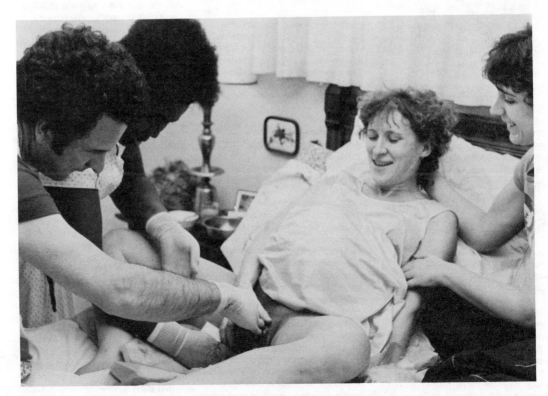

"Feel your baby!" said Mabel Dzata to Robin Dewhirst as Robin's husband prepared to catch baby Hannah. Photo by David Smith from *Mabel: The Story of One Midwife*, Red Lyon Publications.

THE FARM MIDWIVES

THE FARM
156 Drakes Lane
Summertown, TN 38483
615/964-3574 main switchboard

The Farm is an extraordinarily unique and successful experiment in responsible, progressive, communal living. The Farm was founded over 10 years ago when spiritual mentor Stephen Gaskin led a band of hippies from San Francisco to Tennessee, in search of land. Today The Farm has over 1200 members living on 1750 acres, with many sister Farms and City Centers around the country, and The Farm's projects and concerns have had an impact far beyond its own members. The Farm operates a volunteer ambulance service in the South Bronx which is considered a model of compassion and efficiency; Farm members are complete vegetarians and their reliance on soybeans as a staple protein source (and their many cookbooks) has influenced the resurgence of

interest in soybean foods like tofu and tempeh; The Farm operates its own "peace corps" called Plenty, which began with disaster relief and now conducts agricultural projects in South America; The Farm's Book Publishing Company used The Farm's own sophisticated print shop to produce over a dozen books on Stephen's philosophy, soybean cookery, health, CB radio, and the dangers of nuclear power. But perhaps most significantly, The Farm has reclaimed and developed the skills of midwifery so that Farm babies could be born safely and inexpensively at home. Under the leadership of Ina May Gaskin, the birthing practices of The Farm's team of "empirical" midwives and the concepts of "spiritual midwifery" have spread throughout the country and had a profound influence on the home birth movement and on newly emerging lay midwives.

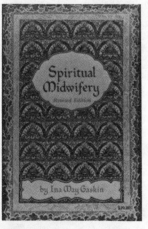

SPIRITUAL MIDWIFERY (Revised Edition)
by Ina May Gaskin
1978, 480 pages, Illus.

from
The Book Publishing Company
c/o The Farm
$10.00 pap.

The first Farm babies were born on the bus caravan enroute to Tennessee and Ina May immediately realized the need for midwifery skills. Once settled on the land, she began to read and study about birth. Two important circumstances influenced the future of midwifery on The Farm: first, the practice of lay midwifery is legal in Tennessee, and second, a friendly local doctor was willing to help and share his knowledge with the midwives. Soon The Farm was experiencing a "baby boom" and the midwives found themselves with lots of opportunities to assist at births and learn. The

midwives kept records of the births and soon noticed that their statistics were very good, with fewer complications than the national averages. Ina May was also very impressed by the emotional quality of the birth stories which some of The Farm women had written. So some of these stories and Ina May's birthing "instructions" were included in The Farm's first book, *Hey, Beatnik*, published in 1972. The response was tremendous; soon people from all over the country were writing to The Farm for more information about birth. In 1975, the first edition of *Spiritual Midwifery* was published.

Spiritual Midwifery, now in its second, revised edition, contains 200 pages of "Amazing Birthing Tales" describing home births on The Farm. Taken all together, these tales create a very positive and healthy picture of normal childbirth, in which each individual birth is unique and yet the same as all the others. The particular personality and circumstances of each family and set of midwives overlay a firm biological foundation of normal reproductive processes, giving a good sense of birth as a healthy and very *accessible* process.

After the birthing tales, Ina May presents her instructions for midwives, based on The Farm's experience with over 1000 births. She covers the anatomy and physiology of pregnancy, prenatal care, and complications. A set of appendices includes a reading list, suggested equipment and supplies, sample birthing records, and The Farm's own detailed birth statistics. Many lovely photo-

graphs are included along with spirited art work and clinical drawings.

The most important factor in all of this is, of course, the element of spirituality in The Farm's practice of midwifery. Birth is seen as a spiritual event for the mother, the family, and the attendants. Emotions and communication are viewed as highly significant factors in the conduct and progress of labor. The midwives attribute many cases of slowed or prolonged labor, for instance, to emotional stresses. An important part of their care consists in helping the mother (and the father) maintain a positive attitude throughout the birth. The midwives have also innovated the use of sexual energy and feeling in birth. Couples are encouraged to "smooch" and fondle each other during labor, and many practitioners are now acknowledging that this kind of stimulation can contribute to an easier, more relaxed labor.

My only quarrel with *Spiritual Midwifery* is with its treatment of pain in labor. Pain is mentioned explicitly only in connection with abnormalities of pregnancy. It is not considered to be a part of normal labor. In the birthing tales, contractions are described as "heavy," "psychedelic," and "strong" but never as painful. I read all this during my first pregnancy, believed in it, and consequently was shocked and unprepared for the amount of *pain* I felt in labor. (To be fair, many of the other home birth and childbirth preparation books I read were also less than honest about pain.) I believe that women can cope with labor pain without drugs. But I think it does women a disservice to obscure the reality of birth. If I had known how painful the contractions of late first stage labor can be, I would have studied the breathing and coping techniques more seriously.

Apart from this, *Spiritual Midwifery* stands as a "classic" work in the new literature of birth and has helped thousands of parents and practitioners to relearn birth as a normal, healthy process.

"We have found that there are laws as constant as the laws of physics, electricity or astronomy, whose influence on the progress of the birthing cannot be ignored.

"The midwife or doctor attending births must be flexible enough to discover the way these laws work and learn how to work within them. Pregnant and birthing mothers are elemental forces, in the same sense that gravity, thunderstorms, earthquakes, and hurricanes are elemental forces. In order to understand the laws of their energy flow, you

have to love and respect them for their magnificence at the same time that you study them with the accuracy of a true scientist. . . .

"During a birthing there may be fantastic physical changes that you can't call anything but miraculous. This daily acquaintance with miracles—not in the sense that it would be devalued by its commonness, but that its sacredness be recognized—this familiarity with miracles has to be part of the tools of the midwife's trade. Great changes can be brought about with the passing of a few words between people or by the midwife's touching the woman or the baby in such a way that great physical changes happen. . . .

"Familiarity with miracles has to be part of the tools of the midwife's trade. Great changes can be brought about with the passing of a few words between people or by the midwife's touching the woman or the baby in such a way that great physical changes happen."

"To one who understands the true body of *shakti*, or the female principle, it is obvious that she is very well-designed by God to be self-regulating. We are the perfect flower of eons of experiment—every single person alive has a perfectly unbroken line of ancestors who were able to have babies naturally, back for several millions of years. We are the hand-selected best at it. The spiritual midwife, therefore, is never without the real tools of her trade: she uses the millenia-old, God-given insights and intuition as her tools—in addition to, but often in place of, the hospital's technology, drugs, and equipment."

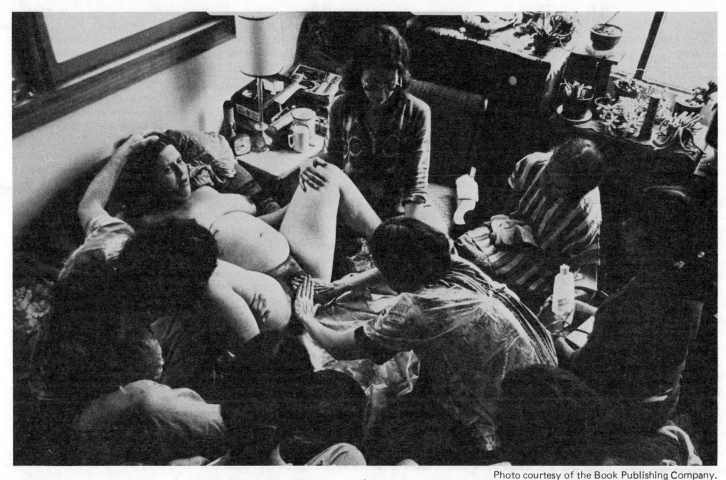

Photo courtesy of the Book Publishing Company.

THE PRACTICING MIDWIFE
c/o The Farm
$8.00 a year

The Practicing Midwife is an excellent, 16-page, quarterly newsletter illustrated in color, and edited by Ina May Gaskin and other members of The Farm midwife team. It contains national childbirth news, useful articles on midwifery skills and techniques (pelvimetry, breech delivery, using oxygen, the safety of Doppler ultrasound, etc.), book and film reviews, and information on breast-feeding and other aspects of women's health.

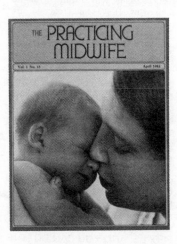

VIDEOTAPES AND FILMS
from VideoFarm Productions
c/o The Farm
Order toll free: 1-800-251-8066

COMMON PROBLEMS OF LABOR AND DELIVERY: A Breech Birth and Shoulder Dystocia
20-minute color film
16mm—$50. rental, $300. purchase
Video—$40. rental, $250. purchase

"A Breech Birth: a 10-minute segment showing the natural delivery of an 8 lb. 6 oz. baby girl, a frank breech presentation. This is the third child of a 34-year-old mother, who needed no anesthesia or episiotomy.

"Shoulder Dystocia: Following the birth of the head, this mother's 10 lb. 4 oz. baby is arrested at the shoulders. The mother is then helped into the hands-and-knees position, from which she quickly delivers with no anesthesia, episiotomy or tear."

THE FARM MIDWIVES—1,000 BIRTHS
$40. rental, $250. purchase

"This video program:
* details the community's role in maintaining a medical support system
* describes prenatal care and screening
* shows a complete natural birth
* includes maternal-infant bonding."

STATISTICS FOR 1200 BIRTHS MANAGED BY THE FARM MID-WIVES: October 1970 to July 1980

This two page sheet of detailed birth statistics is available free from The Farm. Some highlights are listed below:

Total births	1200
Delivered at home	91.3 %
Delivered at Farm Maternity Clinic	4.1 %
Delivered at hospital by doctor or midwife	4.6 %
Vertex presentation	92.3 %
Breech presentation	3.5 %
C-sections	1.8 %
Birth with anesthesia	1.9 %
Maternal Complications of labor	5.5 %
Total Perinatal Deaths	1.3 %
No tear or episiotomy	49.8 %
Tear	27.8 %
Episiotomy	28.0 %
Nursing mothers	99.0 %
Births without continuous fetal monitoring	99.9 %

PRENATAL AND BIRTHING RECORDS

Six-page sets are available for:
25 sets for $5.00
50 sets for $8.00
(see index for description)

The following books are available from the Book Publishing Company of The Farm. See the index for reviews in this *Catalog*.

A COOPERATIVE METHOD OF NATURAL BIRTH CONTROL
by Margaret Nofziger, 1979
$5.00

THE FERTILITY QUESTION
by Margaret Nofziger, 1982
$4.95

BABIES, BREASTFEEDING, AND BONDING
by Ina May Gaskin, 1983
$8.95

Home Birth

About 80% of the world's population is born at home today. Birth at home—that is, birth outside of an institution and within a social family setting, is the way human beings and all animal species have reproduced themselves through our millions of years' residence on this planet. It was not until this century that the trend toward hospitalization for birth began and it was most successful in the United States, when hospital births reached a peak of about 99.4% in 1970. Since then the trend has begun to reverse itself, slowly. As home birth becomes more common, many people innocently ask, "Is it safe?" In fact, the question should be "Is hospital birth safe?" since it is hospital birth which represents a tiny aberrant spot on the long ribbon of history of childbearing.

Doctors claim that hospital birth is safer than home birth because infant and maternal mortality rates have gone down during the period since hospitalization began. Home birth advocates point out, however, that many other factors have been involved in lowering the mortality rates, including improvements in public health, better nutrition, improved sanitation, increases in standards of living, the availability of birth control and abortion, and the improved status of women. No studies have ever shown that hospitalization per se or any particular medical treatment given in the hospital improves the statistical outcome for normal pregnant women. It is also the case that many studies *have* shown consistently lower mortality rates for home births throughout the period of transition to near-total hospitalization. The spectre of death and damage in childbirth which appears to haunt so many parents and which propels them into hospitals, probably has more to do with the poverty and malnutrition of the past rather than its lack of hospitals and doctors. A woman who is healthy and well-nourished will give birth success-

fully in the vast majority of cases (at least 95%) no matter *where* she is or *who* is in attendance.

During the past decade the percentage of home births in the U.S., while still quite small, has gone up dramatically. Though the decision to give birth at home is always deeply personal and unique to each family, three major concerns often arise: safety, emotional needs, and questions of control and autonomy. Many parents are concerned that the hospital is not the safe place for birth it has seemed. Because so many hospital procedures are either unnecessary or harmful, parents seek to avoid them by giving birth at home (see section on Controversies in Childbirth). Parents are also concerned about the emotional coldness of the hospital and its routines which disrupt the emotional life of the family. Being separated from the baby and from family and friends is very often mentioned by mothers as the most negative part of their hospital experience. In a home birth, the family is never separated and bonding may proceed unhampered and in privacy. In addition, the foreign environment of the hospital, with its many connotations of illness and powerlessness, may be stressful to the mother in a way which inhibits the normal progress of labor. Finally, many parents feel that birth (and death) are life experiences which should fall within the realm of the family rather than institutions. They view home birth as a way of regaining control over significant life events from which many have been alienated. Financial considerations are usually the last to be regarded, if at all. But it is true that home birth is significantly less expensive for society, and in many cases for individuals, than is hospital birth.

In this section we have reviewed and listed many of the books, organizations, and other resources available on home birth. Also see the related sections on lay midwifery, gentle birth and bonding, siblings at birth, and other alternatives.

BIRTH BOOK
by Raven Lang
1972, unnumbered pages, Illus.

Genesis Press, publisher
Science & Behavior Books, distributer
P.O. Box 11457
Palo Alto, CA 94306

This book was the first and I approach it almost with reverence. It was the first book on home birth, the first to bring the images and philosophy of its practice into the public realm. Raven Lang is a lay midwife and she documents the return to self-determined birth which grew from the pro-feminist, pro-natural life-styles, anti-war, and anti-establishment climate of the counterculture of Northern California in the late sixties. Her presentation is beautiful on many levels: physically, in the dignity of the many photographs; and intellectually, in the quality of the book's ideas and feeling.

First of all, *Birth Book* is political. This is not a product of the "me generation." The strong sense of community and political responsibility which permeated those times is captured in this book. In her introduction, Raven Lang says: "We have been asking and asking the people in positions of responsibility to respond to our needs and the needs of our children. Now we realize that we must do more than just ask, so we have joined hands in a struggle for

human birth and this is what's happening in this book." Community action began in 1971 when county doctors decided not to provide prenatal care for women planning home births. In response, the mothers and midwives began their own birth center in Santa Cruz to provide care, learn about birth, and assist each other. They studied the history of childbirth to gain a perspective for their current situation. Contributor Jodi Frediani presents an excellent, illustrated overview of the people and practices which have contributed to the "progress" of obstetrics. Soon the birth center women were giving birth and attending births at home, and their birth stories and photographs are the heart of *Birth Book*. The births are attended by lay midwives and often the baby is "caught" by its father. No drugs or fancy equipment are used. Often the mothers are in a hands and knees position for delivery. We see a way of birth which is totally within the realm of the family, and, significantly, is also a social event. As in many "pre-industrial" societies, these home births are attended by many friends, who view the process of birth as a joyous and privileged celebration. These images of birth—the smiles, the informal surroundings, the close support from family and friends, the intimacy and interaction between parents and infants—have a powerful effect and

make an extraordinary contrast with scenes of conventional hospital delivery.

Interspersed between these birth stories are short essays and instructions. Raven Lang talks about imprinting (it's called "bonding" now), about the sexuality of the reproductive cycle, and about confronting fear. She gives instructions for prenatal care, comfort in pregnancy, nutrition, lists birth supplies, and describes what to watch for in labor and birth. There is even a recipe for placenta stew, for those who want to ritually eat this organ after the birth. Finally, there is a transcript of a seminar on home birth, held by the Santa Cruz birth center in 1972.

Critics of home birth have called all of this "romantic"—the work of young, "earth-mother" hippies who innocently assume that birth will always be normal for them. Perhaps the criticisms which have been made against the counterculture youth, the children of affluence, can also be made here. Home birth was and still is a very white, middle-class phenomenon. The benefits of a more natural approach to birth have not yet reached women who are less privileged economically. But I admit gladly to falling under the spell of this "romanticism," with the result that my babies really were born without drugs, without doctors, without medical technology and are alive and very

healthy today, and that success is not inconsequential. Though we have never met, I feel I owe a great deal to the women who made *Birth Book*. I would like to thank them for sending me an important message from afar, so that I could also relearn and reclaim birth.

"During the months that this book was being made we became very social. We challenged the hospital's methods of handling the family as a unit, we challenged the denial of the rights of individuals, we dealt with the community and educated people so that the awareness of birth reaches many, which it must for the sake of us all. We have reached out past our own community, touching people and places far beyond it. People from all over come to observe, teach, learn, and exchange ideas. All this increases our strength. We have built a sisterhood and brotherhood that is real and powerful, along with children who are strong and free. We began the center because we as women understood it to be a necessary and a good step in the liberation of women.

"None of this would have happened if we had waited for organized medicine to come around, or if we had been scared of the laws we break, or if we had waited for money. I want now to say POWER TO THE PEOPLE, AND YOU CAN DO IT IF YOU WANT."

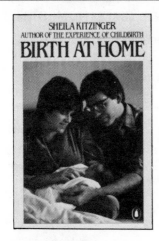

BIRTH AT HOME
by Sheila Kitzinger
1979, 156 pages, Illus.

from
Penguin
625 Madison Avenue
New York, NY 10022
$3.95 pap.

Sheila Kitzinger, British childbirth educator, is a staunch supporter of natural childbirth and home birth (all of her five children were born at home). Several of her many books are reviewed in this *Catalog* (see index). In this book, devoted especially to home birth, she brings her special experience and insight to bear on a delivery practice which is, unfortunately, losing ground in Britain.

Kitzinger discusses the growing home birth movement as part of a general attempt in Western societies to "demedicalize" life, especially birth and death. She describes candidly the many hazards of hospital birth, including both the emotional effects of the hospital environment and the risks of drugs and medical interference. She also provides a reassuring and honest appraisal of the safety of home birth, stressing the importance of good health, a low-risk pregnancy, and skilled attendants. The advantages of home birth for the baby are described. She emphasizes the opportunities for uninterrupted contact and bonding. Kitzinger's chapter on "arranging a home birth" describes the difficulties couples often encounter, and provides suggestions for getting help both in England and America. She lists useful supplies and equipment and also discusses the importance of arranging for home help after the birth. Also included are chapters on the importance of good diet and avoidance of drugs in pregnancy, preparation of siblings for birth, the father's role in labor, a very useful outline of helping techniques for labor, and a description, with quotes from mothers, of what home birth is like. A center section includes photographs of home births by Suzanne Arms.

"In many ways in the West we have lost this awareness of themes of birth and death throughout life. We have turned childbirth and dying into medical conditions which are intended to take place outside the home in special institutions where they are managed by professionals who are not emotionally involved.

Yet birth and death are the two things we must all inevitably confront. They are part of the ebb and flow of life itself. Perhaps we ought to ask how these universal human experiences can have meaning for us all. Only when basic human experiences like these have significance can we feel that we are creators instead of merely being at the mercy of fate, or of doctors, the 'them' who do things to us, and helpless in the cats' paws of large hierarchical organizations . . . .

"One of the reasons why some women want to give birth at home is that many hospitals are not good enough. They are not good enough to provide an environment suited for a peak experience of one's life, nor for the birth of a family. But more than this, they are sometimes frankly dangerous places in which to have a baby . . . .

"Much of what passes for childbirth education today in the United States is instruction to help women face the challenge of being in the alien environment of a hospital, to learn how to be tactful and 'sensible' in their requests and tolerate with equanimity the many assaults on the person which are a standard part of obstetric care . . .

"Obstetric textbooks set out a long list of things that go wrong during and after labour, but although doctors and midwives need to understand these, going into labour burdened by a sense of possible pathology can do the pregnant woman nothing but harm. If a sailor spent his time reading about shipwrecks and disasters he might never summon up the courage to go to sea . . .

"Good health, common sense, a calm mind and careful, observant birth attendants go a long way toward avoiding complications. They cannot rule them out entirely. There remain three kinds of emergency which occasionally happen without prior warning, all of which are far less common at home than in hospital, and which are very unlikely to occur after a normal pregnancy, labour, and delivery but of which the woman should be aware. They are prolapse of the cord, the baby not breathing at delivery, and heavy bleeding in the mother . . . .

"It is taken for granted by most practitioners when the pregnancy is first confirmed that a woman will be automatically booked into hospital. This occurs at a time when the woman is just beginning to get used to the idea that she really is pregnant and is not yet making any detailed plans. So if you think you may want to have your next baby at home, think about it before you become pregnant, and make it clear to your doctor when you first attend for care.

"You are not alone in this. The home birth phenomenon is not a fad or a local, or even a national, reaction to inadequate maternity care and poor quality hospitals. It is becoming a strong movement throughout the Western world. In the United States and Canada, in Britain, and now in Scandinavia, France and Germany women are demanding home births and pressure groups have been formed."

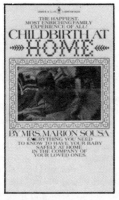

CHILDBIRTH AT HOME
by Marion Sousa
1976, 211 pages

from
Bantam Books
666 Fifth Avenue
New York, NY 10019
$1.95 pap.

I've heard several people say, "This is the book to give your parents when they worry about your home birth plans." Marion Sousa explains why in her introduction:

" 'Have a baby at home? Isn't that what some of those hippies do in California?'

"They certainly do, but so do an increasing number of women from upper- and middle-class America. I'm one of them. As the wife of an Air Force officer and the mother of five young children, I hardly qualify for membership in the counterculture. Yet we had our last two babies at home—by choice, not by chance. Furthermore, only my husband was present when the babies were born. Childbirth, we thought, should be a family affair."

Sousa goes on to give a very good introduction to the home versus hospital controversy, by explaining why people are returning to the home for birth and by describing the hazards of "the American way of birth" in the hospital. She also provides very concrete advice to help couples who have been persuaded and are planning a home birth. She gives specific suggestions for finding and evaluating a birth attendant, and on arranging for prenatal care. But even if no attendant can be found, Sousa does not balk at suggesting that couples can go ahead on their own. She devotes a chapter to describing the management of "do-it-yourself" home birth.

"In an era of growing desire for both consumer and feminine rights, American women are beginning to demand more control over their own deliveries. . . . This trend, although a healthy one, can give rise to paradoxical situations. More and more young couples, well-read and well-prepared for childbirth by prenatal classes, encounter doctor and hospital resistance to the kind of birth experience they desire. The results can be compared to the irresistible force when it meets the immovable object. Disillusioned and bitter, these young parents-to-be must choose between sacrificing their natural childbirth ideals and dropping out of the medical care system completely. This is just what happened to my husband and me. We chose home childbirth only after exhausting every possible avenue of compromise with the medical establishment. . . .

"Women who are pregnant or have babies may know where to find a midwife, especially if they look 'hip.' Also, inquiring at food co-ops or health food stores sometimes turns up some information on the home birth scene. People who work in community or underground newspaper offices, 'hip' bookstores, poster shops or even boutiques may turn out to have the necessary leads on locating a midwife. . . .

"If a couple wants a home delivery, and they are unable to locate any help whatsoever, should they still go ahead with it? This decision is one that each couple must make for itself. Increasing numbers of young people, however, are going to physicians for prenatal care, seeking reassurance that their pregnancies are progressing normally, and then going on to have their babies at home.

"Is this fair to the doctor? In some areas of the United States, this is the only way that a mother who plans on home delivery can get prenatal care. If a woman tells her physician at the outset that she wants to have a home birth, most often the doctor will not accept her as a patient. Very, very few obstetricians will even consent to talk to a pregnant woman who plans to have her baby at home."

NATIONAL HOME BIRTH ORGANIZATIONS

H.O.M.E.

HOME ORIENTED MATERNITY EXPERIENCE
511 New York Avenue
Takoma Park, MD 20912
202/726-4664

Home Oriented Maternity Experience (H.O.M.E.) was founded in 1974 by a group of Washington DC-area childbirth educators who wanted to provide education and support for home birth couples. Their idea was to develop a series of home birth classes, to help prepare parents and to provide information on the medical and emotional aspects of home birth. Today the H.O.M.E. series of classes is offered throughout the country by H.O.M.E.-trained and certified local leaders. H.O.M.E. also provides referrals to local home birth resource people and H.O.M.E.-affiliated groups. Yearly membership includes a subscription to *News from HOME*, an excellent quarterly newsletter. H.O.M.E.'s home birth booklet, first published in 1976, is still one of the best guides available.

"People choose birth at home for a variety of reasons. The foremost is that home is where birth belongs. It is an event integral to family life—not isolated and apart. Couples want to give birth together and remain together in this very sensitive and intimate period of the family unit. The mandatory separation as practiced in the routine hospital setting robs them of one of the natural rhythms of this peak experience and leaves instead an anticlimax.

"To meet the growing needs of those who are carefully choosing their options, HOME has come into being. We are devoted to helping expectant couples achieve the optimum—a safe home-birth—and by giving information and bringing together those who have had home-birth, those who want home-birth, professionals and childbirth educators. Having babies at home demands a high degree of participation, responsibility, and personal commitment of the parents to ensure a positive home delivery."

H.O.M.E. Class Series

Classes are offered free of charge, but H.O.M.E. hopes that couples will join H.O.M.E., contributing their membership fee of $12.00.

The series consists of five classes on the following topics:
1. Advantages of Home-birth to Parents and Baby
2. Parental Responsibilities; Equipment and Procedures
3. Emotions and Other Psychological Issues in Home-birth
4. Medical Considerations
5. Transition to Parenthood; Breastfeeding

NEWS FROM HOME
8-page quarterly newsletter
$12.00 a year, included with membership

H.O.M.E.'s quarterly newsletter has evolved from a typewritten, homemade production to a professionally typeset publication, but has always been characterized by informative articles and news items and lively, original artwork.

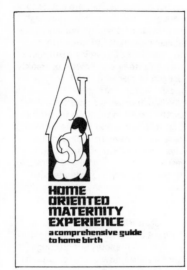

HOME ORIENTED MATERNITY EXPERIENCE: A Comprehensive Guide to Home Birth
by Dorothy Fitzgerald, Esther Herman, Fran Ventre, and Tina Long
1976, 94 pages, Illus.

from
H.O.M.E.
$5.00
bulk rates available

The H.O.M.E. guide covers the same topics as the class series plus information on nutrition, the definition of normal childbirth, postpartum care, and herbs for pregnancy and childbirth. The guide will serve as an introduction for parents who are considering a home birth or as preparation for those who have decided to give birth at home with a midwife or other attendant. For those planning a "do-it-yourself" home birth, it will be an invaluable manual. The guide is illustrated with excellent photographs of pregnancy, labor, and birth.

"There is no way that anyone can absolutely guarantee risk-free birth, at home or in the hospital. Many babies die or are brain damaged in this country because of drugs and unnecessary medical interference imposed upon them in the hospital. Some die because of the lethal germs which would never be encountered at home. On the other hand, a hospital which can prepare for a Caesar-

ean section within five minutes can be a life-saver in those rare instances when dealing with a prolapsed cord or drop in fetal heart rate due to cord compression which does not correct itself.

"If a baby dies in the hospital, even as a direct result of drugs given to the mother, the mother is exonerated from guilt because our society has fully accepted the particular set of risks incurred in the choice of hospital birth. A couple who lose their baby at home will experience deep guilt and regret for their decision unless they have consciously and fully accepted the particular set of risks involved in the choice of home birth. Life is fraught with risk. It is impossible to avoid. At best, we choose one set of risks against another. What is important, what will sustain us in the event of grief is to have deliberately and responsibly chosen the particular set of risks we will take because of our deepest values and convictions concerning life. For the choice of home birth is not just the option for one statistically safer set of risks over another. Concern for physical safety plays a part in the decision, but most people choose home birth because of the deep psychological advantages for their infants and families. Even if all the statistics leaned in favor of hospital births, there would probably be little decline in the home birth movement. For this movement comes, not from a concern for sheer biological survival, but from a commitment to the highest quality and richness of life to be given our children. . . .

"Failure of the baby to breathe at birth is the one condition that causes the most anxiety in parents approaching home birth. . . . Normally, the infant breathes spontaneously immediately after birth. Sometimes there is a delay of 30 to 60 seconds; but, as long as the cord is intact and pulsating, the baby is getting oxygen via the mother's circulation and can go for 3 to 4 minutes without breathing. Therefore, the cord should not be cut except under certain conditions (see "Cord Around the Baby's Neck"), until the baby is breathing on its own and the cord has stopped pulsating.

"One of the major causes of respiratory distress in infants is the use of sedatives, anesthetics, and pitocin during labor, and therefore resuscitation is commonly required in the hospital. Prolonged and difficult labor, malpresentation of the baby, and difficult operative delivery procedures may also cause distress in the infant. At home, where there are no drugs or unnecessary intervention, measures other than simple suctioning are rarely needed."

INFORMED HOMEBIRTH

INFORMED HOMEBIRTH
P.O. Box 788
Boulder, CO 80306
303/449-4181

Informed Homebirth (IH) was founded in 1977 by childbirth educator and midwife Rahima Baldwin. IH offers classes to prepare parents for home birth, teacher training (through attendance at a 5-day intensive workshop or by correspondence), midwifery skills intensive workshops, a cassette tape course in home birth preparation, *Special Delivery*, a guide to home birth, and a quarterly newsletter.

INFORMED HOMEBIRTH CLASSES

Series of seven weekly classes is taught by IH-trained teachers throughout the country and covers the topics listed below. Contact IH for the address of an IH teacher in your area.
1. Choices in Childbirth
2. Attunement with Pregnancy
3. Understanding Giving Birth
4. Attunement during Labor and Delivery
5. When Giving Birth is Difficult
6. Focusing on the Baby
7. Giving Birth to Yourselves as Parents.

CASSETTE TAPE COURSE
$49.75

Course includes a series of 12 half-hour classes on six cassette tapes, a copy of the book *Special Delivery*, and a year's membership in Informed Homebirth which includes a subscription to the quarterly newsletter.

MIDWIFERY SKILLS AND TEACHER TRAINING WORKSHOPS

Five-day intensive workshops for midwives and teachers are offered regularly in various locations throughout the country. Write for a descriptive brochure and current calendar schedule.

Midwifery workshop fee is $175. and includes hand-outs and materials.

Teacher training workshop fee is $325. and includes a teacher's manual, the Cassette Tape Series, a copy of the book *Special Delivery*, a year's membership in Informed Homebirth with newsletter, and a set of five large-size Suchard charts of pregnancy. Teachers will also receive a color slide set of two home births and a nutrition slide series when they begin teaching.

SPECIAL DELIVERY
quarterly newsletter, 16 pages
$10.00 a year, with membership

This 16-page newsletter features good articles and news updates on childbirth and the home birth movement.

Informed Homebirth, cont'd

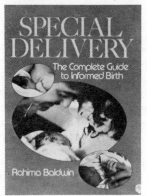

SPECIAL DELIVERY: The Complete Guide to Informed Birth
by Rahima Baldwin
1979, 169 pages, Illus.

Published by
Les Femmes
231 Adrian Road
Millbrae, CA 94030
quality paperback
Also available from
Informed Homebirth
$9.95 plus $1.00 postage
(10% discount to members)

Rahima Baldwin's informed birth "how-to" book is probably the best single source available to prepare parents for home birth. It is a "do-it-yourself" birth guide par excellence—very well organized and clearly written with lots of drawings, photographs, check-lists, reading lists, charts, forms, and birth stories. The book begins with an introductory overview of the "new" home birth movement, provides information on prenatal care and pregnancy nutrition, and outlines the careful preparation which must be made for a successful home birth. Baldwin describes the course of normal labor and delivery, talks about labor pain and methods of handling it, and provides a helpful summary of checkpoints for use during actual labor. The possible complications and emergencies which might arise are discussed as well as the spiritual and psychological aspects of pregnancy and birth. There is also a section on the newborn and another on postpartum care of the new family.

"The driving force behind the new homebirth is the realization that, in order to be fully alive, it is necessary for us to participate actively in what we do, to bring our consciousness, feelings, sense of responsibility and decision-making ability to bear as fully as possible in every action of our daily lives, and especially in an event as momentous as birth. . . .

"You don't have to have your baby at home to participate in this new consciousness. Some women or couples may choose to deliver in a birth center or hospital, either because of risk factors or because they feel more comfortable in an environment where many factors are predetermined and emergency equipment is close at hand. Wherever you give birth, I urge you to explore what it means to take responsibility and to be an informed medical 'consumer.'.

"As the baby starts to crown, you gradually feel yourself opening up, and you may get a warm tingling sensation (like stretching the corners of your mouth very wide). Many prepared women find the crowning intensely pleasurable and very exciting. With a second or smaller baby, it is often possible to be sensitive to each part of the baby as it emerges from the birth canal.

"By the time the head crowns (when the largest part stays at the vaginal opening), you should make sure you have stopped pushing and breathe through the contractions, no matter how strong the urge to push is. The force of your uterus alone is enough to bring your baby out. Adding extra force at this point can result in tearing of your tissue and isn't particularly good for the baby, either.

"There is a tremendous feeling of release as the head slips out. Continue to breathe through the next contraction as the shoulders emerge unless you are told by your attendant to give a gentle push. Again, if there has been no sign of fetal distress, it is not necessary to hurry this stage. Feel and savor it! Touch your baby, even before he is completely out, helping him to come up onto your belly once the shoulders are born."

"The driving force behind the new homebirth is the realization that, in order to be fully alive, it is necessary for us to participate actively in what we do, to bring our consciousness, feelings, sense of responsibility and decision-making ability to bear as fully as possible in every action of our daily lives, and especially in an event as momentous as birth."

DISCOUNTS

Informed Homebirth members receive a discount on books and birth supplies ordered from Childbirth Education Supply Center (see index) and from Moonflower Birthing Supply (see index).

ACHI

ASSOCIATION FOR CHILDBIRTH AT HOME, INTERNATIONAL
P.O. Box 39498
Los Angeles, CA 90039
213/667-0839

Association for Childbirth at Home, International (ACHI) was founded in Boston in 1972 by lay midwife Tonya Brooks and later moved with her to California. ACHI offers a variety of publications, workshops, and classes for parents, childbirth educators, and midwives. Write for more information on the services listed below.

ACHI also provides home birth buttons and pamphlets and reprints on aspects of childbirth. Write for a publications list.

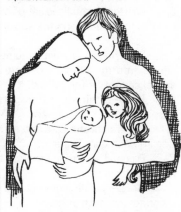

"ACHI is an international training and research organization which has taught over 30,000 couples childbirth classes throughout the United States and Canada and has teachers in Puerto Rico, Japan and South Korea. ACHI has trained nearly 1200 childbirth educators and in 1975 began training midwives. ACHI is developing midwifery training programs to comply with state laws throughout the U.S. and Canada, and will take its midwifery programs to the Third World in 1982. ACHI also holds conferences and professional seminars to acquaint physicians and hospitals with their natural approach to obstetrics. . . .

"The goals and purposes of ACHI are to improve the quality of life in the world by improving maternity care through indentification and implementation of correct obstetrical and pediatric technology. By establishing support and back-up for home births in developed countries, and combining the best of Eastern and Western medical information for the Third World countries, these improvements can be made throughout the world."

TEACHER TRAINING AND CERTIFICATION PROGRAMS

ACHI provides teacher training through a program of directed self-study and traveling intensive seminars. The total cost for training is about $725. Teachers are certified to teach a standard ACHI course in home birth preparation for parents and may also offer the CHOICE Seminar for couples who plan a hospital birth. The Home Birth Series covers the following:
Advantages of Home Birth
The Normal Birth
Psychological Issues
Medical Considerations
Preparation for Birth
The Newborn

MIDWIFERY TRAINING

ACHI provides midwifery training through its "Intensive Seminars in Midwifery Science and Skills," which cover "hands-on" practicals, in-depth labor management, preventing and dealing with complications, and postpartum. Training is also available for advanced and very experienced midwives. ACHI is currently working to establish midwifery training schools in Los Angeles and Seattle.

GIVING BIRTH AT HOME: Parent Information Handbook
by Tonya Brooks and Linda Bennett
1976, 108 pages, Illus.
$10.00 pap. plus 15% shipping

This covers the psychological and medical issues of home birth, what to do if you have to go to the hospital, the prenatal period, labor and birth, the postpartum period, and provides reference information and a description of ACHI classes and services.

"Ten Cardinal Rules for the Laboring Woman"
1) REST EVERY DAY so that you don't go into labor when you're tired. . .
2) During a long 'stop-start' labor, a woman should eat something, but it should be clear broth (natural gelatin with juice, or the like,) NOTHING SOLID OR HEAVY.
3) In early labor, continue pleasant activity (like walking, talking, baking cookies) as long as possible unless tired, then REST.
4) Use the breathing technique THAT WORKS
5) Expend the LEAST amount of energy possible to get you through each contraction.
6) Find your own body rhythm and fit breathing techniques to it.
7) *RELAX!* relax relax relax. . .
8) Stay in PRESENT TIME—Confront each contraction and handle it.
9) DO NOT PUSH WHEN BABY'S HEAD IS CROWNING. RELAX PERINEUM!
10) Keep labor room calm and quiet."

IS HOME THE PLACE FOR BIRTH?
by Sue Baker
1980, 3 pages
(in *ICEA News*, May, 1980)

from
International Childbirth Education
Association
P.O. Box 20048
Minneapolis, MN 55420
$1.00 plus 60 cents for back issue
copies

For this article Sue Baker asked eight people, representing differing points of view, to comment on the advantages and disadvantages of home birth. The commentators include Derrick Jelliffe, MD, of the Division of Population, Family and International Health, UCLA; Henny Ligtermoet, a Dutch midwife currently practicing in Australia; Ina May Gaskin, author and lay midwife of The Farm; Warren H. Pearse, MD, executive director of the American College of Obstetricians and Gynecologists; Julie Butler, editor of *The Partal Post*; Mayer Eisenstein, MD, home birth physician; Janet Leigh, home birth attendant; and Martin Richards, researcher in psychology and human development at Cambridge University. Their comments will be very useful for parents who are considering home birth. Also included is a notice of how to contact home birth organizations through ICEA, a list of home birth books available through the ICEA Bookcenter, and the ICEA Position Statement on home birth, excerpted from the *ICEA Position Paper on Planning Comprehensive Maternal and Newborn Services for the Childbearing Year* (see index).

"Which risks pose the greatest threat to those choosing homebirth?"
Henny Ligtermoet: The greatest threat to those choosing homebirth is the attitude of the medical profession, cajoling and threatening mothers into hospitals. Homebirth done responsibly carries no risk. Irresponsible homebirth is that done without medical attendants and is often due to the medical profession's refusal to acknowledge homebirth. This is a dangerous situation.
Warren Pearse: The general threats to those choosing homebirth are increased maternal morbidity and newborn morbidity and mortality. Among these, the greatest risks are complications of advanced labor contributing to stillbirth and to neonatal hypoxia, and maternal hemorrhage which has been responsible for most of the reported maternal deaths.
Janet Leigh: Assuming excellent nutrition, careful screening and prenatal care, skilled attendants, good medical back-up and labor without drugs and interference with the natural process, I don't really see significant risks. The absence of *any* of the above factors poses significant risk."

HOMEBIRTHS*—ICEA'S POSITION

Excerpts from *ICEA's Position Paper on Planning Comprehensive Maternal and Newborn Services for the Childbearing Year.*

An increasing number of expectant parents are deciding to give birth at home, necessitating the provision of safe, homebirth services for those healthy childbearing women and their families who choose this alternative.

The following features are recommended:
1. Attendance by certified midwives[†] or physicians in consultation with obstetric and pediatric specialists.
2. Written, formalized set of criteria and procedures for consultation with, and referral to, back-up physicians and other professionals.
3. Written, formalized set of criteria and procedures for referral and transport to backup hospital.
4. Provision of written statement to homebirth clients, informing them if backup services (2 and 3 above) cannot be formalized.
5. Home within short transport distance of a hospital.
6. Prenatal health care and education program (see Prenatal Care System).
7. Prenatal screening program to ensure that homebirth clients:
  a. Are personally comfortable with their decision to give birth at home
  b. Are low risk
  c. Are receiving regular, appropriate prenatal care

  d. Have attended prenatal childbirth education classes (or received private instruction) with their chosen support companion.
8. Home visit with family's consent during prenatal period.
9. Advance instruction concerning preparation of home to ensure necessary labor and birth area, bedding, supplies, equipment, and transportation.
10. Newborn evaluation and examination.
11. Arrangements for newborn follow-up that ensure required screening tests and assignment of needed laboratory work and treatment.
12. Home visit and follow-up maternal and newborn postpartum program (see Postpartum Care System).

*Some features modeled after the professional homebirth services of Maternity Center Associates, Washington, D.C.

†As accepted by the International Confederation of Midwives, the international definition of midwife will be used in this Position Paper: A midwife is a person who, having been regularly admitted to a midwifery education program fully recognized in the country in which it is located, has successfully completed the prescribed course of studies in midwifery and has acquired the requisite qualifications to be registered and/or legally licensed to practice midwifery.

ALTERNATIVE BIRTH STUDY
Dr. Queta Bond, Project Staff Officer
Institute of Medicine
National Academy of Sciences
2101 Constitution Avenue
Washington, DC 20418

The Institute of Medicine, with funding from the Health Services Administration, is conducting a study of alternative birth settings. Dr. Queta Bond, director of the study, says: "the major task for the committee, given the limited scientific literature, is to examine *how* to acquire the information to assess alternative birth settings. This will be done by posing important research questions and outlining what research is needed. Further, the committee will suggest the investigational techniques and research designs that will produce the most reliable results. In order to do this, the committee will review what data is already available. . . . I don't know how many questions our study will answer, but we hope the report will stimulate and make possible some research on this important topic." To obtain a copy of the project's final report or to contribute information, contact Dr. Bond.

POLICY STATEMENT ON HOME DELIVERIES OF THE AMERICAN ACADEMY OF PEDIATRICS AND THE AMERICAN COLLEGE OF OBSTETRICIANS AND GYNECOLOGISTS

"Labor and delivery, while a physiologic process, clearly presents potential hazards to both mother and fetus before and after birth. These hazards require standards of safety which are provided in the hospital setting and cannot be matched in the home situation.

"We recognize, however, the legitimacy of the concern of many that the events surrounding birth be an emotionally satisfying experience for the family. We support those actions that improve the experience of the family while continuing to provide the mother and her infant with accepted standards of safety available only in hospitals which conform to standards as outlined by the American Academy of Pediatrics and the American College of Obstetricians and Gynecologists."

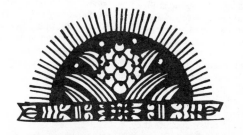

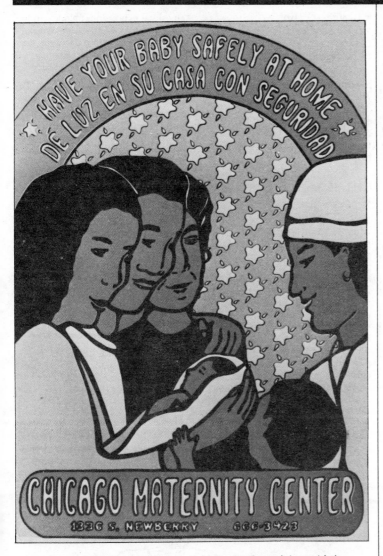

This poster in support of the Chicago Maternity Center's home birth service was produced in 1972 by the Chicago Women's Graphics Collective.

THE CHICAGO MATERNITY CENTER STORY
60 min. 16 mm, black and white film
1976

from
Kartemquin Films Ltd.
1901 West Wellington
Chicago, IL 60657
312/472-4366
Purchase: $500.
Rental: $75. for hospitals and Universities; $60. for high schools and churches; $40. for community groups.

This documentary film was produced by a collective of independent filmakers which specializes in socially progressive films on health, racism, and the labor movement.

"Part I: Healthcare Worth Fighting For"

"For more than 75 years the Chicago Maternity Center delivered babies at home to thousands of mothers. In 1973, plans for an expensive new women's hospital threaten the Center's future. A group of mothers dramatically tell why the low-cost, preventive care the Center provided is worth fighting for. We see footage from a famous 1930's documentary about the Center, and a moving sequence of the Center in action during a difficult home delivery."

"Part II: The Struggle for Control"

"Who controls healthcare in America? A concrete historical analysis shows why modern medicine rejects the Center's approach in favor of high-cost, hospital-based care. The Black, Latina, and White mothers who use and need the Center vocally confront its Board of Directors. Though supported by the community and the staff, the women fail in their effort to keep the Center open. But the struggle for good health-care continues."

"Who controls health care in America?"

THE TRANSITION FROM HOME TO HOSPITAL BIRTH IN THE UNITED STATES, 1930-1960
by Neal Devitt
1977, 16 pages

from
BIRTH Reprints
110 El Camino Real
Berkeley, CA 94705
$1.50

Before 1940, more than half of all American births took place at home. In fact, most people in their 50's or older today were born at home. Hospitalization for all normal births is a very recent development, yet many people take hospital birth for granted, as though it had always been the norm. Obstetricians like to point out that infant and maternal mortality have decreased as hospitalization has increased. However, this article disputes the claim that these two phenomena are related in a positive way and questions the common assumption that the hospital is the safest place for birth. The most startling fact presented is that throughout the transition period from 1930-to-1960, birth mortality and morbidity rates were *lower* for home births than for hospital births.

". . . home birth was not less safe than hospital birth from 1930 to 1960."

"While the techniques of modern hospital obstetrics have saved the lives of many women and infants from genuine pathologies of birth, the literature of obstetrics in the United States from 1930 to 1960 does not show that healthy women with normal pregnancies benefited from hospital obstetric care. Although statistically inconclusive, most of the comparative studies of home and hospital birth from the period show that the incidence of birth injuries and obstetric mortality was greater in hospitals, probably due to interference in the normal birth process. These studies suggest that, despite the poverty, ill health and frequent high risk conditions of women who delivered at home, and despite the frequent poor training of attendants, and the operations and anesthesias used—often in crowded unsanitary settings—home birth was not less safe than hospital birth from 1930 to 1960."

BIRTH GOES HOME: A Study of Couples Electing Home Birth
by Lester Dessez Hazell
1978, 58 pages

from
NAPSAC
P.O. Box 267
Marble Hill, MO 63764
out of print

Lester Hazell is the author of *Commonsense Childbirth* (see index) and this book on home birth grew out of her research for a master's degree in anthropology. Hazell studied the characteristics of 300 home birth couples in the San Francisco Bay area and developed a profile of the typical home birth couple. She found that outwardly home birthers were very similar to their white, middle-class peers, but had certain inner qualities which were distinctive, including the view of birth as a peak experience, an emphasis on good nutrition, acceptance of death as a normal part of life, liking to spend leisure time in family-centered pursuits, valuing breastfeeding, and feeling anger at the medical profession for the "usurpation" of normal birth. Hazell's findings are presented in the form of a research paper; included are a description of methodology, data, summary and conclusions, references, and copies of forms used for evaluation.

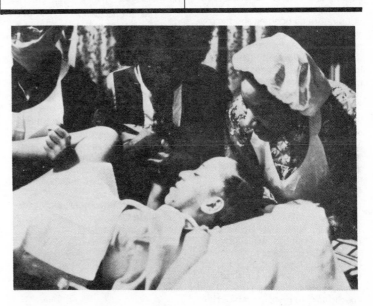

BIRTH AND THE DIALOGUE OF LOVE
by Marilyn Moran
1981, 228 pages, Illus.

from
The New Nativity Press
P.O. Box 6223
Leawood, KS 66206
$10.95 plus $1.00 postage

This book is one of the most interesting and thought-provoking documents to issue from the home birth movement and highlights the contrast between feminist and "traditionalist" thinking about birth. Feminists view home birth and the struggle for childbearing rights as an integral part of the effort by women to regain control over their own bodies. Traditionalists see home birth more as a struggle to bring birth back to the patriarchal family, restoring a measure of authority to the father which has been usurped by the obstetrician and the medical establishment. It is out of this latter mileau that Marilyn Moran's book has grown. She redefines birth as a "love encounter" between husband and wife and elaborates a theory of reciprocal marital "gift-giving" in which the wife's expulsion of the baby into her husband's waiting hands is the literal equivalent and balancing complement of his ejaculation of sperm nine months before. In this way the couple achieve true "sexual equality." Ideally, this exchange can best take place at home, preferably in the privacy of the couple's own bedroom, from which friends, midwives and doctors are excluded. Moran's main argument against hospital or medically-managed birth is that it disrupts the communication and bonding between husband and wife during the "climax" of their marital relationship.

Moran presents these ideas in graceful and compassionate language, backing up many of her assertions with references to the growing body of literature on bonding and the psychological aspects of childbearing and sexuality. She presents her own version of "do-it-yourself" home birth, including suggestions for birth supplies and preparation and instructions to husbands for perineal massage. She concludes with a selection of nine birth stories which illustrate her ideas. Regardless of a couple's religious or political convictions, this book will help stimulate much-needed thought about the emotional aspects of birth for the mother and father.

"In many childbirth manuals the husband is spoken of as a coach, a trainer who carefully watches, exhorts, and criticizes, while his wife conditions and learns to control her body during labor and delivery. Using this comparison Dr. Bradley states, 'your duties as a husband and coach [are] to prepare your obstetrical athlete properly for the great event—labor and the birth of your child.' He even entitled his book *Husband Coached Childbirth.*

"The woman in childbirth is not swimming the English Channel! Rather, she is performing a cosmic dance, and it is not a solo performance. She is engaged in a *pas de deux* and her husband is her partner in the event. What he does, and does not do, affects her conduct, rendering it either spectacular or mediocre. By being lovingly sensitive to each other's needs a husband can bring out the best in his wife, as she brings out the best in him. The moment of childbirth is their command performance, for which the two have long been waiting and preparing . . . .

"When an obstetrician steps in between the lovers at the moment of birth to catch the baby, the cyclic giving and receiving of significant genital gifts is shattered.

"There is nothing in the intellect which is not first learned through the senses. It is not enough that an obstetrician tell a man he has a fine, new son. It is not enough that a man see his child emerge from his wife's body. For a man to really be open to the action of love he must personally participate, with his own hands.

"Human sex is an act of gift-giving. This is what distinguishes human sex from animal copulation. And it is also what distinguishes human birth from that experienced by animals. In coitus a man volitionally bestows upon his beloved his most precious gift from which he relinquishes all possession. The cycle of gift-giving becomes complete at the moment of birth if the woman is able to personally give back to her beloved that which had originated with him nine months earlier, and to which she has added something of her own. This simple fact is the core of the mystery of marital love . . . .

"It is not necessary to try to become an instant-obstetrician by mastering medical (or midwife) texts in order to give birth in a fully humanized manner. Childbirth is a normal, womanly, physiological function. What's more, it *is* a genital expression and if a man and wife approach birth as a love encounter, in the same manner as they approached that other genital expression nine months earlier, then their baby will be born quite effectively. And the event will bring greater satisfaction to the new mother and dad than they had ever known . . . .

"One final reminder—*Don't forget to kiss!*"

THE NEW NATIVITY
P.O. Box 6223
Leawood, KS 66206
$8.00 per year

Since 1977 Marilyn Moran has published a quarterly newsletter, *The New Nativity,* which is mainly devoted to printing personal birth accounts by do-it-yourself home birth couples and which also contains news and updates on issues in home birth.

"*A note to Catholic theologians, moralists, and other interested parties:*

"The Catholic church has insisted that there should be no interference with the normal sexual behavior of married couples. For instance, artificial insemination, even when the husband is the donor, is condemned because there is a unitive aspect as well as a procreative aspect to marital love making, and these two aspects cannot be separated. . . .

"Well, from the stories which have appeared in *The New Nativity* for the past five years, it would appear that there is a unitive aspect to childbirth, as well as a procreative aspect, and contemporary birthing practices in hospitals shatter this unitive aspect. This is an intolerable situation. It is a violation of basic human rights, and the enforced institutionalization of birthing women must cease.

"Furthermore, the *Vatican Declaration on Sexual Ethics* states that all genital expressions belong within the framework of marriage. When a woman goes to a third party for the 'birth climax' (as Robert Bradley, M.D. calls it) she has gone *outside* the framework of marriage.

"You boys have a lot of homework to do on this subject. May I suggest that you start with the Vatican II document, *The Church in the Modern World,* which speaks of 'that human act whereby spouses mutually bestow and accept each other,' 'perpetual fidelity through mutual self-bestowal,' and 'a mutual gift of two persons.' Mutuality in sexual gift-giving is a reality for those couples who give birth in an intimate love encounter manner. It cannot be said for others.

"As Fr. Andrew Greeley once wrote, 'Marriage is still in the primitive stages.' Do-it-yourself home-birth couples are doing their best to change that, however. Thanks be to God!"

BIRTH AT HOME LEAGUE LEADER'S GUIDE
by Marilyn Moran
1981, 16 pages, Illus.

from
The New Nativity Press
$4.00 including class hand-outs

This booklet contains an illustrated class outline for a series of four parent classes in preparation for home birth.

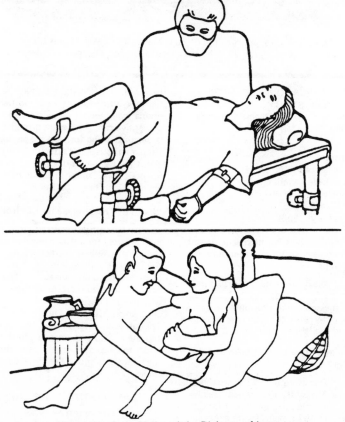

Illustration from *Birth and the Dialogue of Love*

MORE RESOURCES

THE PARTAL POST
c/o Julie Butler, editor
906 Colony Ave.
Kinsley, Ks 67547
316/324-5449
quarterly newsletter
$5.00 a year

The Partal Post is written and published by editor Julie Butler and she describes it as "a Kansas newsletter for people interested in pregnancy through parenting, with an emphasis on home birth and midwifery." Issues typically include birth stories, letters from readers (1981 issues included a letter debate on abortion), articles and short notices on birth and birth resources, and personal commentaries from the editor ("personal partal postscripts").

"Joe and Linda Lenz of Spearville, KS, gave birth at home to Andrew Chauncey, 8 lbs, 6oz, 21½"

long, on May 30, 1981. Linda came over to my house for a nice visit when little Andy was less than a month old, and she told me about her beautiful birth experience. The only thing that marred it was a trip to the local hospital for stitches received from a tear down an old episiotomy scar. She said the doctor was unnecessarily rough and caused her to bleed more after his suturing and abdominal massage than she had bled any time before. The pain from the abdominal massage was excruciating. And all the time he was massaging he was complaining about 'these home delivery patients' and wished they would stop. He wanted to admit her and the baby to the hospital, but she chose to go home where she could receive good care from people who loved and cared for her and her baby. . . .

CHRISTIAN HOMESTEADING SCHOOL
RD 2
Oxford, NY 13830

The Christian Homesteading School offers two Homebirth Courses—an intensive week-long course for expectant parents and aspiring midwives ($120) and a 2-afternoon short course for parents who plan to have a midwife in attendance at their home birth ($25). "We believe and have found through our experience that most births belong at home and that parents can learn all they need for safe homebirth. We have especially tailored our course to meet the needs of expectant parents who may lack support in their areas as well as those who want to become midwives." Write for information on current class schedules.

"The Homebirth Courses are held at the Christian Homesteading School. If you have never been here don't expect brick buildings with manicured lawns. All we have are a few small log buildings surrounded by woods and meadows. Yet we know you can learn more in a week here about having a baby than anywhere else.

"When you are at The Christian Homesteading School, we ask that you respect the general rules here. We ask you to refrain from alcoholic beverages, profanity, non-marital sex, drugs, and the use of such gadgets as transistor radios, recorders, flash lights and cameras. We also ask men to wear long pants and women ankle length dresses.

"You will probably be happily surprised to see how the keeping of these rules gives a spirit of serenity and beauty to our time together."

CHRISTIAN HOME BIRTH: A Preparation for Spirit, Soul and Body
by Joy Young
1980, 208 pages, Illus.

from
Joy Young
P.O. Box 33512
Detroit, MI 48232
$6.00 plus $1.00 postage

"*Christian Home Birth* is unique in its combination of spiritual wisdom and practical information. It shows the Christian woman how to thoroughly prepare her total being for birth and motherhood. Detailed information is included on nutrition, exercise, home birth, hospital birth, breastfeeding, family planning and infant care. There are discussions of delicate, controversial, but very important issues not covered in other childbirth books."

AMERICAN COLLEGE OF HOME OBSTETRICS
664 N. Michigan Avenue
Chicago, IL 60611
312/642-6414

The American College of Home Obstetrics is an association of home birth physicians in the Chicago area who provide support for doctors who attend home births. Director Robert Mendelsohn writes that the College provides a free legal consultation service, offering referrals to helpful lawyers and information on court cases for doctors who are being prosecuted or harrassed in connection with their home birth activities.

FOUR HOME BIRTHS:
A PICTURE ESSAY OF COMMUNITY BIRTHING

The photographs shown on the following pages were taken at four home births which occurred over a period of about one year from June, 1980, to June, 1981. The women giving birth are myself and three of my friends and you will notice in the photos that several of us attended each other's births, along with another friend who is a childbirth educator. Two of the births were medically "unattended" and two were attended by a lay midwife team. The photographs of Ruth and Kate were taken by me, except as otherwise noted; the photographs of Debby were taken by me and Ronda Brooks; and the photographs of me were taken by Sam Aronson. Below are brief descriptions of each mother's labor.

Janet—This is the birth of my second child, my daughter Florence Jean. The birth was my second at home and was attended by my husband Vic (as midwife), my son Rufus, three and a half years old, and a group of friends. I was 31 years old at the time of this birth. My labor began at about 11 A.M. with mild contractions and became active with strong contractions at around 7 P.M. My membranes broke spontaneously at the end of first stage around 11 P.M. and Florence was born at 11:45 P.M. We were concerned because the amniotic fluid was stained with green meconium, but Florence was vigorous and healthy at birth and required no treatment. She was full-term (born on her due date!) and weighed 8 pounds, 4 ounces. She was in a normal head-down position throughout labor (left occipital anterior). I did not have any perineal tears. The placenta delivered spontaneously three hours after birth with no significant bleeding.

Debby—Debby attended Florence's birth in preparation for her own home birth two months later. Her birth was attended by her husband

Jim (as midwife), and a group of friends including myself. Debby was in labor for about eight hours. Her baby was in a persistent posterior position, which was not known until Emily was actually born face up. She had the molded head characteristic of this kind of birth, but the molding quickly subsided. Emily was full-term and weighed 8 pounds, 8 ounces. Debby did not have any perineal tears. The placenta delivered spontaneously after about 10 minutes. Debby was 24 years old at the time of this birth.

Kate—Kate's first baby was born in the labor room of a hospital after a very long labor (60 hours) at home. The baby had been in a posterior position but rotated prior to birth. Kate's second baby was born at home, assisted by two lay midwives, with her husband Tony, daughter Vanessa (18 months old), mother, two step sons and me in attendance. Kate was 23 years old. Her labor lasted about ten hours and Matthew was born in a normal, head down position. He was full-term and weighed a little over 9 pounds. Kate did not have any perineal tears. The placenta delivered spontaneously about half an hour after the birth.

Ruth—Ruth's first three children were born in hospitals (see her story under "Hospital Birth Check-List"). Ruth had previously suffered two miscarriages and her second child was born prematurely. Her pregnancy with her fourth child was normal and the labor was attended by two lay midwives, her husband Ron, her three sons, and a group of friends including myself. Ruth was in labor for about 10 hours, and delivered Rosa in a normal, head-down position. Rosa was full-term and weighed 7 pounds, 4 ounces. Ruth tore on her old episiotomy scar and required a few stitches. The placenta was delivered after about 10 minutes. Ruth was 37 at the time of this birth.

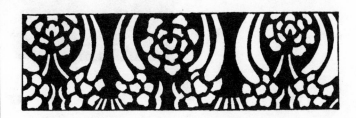

EARLY LABOR

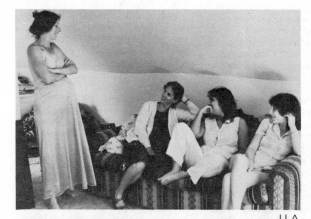

J.I.A.

In early first stage labor, Ruth walks and chats with friends between contractions (left).

Later on, she wants to be close to her husband, Ron (below).

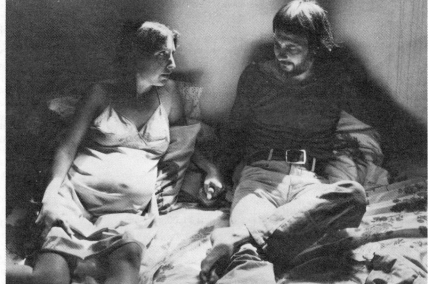

J.I.A.

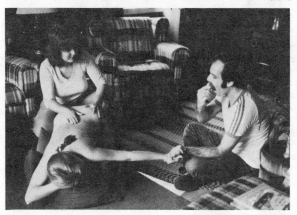

J.I.A.

In early labor Kate felt comfortable in the hands and knees position on the floor, supported by pillows. Her husband Tony holds her hand and her midwife massages her back during a contraction (above).

Later on Kate needed strong counter-pressure on her lower back from Tony, to help relieve the pain of her "back labor." Her midwife provides encouragement and support during a contraction (right).

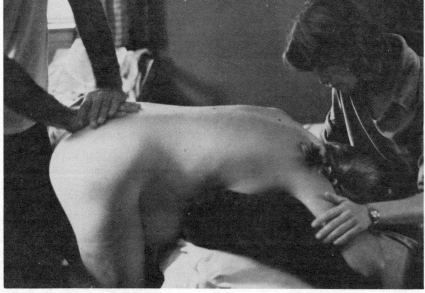

J.I.A.

ACTIVE LABOR

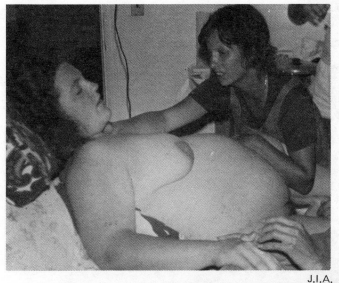

J.I.A.

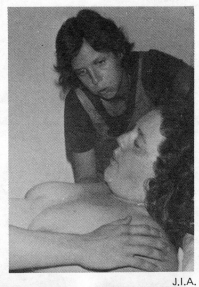

J.I.A.

In the active phase of first stage labor, labor coach Nan helps Debby to breathe through her contractions (left).

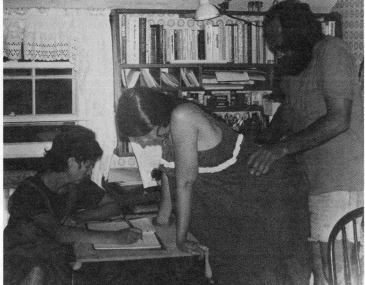

Sam Aronson

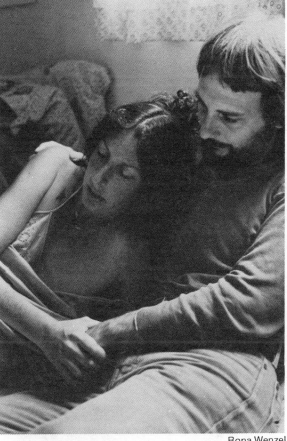

Rona Wenzel

As labor progressed, Ruth wanted to be alone with Ron and her midwives, and asked the rest of the birth crew to leave the room for a while (above).

In mid-first stage I stayed on my feet and leaned over during contractions while Vic pressed on my lower back. Nan recorded each contraction in a "labor log" (above left). Later in the first stage, I leaned over a stack of pillows on the bed and appreciated having my son Rufus with me between contractions (left).

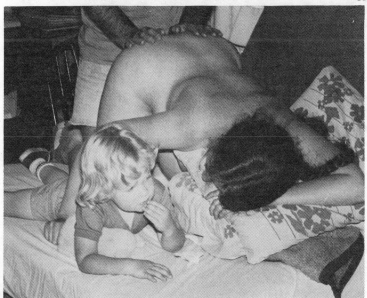

Sam Aronson

SECOND STAGE

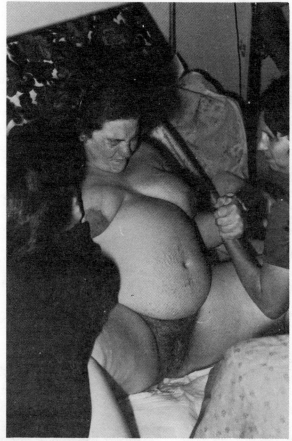

Ronda Brooks

Debby pushes hard to bring the baby's head down through the birth canal. The head is not yet visible. Nan and Ruth hold Debby's hands and "push" hard with her (right).

The midwife slips a length of umbilical cord over the baby's head just before the next contraction. Ron is already smiling over the sight of his new baby.

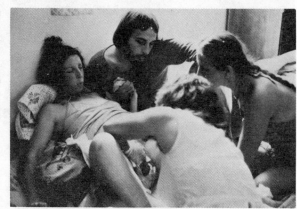

J.I.A.

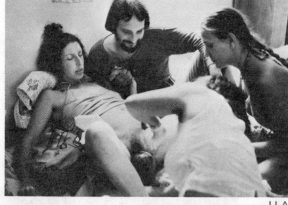

J.I.A.

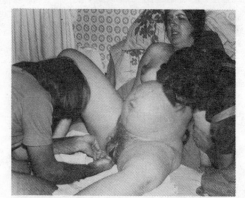

Sam Aronson

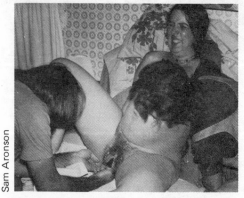

Sam Aronson

My baby's head is visible now and will soon be crowning. I rest between contractions and then push hard to bring the head forward. Vic keeps his hands gently on the advancing head and Nan keeps one arm around me (above).

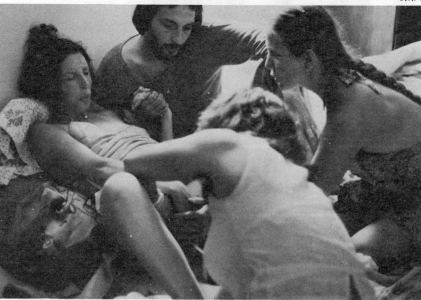

The baby's head is crowning. Ruth and her midwives cooperate to achieve a slow, gentle delivery of the head. When the head is all the way out, Ruth reaches down to touch her baby.

J.I.A.

BIRTH

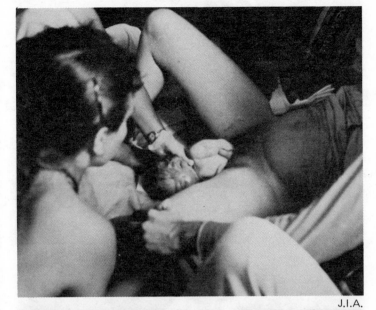

J.I.A.

Rosa is born. Ruth's midwife supports Rosa's head as her shoulders and body slip out (left).

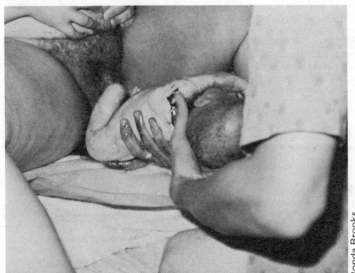

Ronda Brooks

Emily is born face-up. Jim supports his daughter's body as she is born (above).

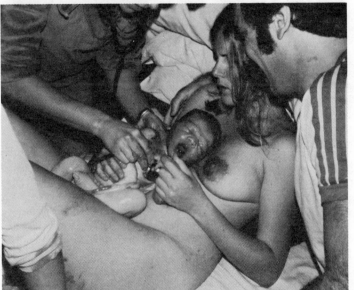

J.I.A.

Matthew is born and laid upon Kate's belly. He cries and the midwives check his heartbeat (above).

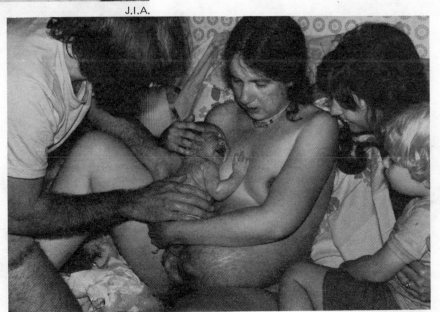

Sam Aronson

Florence is born and cries loudly. Vic lifts her onto my chest and we both cover her with our hands. Her brother Rufus and our friend Nan are happily looking on (right).

THIRD STAGE

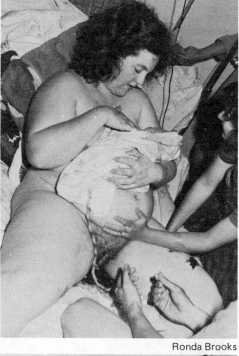

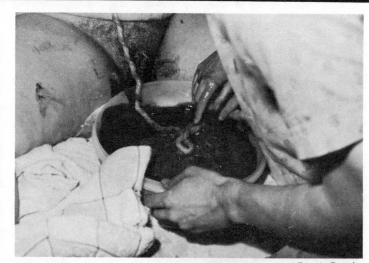

Ronda Brooks

Debby holds Emily to nurse, Nan checks for contractions of Debby's uterus, and Jim waits with outstretched hands for delivery of the placenta (right).

Ronda Brooks

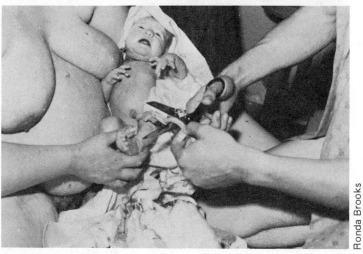

Ronda Brooks

Jim catches the placenta in a shallow plastic bowl. Then he clamps the umbilical cord with plastic clamps and cuts the cord with a pair of scissors sterilized in boiling water (above).

A few minutes after Florence is born she begins to nurse (left).

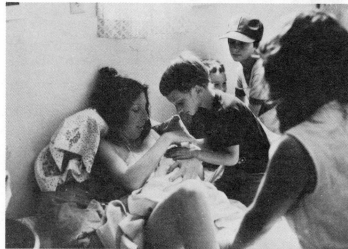

J.I.A.

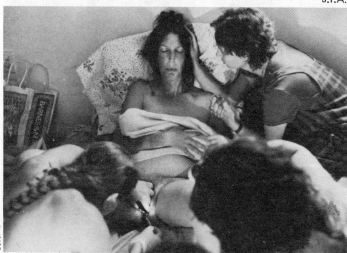

J.I.A.

Right after birth, Rosa's brothers come to greet her. Then Nan holds Ruth's hand and comforts her while the midwives begin to repair a perineal tear (above).

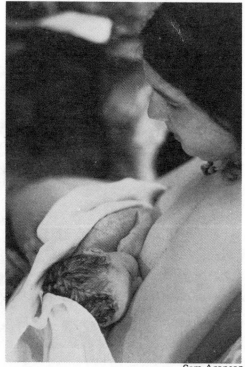

Sam Aronson

AFTERWARD

Now the fathers are able to hold their new baby daughters. Vic holds Florence (below) and Ron holds Rosa while Ruth and brother Jesse look on (left).

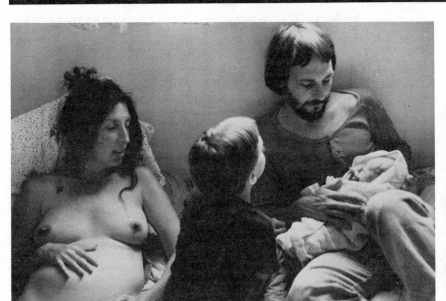
J.I.A.

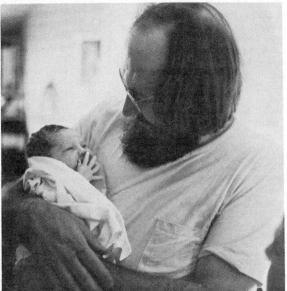
Sam Aronson

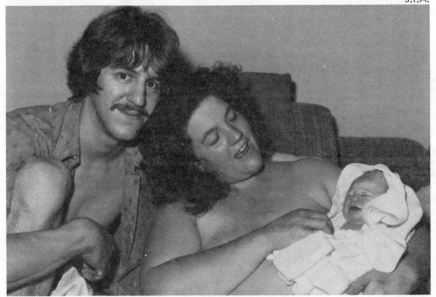
Jim, Debby and Emily pose for their first family portrait (above).
Ronda Brooks

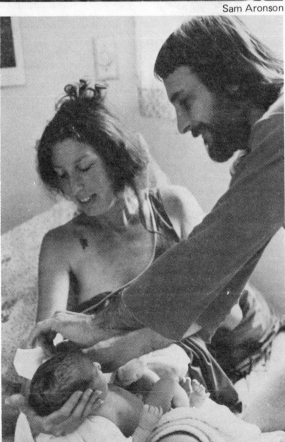
Ron helps Ruth dress Rosa in her very first clothes (above).
J.I.A.

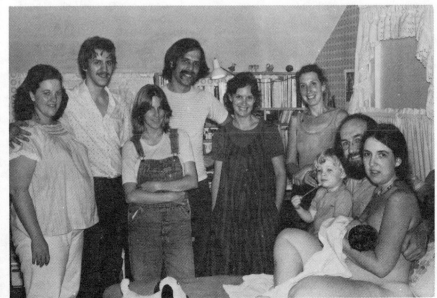
Sam Aronson

Our family and our birth crew at Florence's birth. Debby gave birth to Emily about two months after this picture was taken, and Kate and Ruth gave birth about a year later (left).

ALTERNATIVE CHILDBIRTH SUPPORT GROUPS

Many small, local childbirth groups exist across the country, working to provide information and support in their area. Some are independent, some are member groups of larger organizations like NAPSAC or ICEA and are listed in those groups' directories. To find a support group in your community, contact your local library, women's health organization, women's center, La Leche League leader, or health food store. Listed below is a sampling of local organizations which also provide informative newsletters or other materials to people outside their area.

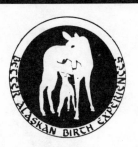

BETTER ALASKAN BIRTH EXPERIENCES (BABE)
Box 4-381
Anchorage, AK 99509

BABE works to promote home birth, birth centers, family-centered maternity care, and the legalization of lay midwives in Alaska. BABE publishes a good newsletter which is available to non-members for $4.00 a year.

"There are many articles written pro and con regarding episiotomies. I'm convinced that most women can deliver safely without tears or with a minor tear, even after a previous episiotomy. This takes preparation on the parents' part and usually some skill on the attendant's part.

"The first thing to do is to find a midwife or doctor that has a history of no episiotomies or very few and uses or advocates massage, warm compresses and warm oil during the birth. If you are planning a hospital birth, you should have someone with you to apply the compresses, warm oil or K-Y jelly if they won't allow oil and do massage of the perineum. . . .

"If a tear does occur an herbal bath can be taken after the birth. It consists of equal parts uva ursa, comfrey, shepherds purse, garlic and 1/4 cup sea salt and is very soothing and healing. Little 4 X 4 herb packs made out of cheesecloth and with comfrey, golden seal, chamomile, and ginger root soaked in hot water and applied to the perineum is very soothing also."
—from "Reducing Perineal Tears" by Chris Rushing in *The BABE Delivery* Fall/Winter 81-82.

BIRTH DAY
P.O. Box 388
Cambridge, MA 02138
617/354-2385

Birth Day provides referrals, childbirth classes, VBAC (vaginal birth after cesarean) classes, breastfeeding counseling, referrals for home birth, postpartum discussion groups, and other services in the Cambridge area. In addition, Birth Day offers the following reprints for $1.00 each. Bulk rates are available.

1. Herbal Guide for Pregnancy and Birth
2. A Labor Guide
3. A Guide for Preparing Children for Birth
4. Childbirth in the Hospital: A Guide for a Planned Hospital Birth or Home Birth Emergency
5. Getting Started with Breastfeeding
6. Starting a Home Birth Group in Your Area

"Home birth becomes a considered alternative when one finds medicalized childbirth in a hospital abhorrent. That is where most of us begin. And most of us begin alone—pregnant and fearful, questioning in isolation the routines so intimately associated with birth in our culture that at times one feels like a heretic daring to question the sacred. We wonder, in despair, how it is that the rest of the country accepts outrageous procedures, the mere thought of which causes us to stiffen in revulsion. . . .

"But no matter how isolated you feel, you are not alone in your questioning, even if you live in a small community. Most of us are products of the same culture, and often come to new and seemingly unique ideas simultaneously, so the odds are on your side sociologically. Perhaps more encouraging is the growing number of expectant parents nationwide who have finally begun to re-examine birth along with other aspects of our lives which

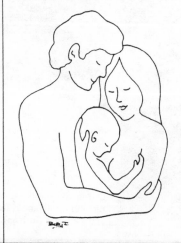

have been co-opted by technology.
"The problem, then, in starting a home birth group is not so much one of 'turning people on' as it is one of finding an occasion to bring others out of isolation. . . ."
—from "Starting a Home Birth Group in Your Area," 1976, by Susan M. Basham for Birth Day.

BIRTH ALTERNATIVES, LAPSAC
4603 Beaver Rd.
Louisville, KY 40207

Birth Alternatives works to support home birth and midwifery in Kentucky. Their newsletter, *Birth Write,* provides updates on efforts to reform midwifery legislation in Kentucky. It also includes an insert from the Sunhillow Home Birth Center which provides childbirth education, home birth services, and teacher training. Subscriptions are $10. a year.

"Senate Bill III, the midwifery bill, passed the Senate and was well established in the House of Representatives when this year's meeting of the General Assembly came to a close. The focus of SB III was to insure education and training for midwives in Kentucky. This is important because many practicing midwives do not have adequate expertise and most citizens look at their laws for guidance. Nationally, Ky. is looked to as a leader in midwifery.

"As a lobbiest for SB III I was privileged to experience the workings of law making . . .

"Initially apprehensive, I found it difficult to conceive that I could be an effective lobbiest. However, I felt that as a citizen of Kentucky I did have a right to discuss my views and all I requested was a chance to be heard. I was treated in a most respectful manner by every legislator.

"The midwifery bill did not pass the 1982 General Assembly. But through our presence at the Capitol many of the ideas were given favorable publicity.

"Natural childbirth, midwifery and home birth are desirable among today's childbearing women and those women should be allowed competent attendants.

"Women, even with babies in arms, can lend pertinent input to relevant issues.

"Nursing mothers can be both good mothers and hard workers simultaneously.

"The medical community is not so powerful that it can buy its laws or votes. Today's legislators are independent, free thinking professionals who represent the needs of the 'folk back home.'

"We have received many compliments on our presence in Frankfort. As concerned parents we should continue to let our voices be heard."

from "Midwifery Legislation—Kentucky 1982" by Nancy Singler, in *Birth Write,* Summer, 1982.

CONCERNS OF MOTHERHOOD
7058 S. Chappel Avenue
Chicago, IL 60649
312/667-3429

Concerns of Motherhood, directed by Rasheedah Mujtabaa, offers childbirth classes, counseling, film showings, lectures, and other services to women in Chicago. Materials are especially geared to the concerns of minority women. The following publications are also available:
Breastfeeding in the African-American Community (pamphlet) $.75
Midwifery (pamphlet) $.75
Nutrition and Pregnancy (pamphlet) $.75
Suggestions for Choosing a Midwife (fact sheet) $.25
Bi-monthly Newsletter—$10. a year

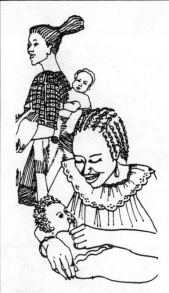

TRADITIONAL CHILDBEARING GROUP
P.O. Box 101
Boston, MA 02121
617/445-9521

This group provides information and support for home birth and midwifery in the Boston area. They are also concerned with issues in maternity benefits and day care. Yearly membership of $5.00 includes newsletter subscription.

"There are several reasons why people choose to birth at home. Birth at home (where it should be) allows one to choose the manner of their birth with the opportunity to labor in familiar surroundings, to have a shared family experience, a sense of being in harmony with one's own body, a chance to practice rituals and necessary measures of comfort and relaxation, and to choose one's own birth attendants.

"The group supports the family structure and the concept that women share expertise in assisting one another in childbearing. We further recognize the special needs of pregnant teenagers and adolescents."

—from Statement of Philosophy

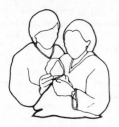

MID-HUDSON AREA MATERNITY ALTERNATIVES (M.A.M.A.)
26 Cortland Street
Middletown, NY 10940
914/342-5920

Mid-Hudson Area Maternity Alternatives (M.A.M.A.) provides information and support for home birth and other alternatives through referrals to birth attendants, film showings, workshops, and regular monthly meetings. "We believe that parents have the right to give birth in a peaceful, supportive environment with loving people. Because of the vulnerability and yet great strength of a laboring woman (family) they must open themselves up to rejoice in their new experience. People who have chosen to attend births should bring a profound respect for the normalcy of the majority of births with them. Attendants must further respect the need of the family to maintain control over their birthing through education and informed choices because the ultimate responsibility is theirs alone." M.A.M.A. publishes an excellent 12-page newsletter with local and national news about childbirth alternatives, schooling, pregnancy, and parenting. Subscriptions are $6. a year.

"Consider how you were counseled (or not counseled) regarding

pregnancy, and the risks associated with routine diagnostic testing.

"Were all procedures and their risks thoroughly explained to you and was your permission asked before they were performed?

"How were you treated by hospital staff—administrative personnel, nurses, doctors, extras? Did they answer your questions satisfactorily?

"Did they respect the rights of your mate?

"Were your feelings, emotions, and intuitions about your family, baby, birth and postpartum care considered? Ridiculed? Abided by?

"THESE THINGS COUNT!!!

"You are the consumer. You have the checkbook and the clout.

"Use it. Don't be intimidated. NOTE: Always remember the *Golden Rule* when dealing with doctors and hospitals is to GET IT IN WRITING! Don't rely on remembering all your requests or on people adhering to them out of the goodness of their hearts. Write them all down. Have a copy attached to your medical records. Bring several with you to the hospital for your husband/coach and the nursing staff. Carry a copy with you in your wallet.

"Always write in a clause protecting your right to *Informed Consent* . . . on your list of requests and on all hospital consent forms. Something like this: "We reserve the right to be informed immediately prior to any procedure (medical or non-medical) and we reserve the right to refuse any such procedure or medication."
—from "Help Our Hospital Reform Project" by Marianne Rahn-Erickson in *M.A.M.A.*, Winter 1981

MAINE ACCESS TO ALTERNATIVES IN CHILDBIRTH CARE
c/o Ariel Wilcox
RFD 1, Box 74
Dixmont, ME 04932
$4.00 per year (6 issues)
$.75 per back issue

Maine Access provides information and referrals for home birth and alternatives in Maine and also publishes a good bimonthly newsletter. Issues usually focus on a single theme. Back issues available include:

No. 1 Safe Alternatives
No. 2 Home Birth and Midwifery
No. 3 Alternative Birth Rooms
No. 4 Women's Health Concerns
No. 5 Home and Hospital, Obstetrics and Midwifery
No. 6 Attaining the Ideal Birth
No. 9 Legislative Attempt to Prohibit Lay Midwives
No. 10 Conference Update on Birth Alternatives by Experts
No. 11 Midwives Speak at Maine ACOG Meeting
No. 12 A Survey of Current Midwifery Legislation Activity in the U.S.
No. 14 Cesarean Birth

"To meet the need for home birth attendants, lay midwives became more numerous and active. Matching the new impetus of the home birth movement, lay midwives have new motivations. Most are concerned with providing skilled and competent care, combining the knowledge and resources of modern obstetrics with the new speciality of alternative birthing. Responding to and protecting the rights of parents and functioning in a non-interventive, participating rather than controlling role are basic principles of contemporary midwifery practice . . . .

"Opposition to home birth is behind recent legislative attempts to outlaw lay midwives, the intent being that home births will stop when there are no attendants available. Unfortunately, the result appears rather to be increased unattended home births. The rationale of the movement to eliminate home births is safety; however, it has never been scientifically proven that hospital birth is safer than birth at home. It would seem to be in the state's interest for public safety to assure a supply of competent caregivers for every consumer choice in childbirth."
(Issue No. 12, August, 1980)

RHODE ISLANDERS FOR SAFE ALTERNATIVES IN CHILDBIRTH
P.O. Box 2593
Providence, RI 02906
401/438-2427 or 438-4909

Rhode Islanders for Safe Alternatives in Childbirth (RIFSAC) provides information, referrals, and support for home birth and other alternatives. The following products are also available.
Bumper Stickers:
    "Support Your Local Midwife" $1.25 each
T-Shirts:
    "Daddy helped born me," children's sizes 2-14, white, $3.50 each
    "Born at Home," children's sizes 2-14, white, $3.50 each
    "Prepared Homebirth" children's sizes 2-14, $4.50 each, adult sizes S, M, L, $5.50 each, blue or yellow
    "The Midwives-Daughters of Time" adult sizes S, M, $6.50 each, yellow or green

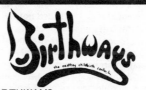

BIRTHWAYS
3127 Telegraph Avenue
Oakland, CA 94609
415/428-1446

Birthways offers a variety of workshops, classes, and support groups for the childbearing year, including birth alternatives, siblings at birth, pregnancy after 30, becoming a father, prenatal yoga, and bellydancing. Birthways' quarterly newsletter, *Umbilicus,* is included in the $15. annual membership fee. Interesting ideas mentioned include pregnancy dream research, baby massage, labor coaching service, and postpartum mother's helper service.

"Pregnant and lactating women and infants, have special nutritional needs. Government assistance and educational programs, such as W.I.C. and A.F.D.C., are vital, in order that all mothers are able to maintain healthy pregnancies and well-nourished babies. We are strongly opposed to the proposed cutbacks in these programs . . .

"All perinatal services should be equally accessible to all birthing women, regardless of financial, cultural, or language barriers.

"Each expectant and new parent has the right to dignified and respectful medical treatment . . . .

"We recognize that the issue of abortion is so ethically and emotionally complex that each woman must decide for herself when and if she will bear children. Therefore, we oppose any political interference which would curtail women's right to control their own bodies . . . ."

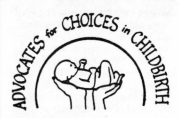

ADVOCATES FOR CHOICES IN CHILDBIRTH
100 Berkley Drive
Syracuse, NY 13210

Advocates for Choices in Childbirth (ACC) is a consumer action group for concerned parents and providers of maternity care. "Primary functions of ACC are to educate the community concerning childbirth choices (including home birth and maternity center births) and to act as a support group for midwives and doctors aiding parents in these choices, to investigate legislation concerning childbearing (i.e. midwifery, silver nitrate), to strive for improvement in existing community birth programs and to provide resource materials related to childbirth issues to the public."

ACC publishes an excellent 12-page quarterly newsletter, *The Advocate,* which is available for $15.00 a year and includes membership in ACC and a subscription to *NAPSAC News.*

The Advocate contains a mini-newsletter from the Cesarean Prevention Movement, also headquartered in Syracuse (see index).

"Why are an ever increasing number of women having 'abnormal labors'? First one has to realize that abnormal length of labor as opposed to normal length is determined in the medical community by the Friedman curve. The use of this graphic representation of labor is greatly disputed. It should be remembered the Friedman lab curve provides a *mean,* not a *norm.* There is a *normal human variation* in length of labor. However, today if labor stops or slows down, (even with no apparent fetal distress) for a period of time there is an increasing possibility a mother will be told she is 'failing to progress' or perhaps she has an 'inadequate pelvis'!?

"The increased use of cesarean section for the indications of 'failure to progress' or CPD or dystocia or a number of other vaguely labeled conditions is how the technological grip on birth is robbing women of their belief in their body to give birth and ultimately robbing them of a vaginal birth."
—from "CPD—A Vague Label" by Esther Zorn in *The Advocate,* Winter, 1982

"WHEN I WAS PREGNANT I PAID such close attention to every little pain that each twinge seemed magnified one hundred times and I thought to myself, 'Will I be able to stand pain worse than this?' That was how I imagined the pain of childbirth. That was how I prepared myself.

"I read books that told of the exhilaration of giving birth naturally yet I also heard many personal accounts given to me by women who tried but just couldn't make it without some sort of medical interference. Natural childbirth didn't have a very good track record around here.

"One woman said to me, 'My three deliveries were no big deal but why torture yourself? I felt safe in the hospital—and god knows, there's enough pain even before they'll give you anything anyway. Don't put yourself through all that, dear.'

"So I wasn't sure of myself, but I did want to try for natural childbirth. After all, to admit that you don't want anything to do with the birth of your baby in this day and age is like admitting to being a racist. So I put up a brave front and when asked said, 'Oh yes, I'm going to have natural.' I only half believed myself.

"I spoke my intentions to the doctor, who smiled and seemed very pleased. He told me that 'natural childbirth' was very much encouraged in this hospital and he and the staff would do everything possible to help me achieve it.

"At first I thought I misunderstood. I couldn't see what the doctor or the staff had to do with a natural childbirth. I was five months pregnant and so naive that I really thought I was going to be allowed to just give birth spontaneously in a hospital bed with the doctor looking on ready to step in only if something should go wrong.

"Then I found out about the shave ('only a little trim, just where your stitches will be'), the enema, the rectal exams during contractions, the move to the delivery room at a most inopportune moment . . . I could hardly believe it. I saw nothing 'natural' in any of this but when I protested that I really meant to have natural childbirth I was assured that I would be given no drugs against my will, therefore I would be having 'natural childbirth.'...

"I had been worried about going through labor from the beginning of my pregnancy, but now I was worried about what was going to be done to me when I got to the hospital. I couldn't see that anything that would be done to me there was going to make me more comfortable. I even doubted that it would make childbirth safer. Now I understood why so few women ever have their babies without drugs. Being poked, probed, and moved all for the sake of routine was bound to produce failure. Hospitals are not the place for truly natural childbirth.

A HOME BIRTH STORY
by Debbie Fields

"I told the doctor that he could not do an episiotomy on me. At first he took my request so lightly that I immediately realized that he did not take me seriously. I pressed stronger, stating that he absolutely could not cut me up. (I was dumb enough to think that I had the option of refusing these procedures. After all, no reputable surgeon will operate without consent.) The doctor got angry and said that if I didn't have an episiotomy, when I was 40 years old my 'organs would fall down.' I did not believe that and told him outright that I didn't. I left the office wondering what sort of jerk he was and I'm sure he thought me insane.

"It was too late to change doctors. Anyway, I didn't feel I could trust the medical establishment. My doctor had maintained all along that I could have 'natural childbirth,' yet we were obviously thinking of two different things. I decided not to have my baby in a hospital....

"I sought out a midwife and after two months of searching I only found one by accident. (I learned later that someone in the La Leche League could have referred me, although this is not true everywhere.) She was a lay midwife (California does not license or recognize lay midwifery at this time.). She had had her first child in a hospital and the second at home. She had learned her trade by apprenticeship and on-the-job experience.

"When I went to talk to her I really didn't know what I was looking for. I'd done a lot of reading and felt that I understood and agreed with the physical and emotional merits of home birth. But I wasn't totally against doctors and hospitals either. If she had turned out to be a fanatic who dwelled on the mistreatment of women and children in the hospital, I probably would have got up and left. After all, if you need one what could be more wonderful than a hospital?

"I discovered the midwife to hold many of the same views as I did. We agreed that childbirth is a natural function, that in most cases cannot be improved upon and therefore should not be interfered with. She agreed to attend my birth, which would be directed any way that I wanted and I reserved the right to change my mind at any point. (I was pre-registered at the hospital and got the doctor to agree to meet us at the hospital if his services should be needed.) Although the doctor did not approve of home birth and tried his best to dissuade me with scare stories of hemorrhage and shock, at least he continued prenatal care and gave me free access to my records (the midwife wanted certain information, such as the results of blood tests, etc.) which is not true of many doctors. Frankly, I think he thought I would change my mind after I was overcome by the pain of labor. He told me that 'first time mothers are often surprised by the pain involved' in childbirth. I told him that he wasn't in any way qualified to tell me about 'pain' in childbirth. After he'd given birth to his first child himself, I might listen, but until then I decided to wait and see for myself.

"The midwife held classes to prepare us. She showed slides of many of the births she'd attended. Now, I'd seen films of childbirth before and thought I knew what giving birth would be like. But what I'd seen before were hospital deliveries with lots of sheets covering up most of the action. The midwife showed us the real story—no antiseptic hospital cover-up. The blood was bright red and the faces of the birthing women were agony to look at. It was so different from the sterile hospital films made for delicate students that I almost couldn't handle it. I left her house very worried. I didn't think I could do THAT . . . and it was all the more frightening because there was no 'official' looking equipment around or important looking people wearing scrub suits and masks. Only a hard working, laboring woman in a pajama top (or nude) squatting on the floor, with Donna dressed in blue jeans with a scarf on her head, holding out her hands to catch the newborn child.

"I wasn't at all comfortable thinking that it might happen to me that way, yet that was supposed to be the beauty of it all. In spite of all my nonchalant airs and talk of childbirth as a natural function, it looked like something that I still wanted to be protected from.

"I spent several sleepless nights wondering if I should even try to have the baby at home. I wasn't especially worried about anything happening to me. I truly believe that the dangers of childbirth are over dramatized. Nor did I worry about the baby. I figured that if the child was healthy, it would survive an uncomplicated birth. My biggest concern was, what if I should completely blow my cool? The thought of losing control and dignity in front of witnesses is what bothered me most.

"I was sure that all would turn out well in the end, but it was how I would manage to handle myself during the middle that worried me. Of course, I realized that I had a better chance of keeping calm at home than I would in the hospital, where unspeakable, random things would be done to me. But if I failed in the hospital, I could blame someone. At home I had to depend solely on my own resources and what if I discovered that I didn't have any?

"The best way to deal with this fear was, of course, to discuss it with those involved. My husband, Joe, said something like, 'Of course, it will be understood that you'll be under a lot of stress.' The midwife assured me that just about any sort of behavior was acceptable. 'If a good yell will make you feel better, by all means, yell.' And Francine, a friend who would be there, also seemed to expect a certain amount of irritability on my part. 'The only one who hasn't accepted it yet is you,' she told me.

"INEVITABLY MY TIME GREW closer and my moods alternated between hope and despair. Every time I heard about an easy, short delivery, I become lighthearted. Every time I heard about a long, difficult one, I lost confidence.

"In the daytime, or when I felt rested, I was very excited about the possibility of a home birth. It was an ego thing, for sure. Maybe deep down I wanted something to confirm my femininity to others and my strength to myself. I do not look 'built' to have babies. During my pregnancy people would look at me and say something like, 'But you're so tiny!' meaning, 'You're in for a lot of trouble!' And to have a baby really naturally seemed to me to require bravery, strength, and determination under great duress. It would be nice to think that I had such attributes. But at night, or when I was tired after working all day, I wondered where I would come up with the energy to sustain myself through such an ordeal as childbirth. I wondered if maybe I was fooling myself. Sure, I said I wanted 'natural childbirth,' but in the hospital I could always change my mind. At home I was really committed.

"IT WAS THE MIDDLE OF THE night and I was too restless to sleep. I was having Braxton-Hicks contractions. My baby wasn't due for another two weeks so I doubted that I was in labor.

"In the morning I got dressed for my regular doctor's appointment. I was still experiencing some cramping off and on, but nothing that would prevent me from doing what I had planned that day.

"The doctor examined me and said, 'Well, are you all set to have your baby?' When I told him that I was all ready, he said, 'Good, because it's going to be soon—like tonight.' I was totally effaced and dilated 2 centimeters, but the real sign was that my 'membranes bulged' during a contraction. I left the office confused. Certainly I wasn't in any pain.

"I stopped off at the restroom on my way out because the exam had

Home Birth Story, cont'd

caused a little bleeding and I wanted a sanitary pad. I was on my way to lunch with a friend. But as soon as I sat down on the toilet a thick discharge dropped out. It was like a clot from a period. I jumped up and stood there looking at it. Was this the 'bloody show' or had the doctor's probing fingers done me some damage? I nervously cleaned myself up. There was not much blood, not even enough to bother with a pad. I wondered what I should do.

"I had my delivery all planned and rehearsed, but now that I appeared to be in labor, I went through some moments of panic. Not because of any pain that I was in—I was only mildly uncomfortable—but in anticipation of the pain that I thought might be ahead of me. What if having a baby is really as awful as everyone says it is? Maybe I should just go back upstairs to the doctor and ask him what to do . . .

"After a few deep breaths and a little reasoning with myself I decided to go home. This must be a false alarm. I wasn't due for two weeks, I felt OK, I wasn't in pain, so this wasn't labor.

"I called my friend and told her I wouldn't be there for lunch and I explained to Joe just what the doctor had said. He convinced me to call the midwife and Francine, my friend who was coming to the birth. I told everybody that I thought it was only a false alarm, though somehow I knew it really wasn't and I was scared to death.

"WELL, IF THIS WAS IT, I DECIDed to get ready and put up as brave a front as I could muster. I ate a small lunch, took a shower, and made myself a cup of tea with honey. Then I covered the seat of my rocking chair with plastic and a towel (in case of membranes breaking), put a clock nearby, and sat waiting for something to happen.

"I would time three contractions in a row, each lasting 60 seconds, about five minutes apart, but then nothing would happen for awhile. This irregularity went on until late afternoon when I was so tired that I fell asleep on the couch.

"When I awoke I felt perfect, no more cramps or tightness in my back and I was convinced that I'd been a victim of false labor. The midwife came by and confirmed that labor had started but seemed to have stopped for the time being. The only thing to do was wait and I breathed a long sigh of relief at having been spared a little longer.

MARCH 15, 1977

"I slept well and was dressing to go out when the contractions started again. They weren't much, the same as the day before, but this time I decided to keep it to myself. It was too embarrassing to have everyone hovering around expecting a baby to pop out any minute.

"But just to be on the safe side, I took it easy, ate lightly, and drank lots of fluids just as the midwife instructed.

"The entire day passed like this. Contractions off and on but with no more intensity that a period cramp. At 10:30 P.M. I was in bed reading when I heard a strange popping noise—like knuckles cracking. I sat up wondering if the sound could have have come from me. I felt a gush of wetness and rushed to the bathroom thinking that I was wetting my pants. More wetness leaked out.

"I went downstairs to consult Joe on this new development. He suggested that I collect a bit of the fluid so that we could check it better. I did this, leaking more all the while, and we found it to be clear with bits of white in it. (We later learned that this was vernix.) But since I was expecting totally clear liquid, I still wasn't sure if my water had broken or not.

"I went to bed while Joe called the midwife. Now the contractions were strong, although not painful. I sat cross-legged on the bed, alone in the room, looking at all my little things on the dresser. Perfume bottles, jewelry . . . the hall light was on and I wanted it off, but not enough to get up and do it myself.

"So this was labor. Now I was sure. There was nothing vague about the hardness of my stomach or the pull in my lower back. But now I wasn't afraid. I don't know why because, god knows, I spent many hours worrying about this moment. I can only think that it's the waiting and imagining that is worse than the reality.

"The midwife arrived shortly and did an examination. I was 3 cm. with regular contractions. The baby's heartbeats were good and the head was dropped and moveable in my pelvis. She reminded me to go to the bathroom often, drink fluids, and relax. Then she left to attend another birth that was happening at the same time. We all assumed that there was plenty of time left before we would meet this child.

"Joe put a chair near the toilet so I could lean forward and relax while sitting there. I didn't want to stay in bed. I'd walk up and down the hall until I felt a contraction coming on, then I'd rush back to bed or to the toilet and sit down. I wanted and expected complete silence during a contraction. Since Joe was the only one with me (Francine did not arrive until later) this was not difficult to get.

"As long as there was a space between the contractions I was not bothered by them. I consciously made an effort to relax but did nothing more. I was slightly uncomfortable, nothing more.

"But suddenly—or so it seemed to me, anyway—I was getting barely any rest between contractions. They were coming right on top of one another. I asked Joe to time them and snapped at him as though it were his fault that I couldn't tell where one ended and another began.

"I felt the need to go to the bathroom. I looked at the clock. It was 1:30 A.M. It had only been three hours since my water broke, so I assumed that I really did have to go. I pulled myself up and hobbled down the hall. I got caught midway by the most horrendous contraction which doubled me over and sent me crawling back to the bedroom. This was the only real pain I experienced during my entire labor and delivery.

"I gave up the idea of going to the bathroom. The bed wasn't comfortable, so I rolled down to the floor. I lay on my side in the doorway feeling confused and miserable. Not that the pain was so awful, but because I was on my threshold of tolerance, and was expecting many more hours of labor. If it got any worse I didn't feel that I could make it.

"A tingling sensation came over me and for an instant I felt faint. Then all of a sudden my abdomen gave a gigantic heave and I felt a great mass move and drop downward. The quality of this last contraction was so different from the others that I immediately took notice. When the next one came (for now there was a break between contractions) there was no doubt in my mind. This was the 'urge to push.'

"I called to Joe, who was bringing up my beanbag chair. I didn't want to lie in bed, yet needed a little support for my back. We put a sheet over the chair and Joe helped get me positioned before running downstairs to call the midwife.

"I no longer felt confused or miserable but clearheaded and strong. Somehow I had been counting on a burst of instinct and that's exactly what I got. I felt I knew just what to do.

"Francine came in at this time and urged me to blow out rather than push. But although I made a disorganized effort to comply, my body was going against my will and pushing anyway. I discovered that the harder I pushed, the better I felt—and I did feel good at this stage—lots of energy and enthusiasm. And I discovered that if I pushed real hard there was absolutely no pain, not even mild discomfort.

"The midwife hurried in, pulled on her gloves and said, 'OK, let your baby come down.' Joe sat behind me and I used his bent knees for grips. I could feel the baby sliding down and it was a strange sensation, but in no way painful.

"I rested between contractions and everyone was quiet and smiling as we waited. When the head crowned, a mirror was brought in so that I could see, but I was only interested in catching my breath so that I could push even harder when the next one came.

"After a few good, hard pushes Francine said, 'There's an ear!' She was sitting on the bed. And the midwife said, 'Touch you baby's head.' I started to reach down, but really wanted to rest. It felt so strange having that head stuck between my legs that I eagerly waited for the next contraction. While this felt strange, it did not hurt.

"Once the head was born the rest just slid out. She kicked as she was born and the midwife announced, 'A baby girl!'

"Emily gasped a bit and whimpered but never really screamed. She was put on my stomach, cord still attached, while the midwife massaged her limbs to get a pinker color. She just looked around bewildered. Joe brought up a blanket that had been heated in the oven and this was put over us both.

"The cord was cut after all the blood had gone through and Emily was put to my breast to nurse and help bring on the contractions that would expel the placenta. It surprised me that such a tiny person knew how to nurse, but she did and she grabbed right on and sucked so vigorously that it hurt. The placenta came twenty minutes later.

"I rested a while in the beanbag chair where Emily was born, nursing her and checking to make sure all her parts were there. Francine held her while Joe helped me take a shower. I was concerned about the amount of blood that dripped out when I stood up, but the midwife assured me that I hadn't lost very much.

"When I returned to the bedroom all evidence of a birth had been removed and the bed had been turned down for me. I propped myself up with a few pillows and sat on a "chux" pad with an "ice bag" (a rubber glove filled with ice) on my swollen perineum. The midwife inspected for tears, found none, then asked me to do a Kegel exercise. Everything was in good order.

"I nursed Emily and Francine brought me orange juice, toast and a scrambled egg. It was now about 3:30 A.M. My entire labor, from the time the water broke until delivery, was four hours. Emily weighed six pounds, ten ounces at her newborn exam, which took place the next day or when she was about 12 hours old.

"DOWNSTAIRS THERE WERE blood spots on the kitchen floor. The midwife had inspected the placenta there and a bit of the mess had gotten spread around. I cherished those spots and never washed them up. Having Emily had been such a great experience that I wanted to remember every detail."

Gentle Birth and Bonding

An important element of family-centered birth concerns the way in which the newborn is welcomed into the family. Handling the baby gently and with respect for its very well-developed senses and needs can ease the transition to life outside the womb and early, intimate contact between mother, father and baby helps ensure a strong family bond.

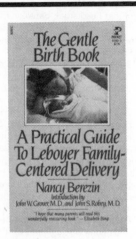

THE GENTLE BIRTH BOOK: A Practical Guide to Leboyer Family-Centered Delivery
by Nancy Berezin
1981, 217 pages, Illus.

from
Pocket Books
1230 Avenue of the Americas
New York, NY 10020
$2.95 pap.

This book serves as a 'good introduction to the concept of gentle birth as it is applied in the hospital environment. Medical writer Nancy Berezin provides an overview of the psychological theories of birth trauma which combined with current dehumanized practices in obstetrics to set the stage for the tremendous response to Leboyer's theory of "non-violent" birth. She explains how Leboyer's ideas came to be applied in the U.S., giving detailed descriptions of the baby's handling under both conventional and "gentle" systems. She discusses the new knowledge of infant responsiveness and bonding and goes on to provide a very detailed description of how nonviolence works in practice; that is, how the concepts of gentle birth can be meshed with the hospital system (home birth is dismissed as too risky). Berezin discusses the impact of the birth experience on the baby's later behavior, particularly with regard to crying, and concludes with advice on how to choose a "sympathetic practitioner" for gentle birth. Unfortunately, the concepts of gentle birth come to seem like palliatives applied to ease the trauma caused by harmful obstetrical practices (being drugged for birth, rapid clamping of the cord, early separation of mother and infant) which should never have become routine for normal births in the first place. Home births, without medical intervention, are already by definition "gentle," without need for compensating treatment or theory.

"What makes a gentle birth? Nine elements spring to mind:

"A nurturing, family-centered setting for birth, with avoidance of unnecessary medical intervention.

"Preparation for childbirth and minimal use of sense-deadening medication.

"A subdued environment—darkened and quieted to the extent that this is feasible.

"Delayed clamping of the umbilical cord until pulsations have ceased.

"Placement of the newborn in a postural drainage position in direct skin-to-skin contact with his mother.

"Gentle massage of the baby by both parents.

"A water bath in which the father's role predominates.

"Laying the baby at his mother's breast to nurse.

"Extended contact, with opportunities for parental-infant visual, auditory, and tactile exchanges, during the recovery period and throughout the hospital stay. . . .

"For some practitioners, the changeover from the traditional, paternalistic doctor-patient relationship to one of mutual respect and cooperation has come naturally—almost as a relief. For others, it remains an impossibility. For the majority, those who already advocate childbirth education and the couple approach but are reluctant to make waves among their colleagues by trying a new technique of delivery, or who regard the additional minutes spent in the labor room and overseeing the massage and bath as a useless waste of their time, a campaign of friendly-but-stubborn persuasion works best.

"The patient who arrives at her first prenatal visit with a list of demands a mile long and loudly threatens to go elsewhere if the doctor does not immediately agree to meet every one of them will probably be advised to do just that. On the other hand, the patient who proceeds tactfully—having judged that this is an individual with whom she can work, one who is already in agreement with her on the majority of issues and is willing to give her views a fair hearing—stands a good chance of persuading her physician to try a nonviolent birth."

BIRTH WITHOUT VIOLENCE
by Frederick Leboyer
1975, 115 pages, Illus.

from
Alfred A. Knopf, Inc.
201 East 50th Street
New York, NY 10028
$9.95 hd.

When I was pregnant with my first child, one of my friends told me of a local doctor who practiced "Leboyer" birth in the hospital. My friend hoped that this kind of option might make me change my mind about wanting a home birth. At her urging, I called one of the doctor's recent patients, who was very enthusiastic about the method. "Oh, it's really wonderful," she said. "The doctor lets your husband bathe the baby. She has a special pan of warm water right there in the delivery room. She has the lights low and everything!" This sounded innocuous but somewhat odd to me. I had been reading in my obstetrics texts about the importance of keeping the baby warm right after birth. Why risk chilling the baby in a bath? Why remove the creamy coating of vernix right away? I wondered why bathing was necessary at all and why the baby wasn't being held in its mother's arms.

Sometime later I came across a very strongly worded critique of Leboyer in the *Monthly Extract*, a woman's health newsletter ("Birth Without Mothers: More Violence Against Women," by Judith Dickson Luce in *The Monthly Extract*, May/June 1976). The author claimed that Leboyer's method is artificial and anti-woman. Leboyer's book, she said, "is an indictment of the inhuman and violent manner in which babies are delivered in hospitals. But the enthusiastic and uncritical reception of his work by child-bearing women and the wider community can be taken as an indictment of our own level of consciousness. Only in a culture so far removed from the natural experience of birth could his work and techniques be considered 'revolutionary.' We are so removed from the experience of birth that we cannot even recognize a gimmick." Luce accuses Leboyer of being "contemptuous of women." She says, "he does not trust us to respond in a tender loving way to our own newborn. It is left to a male, medical professional to create an artificial rite of passage for the natural one we could create if we were not denied the opportunity."

I went right to the library and checked out a copy of *Birth Without Violence*. I had skimmed through the book once before, looking at the nice photographs of happy babies. This time I read every word and was surprised and shocked, and still am, by what I found.

First of all, the Leboyer "method" itself is quite simple. It consists of delivering the baby in a hospital room which is quiet and dimly lit; delaying cutting the cord until the baby's breathing is well established; handling the baby very gently; and immersing it in warm water soon after birth to ease the transition from the watery womb. This treatment, in itself, does not seem either outrageous or dangerous, as some critics have claimed. Leboyer's insistence that the cord be left intact is admirable, since rapid clamping is "unphysiological" and prevents the baby from receiving the full complement of blood it needs from the placenta. But Leboyer's call for gentle handling and bathing of the newborn is based, not on a simple respect for the needs of the baby, but on the theory that normal birth is such a traumatic, intolerable experience that its effects will scar the infant's psyche if not immediately remedied. Leboyer's vision of the process of birth—revealed in his remarks on the nature of labor, its effects on the baby, and the subsequent relation between mother and child—is so exaggerated that it borders on the perverse. For example, this is the way Leboyer describes normal labor:

"One day, these contractions are no longer a game. They crush, they stifle, they assault.

"One day labor starts. The delivery has begun.

"An intransigent force—wild, out of control—has gripped the infant.

"A blind force that hammers at it and impels it downward.

"It is no longer enough for the infant to bend its back.

"Overpowered, it huddles up as tightly as it can. With its head tucked in and its shoulders hunched together, it is hardly more than a little ball of fright.

"The prison has gone berserk, demanding its prisoner's death. The walls close in still further. The cell becomes a passageway; the passage, a tunnel.

"With its heart bursting, the infant sinks into this hell.

"Its fear is without limit.

"Then, suddenly, fear changes to anger.

"Enraged, the infant hurls itself against the barrier. At all costs, it must break through. Free itself.

"Yet all this force, this monstrous unremitting pressure that is crushing the baby, pushing it out toward the world—and this blind wall which is holding it back, confining it—

"These things are all one: the mother!

"She is driving the baby out.

"At the same time she is holding it in, preventing its passage.

"It is she who is the enemy. She who stands between the child and life.

"Only one of them can prevail; it is mortal combat.

"The infant is like one possessed.

"Mad with agony and misery,

alone, abandoned, it fights with the strength of despair.

"The monster drives the baby lower still. And not satisfied with crushing, it twists it in a refinement of cruelty. The infant's head and body execute a corkscrew motion to clear the narrow passage of the pelvis.

"And the infant's head—bearing the brunt of the struggle until it is almost forced down between the shoulder blades, down onto the chest—why doesn't the head give way?

"The baby is now at the height of its travail. The effort required is too great. The end is surely near. Death seems certain.

"The monster bears down one more time, and it is then that. . ."

What an extraordinary description of normal labor! To say that it smacks of misogyny is an understatement. As a mother, I profoundly resent being referred to as a "monster" and having my body called a "prison." It is amazing to me that these ancient male fears of "containment" and of ambivalence about women's reproductive capacity have found their way, unquestioned, into a modern theory of "non-violent" birth.

Apparently, the evidence for Leboyer's assertions and for his attribution of complex, sophisticated emotions to the newborn, consists of his own "memory" of his own birth, recalled through psychoanalysis. As evidenced by his writing, Leboyer's birth memory must be colored by some fairly negative feelings about his mother and himself, for his image of the role of women in childbearing and their reaction to their offspring is very ominous.

"Whose hands should hold the child? The mother's, naturally, provided that these hands know. . .everything we have been saying.

"But that cannot be taught. Although it can be forgotten. . . ."

In practice, this means that Leboyer himself is usually the one deemed most qualified to soothe the child and his hands, not the mother's, appear in most of the photographs which accompany his text. He goes on:

"Many mothers do not know how to touch their babies. Or, to be more exact, do not dare. They are paralyzed. . . .

"There is something that restrains these mothers. Some profound inhibition.

"This new body has emerged from what modesty has led us to call, by a curious euphemism, the 'private parts.'

"Whatever circumlocution we use, our education has still conditioned most of us to consider these parts of the body as dirty. To reject them. Not to mention them.

"But the baby has come from there.

"From this region of the body that we are meant to know nothing about, that we don't examine, that we don't display or touch. That we would deny.

"Now this something has emerged from 'there.' Something warm and sticky. And the result of muscular efforts that resemble those we use in excreting."

I don't think I have ever encountered a more extreme example of "projection." Never have I read or heard or imagined that there could be a confusion in women's minds between babies and excrement. Perhaps I have not had enough experience in obstetrics to have encountered women with such feelings, but my sense is that the response of a newly-delivered, undrugged human mother is to reach for and hold her baby. The revulsion at the genitals and at the baby which Leboyer describes so vividly may bear more relation to his own feelings than to those of the mothers he attends. Strikingly, Leboyer does discuss the tendency to project one's own feelings onto others, but without recognizing that he shares in this phenomenon in his own writing.

"Anyone present at a birth has got to be profoundly unsettled—whether obstetrician or attendant, whether having witnessed ten births or ten thousand.

"No doubt this is because we have all experienced birth. And the experience echoes deep inside us, as potent as it is suppressed.

"Nothing is forgotten—birth least of all. Only its immediate imprint has been blurred.

"Thus the doctor and his associates find themselves profoundly but unconsciously involved in every birth they participate in. . . ."

"When the infant makes its first appearance, emotion is at its height. And everyone's breathing—already tight—chokes, stops altogether.

"Will the baby breathe?

"We are holding our own breath. Identifying with the baby, however unconsciously.

"We have all returned to our own births—fighting for breath just like this newborn baby; close to suffocation.

"And we don't have the umbilicus to supply us with oxygen. So things quickly become unbearable.

"It's necessary to 'do something.'

"The easiest, the most sensible, the most obvious thing for the onlooker to do—would be simply to breathe.

"Instead of which, he cuts the baby's umbilicus.

"His own emotional involvement has made him irrational.

"Naturally, the infant howls.

"Each person present exclaims in relief: 'He's breathing!' . . .

"Without knowing it, he has made a transference. He has rid himself of his own anguish by projecting it onto the child."

It is precisely this attempt to relieve the anxiety of the onlookers—the birth attendants and perhaps also the parents—which shapes Leboyer's method; much more so, I think, than the actual needs of the baby.

Is the womb really such a blissful place? Is the passage through the birth canal really so traumatic? I think both concepts are exaggerated and are expressions of people's deep feelings about women. Sociologist Barbara Katz Rothman sees Leboyer birth as an aspect of men's desire to participate in birth and perhaps to improve on the woman's role. In *In Labor* (see index) she says, "[Leboyer] seems to try to make amends for the supposed nightmare of being born by repeating the birth more 'gently.' Shortly after birth the baby is placed in body-temperature water and then massaged. The bath and massage are done by Leboyer himself, as he describes it, but in this country the Leboyer bath is typically done by the father. The symbolic reemergence from the amniotic fluid and the rebirthing by the father's hands is the male improvement over the female's birthing."

Many doctors think Leboyer is a "crack-pot" and I can understand why, though perhaps our reasons for thinking so are different. But some doctors are promoting Leboyer's method in a way which Judith Luce finds detrimental to women. She says, ". . . in one week two women told me that they had decided on 'Leboyer births' as substitutes for the home births they had wanted but had not been able to arrange. In the same week another woman told me that a prominent obstetrician had offered her a 'Leboyer birth' as an alternative to keeping her baby with her after birth, which is what she had originally wanted. . . .

"Unfortunately, Leboyer in no way challenges the current practice of obstetrics. The band-aid approach he takes leaves itself open to being coopted and parodied out of any meaning. It is possible right here in Boston to have a 'Leboyer birth' (quiet, dimly lit room, massage, bath to relax and recreate the womb experience) along with an epidural, fetal monitor, and perhaps your 'drug of choice.' "

NATIONAL ASSOCIATION FOR THE ADVANCEMENT OF LEBOYER'S BIRTH WITHOUT VIOLENCE, INC.
P.O. Box 248455
University of Miami Branch
Coral Gables, FL 33124
305/665-9506

This organization is devoted to promoting public awareness of Leboyer's gentle approach to birth. The Association sponsors a film showing and provides counseling in Florida and also provides publications on gentle birth. The articles listed below are available for 40 cents each.

The Association also provides an informational brochure (please include a SASE with your request) which describes the basic elements of gentle birthing.

"Gentle birthing is merely an extension of the awake and aware methods, which usually end once the baby is born. The Lamaze, Bradley or other techniques focus on the mother: Leboyer focuses on the baby. Prepared childbirth helps lessen the pain of delivery for the mother. Leboyer's approach seeks to remove the pain of birth for the infant."

1. *When Patients Ask About Gentle Birth*, by Charles Mahan

A very informative description of the gentle births at Shands teaching hospital in Gainesville, Florida.

2. *Birth Without Violence: A Medical Controversy*, by Alice Salter

A study of the Leboyer approach to childbirth using six control infants and six experimental infants is presented. The hypothesis, increased alertness will be observed in Leboyer infants in the immediate post-delivery period, was upheld.

3. *The First Day of Life*, by Charles Spezzano and Jill Waterman

The authors explain how hospital procedures interfere with and sometimes prevent early infant/parent bonding, and they stress the importance of bonding for the welfare of the entire family.

4. *Frederick Leboyer—Welcoming the Newborn*

Dr. Leboyer explains gentle birth and its underlying rationale.

5. *Gentle Birth: Its Safety and Its Effects on Neonatal Behavior*, by Charolette and George Oliver

Twenty Leboyer babies were compared to 17 born in the traditional manner. The conclusion was that the infants receiving gentle birth were significantly more relaxed. Temperatures and hematocrit were also compared.

6. *The Physiological Basis for the Leboyer Approach to Childbirth*, by Jeffrey Gimbel and James Nocon

The psychological and physiological foundations of gentle birth are explored. The authors conclude that gentle birth is valid and based on accepted physiological principles.

7. *Bonding*

A 12-page booklet discussing how parents become attached to their babies. Kennell, Klaus, Montagu, and others are quoted.

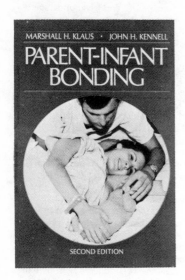

PARENT-INFANT BONDING
by Marshall H. Klaus and John H. Kennell
1982, 314 pages, Illus.

from
C.V. Mosby
11830 Westline Industrial Drive
St. Louis, MO 63141
$17.95 hd.

Animal studies have shown that mammals exhibit certain "species specific" behaviors during birth and in caring for their newly delivered offspring. Typical behaviors include seeking a safe, secluded place for birth, licking the newborn, and adjusting the body to facilitate nursing. Studies have also shown that when these natural behaviors are disrupted by early separation, the mother-infant bond suffers. "Separation of a newborn or young animal from its mother during the formation of the maternal bond. . . significantly alters maternal behavior," say the authors. "The sooner after birth the separation occurs the stronger are the effects. For each species there seems to be a specific length of separation that can be endured. If separation extends beyond this sensitive period, the effects on mothering behavior during the breeding cycle are often drastic and irreversible."

The significance of these findings for human mothers, fathers, and infants is now being widely discussed and the term "bonding" has become well known. In this second edition of *Parent-Infant Bonding* (the first edition was titled *Maternal-Infant Bonding*), Drs. Klaus and Kennell, pioneers in this field, present what they have learned about the mechanisms of attachment during pregnancy and birth and what the implications may be for the medical care of pregnant women. They describe the important factors in pregnancy which influence the formation of a mother's bond with her infant and discuss the specific effects of obstetri-

cal practices on the physical and psychological outcomes of birth, paying particular attention to the effects of a supportive companion for birth, bonding in home birth, drugs in labor, the evidence for a "sensitive" period in the early time after birth, the effects of early sucking on later breastfeeding, the role of fathers in birth, and the specific mechanisms which bond parents and infants (touch, eye contact, voice, etc.). The authors present recommendations for changing hospital birth care in order to enhance bonding. These recommendations include: individualized and respectful care, childbirth education in pregnancy, a companion in labor, privacy and time for close contact immediately after birth, delaying the use of eye medication for the baby, rooming-in, early discharge, frequent breastfeeding, family visitation, and sympathetic care from medical staff.

A group of contributors describes the "alternative birth center" program at Mt. Zion Hospital in San Francisco as an example of an attempt to respond to the needs of parents for humanistic birth care. Mary Anne Trouse and Nancy A. Irvin also discuss the special needs of the sibling, considering the effects of separation when the mother goes to the hospital, the issue of siblings witnessing birth, and recommendations for easing the adjustment of children and parents to the birth of a new family member.

Much of Klaus and Kennell's interest and work in bonding was stimulated by their experience with the care of premature and sick newborns and the effects of early separation in the hospital nursery. So they have included important chapters on caring for the parents of infants in the intensive care unit, parents of children with birth defects, and parents of children who are stillborn or who die in infancy.

"We faced a real dilemma in deciding how strongly to emphasize the importance of parent-infant contact in the first hour and extended visiting for the rest of the hospital stay, based on the available evidence. Obviously, in spite of a lack of early contact experienced by parents in hospital births in the past 20 to 30 years, almost all these parents became bonded to their babies. The human is highly adaptable, and there are many fail-safe routes to attachment. Sadly, some parents who missed the bonding experience have felt that all was lost for their future relationship. This was (and is) completely incorrect, but it was so upsetting that we have tried to speak more moderately about our convictions concerning the long-term significance of this bonding experience. Unfortunately, we find that this has led some skeptics to discontinue the practice of early contact or to make a slapdash,

rushed charade of the parent-infant contact, often without attention to the details necessary to the experiences provided for mothers in the studies. There are still large hospitals that have never provided for early and extended contact, and the mothers who miss out are often those at the limits of adaptability and who may benefit the most—the poor, the single, the unsupported, the teenage mothers . . . .

"We believe that there is strong evidence that at least 30 to 60 minutes of early contact in privacy should be provided for every parent and infant to enhance the bonding experience. Studies have not clarified how much of the effect may be apportioned to the first hours and how much to the first days, but it would appear that additional contact in both periods will probably help mothers to become attached to their babies. For some mothers one period may be more important than

the other. If the health of the mother or infant makes this impossible, then discussion, support, and reassurance should help the parents appreciate that they can become as completely attached to their infant as if they had the usual bonding experience, although it may require more time and effort. Obviously the infant should only be with the mother and father if the infant is known to be physically normal and appropriate temperature control is utilized. We also strongly urge that the infant remain with the mother as long as she wishes throughout the hospital stay so that she and the baby can get to know each other. We believe that in the near future, placement in the large central nursery will be phased out for most babies. Allowing the infant to be with the mother will permit both mother and father to experience longer periods to learn about their baby and to develop a strong tie in the first week of life."

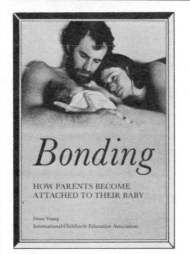

BONDING: How Parents Become Attached to Their Baby
by Diony Young
1978, 12 pages, Illus.

from
Int'l Childbirth Education Association
P.O. Box 20048
Minneapolis, MN 55420
$.50 plus .60 postage
bulk rates available

Diony Young has long been active in educating parents through ICEA and also served as manuscript editor for Klaus and Kennell's *Parent-Infant Bonding*. In this booklet, she describes the essential elements of the bonding theory and process in a way that will be immediately useful for parents. She discusses what bonding is and what factors influence bonding, including prenatal influences, labor and birth, obstetrical medications, the sensitive period, the role of the father, breastfeeding, rooming-in, siblings at birth, high-risk birth, and care from the hospital staff.

"For most babies the primary caregiver or 'need satisfier,' is the mother—the source of food, protection, warmth, stimulation and affection. The bond, or attachment, that she forms with her baby begins during pregnancy, possibly when she first feels the fetus within her body. It is a gradually unfolding relationship that blossoms with the baby's birth as the mother and baby exchange messages and feelings with all of their senses—with the meeting of their eyes, through skin-to-skin contact, with body warmth and movements, by smell, and by sound. In fact, the first minutes and hours of life may be especially, perhaps critically, influential for the initiation of the maternal bond, triggering a sequence of nurturing responses that may have long-lasting effects on the mother-child relationship. It is important to realize, however, that this is not necessarily the only stage in a baby's life during which the strong mother-to-baby bond is established. Most mothers who have been separated from their newborn babies in the hospital, as well as adoptive mothers, do develop a close, loving maternal bond with their babies in the early weeks and months.

"Drugs used by the mother tend to concentrate in the baby's bloodstream and central nervous system, leading to less responsive behavior, depressed respirations, and poor sucking ability in the first few days after birth. The responses of a depressed baby may be dulled by the effects of the drugs, and he will be less able to interact with his parents who, in turn, will be less spontaneous in their responses to him. Thus a chainlike series of events can occur with drug use, ultimately affecting the mother's, father's, and baby's responses to each other."

PARENT TO INFANT ATTACHMENT
Edited by David Klaus
1978, 71 pages
(Winter, 1978 issue of *BIRTH*)

from
BIRTH
110 El Camino Real
Berkeley, CA 94705
$4.00 single issue

This issue of *BIRTH* presents a group of papers given at a conference on parent-infant attachment held in November, 1977, by Rainbow Babies and Childrens Hospital, Cleveland Regional Perinatal Network, and Case Western Reserve University School of Medicine. Below is the complete list of contributions.

Preface
John H. Kennell, M.D. and Marshall H. Klaus, M.D.
Introduction
Richard E. Behrman, M.D.
The Remarkable Talents of the Newborn
T. Berry Brazelton, M.D.
An Anthropologic Approach to Infant Care
Betsy M. Lozoff, M.D.
Evolutionary Background of Human Maternal Behavior—Animal Models
Jay S. Rosenblatt, Ph.D.
The Biology of Parent to Infant Attachment
Marshall H. Klaus, M.D.
Prolonged Hospitalization of Pregnant Women: The Effects on the

Family
Ruth Merkatz, R.N., M.N.
Birth in the Hospital—The Effect on the Sibling
Mary Anne Trause, Ph.D.
The Father's Role in Infancy: A Reevaluation
Ross D. Parke, Ph.D.
The Death of a Newborn: Care of the Parents
Erna P. Furman
Birth of a Malformed Baby: Helping the Family
John H. Kennell, M.D.
Parenting in the Intensive Care Unit
John H. Kennell, M.D.
Intervention and Failure to Thrive: A Psychiatric Outpatient Treatment Program
Selma Fraiberg, Ph.D. and John Bennett, M.S.W.
The Effect of Extended Postpartum Contact on Problems with Parenting: A Controlled Study of 301 Families
Susan O'Connor, M.D., K.B. Sherrod, Ph.D., H.M. Sandler, Ph.D., and P.M. Vietze, Ph.D.
Home-like Deliveries in Hospital
John Franklin, M.D.
Future Care of Mothering Disorders
Selma Fraiberg, Ph.D.
Future Care of the Infant
T. Berry Brazelton, M.D.
Future Care of the Parents
Marshall H. Klaus, M.D.
The Family in the Swedish Birth Room
John Lind, M.D. (Sweden)

TOUCHING: The Human Significance of the Skin (rev. ed.)
by Ashley Montagu
1978, 406 pages

from
Perennial Library
Harper & Row
10 East 53rd St.
New York, NY 10022
$5.95

Skin to skin contact is considered an important part of the bonding process. In this book, anthropologist Ashley Montagu discusses the importance of close physical contact between mother and infant during the first months of "extrauterine life."

"What the child requires if it is to prosper . . . is to be handled, and carried, and caressed, and cuddled, and cooed to, even if it isn't breastfed. It is the handling, the carrying, the caressing, and the cuddling that we would here emphasize, for it would seem that even in the absence of a great deal else, these are the reassuringly basic experiences the infant must enjoy if it is to survive in some semblance of health. Extreme sensory deprivation in other respects, such as light and sound, can be survived, as long as the sensory experiences at the skin are maintained."

BONDING: As Love and Trust Unfold
1981, 8 pages, Illus.

from
Snugli Inc.
1212 Kerr Gulch Road
Evergreen, CO 80439
free

This booklet, from the makers of Snugli baby carriers, describes the process of bonding at birth and how bonding continues through close physical care and contact with the new baby.

"Interest in bonding seems to come from two sources—study of newborns and study of other cultures. Sociologists and anthropologists in the last 20 years have been impressed with the remarkable composure of babies in other, 'primitive' cultures.

"Many, many experts and casual travelers alike have remarked that, in these cultures, you do not see crying babies. A Peace Corps worker, in Africa in the 60's, recalls that in a marketplace with perhaps 50 babies present—each carried high on his mother's back, held in place with a knotted shawl—not one would be crying."

MOTHER-INFANT BONDING
Computer search bibliography
August, 1981, 13 pages

from
Clearinghouse on Child Abuse and Neglect Information
P.O. Box 1182
Washington, DC 20013
703/558-8222
free

In response to my request for information on the effects of bonding on child abuse, I received this bibliography of fully annotated citations for 28 sources. The bibliography was drawn from a computerized database containing descriptions of about 10,000 documents, research projects, programs, audiovisual materials, and state laws about child abuse and neglect. This bibliography is one of a series prepared on frequently requested subjects. Bibliographies are updated semiannually. There is no charge for this bibliography service. A sample entry is given below.

BONDING, BIRTH AND VIOLENCE

Assemblymember John Vasconcellos, of the California State Assembly, has become interested in the way birth practices may effect later violent crime. In January, 1982, the California Commission on Crime Control and Violence Prevention released its first report on the causes of violence *(An Ounce of Prevention)*. The birth experience and parental-infant bonding were included among factors which have been associated with later behavior. The following are excerpts from a press release issued by Vasconcellos.

". . . a positive birth experience—one that is gentle, loving and non-traumatic—increases the likelihood of healthy child development."

For more information contact Margaret O. Prado at 916/445-4253.

"Although no direct link is known to exist between the birth experience and violent behavior, the events surrounding birth influence subsequent relations between parent(s) and child, and thus affect the child's emotional, cognitive and behavioral development. Accordingly, the Commission believes that a positive birth experience—one that is gentle, loving and non-traumatic—increases the likelihood of healthy child development.

"Early parent-infant bonding is facilitated by a healthy birth experience. An optimally healthy birth experience is family-centered, loving, natural, gentle and non-traumatic; actively involves parents in their child's birth, its planning and facilitation; and includes the presence of a supportive person for the woman in labor—be it father, friend, or trained assistant."

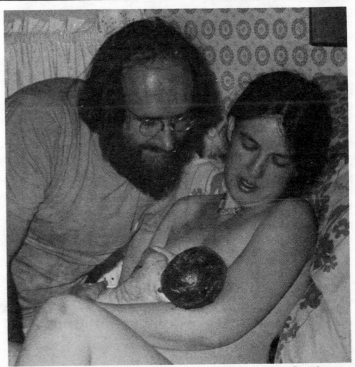

Sam Aronson

Siblings at Birth

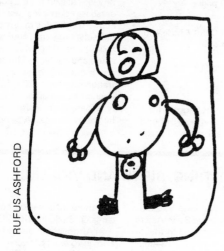

RUFUS ASHFORD

Many parents are involving their children in the births of new siblings, just as fathers were brought into the birth room some twenty years ago. Of course, birth has been and is a family affair in many cultures and times.

My son was almost three years old when I became pregnant for the second time and I began preparing him for the birth right away. One of our favorite activities was looking together at picture books of pregnancy and birth. Rufus especially liked the illustrations in **A Baby is Born** by the Maternity Center Association (see index for review). We also looked at our own color photographs of Rufus himself being born and listened to the tape made of his birth. Rufus was alarmed at first by the sounds of my heavy breathing and groaning on the tape, so I "practiced" making these sounds for him until he was more comfortable. Towards the end of the pregnancy, when my belly was very big, Rufus and I talked a lot about the coming birth, usually at going-to-bed time. We felt the baby move inside me and really felt its presence in the room. We called the baby by the names we had chosen for a boy or a girl. I remember this as a very happy, quiet time for me and Rufus.

We arranged for a couple whose birth we had attended to attend our birth as Rufus's special caretakers. When labor began and people began to arrive at the house, Rufus was excited by the "party" atmosphere. He knew there was cake and ice cream in the house for after the birth. During most of first stage labor, Rufus wandered in and out of the birthing room, not very interested in the progress of labor. But he was close by on the bed and watching very intently as I finally pushed his sister Florence out. He was glad to see her but did not want to hold her because she was too "gooey." He wanted to have the "birthday present" we had promised him and soon became absorbed in playing with his new pencil box and colored pencils while the afterbirth activities went on around him. He went to bed fairly soon after the birth because it was quite late when Florence was born.

The next morning, when we were all together in the big bed, we asked Rufus what he thought about the birth. He said, "When her head was coming out it was like a flower blooming." We were astounded at such a poetic response and asked among the birth crew to see if anyone had mentioned this metaphor to Rufus, but apparently it was his own creation.

Two years later, in preparation for this book, I asked Rufus again about the birth:

Q. What did you think about watching Florence be born?
A. When her head was coming out it was like a flower blooming.
Q. What do you mean?
A. Well, her head coming out was like the middle of the flower and the vagina around it was the leaves.
Q. Was it pretty?
A. No! It was yucky.
Q. But a flower is pretty.
A. Yes.
Q. Some people think that children shouldn't be allowed to watch babies being born. Did you know that?
A. No.
Q. Do you think children should be able to watch babies being born?
A. Yes.
Q. Why?
A. Because.
Q. Because why?
A. Because children *like* babies.

Tracy Scott was 5 years old when her brother Morgan (Muffy) was born at home. Mary Scott (who reviewed materials on baby and child care for this *Catalog*) made this interview with her daughter Tracy when Morgan was about one year old.

Mary: Did you know what was going to happen just before Morgan was born?
Tracy: No.
Mary: What did happen?
Tracy: It turned out to be a boy. First Mom was 'practice breathing.' Doing that funny breathing. Then Morgan's head popped out. Then his body. Then finally his legs. Then his feet. He was all covered with a cream cheese, like jelly.
Mary: How did you feel about what you saw?
Tracy: I felt too bad because Mom's vagina was burning right before his head popped out.
Mary: Then how did you feel?
Tracy: Glad that it was a brother!
Mary: What would you tell your friends about the birth?
Tracy: I don't know.
Mary: What was the most exciting part?

Tracy: Mom in the spice bath. That was the most fun. I love it. It smelled so good. Basil and other good spices. [Mary's postpartum bath]
Mary: What was the strangest part?
Tracy: Mom's practice breathing. It sure sounded strange.
Mary: What was the scariest part?
Tracy: When Mom's vagina was burning.
Mary: What was the funniest part?
Tracy: When I saw Muffy with all that cream cheese over him. I've never seen a little kid with all cream cheese over him . . . or her.
Mary: Do you want to have babies?
Tracy: Of course! But all home births.
Mary: Why all home births?
Tracy: Because it's more fun, and you get your family to see everything that's going on, and hear everything that's going on. I wouldn't be scared because it was everything that Mom did. I would do everything that Mom did.
Mary: Do you think everybody should have babies at home?
Tracy: No, they can do what they want for births.

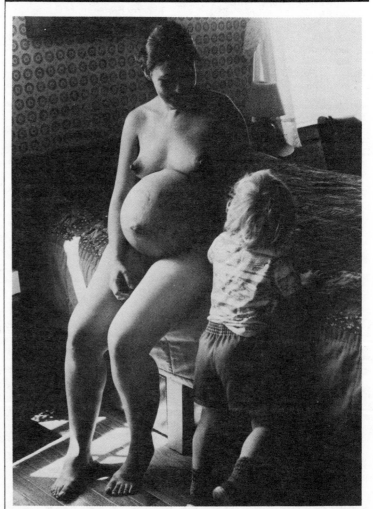

VIC ASHFORD

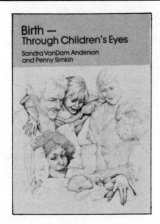

BIRTH—THROUGH CHILDREN'S EYES
by Sandra VanDam Anderson and Penny Simkin
1981, 141 pages, Illus.

from
the pennypress
1100 23rd Avenue East
Seattle, WA 98112
$10.50

Sandra Anderson is a doctoral student in nursing anthropology and has studied children at birth for some years. Penny Simkin is the director of the pennypress and author of many pamphlets in her excellent *Better Baby Series.* Together they have produced a lovely and informative book which will be of interest to parents who are preparing a child for the birth of a sibling, and also to staff who want to facilitate sibling programs in their institutions. The first three chapters present an overview of the subject, results of a comparison study of children present and absent at siblings' births, and an analysis of children's perceptions of birth based on interviews and children's drawings, many charming examples of which are reproduced in color. Contributors Susan Parma and Sara Pitta describe their prenatal preparation classes for siblings. Paulina Perez discusses implementing sibling programs in a birthing center and includes many excellent photographs of births with children present. Ann Armstrong Scarboro and Penny Simkin discuss explaining cesarean birth to children. Lester Hazell provides a foreword and David Stewart of NAPSAC concludes with an afterword.

"From our observations, several recommendations can be made. If children are in fact going to be present at birth, it is essential that they be prepared for this experience. In order to provide adequate prenatal preparation to facilitate a positive experience, and to anticipate concerns of the child during labor and birth, I suggest the following guidelines for the parents:

1. Tell the child as early as possible about the anticipated birth of a sibling.

2. Take the child to at least one prenatal visit with the doctor or midwife, to enable the child to meet the provider of care and to listen to the fetal heart beat.

3. Show the child colored pictures in books, slides, films, and videotapes to acquaint the child with the sights and sounds of labor and birth. Specific attention should be given to blood, which will be noticed on the mother and baby, and also to the sounds of work and/or pain emitted by the mother in the process of birthing the baby.

4. Discuss with the child the appearance of the newborn, with special attention given to the umbilical cord and the placenta. The child should realize that the cord will be cut, which will not be painful to the baby or mother. The child should know that the baby might cry, and that he or she will not be the ideal playmate immediately.

5. Try to be comfortable around the family, at least on occasion, without clothes on . . . .

"The children who were present at births generally drew a family scene for the birth setting, which often included other people, usually the father and/or children. Other items which are noteworthy in several pictures are furniture, patterned sheets, smiles, and bright colors. There seems to be an atmosphere of joy and celebration. In contrast, the pictures drawn by children not present rarely included other family members. They tend to have less detail and less color. Often the woman giving birth is alone, or attended by a nurse or doctor with a mask on. In only one drawing is a father included in a picture of a baby being born. None of the drawings by children absent at births include children in their pictures. However, some of the children who were not present at the hospital births of siblings drew detailed pictures of the scene of birth in the hospital, of the doctors and nurses, and of the equipment used. . . . It is interesting that most of the technically oriented pictures have been drawn by children who were ten years old or older and were not present at the birth. Their perceptions are probably based on books, films, television, conversations and their fantasies. They are remarkable in their accuracy. In contrast, children present at home births seemed to focus on the people present rather than on equipment . . . .

"As vaginal exams are done, the nurse can remind the child that she is trying to feel the baby's head and that when she feels a lot of it the mom can begin to push the baby out. When pushing begins she can comment to the child that pushing is very hard work. I often tell the child that pushing the baby out is a little like climbing a mountain. It is very hard while you're doing it but you are very happy when you've finished it. Birth is often not quiet. The child has been taught about the noises of childbirth but I often find it helpful to remind the child of the film he/she saw. I also comment that the mom is OK and that her body is made so that it can stretch as she pushes. Often, between pushes the mother will comment to the child about what's happening. One mother said, 'The baby's head is making my bottom burn but that's a sign it will be born soon.' Another commented, 'Mom is hurting now but I'm OK and the baby will be born soon.' When one mother was pushing and making noises her three-year-old asked, 'Is mom crying?' She was reminded that those were pushing noises. As the baby began to crown she excitedly announced, 'Oh, it's a BABY!'. . . .

"During the delivery itself the physician, the nurse, or the child's support person may "talk the child through the birth." The nurse should allow the child to relate to the birth in any way he/she chooses. Some children are very verbal and involved. In one birth such a child told the physician he was 'wasting those gloves by using them just once.' Another commented, 'I can't see—the doctor is in the way.' Other children are very quiet and somewhat awestruck. As one mother explained, 'It wasn't what she said at the birth but how she looked.' The nurse or doctor often makes comments such as, 'Mom is blowing so the baby's head comes out slowly,' or 'It's hard work to push the baby's head out.'

When the baby's head is delivered the children are most excited. One three-year-old who badly wanted a baby sister exclaimed, 'It's my baby Holly!' when only the head was born. When one baby opened his eyes before the body was born his brother said, 'He's looking at me. I think he likes me'. . . .

"Adults can learn a great deal about life by working with children when life begins. Children can add such joy to our lives—sometimes with a simple comment. After the birth of her sister one three-year-old approached her mother, gently patted her on the cheek and softly said, 'Thank you, Mom.' What can replace the feeling you get while watching a child hold and rock his new sister fifteen minutes after her birth? One three-year-old sat and sang songs to his new brother. Watching a child begin to attach and form a bond with their new siblings is most touching. But the feeling is much stronger when you begin to realize what an impact these moments may have on their relationship. Eleven months after his brother's birth one seven-year-old child commented: 'Sometimes when he gets into my toys and messes them up he drives me crazy but I just love him so much.' Moments such as these are the reasons I am enthusiastic about working with children and their families. Sharing births with children has helped me to truly appreciate the miracle of birth. Seeing birth through a child's eyes has helped me to see the wonder and beauty of life."

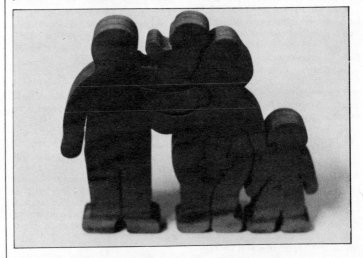

CHILDREN AT BIRTH
by Marjie and Jay Hathaway
1978, 180 pages, Illus.

from
Academy Publications
Box 5224
Sherman Oaks, CA 91413
$5.95 pap.

Marjie and Jay Hathaway are the directors of the American Academy of Husband-Coached Childbirth (see index) and have taught the Bradley method of childbirth preparation to many thousands of couples and teachers. They are also good friends of David and Lee Stewart, directors of NAPSAC (see index) and this book features photos taken by Jay of the Stewart's home birth of their fifth child.

Based on their own experience and reading, the Hathaways believe that children should be present at birth and they present a good discussion of the important issues in this area: the advantages and disadvantages of having children at birth, how to decide if your own child should be present, preparing your child for birth, and how to handle the actual birth. There are several interviews with medical professionals and with parents and children. Many excellent "photo essays" of sibling-attended birth are included, which show clearly what birth really looks like. There are also extensive chapters on childbirth preparation and nutrition based on the Bradley method and on consumer issues in birth, so this book will be helpful even for parents who are expecting their first child.

(Jay Hathaway has also produced several films on alternative birth, including children at birth, which are distributed by Cinema Medica, see index.)

"Our daughter Susan, having attended many births, wrote 10 points on how to prepare other children for attending births. At the time she wrote this she was 13 years old.

1. Keep in mind that each situation is different. Be prepared to be flexible.
2. The parents must decide if they want the children there first. Then they can be part of the following decisions.
3. Prepare your children:
   a. So they know in reality, what will happen.
   b. Watching childbirth movies helps prepare.
   c. Some kids have said the things that scared them were:
      The baby was blue when it was born.
      The baby didn't cry right away.
      I thought it was too bloody.
   These things should be discussed.
4. Keep things positive.
   a. Avoid medicated birth films. Avoid mechanized medicated birth, because medicated births are out of control and unnatural and frightening. I think it would do more harm than good for a child to be present at a medicated birth.
   b. Parents should be open and willing to talk about birth.
5. Make the children feel important, useful and wanted.
   a. Give them some sort of job to do.

1) Getting ice chips
2) Help time contractions
3) Have them squeeze orange juice
6. Children need a caretaker. Even older children need someone whose job it is to explain what is happening. This person should be willing to take care of the children if something goes wrong and parents have to leave.
7. Don't neglect other children after the baby is born. They should be part of the bonding process.
8. Don't force anyone especially children to be at a birth.
   a. Some children aren't ready.
   b. Some adults can't take it either.
   c. Depends on their background.
9. You can make a party out of it.
   a. Freeze a cake.
   b. Have orange juice.
   c. Ice Cream.
10. Most of all, please remember that this is a joyful event—a miracle and that whoever is there will remember it for the rest of their lives. So make it as joyful as possible for all concerned."

CHILDREN AT BIRTH
Rosemary Cogan, editor
1981, 8 pages, Illus.

from
Int'l Childbirth Education Association
P.O. Box 20048
Minneapolis, MN 55420
$1.50 plus $1.00 postage

This issue of *ICEA Review* (December, 1981) features an introduction, and abstracts of literature on children at birth, birthing room programs for children, preparation of children, and sibling visitation. Sandra VanDam Anderson, co-author of *Birth Through Children's Eyes,* provides an excellent concluding commentary.

"Little more than a dozen years ago, debate raged as to the suitability of permitting husbands to be present at birth. It was argued by some that women who wanted to have their husbands present at birth were undoubtedly neurotic and that if husbands were permitted to be present during birth, they would lose all sexual interest in their wives. At the same time, many people felt that birth was a deeply meaningful event in the lives of the whole family and that when husbands and wives mutually chose to share birth together it could be an exceptionally positive experience for both . . . .

"Just as it was important to understand the medical-legal issues associated with husbands or partners at birth not long ago, it is important now to understand and explore the issues and data associated with children at birth."
—Rosemary Cogan

MONKEY BUSINESS
Box 20001
Tallahassee, FL 32304
904/576-7406

Natalie birthing doll

Completed doll with gown	$35.00
with cesarean option	3.00
dressing gown	4.00
kit	14.00

Jan Alovus made her first "birthing doll" in 1977 as a gift for a child who was expecting a new sibling. The original doll was called "Bertha" and was made from red-ball socks. Soon friends wanted birthing dolls, others began to hear of Bertha, and Monkey Business was launched. The doll became popular with childbirth educators involved in the new field of preparing siblings for birth. In 1979, Jan introduced Natalie, a 22 inch human rag doll who gives birth to a cloth baby with detachable cord and placenta and with a cesarean option, if desired. Now Bertha is being redesigned and Natalie is available as a completed doll or as a kit. Natalie has velcro on her hands and legs so she can hold her legs during labor and hold her baby after birth. She comes with a dressing gown and is the right

size to wear infant clothing. The kit includes printed material and directions, stuffing, and velcro.

Monkey Business is a cottage industry which is part of the "cooperative community." Dolls are sewn by Tallahassee-area seamsters and Monkey Business also sells the kits by wholesale for those who want to sew and sell the finished doll locally (write for wholesale prices). After *Ms.* magazine featured Natalie in their December, 1981 issue, orders began flooding in and Jan has been working hard lately to keep ahead of the business. She believes strongly in the concepts of "right livelihood." She says, "We in the cooperative community are in a unique position. For years many of us have seen that big changes in the economy were coming and have begun to live our lives accordingly. The attitudes, skills, and tools we've developed are important resources for decentralizing our society. Now, with thoughtful marketing, we can make our discoveries available to a wider range of Americans and even get paid, at least minimally, for doing what we like best."

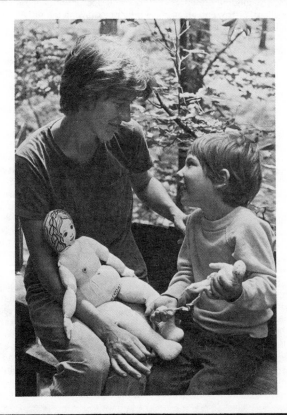

RUFUS AND HIS SISTER'S BIRTH

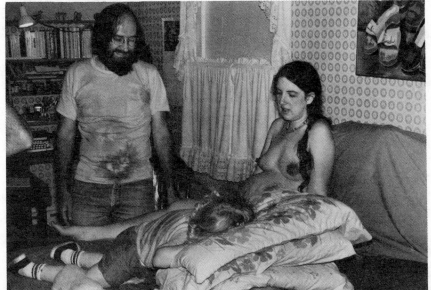

Sam Aronson

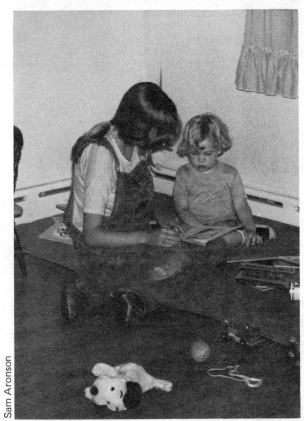

Sam Aronson

During much of the labor Rufus enjoyed playing with his special caretaker, Kate.

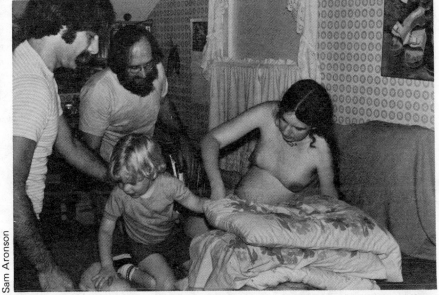

Sam Aronson

Sometimes Rufus came into the bedroom to be with me and his father during labor. He lay on my stack of pillows while I rested between contractions. But when the next contraction started Tony helped Rufus get out of the way *fast* so I could lean over in my comfortable position.

RUFUS AND HIS SISTER'S BIRTH

When Florence was born Rufus was right next to us on the bed, watching intently with our friend Nan. He was happy about Florence.

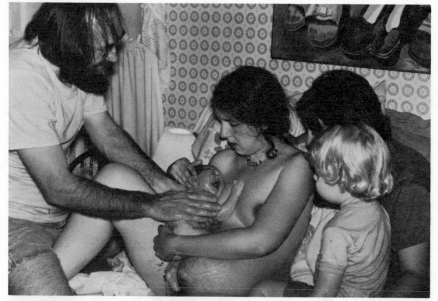

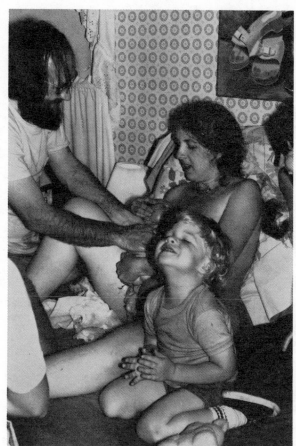

Sam Aronson

Sam Aronson

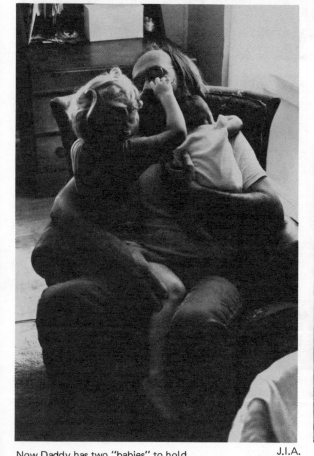

Now Daddy has two "babies" to hold.   J.I.A.

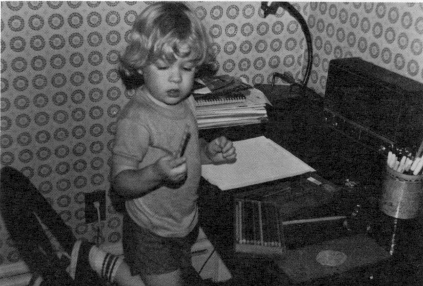

Soon Rufus remembered the "birthday present" he'd been promised. He got a new pencil box with his name on it and a set of colored pencils. He wanted to do some drawing right away, while the after-birth activities proceeded around him.

Sam Aronson

Grandma Lucy (Vic's mother) came to stay with us for two weeks after Florence was born. Rufus enjoyed doing artwork with her.

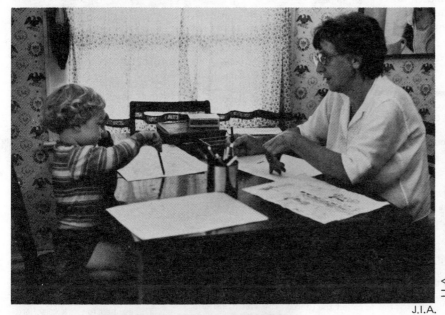

J.I.A.

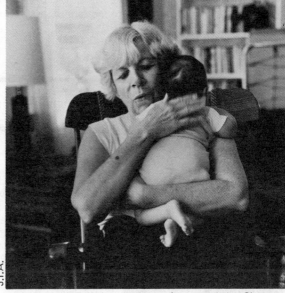

J.I.A.

Next Grandma Alice (Janet's mother) came to help. She comforted colicky Florence. It helped us and Rufus a lot to have our grandmothers come to stay.

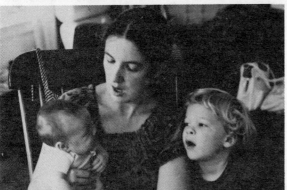

Alice Isaacs

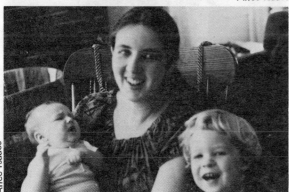

Alice Isaacs

Florence cried a lot in the first months of her life. But Rufus and I liked her anyway.

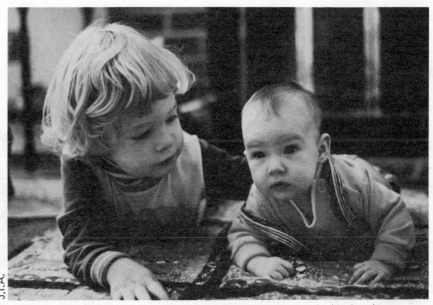

J.I.A.

Rufus rarely speaks of Florence's birth. But he shows his affection for his sister in many ways.

PREPARING CHILDREN FOR BIRTH

The following books will help parents prepare their children for the birth of a sibling. These books will also help first-time parents prepare *themselves* for birth, since the careful descriptions for children of the sights and sounds of birth are sometimes more honest and explicit than those written for adults.

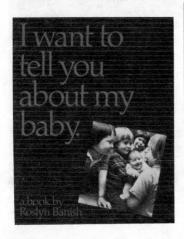

I WANT TO TELL YOU ABOUT MY BABY
by Roslyn Banish
1982, 56 pages, Illus.

from
Wingbow Press
2940 Seventh Street
Berkeley, CA 94710
$5.95 pap.

This book will help prepare children whose mother will give birth in a hospital. Written in the first person voice of a little boy, the simple text and photographs describe pregnancy and its effects on the mother and family, the arrival of grandparents, birth (hospital scenes are included but do not show the actual birth of the baby), visiting mother in the hospital, coming home, the demands of new baby care, and the adjustment and growing pride of the big brother. Both text and pictures are very warm and sensitive and the sections on breastfeeding and the first days with the new baby are especially good.

"My Mom gave a big push. The baby comes out an opening between her legs. The doctor catches it and says it's a boy. My Dad says that is how I was born too."

"My Grandpa takes me to the hospital. Here I'm waiting to see the baby. Where is my Mom? Where is the baby?

"Here she is! My Mom gives me a great big hug and says 'I love you.' I tell her to come home."

MY CHILDBIRTH COLORING BOOK
by Laurence K. Scott and David Baze
1977, 32 pages, Illus.

from
Academy Press Limited
360 N. Michigan Avenue
Chicago, IL 60601
$2.95 pap.

The sex of the child who narrates this book is not revealed, "so that both boys and girls can feel at home with the voice that tells the story." The text is suitable for parents to read aloud to young children or for older children to read themselves. It covers the growth and development of the narrator's mother and father from infancy to adulthood; their falling in love, marriage, lovemaking, and pregnancy; birth and breastfeeding. The book is exemplary in its nonsexist treatment of sex differences and development, and the line drawings are very clear and elegant.

"When Mom and Dad were about twenty-five years old, they decided it was time for Mother to become pregnant. Until then they had used birth control, which means a way of making sure a baby isn't begun before the parents are ready. They didn't need to use birth control again until after I was born nine months later, because once a baby is started no new ones can be started until after the first is born."

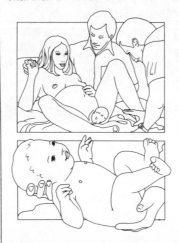

DID THE SUN SHINE BEFORE YOU WERE BORN?
by Sol and Judith Gordon
1982, 40 pages, Illus.

from
Ed-U Press
P.O. Box 583
Fayetteville, NY 13066
$4.95 pap.

This is a beautifully illustrated book for children between the ages of 3 and 7. It can be used as a base for parents to start from or as a supplemental explanation when children wonder about where they came from and how babies come to be. It is primarily intended as a read-aloud book, but much of it can be read by a beginning reader.

The illustrations clearly show many different kinds of families (varied lifestyles and cultures) and non-sexist behavior (e.g. both fathers and mothers hugging their children, a boy playing with a doll, a girl with a pair of pliers). This is an open-ended book which will help to stimulate questions and thoughts in families with young children, as well as simply answer some basic questions.

(Susan Ritchie)

"The baby grows in a special place inside the mother. This place is called the uterus. It is warm and safe there. The food the mother eats helps the baby to grow.

"It takes a baby about nine months to grow large enough and strong enough to be born. That's almost as long as from your last birthday to your next birthday."

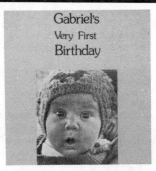

GABRIEL'S VERY FIRST BIRTHDAY
by Sherrie Farrell
1976, 40 pages, Illus.

from
Pipeline Books
Box 3711
Seattle, WA 98124
out of print

Written in the form of a letter, this book tells the story of Gabriel's midwife-attended home birth in a log cabin in the mountains. The black and white photographs which accompany the simple text are very explicit, showing in detail the effort of second stage labor and the birth of the baby. The father's support in labor and early nursing and bonding are also clearly shown.

"Therese had to work very hard so that you could be born.

"She pushed and pushed, pushed and pushed.

"She pushed again . . . and we saw you!

"You took your first breath.

"She pushed again . . . and your shoulders were free!

Then you just slipped out. You were born."

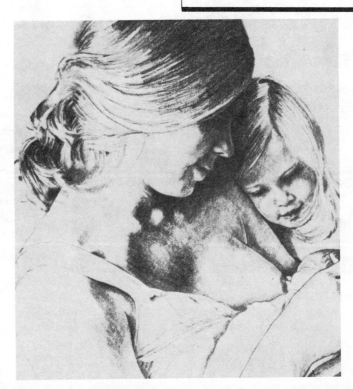

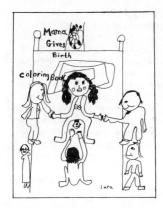

MAMA GIVES BIRTH: Coloring Book
by Gina Kaefring
1978, 28 pages, Illus.

from
Emma Goldman Clinic for Women
715 N. Dodge St.
Iowa City, IA 52240
$2.50 pap. plus $.75 postage

The Positive Experience Pregnancy Group of the Emma Goldman Clinic and the Sophonisba artist's group of Iowa City joined together to produce this coloring book. It includes drawings by eight different artists depicting pregnancy and birth in a non-traditional extended family. The text is simple and the drawings are exuberant and fanciful.

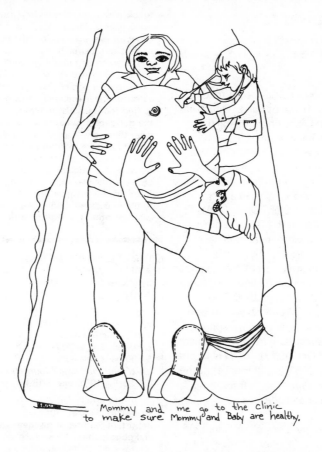

Mommy and me go to the clinic to make sure Mommy and Baby are healthy.

MAKING BABIES
by Sara Bonnett Stein
1974, 47 pages, Illus.
$7.95 hd.

THAT NEW BABY
by Sara Bonnett Stein
1974, 47 pages, Illus.
$7.95 hd.

from
Walker and Co.
720 Fifth Avenue
New York, NY 10019

These two books are part of the *Open Family* series for parents and children to use together. Each page spread features a large black and white photograph, a simple text for children and a parallel text for parents to help them explore with their children the important concepts and feelings being presented. *Making Babies* talks about human reproduction using photographs of animals giving birth, nursing, and mating along with pictures of pregnant women, babies and children. *That New Baby* features a black family with two older children as they go through pregnancy and the birth of a new baby brother.

MOM AND DAD AND I ARE HAVING A BABY: A Book for Children About Childbirth
by Maryann P. Malecki
1982, 70 pages, Illus.

from
the pennypress
1100 23rd Avenue East
Seattle, WA 98112
$6.95

Maryann Malecki is a nurse, childbirth educator and birth attendant. Her book is especially designed to help prepare children who will participate in a home birth. Aspects of birth which may be upsetting to children (blood, the placenta, the mother's grunting and pushing efforts, the appearance of the baby) are discussed. The text is written in a child's voice and Malecki's pencil drawings are very soft with important features highlighted in color.

SPECIAL DELIVERY: A Book for Kids About Cesarean and Vaginal Birth
by Gayle Cunningham Baker and Vivian M. Montey
1981, 63 pages, Illus.

from
The Chas. Franklin Press
18409 90th Avenue W
Edmonds, WA 98020
$5.95 paper

Three cesarean mothers wrote and illustrated this book to help explain cesarean as well as vaginal birth to children. Line drawings and split text (large type in simple language for small children, a more detailed text for older children) are used to describe basic anatomy and conception, pregnancy, vaginal birth, cesarean birth, recovery and going home.

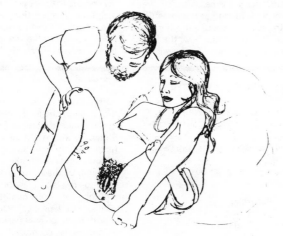

Somebody said that he could see the baby's head. That doesn't look like a baby's head to me!

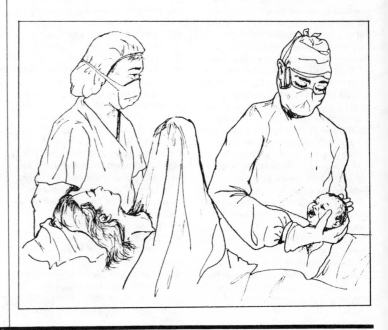

More Alternatives

MICHEL ODENT

Michel Odent is a French surgeon who directs a special maternity unit at the public hospital in Pithiviers, outside of Paris. Odent has developed (or perhaps rediscovered) ideas about how the birth environment affects the mother and can hamper or facilitate her labor. At Pithiviers, labor progresses without any obstetrical intervention. Women are encouraged to choose any position, change positions, walk, or relax in warm baths or swimming pools. Delivery often takes place in a "supported standing-squat," or in a birth chair, while kneeling, or occasionally in the water. Dr. Odent is particularly interested in birth position and in the way the birth environment may help women regress to a more instinctual level of feeling, in which labor can proceed more smoothly.

Michel Odent's work has attracted the attention of many women in the alternative childbirth movement. Sheila Kitzinger sponsored a study day with Odent at her home in England, in 1980. Odent has also visited with members of the Boston Women's Health Book Collective (BWHBC). An article describing Odent's work appeared in the October 27, 1979 issue of *The Lancet* (Gillett, J.: Childbirth in Pithiviers, France. Lancet II:894, 27 Oct. 1979). *BIRTH* journal published an article by Odent in Spring, 1981 (see this page). Jane Pincus, childbirth editor for *Our Bodies, Ourselves*, is translating Odent's books from the French and American editions are planned by Schocken and Pantheon.

Below is an exerpt from an "abridged paraphrase" of Odent's book, *Genese De L'Homme Ecologique: L'Instinct Retrove*, published in Paris in 1979 by Epi publishers, translated by Jane Pincus and made available by the BWHBC.

For further information on Odent's methods, readers may contact:

Jane Pincus
c/o The Boston Women's
Health Book Collective
Box 192
West Somerville, MA 02144

Dr. Michel Odent
Centre Hospitalier General de
Pithiviers
45300, Service de Maternite
Pithiviers, France

"Human beings have roots. We are tied to the earth, to our collective animal phylogenetic past. Childbirth can be a magnificent opportunity to evoke, to awaken our awareness of these roots. But childbirth practices in industrialized countries, which involve routinized mechanized interventions during labor and birth, artificial birthing environments, and separation of mothers from newborns after birth, only serve to alienate and dehumanize us, to make us lose contact with our 'ancient memory.' Mothers in other than 'modern' medicalized surroundings can be in touch with the rhythm of their own labors, find the best positions to labor in, have immediate skin-to-skin contact with their newborns, and breastfeed right away. Freed to live these processes in their own ways, they get in touch with ancient reflexes, ancient memories, and their newborns make immediate, profound contact with them. . . .

"For one thing, it is especially important for the father to be present at childbirth. In past and present cultures, women's and men's worlds have been kept separate, a separateness expressed and emphasized by rituals. But we believe that the father's presence is one of the keys to the fusion of male and female worlds. When men are involved in labor and childbirth, they become familiar with female genital life. They immerse themselves in the humanity of women. The feminine world opens to them, and they can be liberated from their exclusive roles as traditional men. There will be a new paternal image of men who are both sweet and strong.

"In our '*salle sauvage*,' our birthing room at Pithiviers, the dorsal position seems out of place (though three centuries have sufficed to make dorsal childbirthing a cultural characteristic, and some women have ended their labors in that position). The dorsal position is harmful because it compresses important veins, goes against gravity, doesn't allow for pelvic expansion, the perineum doesn't stretch as it should, and retained amniotic fluid can be a source of infection. Women who listen to their bodies (*qui se mettent a l'ecoute de leur corps*) know how to find spontaneous alternatives to the dorsal position as they 'forget' what they have learned and 'remember' old familiar positions. There is an infinite scale of possible positions in no particular chronological order. After two years of learning from these women who are attuned to their needs and bodies, we in turn can help other women find efficient birthing positions. To sum up our observations in a general way, we've noticed that for the first phase of childbirth, dilation, standing and walking are common. In the second phase, women kneel and stand with bust forward to facilitate rotation. For pushing, supported squatting is most useful and least painful. With these ideas as guides, we have seen a spectacular lowering of Cesarian rates (down to 6 percent)."

THE EVOLUTION OF OBSTETRICS AT PITHIVIERS
by Michel Odent, M.D.
1981, 9 pages, Illus.

from
BIRTH
110 El Camino Real
Berkeley, CA 94705
$4.00 per single issue
(*Birth and the Family Journal*, Vol. 8:1 Spring 1981, pgs. 7-15.)

In this article, Dr. Odent describes his clinic at Pithiviers and the important features of his methods and philosophies. Many excellent photos are included of under-water births and birth in the standing-squat position.

"These last years, we understood better and better what to do to help the mother become more instinctive, to forget what is cultural, to reduce the control of the neocortex, to change her level of consciousness so that the labor seems to be easier. For example, assistance by a female is always beneficial. Not all women can be effective as midwives. Women must engage themselves effectively to bring love, and at the same time to bring experience, as a mother would. We sometimes have the feeling that the presence of a male is negative. Of course, it is not so simple. Nobody is just negative or positive; nobody is just a man or just a woman. But sometimes I feel I must not be present during the delivery. The father, who is a male and a familiar person, may or may not have a negative effect—it is not a simple problem. . . .

"We have also discovered the efficiency of water in the first stage. The reason why kneeling or immersion in water during labor is so helpful is mysterious. Sometimes just a shower is sufficient to relieve an inhibition in labor. We know that delivery and the first sucking are events belonging to a woman's sexual and affective life. That means that sometimes there are inhibitions that we cannot always appraise. On the other hand, we sometimes see inhibitions thrown off without understanding why. What is sure is that water is often the way to reduce inhibitions. Of course, there are many ways to use water. Some enter a different level of consciousness in water. And we observe that, during such immersion in warm water, semi-darkness is the best way to reach a high level of relaxation, a degree of relaxation that can be reached by many women without any preparation, without any classes."

VIDEOTAPE OF DR. MICHEL ODENT
50 minutes, black and white
(VHS 3/4 industrial or ½ inch cassettes)
Rental fee: $40. prepaid plus $3. postage
Purchase Price: $135.00

from
Nancy Bardacke
6536 Dana Street
Oakland, CA 94609
415/655-2252

"This videotape was made during Dr. Odent's recent visit to the United States. It shows his Grand Rounds presentation to the students and faculty at the University of California, San Francisco, Medical School on November 4, 1980. In the presentation Dr. Odent describes the evolution of the birth practices used in the maternity unit at Pithiviers. Slides are shown of their alternative birth environment, of the midwives, of alternative positions used for birthing, of the warm pools of water used for the laboring woman, and of a number of unplanned 'underwater' births. The tape also includes a question and answer period. This videotape has been used successfully by nurses, doctors, and OB-GYN residents, as well as by childbirth educators for their own training and for viewing in childbirth preparation classes."

—Nancy Bardacke

LOTUS BIRTH

CLAIR LOTUS DAY, who describes herself as "a clairvoyant, nurse and teacher," believes that the umbilical cord should not be cut at birth but allowed to fall off naturally with the placenta at around the 7th day after birth, the time when the umbilical stump of a cord which has been cut will usually shrivel and fall away. Clair calls this way of birth "Lotus Birth" and has developed very elaborate written material describing the spiritual benefits of this method and the psychological harm which may result from cutting the cord. Below is an excerpt from this material. For more information on Lotus Birth, readers may write directly to Clair Lotus Day. When requesting information, please include a donation to cover the costs of duplicating materials and postage.

Clair Lotus Day   or
c/o Open Eden   c/o Open Eden
P.O. Box 737   1007 Addison
Bolinas, CA 94924   Berkeley, CA 94710

"I have been clairvoyant now for about ten years, and after the birth of my second child my clairvoyance led me more into sightings dealing with health. On more than a hundred occasions I have seen the astral vibration of the umbilical cord being severed and on many different times this vibration occurred when the person was in what one might call a negative state. . . . All of these hundred and more instances led me to the belief that possibly the umbilical cord did not necessarily have to be severed. I began thinking more and more about the possibility. I also contacted twenty doctors in obstetrics departments in San Francisco and the government with replies that severing was done because of custom and cleanliness. We can change the custom and be clean. I talked with a doctor at the maternity section of Public Health in Berkeley who referred me to the book *In the Shadow of Man,* by Jane Goodall, who states that the chimps seem to keep the placenta intact until it comes off naturally and at the back of the book it raises the question of why are they as adults so family-oriented? I, of course, think it is because the cord was not severed at birth, keeping the unity of the pregnancy, mother and child.

"In the Old Testament in Ezekial 16, verse 6 it says: 'In the beginning thy navel was not cut thou was cast out into an open field where none pitied thee. . .'' and goes on to say 'a sapphire was given for thy third eye and a crown for thy head.' Sounds like the people achieved enlightenment through the vivification of the chakras. . . .

"I then became pregnant for the sole purpose of having a child in this way.

"The doctor whom I worked with for eight and a half months on it, at the last moment before and during my labor (near transition) wanted to take me to the hospital and cut the cord. I released him and was guided. I went to Drs.——— and explained my clairvoyance, that I also had two years of nursing with five years experience, that I had a small pyramid at home to cure the placenta in while the cord came off naturally. Dr. ——— said that he would consult with the other doctors, but to get myself to ———Hospital in San Francisco or I would have the baby at the door step, so with hope in my heart and a new being on the way I arrived at the hospital. It was a completely natural birth, the placenta was expelled five minutes after birth. Dr. ——— came up to me and said you look like the kind who would like to go home with the placenta still intact. Praise God. That was the best gift that could ever have been given to me. The only red tape I had to go through was to sign a piece of paper stating why I did not have the blood test done from the cut cord. I said for health and religious reasons. An hour after Trimurti was born I was on my way home, put the placenta in the upper chamber of the pyramid, wrapped his cord with sterile gauze, leaving it straight and horizontal. . . I sat with my heavenly child as his heart system was paved in harmony with what sustained him, I figuratively and symbolically liken to the tree in the middle (the umbilical cord). He is a most harmonious, strong, healthy happy alert child who is bringing completeness and fullness into my life. . . A center opened up in me near the cervix and root chakra, much like a circle—open and full, extending my energy and giving me a total prospectus and naturalness. I did not find this center full with the other ladies whom I came near when I went back for my six week check-up. This centrifugal center has kept my energy full and my Karma my own."

—Clair Lotus Day, from a letter written in 1975.

R.D. Laing, the well-known British psychiatrist, has written about the cutting of the umbilical cord as a source of birth trauma for the infant. His thoughts on this are presented in Chapter 7, "Cutting the Umbilical Cord" in his book *The Facts of Life* (Pantheon, 1976)

LOTUS BIRTH FULLY BLOOMED

by Jeannine Parvati Baker, MA

"I agreed to do the best that I could while planetside. Practicing Lotus Birth is part of that original agreement. As soon as I heard about the Lotus Birth an inner 'truth bell' began to ring. I felt this way upon doing my first asana (yoga pose) and seeing my cast horoscope and conceiving my first baby and hearing Stevie Wonder's music. And many other momentous times in my life where this ring of something true resounds through my being. I have already written in detail about the visitation—a clairvoyant coming to my pregnant home with her message. The missionary shared with me the practice of Lotus Birth and as it made complete sense to me, I agreed to try it. The rest is her story. (See *Hygieia: A Women's Herbal* for the 15 hour deliberation and execution to twin umbilical cords. A new note to that is though my [1st] husband and I were respectful and each of us cut one cord, we later divorced painfully.) It is with much humble joy that we report the full blooming Lotus Birth of my 4th baby, our 1st son 2 years ago (1980). We saw so much value in allowing the cord to break forth on its own! His navel is exceptionally beautiful and his power as a being remains intact. Needless to say, we did not circumcize (or violate in any metallic way his being).

"What we saw was the perfect balance of nature—as the new one, our son came into his body more fully, the old one, the placenta, left this world. When the third day postpartum arrived, the cord was quite crisp and the temptation to help its brittleness along was strong. We mother roasted—that is, had a lying in ceremony of warming up the birth room, like a sauna, and letting both the mama and baby be naked together in warm comfort. However, we didn't break the cord but allowed it to organically fall away. This waiting set the way for subsequent patience in letting old withered parts of the psyche drop off when its inner and organic cycle was complete. A much softer way than the heroic warrior with a sword who cuts away, breaks through defenses and otherwise valiantly wounds the soul. We would allow our son's attachments to let go when their own time was ripe, and the lotus birth was the initial testimony to that promise.

"In the early afternoon, as the scent of placenta wafted richly around our redwood forest cabin, I noticed that the cord right at the umbilical cord looked very different than the last three days. It looked complete. Full and ready to break forth. The old placenta—who was named 'Grandmother' by my five year old daughters—rested in my Blessing Way and Placenta Bowl. It was given to me by my mother when I birthed my first baby and I ceremoniously cared for it. The big ceramic green bowl was on the bed with me and our baby, connecting us three together. We honored Grandmother while she was with us but could see she wanted to rest in her mother, the Earth, very soon. We burned cedar around our son's navel as an incense. And watched, waiting, following closely. Our son's cord came away from his belly-button with his family watching, the same loving sisters and papa who were at his birth. We all said it felt like his second birthing when the cord fell away. Right then he seemed to purposefully grab onto his dried cord. And he grasped it, slowly waving his arms, all the while holding his newly released umbilical cord. A few minutes later, seeming in very slow motion time, our newborn let go his cord and each one of us experienced an incredible energy rush. We felt his solid committment to be HERE at that moment. In his own time. Thank you Clair Day for telling me about Lotus Birth."

(Editor's Note: Jeannine Parvati is the author of *Prenatal Yoga and Natural Birth* and *Hygieia: A Woman's Herbal*, both reviewed in this *Catalog*.)

UNDERWATER BIRTH

IN UNDERWATER BIRTHING, the mother labors and gives birth while sitting in a tub or trough or pool of warm water. The baby is born into the water and may float submerged for several minutes before being brought to the surface for her first breath. Apparently, newborn babies will not attempt to breathe until brought into the air.

This new method of birth has caused quite a bit of controversy and interest recently. Films of underwater births conducted in the Soviet Union have been shown on American television. Newspapers, magazines, and radio and television shows have interviewed the small number of parents in this country who have given birth in this way. The following resources are available for readers who would like more information on this method.

STAR ENTERPRISES
P.O. Box 10205
Austin, TX 78757
512/453-8194

Rima Beth and Steven Star describe themselves as "Certified Rebirthers" and conduct workshops and courses in "rebirthing" techniques, in which people claim to re-experience their birth. The stars gave birth to their second child under water and found it to be a healing experience. The Star's first child had drowned at the age of four, nine years before.

The Stars offer the following booklets and tapes on underwater birthing.

CELEBRATION! The Underwater Birth of Mela Noel
with Rima and Steven Star
1 hour audio tape
$10.00 plus 15% shipping

"How and Why we created an underwater birth and what we have learned since Mela's birth. Also talks about the relationship between 'conscious birthing' and Rebirthing."

HANDBOOK FOR UNDERWATER BIRTH
by Steven and Rima Beth Star
$3.00 plus 15% shipping

"How we prepared for and gave birth to our daughter. Includes technical information as well as affirmations, processes and techniques for personal and group clearing."

DIVINE CHILDBIRTH AND REBIRTHING
by Rima Beth Star
Reprinted from *Mothering* magazine
$1.00 plus 15 cents shipping

"Observations on the first birth I attended other than my own, immaculate conception, the spiritual side of birthing, the unity of masculine and feminine energies and affirmations for divine childbirth."

BIRTH IN THE NEW AGE
30 minute color videotape
Rental: $30., purchase: $225.

"Includes film and slides of two underwater births—Jeremy Lighthouse and Mela Noel Star. Sandra Ray interviews Rima and Beverly (a pregnant woman planning an underwater birth). Very informative, educational, beautiful and heartwarming."

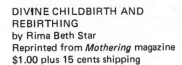

Michel Odent

Underwater births sometimes occur at Michel Odent's clinic in Pithiviers, France, because the mothers become too comfortable to want to get out of the water. In the Summer, 1981 issue of *BIRTH*, Dr. Odent replied to letters questioning the safety of underwater birth for the baby. For more information see the section on Odent, previous page.

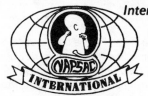

Inter **National Association of Parents & Professionals for Safe Alternatives in Childbirth**

NAPSAC, INTERNATIONAL (NATIONAL ASSOCIATION OF PARENTS AND PROFESSIONALS FOR SAFE ALTERNATIVES IN CHILDBIRTH)
P.O. Box 267
Marble Hill, MO 63764
314/238-2010

The National Association of Parents and Professionals for Safe Alternatives in Childbirth (NAPSAC) is currently the "umbrella organization" for the alternative birth movement in the U.S., bringing together over fifty member groups and many thousands of individual members and supporters across the country. Since 1976 NAPSAC has sponsored major yearly conferences, inviting well-known figures in the alternative birth movement to speak and conduct workshops. The transcripts of some of these conferences have been published in book form and offer a wealth of information on home birth, midwifery, family-centered maternity care, risks of obstetrical practices, and consumer rights in childbirth. NAPSAC publishes a Directory of Alternative Birth Services which lists member groups and individuals offering services and support for birth alternatives. NAPSAC also publishes a very informative quarterly newsletter which provides particularly extensive coverage of cases in which midwives, parents, and physicians have been prosecuted or otherwise harrassed in connection with their home birth activities. NAPSAC representatives have testified at government and court hearings and sit on the advisory boards of several consumer organizations and committees, representing the concerns of parents who want better access to safe alternatives to standard hospital maternity care.

"*Pregnancy and parturition* are unique in health care in that they are *natural* functions, not products of disease. They are events of profound and *lasting emotional significance* in the lives of the families involved. We believe the policies and procedures of the health care community should reflect not only the physical safety of the mother and baby, but also the inseparable and important *psychological needs and desires of parents*. To meet these needs requires flexibility and informed choice in maternity care. . .

"*The responsibility* of pregnancy, childbirth, baby care, and child care ultimately lies with the parents. Personal responsibility of all aspects of parenthood has been gradually relinquished to professionals in many fields. *Rightfully* we depend on professionals for advice, information and expertise *for which they have been trained.* But individuals need to assume *more personal responsibility* in the choices involving their lives and the lives of their families. . . ."

NAPSAC NEWS
$12.00 a year, includes membership

NAPSAC News is a 28-page quarterly newsletter featuring articles on home birth, midwifery, harrassment of alternative birth practitioners, book reviews, letters, notice of resources, and news updates.

NAPSAC DECLARATION OF INDEPENDENCE
single copy free with SASE
10 copies for $1.50

In 1980, the NAPSAC Board approved this declaration to firmly state NAPSAC's position that families and not medical professionals should ultimately determine where and how babies are born. The Declaration was signed by 26 prominent NAPSAC officers and consultants, representing lay midwives, nurse-midwives, childbirth educators, parents, consumer health advocates, and physicians.

"We hold these truths to be self-evident, that all men, women, children, parents and professionals are created equal; that they are endowed by their creator with certain unalienable [sic] rights; that among these are life, liberty, the pursuit of happiness, the right to a safe, natural birth assisted by and in the company of those who love them, the right to be well nourished in their mother's womb, and the right to be breastfed. . .

"The Medical Establishment has sought to limit freedom of choice and the availability of safe, efficacious, beneficial alternatives in health care and has conspired to create and maintain a monopoly in the practice of healing arts by seeking to eliminate midwives and most other potential competitors; seeking to regulate, limit and hold subservient the practices of nurses and all other health professionals; and seeking to force all families into medical centers, hospitals, and routines, by control of how much, to whom, and for what services the payment of insurance and government reimbursements are to be made, as well as by entrenching its authority through the coercion of city, county, state, provincial, and national laws, statutes and regulations."

REFERRAL SERVICES

To people who inquire about alternative birth services, NAPSAC provides an introductory brochure on the organization, a flyer describing their books and publications, an order form for their mail-order book service (over 70 titles are available), and a sheet listing the addresses of all current member groups. Please include a self-addressed, stamped envelope with your inquiry.

NAPSAC DIRECTORY OF ALTER-NATIVE BIRTH SERVICES AND CONSUMER GUIDE
1982, 198 pages
$5.95

NAPSAC's Directory begins with an excellent 37-page consumer guide to choosing and using health care services, written by Penny Simkin. The *Consumer Guide* is also available separately for $2.00 (see index). The Directory itself lists over 4,000 individual and group members of NAPSAC, indicating what birth services they provide. Services include birth centers, childbirth education, home birth care, information and referrals, labor coaching, midwifery, etc. Listings are arranged in zip code order by state (to help readers find the nearest local resources) with a cross-index of names in alphabetical order. Also included is an annotated listing of selected national organizations, journals, periodicals, and other resources in alternative birth.

BOOKS

THE FIVE STANDARDS FOR SAFE CHILDBEARING
by David Stewart
1981, 483 pages

The five standards for safe birth, as ennumerated by NAPSAC director David Stewart, are good nutrition, skillful midwifery, natural childbirth, home birth, and breastfeeding. Stewart elaborates on each of these and presents an especially strongly worded case in favor of midwifery for all normal births, arguing that the more highly specialized the birth attendant (i.e. board-certified obstetrician), the worse the mortality rates for birth. He says, "Between 1940 and 1980, at least a million babies have died in American hospitals who would have lived were it not for the doctor-dominated maternity system that dictates standards for American childbirth. At least 30,000 mothers died from childbirth that should not have died. At least 1.5 million babies were severely brain damaged because of obstetrical procedures. At least 45 million children suffered minor brain damage who would have been normal. These include reading and other educational disabilities, as well as generally lower I.Q.'s. . . . These unnecessary injuries continue to the present day. On an average, at least one baby dies every 29 age, at least one baby dies every 29 minutes in an American Hospital because of doctors—babies that would be born healthy and live under the care of properly trained midwives." Stewart provides extensive documentation for these assertions, citing several hundred scientific and tech-nical sources. Additional chapters have been included by speakers at the 1979 NAPSAC conference held in Nashville, Tennessee, including G.J. Kloosterman on midwifery in the modern world, Ina May Gaskin on lay midwifery, Rhondda Hartman on childbirth education, Yvonne Brackbill on the hazards of obstetrical drugs, Marion Tompson on breastfeeding, and Lewis Mehl on emotional factors in birth. In an appendix, "How to Choose a Safe Birth Attendant," Stewart presents a very useful and candid guide to evaluating the safety of potential birth attendants, comparing midwives, family-practice physicians, and obstetricians.

"The reality of maternity services in today's American system is that the alternatives available to most parents are not ideal. The best and safest birth attendants are either not there locally or, if there, are legally prohibited from practice. For most parents, the choices are between two extremes, both negative: A technologic assembly-line hospital delivery of certain risk or a medically unattended birth at home without back-up. In this situation, the safer of these two negatives is often the UHB [unattended home birth]. This is especially so where the parents are responsible and mature and are willing to put forth a great deal of effort to become informed. . . . Better, in these cases, to accept the slight unknown risk of an informed UHB than the significant and known risk of an interventive, technologic hospital."

"For most parents, the choices are between two extremes, both negative: a technologic assembly-line hospital delivery of certain risk or a medically unattended birth at home without back-up. In this situation, the safer of these two negatives is often the UHB."

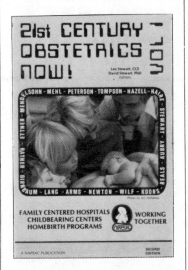

21st CENTURY OBSTETRICS NOW!
Edited by David and Lee Stewart
1977, 625 pages, Illus.
$12.25 (2-volume set)

This 2-volume set features talks presented by over 30 speakers at the NAPSAC conference held in Chicago, in 1977. Topics include safety of home birth, the role of women in birth services, the future of nurse-midwifery, risks of hospital birth, psychological issues in alternative birth, family and infant bonding, birth centers, home birth, nutrition in pregnancy, breastfeeding, lay midwifery, and legal aspects of alternative birth.

COMPULSORY HOSPITALIZA-TION OR FREEDOM OF CHOICE IN CHILDBIRTH? (3 volume set)
Edited by David and Lee Stewart
1979, 986 pages, Illus.
$19.50 pap.

This three-volume set is based on talks given at the 1978 NAPSAC conference held in Atlanta, Georgia. It includes presentations by over 80 well-known contributers on government regulation, perinatal regionalization, obstetric intervention, and hospital practice (Vol. I); midwifery, birth centers, home birth, and legal aspects (Vol. II); and consumer involvement, childbirth education, children at birth, and philosophical topics (Vol. III).

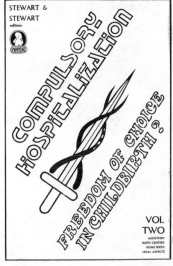

SAFE ALTERNATIVES IN CHILD-BIRTH
Edited by David and Lee Stewart
1976, 193 pages, Illus.
$5.95 pap.

This book is a transcript of the first NAPSAC conference held in Arlington, Virginia, in 1976. It includes presentations by 22 contributors on topics including the trend toward home birth, maternity practices around the world, birth centers, home birth statistics, lay midwifery, parents' reasons for choosing home birth, and legal aspects of home birth.

Herbs and Natural Healing

Many women are using and recommending herbs for the common complaints of pregnancy and childbirth and for health care in general. Herbs can be a good replacement for some more harmful medications, but it's important to realize that herbs also contain chemically active substances which can be harmful. If an herb is potent enough to produce an effect on you, be very careful about its use. Be sure you are certain about the properties of any herbs you use and consult a book on herbal pharmacology if you are not sure.

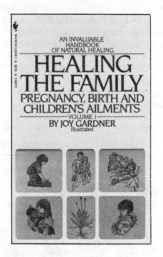

AN INVALUABLE HANDBOOK OF NATURAL HEALING.

HEALING THE FAMILY
PREGNANCY, BIRTH AND CHILDREN'S AILMENTS
VOLUME I
BY JOY GARDNER
Illustrated

HEALING THE FAMILY: Pregnancy, Birth and Children's Ailments (Volume I)
by Joy Gardner
1982, 347 pages, Illus.

from
Bantam Books
666 Fifth Avenue
New York, NY 10103
$3.95 pap.

This book describes natural healing through the use of herbs and nutrition. It includes extensive coverage of pre-pregnancy health concerns, common complaints of pregnancy, nutrition and things to avoid in pregnancy, preparing for birth, labor, after the birth, breastfeeding, and the care of infants and children (including the pros and cons of immunization). Included is a table of "Identification and Safety/Toxicity Status of Herbs which are Listed in this Book" which includes their GRAS status (generally recognized as safe) according to the Food and Drug Administration.
(Editor's Note: The original self-published version of this book, *Healing Yourself,* is available from Healing Yourself, Box 752, Vashon, WA 98070

"... it's important to realize that just because a substance is 'natural,' there is no guarantee that it will be harmless. For example, recent studies have shown that comfrey, the beloved herb of many people, contains cancer-causing substances. I discussed this with Dr. Farnsworth, who has tested many samples of comfrey roots and leaves and has found these cancer-causing substances in most roots and some leaves. His personal opinion is that it probably wouldn't be harmful for an adult male, for example, to drink comfrey leaf tea two or three times a week. However, in the case of a pregnant woman, even a minute amount of a possibly harmful substance could harm the fetus, so he suggests that pregnant women should avoid comfrey tea entirely, though he feels that external use would be all right. In this book, I have recommended several teas for nonpregnant women and children, which contain small amounts of comfrey leaves. None of these teas are taken for more than one week. Comfrey is an extremely healing herb, and I do not want to leave it out of our pharmacopoeia entirely. I think that if we use it carefully and moderately, it can continue to be very useful . . . .

"People who use folk medicine are often cautioned by professionals that we may do harm to ourselves by trying to treat our own illnesses. But I am just as concerned about doing harm to myself by taking a poisonous medicine for what is often a minor complaint. I do not believe in *starting* with highly powerful drugs when there are more benign alternatives that can be tried first. If these are not effective, and the condition grows worse, then we are fortunate to have stronger medicines to resort to.

"Before the advent of modern medicine, most healing was done with herbs, by midwives. When that changed, something was lost and something was gained. Now many women and men are going back, hoping to retrieve what was lost. If we're careful, we may be able to do this without losing what was gained."

HYGIEIA: A Woman's Herbal
by Jeannine Parvati
1978, 248 pages, Illus.

from
Freestone Publishing Company
P.O. Box 398
Monroe, Utah 84754
$10.00

This is a very beautifully illustrated and printed book with lovely drawings and decorative borders and calligraphy. The text was written by Jeannine Parvati in fulfillment of a master's degree in psychology at the University of California (which, after some reluctance from the department chairman, was accepted). She also wrote *Prenatal Yoga and Natural Birth* (see index). Her book covers the use of herbs in menstruation, infertility, herbal birth control, anaphrodisiac herbs, aphrodisiac herbs, herbs for the mind (psychedelic drugs), self health, balancers and toners (herbs for the cycle and reproductive organs), herbs for pregnancy, childbirth, lactation, and menopause. Also included is a whole series of appendices consisting of letters, essays, dreams, meditations, recipes, etc. Jeannine Parvati is an original mind and her ideas are always stimulating. I cannot testify as to the empirical value of her herb lore, but it hardly seems to matter whether the herb remedies work or not. It is a delight just to look at and read this book.

"This is the best of all possible times to begin your herb garden. As a tiny sprout of your love grows within, your days are filled with tender caretaking of herbal seedlings. The daily visit, under Mr. Sun's shining glow, to your herbal garden will help you develop qualities every mother needs—patience, tenderness, unconditional loving, plus discipline—just to get out there each and every day. This is akin to any spiritual practice which requires perserverance—good preparation for tending to the daily needs of a baby. Gardening literally gets you in touch with the Mother, our Earth. It is so much like our own fertile wombs. Enjoy your quiet moments among the herbal flowers—catching fairies out of the corners of your eyes—breathing the freshness of these plant friends. These moments may be your last of sustained silence for quite awhile after your baby is born—savor them. The coming of children are a bouquet of sound; yet silence has its own healing, a special healing . . . .

"I would guess that the majority of newly delivered women might not pay much heed to their placentas, especially *after* it passed from the body. But an ever-growing group of beings devoted to awareness, are obeying very old rituals about placentas. The Salish woman on the coast of British Columbia would bury her placenta with a scallop shell, thusly giving her a few years rest inbetween pregnancies. The Cherokee father would walk over as many ridges with the placenta as years they desired not to conceive children. There he would bury it deep in the ground. A lot of my natural childbirth students, with no placenta recipe to follow, so to speak, spontaneously decide to bury them. It's a rich experience—we buried one deep in the center of a circular garden one summer. However, many others elect to eat their placentas, vegetarians alike, though less likely on the whole. On cooking: prepare the placenta any way you enjoy(ed) the organs of animals. Liver, or better yet, kidney recipes are good starters. Read a few in the natural foods cookbooks and then forget them. When you first encounter the meat, remember to pause—placenta can be sacred food, if you let the meat tell you how to prepare it for the fire. (Raw is possible always—it's up to you.) The Paiute Indians thought that the woman might become barren if her placenta were eaten by an animal (or buried upside down to boot!). Were contraception this easy . . . ."

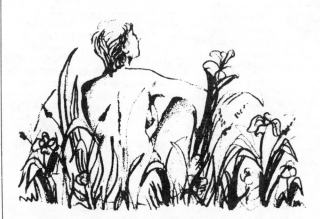

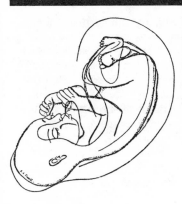

ACUPUNCTURE AND HERBS FOR OBSTETRICS
by Shelley Sovola Francis
1980

from
Shelley S. Francis
2455½ Cheremoya Avenue
Los Angeles, CA 90068
$6.95

"A new text for professionals and lay persons. The book covers Acupuncture/Acupressure Points and Auricular (ear) Points for Pre-Natal thru Post-Natal care of mother and infant. In depth usage of Moxibustion and Herbal formulas that are easily available. Included are charts for accurate Point location. A section is included as a reading list, with suppliers of books, herbs, health care practitioners in the Los Angeles area." (Shelley S. Francis)

HERBS, HELPS, AND PRESSURE POINTS FOR PREGNANCY AND CHILDBIRTH
by Katherine Tarr
1981, 49 pages, Illus.

from
Katherine Tarr
780 North 2250 West
Provo, UT 84601
$3.50 pap.
bulk rates available

Katherine Tarr is a lay midwife practicing in Utah and this booklet is based on her own experience in providing prenatal care and care for birth. She identifies red raspberry, alfalfa, and comfrey as the three most useful herbs for pregnancy, mainly because of their high contents of vitamins and minerals. She briefly discusses diet, weight gain, drugs and exercise in pregnancy and describes the old-fashioned sitz bath as an all-purpose help for many complaints of pregnancy (a sitz bath simply involves sitting in a washtub or bath tub filled with very warm or cold water). Katherine provides advice on natural remedies, including herbs and diet changes for common problems in pregnancy. There is a section on comfort measures for labor, including acupressure points, herbs, and aids for after the birth. There are also sections on breast-feeding, circumcision, natural remedies for common newborn problems, and on bonding.

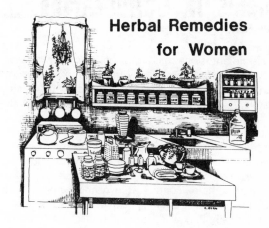

HERBAL REMEDIES FOR WOMEN
by Robin Van Liew
1980

from
Feminist Health Works
325 Spring Street, Room 227
New York, NY 10013
request price information

This revised and expanded booklet provides a self-help approach to women's health concerns, including menstruation, fertility consciousness, menopause, pregnancy, and childbirth. Certain commonplace foods and their therapeutic uses are explained. Information on herbs includes simple recipes, preparations, and where to buy them. Proceeds go to the support of Feminist Health Works (see index).

HERB SUPPLIERS FOR PREGNANCY AND BIRTH

WISH GARDEN HERBS
P.O. Box 1304
Boulder, CO 80306
303/449-0059

Barbara Wishingrad, of Wish Garden Herbs, is Assistant Director of Informed Homebirth (see index). She writes the following about her herb business:

"I have studied herbs and natural healing for eight years, midwifery for two years. Last October (1981) I began to make herbal preparations specifically for pregnancy and birth, combining these two interests with my love for ritual—I do all my herb work on the new moon. By June I had grown into a small mail order business; in July I started teaching workshops to share the recipes and ritual with others who wanted to use herbal combinations made by their own hand. For others, too busy or unable to do so, I offer homemade herbal tinctures, salves, oils and bath herbs made in tune with nature's cycles and love for the herbs and for women and babies. I fresh pick and dry my own herbs whenever possible."

Wishingrad offers an anti-itching Pregnancy Belly Oil and an After Birth Sitz Bath Pak (five individual packages) which includes comfrey leaves, comfrey root, myrrh, garlic, sage, sea salt, uva ursi, shepherd's purse, and osha root.

Write for a complete list of herb products and prices.

PAN'S FOREST HERB COMPANY
Route 1, Box 211
East Jordan, MI 49727
616/536-7445

Pan's Forest offers dried herbs, tinctures, sachets and pillows, bath herbs, and amulet bags. Their Postpartum Bath Blend includes "thyme (reduces swelling and soreness), lavendar (calmative, antiseptic, aids in clearing airways), sage (astringent), comfrey (aids healing), and rosemary (antiseptic and astringent)."

"Pan's Forest Herb Company is located about 60 feet from the goat barn, tucked into the edge of a northern Michigan forest. Because of my background as a midwife, you may notice an emphasis on herbs and herb products that are useful in childbirth and child-raising. As a midwife and mother I have found herbs in tincture form to be particularly helpful. They save time and trouble, take up much less room in a crowded birth kit or diaper bag than do dried herbs, and are palatable, powerful, and easily assimilated by the body. . . . raspberry leaves, shepard's purse, and comfrey have common use in pregnancy and birth."

—Loren of Pan's Forest

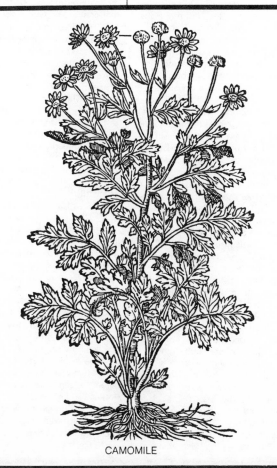

CAMOMILE

Problems in Childbearing

Infants at Risk

Priya Morganstern, editor

A high risk infant is one that has a significantly increased chance of mortality, morbidity, or both, any time within 29 days after birth, or an increased chance of subsequent disability. Each year approximately 250,000 newborns are considered high risk due to structural and/or functional intrauterine growth deviations (IUGD), or inappropriate gestational age (prematurity or postmaturity). Many of these high risk conditions—such as intestinal obstruction or imperforate anus—require immediate surgery but should not otherwise cause critical problems. Others—such as prematurity or spina bifida—are complex conditions involving many different therapies and treatments. Lifelong handicaps may result.

Treating critically ill newborns requires special facilities, highly trained personnel, and tremendous amounts of money. Neonatal Intensive Care Units (NICU's) are developing across the country to offer high technology-high quality care. Neonatology has recently come into its own as a medical specialty, and it is estimated that the United States spends $200 billion a year to treat critically ill babies. As a result, we are seeing an increased survival rate among babies that previously would have died and the babies that do survive are also not as handicapped as was previously expected. However, tremendous legal and ethical issues are frequently involved and the rapidly growing technology is making the situation even more difficult. As treatments improve and become more routine, parent's rights of choice may become eroded. And as treatment starts to occur more frequently during the fetal stage, the entire concept of when the fetus becomes a patient must be explored: (If both fetus and mother are "patients," whose rights take precedence?).

Of the many neonatal high-risk conditions which can occur, only those for which there are support groups or other resources are included here. Information on the other, more unusual conditions can usually be found in nursing or medical texts. See these other sections of the book: "High Risk Pregnancy," "Genetic Testing," and "Parenting." (PM)

PARENT-INFANT BONDING
by Marshall Klaus and John Kennell
1982, 314 pages, Illus.

from
C.V. Mosby Co.
11830 Westline Industrial Drive
St. Louis, MO 63141
$17.95 Hardcover

This recently revised classic contains substantial chapters which are relevant to the study of high risk infants: "Caring for the Parents of Premature or Sick Infants" and "Caring for the Parents of an Infant With a Congenital Malformation," and they all contain a wealth of information that is useful not only to parents, but also to health professionals, counselors and social workers.

The discussions include a brief history of "styles" of neonatology, parent's reactions to premature births, and observations made after discharge. Klaus and Kennell feel that the parents' hospital experience is a very relevant factor in their relationship with the baby, and make several recommendations. These include opening the Neonatal Intensive Care Unit to parents, keeping baby and mother in the same hospital (or transporting one or the other to do so), rooming-in for the parent, early discharge of baby, and use of parent support groups. (PM)

"Had we read closely the first text of neonatology by (Pierre) Budin (1907), we could have foreseen and perhaps avoided the tragic problems that became associated with the care of premature or sick infants. In his book, *The Nursling*, he wrote, 'Unfortunately... a certain number of mothers abandon the babies whose needs they have not had to meet, and in whom they have lost all interest. The life of the little one has been saved, it is true, but at the cost of the mother.'

"The anxieties of a parent about to enter the nursery for the first time, whether in the 1950's or today, are naturally much greater than those of the physician. The average mother who comes to visit her infant—let us say a daughter—was not prepared physically or emotionally for the early birth, and she is still shaky from it. She is extremely anxious about the health of her daughter, wonders about any abnormalities, worries about whether she will be criticized for producing an unfinished, feeble, imperfect product, and fears that she may carry germs which will harm her daughter. She enters the brightly lit, stainless steel and glass citadel, filled with unfamilar sounds and smells, densely populated by intense young men and women who rush from incubator to incubator, manipulate complicated equipment, and spend long periods of time hovering over individual babies with serious expressions on their faces. These activities appear ominous and suggest an air of great tension—even after several visits. It is not until she has been told that her daughter is definitely progressing well or, far better, until she has touched and seen for herself, that she can begin to relax. But there are usually frightening surprises at the early visits. Complicated wires, fine tubes, large tubes, bandages on the head, arms, or legs, and bright lights and bandages on the eyes cover the baby. She is so tiny, so different from a normal baby. Her head is large, her extremities thin, her movements jerky, and her respirations irregular and labored.... At each visit a new problem may be discovered or announced, and with every problem the mother feels a sharp visceral pain. 'Do babies with jaundice live?' 'How will she ever stand the strain of breathing so hard when she is already so small and fragile?' 'Does such a tiny thing ever grow up to be a full-sized child or adult?' 'Are they really telling me the truth?' 'What have I done to my poor child?' "

IS MY BABY ALL RIGHT?:
A Guide to Birth Defects
by Virginia Apgar and Joan Beck
1972, 493 pages, Illus.

from
Trident Press
630 Fifth Avenue
New York, NY 10020

Virginia Apgar, M.D., is an internationally recognized specialist in the problems of newborn infants. She is the creator of the APGAR scoring system (see index), has been involved with over 17,000 deliveries, and is director of the National Foundation-March of Dimes. With Ms. Beck, a syndicated columnist, she has written a classic book dealing with the subject of defects and disorders present in the newborn (or shortly thereafter) due to genetic or environmental causes. "A birth defect will be defined as any abnormality present at birth or immediately afterward which will make a difference in the child's life by affecting his survival or by requiring special attention from parents, family, physicians, teachers, specialists of any kind, or other members of the community." This admittedly broad and humanistic definition reflects the author's attempt to help the largest possible number of families and specialists who work with handicapped children.

Included in the book are defects due to genetic problems, accidents at birth, and lack of adequate diet or prenatal care during pregnancy. A good deal of the book, in fact, is devoted to discussions of "how life begins," "life before birth," and "what can go wrong and why"—the rest of the book discusses, in alphabetical order, dozens of the most common birth defects.

The beauty and real value of *Is My Baby All Right?* lies in its clarity and readability. Although relevant medical terms are included where necessary, most discussions are in lay terms and are easily understood. Many short "case histories" are used. Even difficult genetic concepts are clearly explained.

For parents whose new child has been diagnosed as having a specific disorder, this book is truly an invaluable source of information. (PM)

"So many hundreds of thousands of intricate steps must be taken in precise order in the making of a human baby, the wonder is not that a small percentage of infants are born with defects, but that most children are so nearly perfect.

"Hundreds of different defects are known to occur because there is a mistake in the blueprint contained in the genes which provide the set of instructions for a baby's prenatal growth. This error can be so small that it involves only one of tens of thousands of genes in the egg or sperm that combined to start the infant—a mistake comparable to one misspelled word in a whole book. Or, the abnormality may be caused by an entire chromosome—almost as if there were an extra chapter or some misplaced pages in a book of directions for making a baby.

"Other big groups of birth defects begin during the earliest weeks of prenatal life, when a tiny mistake can occur in the precise timetable of development. Just a few cells may not appear in just the right places at just the right day or hour, or they may not function exactly as they should. Because these key cells direct the growth of many subsequent bits of tissue, what seems to be an exceedingly minor error can result in a major birth defect.

"Most birth defects have already been built inexorably into an unborn infant by the end of the first three months of prenatal life. Only a few begin later on in pregnancy, or result from injuries during the process of birth itself."

BORN AT RISK
by B. D. Colen
1981, 212 pages, Illus.

from
St. Martins Press
175 Fifth Avenue
New York, NY 10010
$9.95 hd.

Born at Risk has a long, but descriptive subtitle: *The Dramatic True Story of the Struggle for Life In an Intensive Care Nursery.* More than a book about high risk infants, it is a paean to the science of neonatology. The book basically describes the art and science of caring for critically ill newborns, the efforts of the doctors and nurses involved, and the dilemmas and choices presented to parents when the prognosis for their child is poor or unknown. By following the events of a fictitious neonatal intensive care unit (NICU) over a period of 24 hours, Colen conveys the amount of skill, technology and heart that is present in a good, critcal care nursery. In fact, the book's greatest asset is that it reveals how large a difference a *good* NICU can make in outcome—both for a society in general, and for a family in particular.   (PM)

''. . . a recent study by the National Capital Medical Foundation

. . . found that over 90 percent of the newborn infants who died in Washington in 1977 weighed less than 2,500 grams at birth. They were, by definition, born at risk. But what was particularly horrifying was the wide variation in mortality rates at different hospitals: The best hospital in the city saved 54 percent of the babies born weighing between 500 and 1,000 grams, while the next-best, a private university teaching hospital, saved only about 33 percent. Another university hospital had less than a 25 percent survival rate for infants in the same weight group, and D.C. General Hospital, the city's municipal hospital, had about an 86 percent *mortality* rate—it saved only 14 percent of the babies in the same weight category in which the best hospital saved 54 percent.

"The study, which examined the care the dead infants received in the hospital, painted a picture that can only suggest that these very low birthweight babies are being written off as unsavable in hospitals just a few miles from the National Institutes of Health, and only blocks from the seat of the federal health establishment."

THE RESULT OF INTENSIVE CARE THERAPY FOR NEONATES
by T. Thompson and J. Reynolds
1977, 17 pages

from
Professional Education Division
The National Foundation/March of Dimes
1275 Mamaroneck Ave.
White Plains, NY 10605
single copy free

This reprinted article is part of the March of Dimes *Perinatal Reprint Series.* The article is from the *Journal of Perinatal Medicine*; both authors are physicians. Thompson and Reynolds examine the impact of the development of Neonatal Intensive Care Units (NICU's) on overall neonatal mortality rates and long term prognosis for low-birth-weight (LBW) babies.

The study is a very detailed, statistical evaluation of selected hospitals and regions. The results led the authors to make the following conclusions:
1) There has been marked improvement in the overall survival rates for neonates with the advent and increasing utilization of NICU's.
2) Current survival rates approach 75% to 95% for LBW infants cared for in NICU's.
3) The long-term prognosis for LBW infants has significantly improved since the introduction to intensive care therapy.

4) The increased survival rate of LBW babies has not resulted in larger numbers of retarded or handicapped infants.

In addition the authors recommend that women in premature labor (especially under 34 weeks) be transferred to a regional high risk perinatal center.   (P.M.)

"There has been a reduction among LBW survivors in the incidence of such disabling handicaps as moderate to severe mental retardation; neurologic or physical sequelae including cerebral palsy or seizures; severe deafness; and blindness. Both growth and development have dramatically improved with better management of LBW infants. Not all survivors are perfect, but the majority do not have incapacitating defects requiring institutional care, and the minor defects do not usually preclude a useful and rewarding life in society. As once feared, *implementation of intensive care therapy for critically-ill neonates has not saved children who are brain-damaged or severely handicapped, but has been responsible for an improved physical and developmental status for survivors. . . .''*

SHELISE
2 lbs, 4 oz. at birth

poked and prodded from your first breath
whisked away and wired to avert death
never held in your mother's arms
why did you want to come so soon

i've never seen anything so small
full of the power of life
struggling to fill your lungs with breath
your mother never held you
you should be held in a jar

do we let you go
or do we try with all of science
to keep you in your body
if you go we still hold you in our souls
if you stay you have lost your mother's arms
does saving you do more good than harm

Karen Hope Ehrlich, from *Birth Song* (see index for review).
© 1979 Karen Hope Ehrlich. Reprinted by permission.

SAVING BABIES BEFORE BIRTH:
The New Promise of Fetal Surgery
by Robin Marantz
New York Times magazine
February 28, 1982
10 pages, Illus., starts page 18

Available on microfilm in your local library. Copies may be made directly from microfilm at a reasonable cost.

With the advent of new methods of prenatal diagnosis, parents of "defective" fetuses are faced with the sometimes agonizing choice of carrying a child who may be severely disabled or having an abortion. There are some who believe that perinatal surgery offers an alternative.

A very new technique, fetal corrective surgery has been performed on 20 fetuses to correct defects that include hydrocephalus ("water on the brain"), hydronephrosis (blockage in urinary tract), and fluid in the lungs. There have been cases where the surgery was successful and prevented the death or disability of the baby; some of these cases are outlined in the article. But fetal surgery —viewed by some as miraculous—also opens up a Pandora's box of ethical problems. Besides the fundamental problem of deciding at what point the fetus can be considered a patient, doctors and parents must grapple with the fact that by the time a defect is diagnosed, it may have caused secondary damage that remains even if the defect is corrected. Also, anomalies frequently come in groups; treating one may merely keep alive a fetus which will be born with

other defects. And finally, the procedure itself may be fatal to the baby.

Morantz clearly presents both sides of the fetal surgery issue. While admiring the technology and acknowledging its potential usefulness, she never loses sight of the moral issues involved.   (PM)

"The prospect of such intervention, risky as it is, raises fundamental questions about when life begins and leads, inevitably, to issues of abortion and the right to life. If the fetus can be treated, then is it a patient? If it is a patient, then is it a person? When is this status reached? How much risk should the fetus, and its mother, be expected to endure—especially when there is no guarantee of a normal outcome? And if the treatment of certain conditions *in utero* becomes commonplace, what are the implications if the parent refuses fetal surgery, or opts for an abortion?"

NEONATAL INTENSIVE CARE:
A Bibiography
prepared by Eileen Koff
1979, 9 pages

from
National Library of Medicine
8600 Rockville Pike
Bethesda, MD 20209
(request Literature Search No. 79-21, Neonatal Intensive Care)

This bibliography is part of the National Library of Medicine's Literature Search Program. It contains 131 citations, all of which are from professional journals.   (PM)

LOW BIRTH WEIGHT

Low birth weight (LBW) babies are those that weigh less than 5½ pounds at birth. The baby may be premature, small-for-gestational-age (SGA), or both. One out of every 13 babies in the United States is born too early, too small, or both. LBW infants account for 70% of all neonatal deaths, half of which occur during the first 24 hours of life.

In the past, weight was thought to indicate maturity and all babies below 2500 grams (5½ pounds) were considered premature. Now it is understood that intra-uterine growth retardation is a separate problem and may require care that is different than that for a "premie." Both types of babies require special attention to thermoregulation (body temperature) and nutrition. The premie in particular is likely to develop respiratory distress syndrome, a very serious condition.

A premature baby will often spend its first weeks, and even months, in an intensive care nursery. Besides the tremendous financial burden this places on the parents and on society, the physical separation itself can also cause problems with the relationship between parents and child. It is believed that prolonged early separation of parent and infant disturbs the bonding process and may have life-long consequences. In fact, studies have shown that an unusually high percentage of abused children were premature babies and/or spent the first weeks of life in a special care nursery.

American women give birth to an unusually high number of low birth weight infants, with small babies being born to black women twice as frequently as to white. Although premature and SGA babies have been born to well-nourished, healthy mothers of all income levels, there are certain maternal factors that do predispose a woman to give birth to a small baby. LBW infants are more often born to women who are: under 16; undernourished; addicted to cigarettes, alcohol or narcotics; or who have not had regular prenatal care. Clearly, most LBW births should be preventable. On a personal level this means good diet habits and regular prenatal care. On a public scale it means increased funding for outreach education, midwifery training, and food supplement programs like WIC (Women, Infants and Children program). (PM)

FOR FURTHER READING

MY BABY IS A SPECIAL CARE INFANT: A Parent's Guide to Neonatal Intensive Care
by M. Jude Langhurst, 1981

from
PFSCI
1452 Mulrose
Wichita, KS 67212

GETTING TO KNOW YOUR PRE-MATURE BABY
by Sharon Cozine Metcalf, 1978

from
Children and Youth Project
Department of Pediatrics
University of Louisville
323 E. Chestnut Street
Louisville, KY 40203

THE PREMATURE INFANT
by Nancy Shosenberg, 1980

from
The Hospital for Sick Children
555 University Avenue, Room 1218
Toronto, Ontario
M5G 1X8 Canada

BREASTFEEDING RESOURCES

BREASTFEEDING YOUR PRE-MATURE BABY
1980, 12 pages
$.50

A MOTHER'S GUIDE TO BREAST-FEEDING AND MOTHERING THE PREMATURE OR HOSPITALIZED SICK INFANT
1979, 4 pages
$.25

BREASTFEEDING THE BABY WITH A CLEFT OF THE SOFT PALATE
1980, 4 pages
$.25

BREASTFEEDING THE DOWN'S SYNDROME BABY
1980, 8 pages
$.75

All available from:
La Leche League
9616 Minneapolis Avenue
Franklin Park, IL 60131

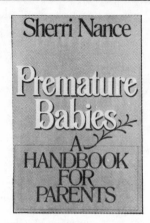

PREMATURE BABIES: A Handbook for Parents
by Sherri Nance
1982, 322 pages, Illus.

from
Arbor House Publishing Company
235 East 45th St.
New York, NY 10017
$15.95 hardcover

In Houston in 1976, five mothers who had given birth prematurely found each other and started to meet as a support group. They were joined by a perinatal social worker, and a few of their husbands, and continued to meet informally in members' homes. The group grew quickly, and the members found that regardless of individual experiences, certain feelings were shared in common. They formed a telephone support group. They gave presentations at hospital staff meetings, school workshops, and statewide conferences. Writing a book was the obvious next step.

Sherri Nance, with the help of other members of her organization, Premature Inc., has written a desperately needed book and has done an excellent job of it. The book is the only one we know of that is specifically designed for the parent of a premature baby. Because it is written by other parents of prematures, the book focuses on exactly what a parent needs to know. In the first half of the book, Nance deals with the hospital experience after the birth of a premature child. She discusses some causes and effects of prematurity, and parents' role in the care of their baby. She gives detailed descriptions of the Neonatal Intensive Care Unit, its equipment, and staff—explaining everything briefly but clearly. She also provides a list of steps that can be taken to cope financially with the child's care. Nance recommends asking questions of the staff and giving the baby as much love and stimulation as possible (and/or permissable). In short, she tries to help parents feel as comfortable with the situation as possible through preparation and knowledge.

The second half of the book focuses on parenting the premature in-

fant. She discusses the reactions of friends and families and the emotional state of the parents, including their fears. A large portion is devoted to feeding the child, with information on breast pumping, care of the breast, and switching from bottle to breast when the baby comes home. She does include information on formulas and instances when formula use would be indicated.

Finally, the book has a very good glossary, and list of other resources, and patterns for making clothing to fit very small babies. (PM)

"Communication is always difficult between a professional and those unfamiliar with the specialized language of that professional's field. Such communication is even more complicated when it deals with such an emotional issue as the health of a child. Confusion can arise when the professionals caring for the child do not agree . . . .

"How do parents react to such a conflict of opinions? The debate concerns *their* child, whom they want to live, grow and thrive. In this particular case, the parents' emotions swayed each time they heard a new report: from a hopeful 'wait-and-see' attitude, to guilt and sadness at the thought of the things their son may never be able to do, to renewed hope when presented with a brighter outlook.

"These parents realized that a matter of judgment was involved and that they should keep asking questions. The doctors who care for premies are faced with life-and-death situations on a daily basis, but the questions that arise change as smaller and smaller babies are helped to survive. A doctor may not know whether a baby can be saved nor the possible long-term effects that may result from that baby's early birth. The doctor can only use past experience to deal with the complications that arise. The doctor has a responsibility to the child to follow the course that seems most logical in the treatment of a particular condition. Parents have the responsibility to continually ask questions about treatment which seems incomplete or inadequate. In some instances, parents may wish to seek second and even third opinions from other medical specialists. As one parent puts it:

'The whole thing boils down to the fact that these doctors bust their butts while having to shoot in the dark. They have to make educated guesses based on a hell of a lot of experience and the available facts. But doctors still are not prophets who predict the absolute future. If your child makes it and how well depends to a great extent on how hard your child is willing to fight to live.'

"Quite often, no one doctor is completely right and no prognosis is completely wrong. Continual reassessment of the situation is called for."

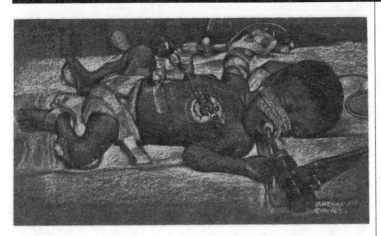

PRE-TERM BABIES
by Marilyn Sargent
1980, 14 pages, Illus.

from
Public Inquiries
National Institute of Mental Health
5600 Fishers Lane
Rockville, MD 20857
free (request DHHS Pub. No. (ADM)
80-972)

Part of the *Caring for Kids* series, this booklet briefly defines and describes prematurity in easy-to-understand terms. It lists possible causes and factors and stresses that smoking is definitely associated with low birth weight babies. The booklet is conscientious in warning of the possible hazards of drugs and medications taken during pregnancy, but less careful about describing the risks of diagnostic procedures like amniocentesis, ultra-sound, and x-rays. In general, however, the emphasis is on good medical care started in early pregnancy and good nutrition to prevent premature births.

The booklet also describes the intensive care nursery, the role of parents, and the special stress they will feel while their child is in ICU. It discusses possibilities of problems in the future, although it states that 75% of

premature babies develop normally. For calming irritable "premies" the author recommends a traditional method (substantiated by research of course): swaddling. (PM)

"One of the simplest and most effective calming techniques is swaddling which involves wrapping a baby securely from shoulders to feet with a small blanket or sheeting, much in the way that Indian mothers wrap their papooses. While parents may feel uncomfortable about restricting the movement of their infants arms and legs in this way [researchers] found that swaddling for limited times seems to soothe babies.

"No one is sure why swaddling is such an effective calmer. Possibly it gives a baby a sense of security to be tightly enwrapped, or maybe it is the sensory stimulation of the blanket or sheet on the baby's skin. Researchers have found that various other types of sensory stimulation—certain sounds and movements, for instance—seem to calm babies. Although parents may not have realized they were stimulating their baby's senses by holding, rocking, singing, and talking to them, they have long used these techniques to soothe their infants."

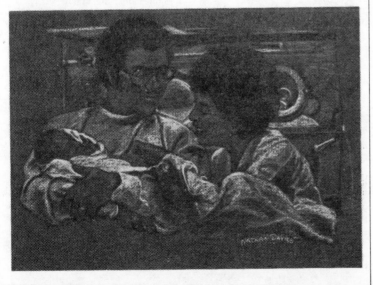

PARENTS OF PREMATURES
13613 NE 26th Place
Bellevue, WA 98005
206/883-6040

Parents of Prematures is a parent support group made up of parents who have experienced the birth and hospitalization of a premature or sick baby, and who share an interest in offering emotional and educational support to others. The organization is supported in part by a grant from the March of Dimes and is an affiliate of the Childbirth Education Association of Seattle.

The group offers telephone contacts with trained outreach parents, guidelines for breastfeeding a premie, a monthly newsletter, parent education meetings, and speakers for classes, meetings and conferences. The group also offers services designed especially for health professionals, such as assistance in developing informal classes for parents of premies within the hospital, and in-service training sessions for the staff.

Parents of Prematures welcomes your story of your "premature experience" for publication in their newsletter, which is available free. A Parent Support Group Packet containing information and guidelines is available for $2.00. (PM)

SPECIAL PATTERNS
by Patricia Silvers
Box 217-WB
Lopez Island, WA 98261
$2.95 plus $.75 postage

Patricia Silvers has designed a layette set for "extra small babies": those who weigh three to four pounds. The patterns are for a drawstring gown, a cap, a long sleeve shirt, a short sleeve shirt, and a footed sleeper. (PM)

"When a parent (especially father) sees the tiny premature baby surrounded by mechanical devices, 'plugged' into sensors and monitors, tubes, etc., and encased in plastic—s/he almost does not recognize the baby as a real human being.

"Clothing—with laces and trims, etc., makes a baby seem more 'real,' to say nothing of clothing being functional; keeping a 3 pound baby's own body heat in is so important. When they can start emerging from their incubators, they are usually wrapped and bundled—because they have no warm clothing that *fits!* They need the freedom of movement for exercise, like any other person.

"Our little caps are especially nice because they are snug as well as cute."

LITTLE BABIES: Born Too Soon, Born Too Small
1977, 14 pages

from
National Institute of Child Health
and Human Development
National Institutes of Health
Bethesda, MD 20014
free (request DHEW Pub. No. (NIH)
77-1079)

The National Institute of Child Health and Human Development is currently involved in research to determine the causes of low birth weight.

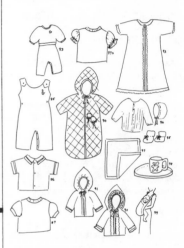

PREMIE PETITES, INC.
c/o Linda Francis
3318 Western, No. 117
Amarillo, TX 79109
806/353-4206
free catalog with SASE

Premie Petites, Inc. manufactures ready-to-wear clothing for premature babies. The catalog is extensive and includes diapers, caps, jogging suits, terry stretchies, dresses, jumpsuits, and overalls. Prices range from about $1.00 to $30.00 (for a long, lace-trimmed christening gown). (PM)

RESOURCES FOR PARENTS WHOSE CHILD IS BORN WITH A BIRTH DEFECT

The following resources and organizations can help with some of the difficult decisions and tasks facing the parents of children born with birth defects. Some of the important issues to consider include: 1) should the fetus diagnosed as defective be aborted or carried to term?, 2) should the baby born with severe defects be treated by "heroic" medical means, treated less "aggressively" or be allowed to die?, and 3) how can parents best care for the child with a birth defect?   (JIA)

DOWN'S SYNDROME CONGRESS
529 S. Kenilworth
Oak Park, IL 60304
and
1640 W. Roosevelt Road, R. 156-E
Chicago, IL 60608
312/226-0416

The Down's Syndrome Congress is "an organization of parents and professionals concerned with Down's Syndrome." By writing for information you will receive membership information, a sample of *Down's Syndrome News*, fact sheets, a listing of items available from the Congress, and an extensive annotated bibliography.

FACTS ABOUT DOWN'S SYNDROME

"Every year the approximate incidence of children with Down's Syndrome is one in every 1,000 births in the United States. Women under 35 years of age bear 80% of these children. In 25-30% of children with D.S. the extra number 21 chromosome is contributed by the father."

NATIONAL ASSOCIATION FOR DOWN'S SYNDROME
P.O. Box 63
Oak Park, IL 60603

CLOSER LOOK
Box 19428
Washington, DC 20036

CLEFT LIP AND PALATE GROUP OF CEA
129 Fayette Street
Conshohocken, PA 19428
215/828-0131

This group provides direct services to parents in the Philadelphia area and may be able to provide information to others.

AMERICAN CLEFT PALATE EDUCATIONAL FOUNDATION, INC.
331 Salk Hall
University of Pittsburgh
Pittsburgh, PA 15261

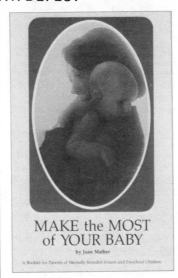

MAKE the MOST of YOUR BABY
by June Mather
A Booklet for Parents of Mentally Retarded Infants and Preschool Children

ASSOCIATION FOR RETARDED CITIZENS
2501 Avenue J
Arlington, TX 76011
817/640-0204

The Association provides the following pamphlets and booklets of interest to parents, including: "Make the Most of Your Baby," 50 cents.

CEREBRAL PALSY: Hope Through Research
1980

from
Scientific and Health Reports
National Institute of Neurological and Communicative Disorders and Stroke
National Institutes of Health
Bethesda, MD 20205
free

This booklet describes some of the causes of and treatments for cerebral palsy.

UNITED CEREBRAL PALSY ASSOCIATIONS, INC.
66 East 34th Street
New York, NY 10016
212/481-6300

A national, voluntary agency which supports research and provides services to parents. Write for more information and for listings of local chapters and clinics.

NATIONAL EASTER SEAL SOCIETY
2023 West Ogden Avenue
Chicago, IL 60612

The Society provides publications on several disabling conditions including cerebral palsy, learning disabilities, speech, language, and hearing problems, and spina bifida.

SPINA BIFIDA ASSOCIATION OF AMERICA
343 South Dearborn, No. 319
Chicago, IL 60604
312/663-1562

The Spina Bifida Association of America is a voluntary, non-profit organization that offers educational materials, media presentations, national conferences and various regular publications for lay and professional persons concerned with spina bifida. The association publishes a large selection of booklets, including: *The Child with Spina Bifida, The Teacher and the Child with Spina Bifida,* and others. There is also a coloring book for young children. Most of these publications are available for $1.00 each. There are over 100 chapters throughout the country and each chapter seeks to offer advice, support and local referrals for parents of spina bifida children.   (PM)

"Spina Bifida is a birth defect which involves damage to the spine and nervous system. The vertebrae of the spine and the spinal cord are not formed properly and surgery is usually required immediately after birth. The long-term effects frequently include weakness or paralysis of the legs and problems with bowel and bladder control. Spina Bifida is often accompanied by hydrocephalus (accumulation of fluid within the brain), which is controlled by a surgical procedure relieving the fluid pressure. Genetic counseling should be sought by all people with any form of Spina Bifida, hydrocephalus or a family history of either condition. Prenatal diagnostic testing for Spina Bifida is available to interested couples."

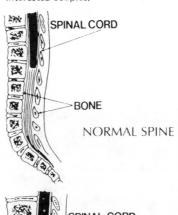

SPINAL CORD

BONE

NORMAL SPINE

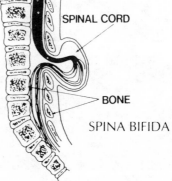

SPINAL CORD

BONE

SPINA BIFIDA

IF YOUR CHILD HAS A CONGENITAL HEART DEFECT: A Guide for Parents
1981, 38 pages, Illus.

from
American Heart Association
7320 Greenville Avenue
Dallas, TX 75231
free

This is an excellent and well illustrated booklet on congenital heart defects. Although the book is designed for parents of older children, the information all holds true for infants and will help parents learn what to expect when their baby gets older.

The first part of the booklet describes operable heart defects. Each description is accompanied by an illustration of a normal heart and of a heart with that particular defect. These drawings are invaluable in understanding the various mechanisms (and their problems) within the heart. The rest of the booklet describes surgery, cardiac intensive care units, and medical follow-up. Also discussed are the various services available to families, including financial, educational and vocational assistance.

A nice touch: on the back page is a diagram of a heart for the doctor to use in showing a parent their child's heart defect, and a check list of questions the parents may want to ask their doctor.   (PM)

The following organizations offer information and referrals of a general nature.

BIRTH DEFECTS BRANCH
Center for Disease Control
U.S. Public Health Service
1600 Clayton Road, NE
Atlanta, GA 30333

DIGHT INSTITUTE FOR HUMAN GENETICS
University of Minnesota
400 Church Street, SE
Minneapolis, MN 55455

ENVIRONMENTAL TERATOLOGY INFORMATION CENTER
Oak Ridge National Laboratory
Bldg. 9224, 4-12
Oak Ridge, TN 37830

NATIONAL FOUNDATION/ MARCH OF DIMES
1275 Mamoroneck Avenue
White Plains, NY 10605

NATIONAL REFERRAL CENTER
Science and Technology Division
Library of Congress
10 First Street, SE
Washington, DC 20540

For more information on birth defects see the resources listed in the section on Genetic Testing in this Catalog.

Stillbirth and Infant Death

Priya Morganstern, editor

In the past, when infant mortality was higher and death in general was a more accepted part of life, a woman who lost her baby in childbirth or shortly thereafter was not without company. She almost certainly knew several other women who had experienced the same thing; perhaps she had even gone through it before. It could be shared. The grief was intense but it was not foreign. Now, gratefully, a woman in Western society does not have to give birth eight times in order to ensure the survival of four healthy children. Newborns almost always live; stillbirth and infant death are rare. As a result, today's bereaved parents not only experience grief and anguish, but they may also experience a strange *silence* on the part of family, friends, and doctors. Dear ones, uncomfortable with the death of a baby, may simply not know how to comfort the parents. Or, as with miscarriages, the severity of the event may be minimized: "You'll get over it soon; you can always have another."

Most of the books reviewed in this section are written by parents who have experienced a stillbirth or the death of a young infant. All of them express frustration that although they wanted and needed to talk about the baby and his or her birth, most friends and family members would carefully avoid the subject. In addition, most parents who never saw or held their baby cannot forgive themselves for not demanding it.

Parents and others have made recommendations about how hospitals can handle perinatal deaths. Many suggest allowing the parents to see and/or hold their child (with needed privacy), and the taking of photographs and footprints. Hospitals can also put the parents in touch with a local support group, and have pamphlets prepared on such subjects as grief, autopsy, funerals, grief and marriage, siblings, and thinking about another pregnancy.   (PM)

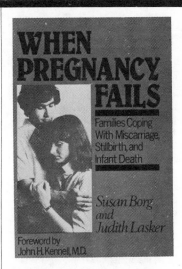

WHEN PREGNANCY FAILS:
Families Coping With Miscarriage,
Stillbirth, and Infant Death
by Susan Borg and Judith Lasker
1981, 252 pages

from
Beacon Press
25 Beacon Street
Boston, MA 02108
$12.95

The very thought of failed pregnancy is frightening for those of us who have experienced miscarriage, elective abortion, premature and stillbirth, and infant death, because of the very real, very deep, sad, and hurtful memories it brings. Whether becoming pregnant is easy or extremely hard—STAYING pregnant long enough to deliver a healthy living baby can be even harder for some of us.

When Pregnancy Fails is a guide to those terrible moments in women's lives when there is nothing that they or anyone can do to save their child-to-be. There is not much guidance, yet, from the medical establishment; we are told facts and percentages, not the "whys" of fetal and infant death. *When Pregnancy Fails* explains through examples of real families' tragedies what hurts and what helps, the impact of a failed pregnancy on the woman, her spouse, their families, and friends. Through the experiences of their own lost pregnancies, Lasker and Borg help us with sections on medical care, grieving, work, the next child, and more.

While it helps to know that we are not alone with our tragedy, and that there are close to 1 million failed pregnancies each year, there are still dark moments for us, wondering what went wrong, how it could have been prevented or handled differently, and whether it will happen again. This book helps us learn about our responses to these issues and provides a state-by-state list of resource groups.   (Abby Pariser)

"Statistics do show that the problem is widespread, but they tell

nothing about the tears, the regrets, the feelings of guilt, the long process of rebuilding hope. They hide the loneliness of those who feel they are the only ones in the world who have failed to become parents. We have written this book in an attempt to help grieving parents break through the barriers of their isolation; to offer them reassurance, information, encouragement, and advice. Our book is also for those professionals who want to understand and to help them and for the families and friends who wish to console them. . . .

"It is especially important for professionals to assist parents in beginning to grieve. They can do this by helping create concrete memories for the parents to hold on to."

"Many professionals who come in contact with the mourning couple —medical people, clergy, funeral directors—often fail to provide appropriate support and counseling. This is true in many situations of death and dying—these are still difficult subjects to talk about. But when a miscarriage, a stillbirth, an abortion of a deformed fetus, or an early infant death occurs, it is especially important for professionals to assist parents in beginning to grieve. They can do this by helping create concrete memories for the parents to held on to. Yet in many hospitals, still, all reminders of the baby are removed quickly, and rarely are parents encouraged to consider a full funeral or other formal mourning practices.

"These parents are further isolated because they seldom know anyone else who has experienced a birth tragedy. They have no assurance that their own feelings and reactions are normal. Hardly a word is written about unsuccessful deliveries in any of the numerous books about childbirth for consumers."
(Editor's Note: This book is one of the finest reviewed in this *Catalog*. Even though I have not suffered a miscarriage or infant death myself, I found the book useful and enlarging. The chapters on "Prenatal Diagnosis and the Unwanted Abortion" and "Possible Causes: Is Progress Killing Our Babies?" deserve a wide audience among pregnant couples. JIA)

AFTER A LOSS IN PREGNANCY
by Nancy Berezin
1982, 170 pages

from
Simon and Schuster
Rockefeller Center
1230 Avenue of the Americas
New York, NY 10020
$9.25

Nancy Berezin is a medical writer and editor specializing in obstetrics, gynecology and pediatrics. She is the author of *The Gentle Birth Book* (see index), as well as many monographs and magazine articles. Her familiarity with women's health issues is evident as she easily shifts from hard, factual information to sensitive examination of the issues surrounding perinatal death. In *After A Loss in Pregnancy*, Berezin describes women's grief, and the many social forces and institutions which work for—or against— her recovery. In particular, she decries the attitudes of friends, family and medical personnel which deny a mother's rightful grief, especially after miscarriage.   (PM)

"Shortly after I began writing this book, I received a telephone call from a friend. 'Nancy,' she said, 'my neighbor has just given birth to an anencephalic child who is not expected to live more than a few

hours. Her obstetrician told her to go home and pretend it never happened, and to try to get pregnant again as soon as possible. She's very upset and wonders whether that advice is really right for her. Would you call her?'

"'I did call, with the address of a local clinic that specialized in family crises of this kind, a list of reading material, and what meager words of sympathy I could offer to a woman I had never met, whose grief was shattering, and whose physician had given her what amounted to a prescription for emotional illness.

"Why? Because no amount of pretending would ever bring this woman's baby back or convince her he had never existed. The obstetrician—also, incidentally, a woman— had been well-meaning, but her advice was founded on the terrible misconception that grief can be side-stepped, that the joy of a successful second pregnancy could miraculously erase the memory of a loss."

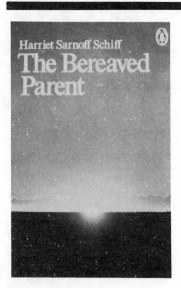

THE BEREAVED PARENT
by Harriet Sarnoff Schiff
1977, 146 pages

from
Penguin Books
625 Madison Avenue
New York, NY 10022
$7.95 pap.

"From here on, will you have a life or an existence?" This is the question Harriet Schiff poses to parents who, like herself, have out-lived their child. Ms. Schiff chose life, and in this very beautiful book, describes how she pulled her life together in the aftermath of her son's death at age 10 of heart disease. She is telling her story to help others who are in the same situation, and by relating her own experiences (including mistakes) as well as those of others, she offers very realistic suggestions on how to cope with life in times of death.

Referring to the death of a child as "the most unnatural of disasters," Ms. Schiff explores its effects on marriage, coping abilities, religious beliefs, and self image. She also discusses funerals, guilt, powerlessness, communication and functioning "normally." Every chapter is insightful and sensitive; the chapters on marriage and siblings are particularly good.

By frequently using fables, metaphors, and proverbs in her writing, Schiff reminds us that issues of a child's death cut across all religious, economic, and cultural lines. Her writing is simple and direct. And by writing in a very personal manner, our hearts are touched; I cried several times while reading the book, but it is hopeful—and this hopefulness is truly a gift to other parents. (PM)

"Do not forget that life goes on and with it come day-to-day problems. Do not sweep them under the rug. Do not fear your mate's anger Tell him to stop avoiding coming home at night. Tell her you expect dinner to be prepared. If you do not take these basic concrete steps you will find yourself walking on separate sides of the river of grief with no bridge upon which to meet.

"Above all and beyond all, remember everyone must carry his own mourning. It is something that cannot be shared. Do not make demands of comfort from your mate when he is feeling the same pain you feel. Recognize that she would help if she could. You must content yourself with this if you wish your marriage to survive.

"Value that marriage. You have lost enough. . . .

"People who are religious are the ones who can ask 'Why did this happen to me,' without destroying themselves emotionally. They can give themselves many answers.

"One ancient example of this is the tale of the wife of a revered and wise rabbi whose twin sons died while he was away from home.

"Knowing how deeply he loved the boys, his wife decided to keep the tragic news from her husband until he could fortify himself with dinner that evening. When the rabbi came home, he asked for his sons repeatedly. His wife always replied, 'They are away from home now.'

"After the meal, she sat with him and said, 'You are a very wise and learned man. Help me with the answer to a problem. If you were lent two precious jewels and told you could enjoy them as long as they were in your keeping, would you be able to argue when the lender asked for their return?'

"Her husband thought for a moment and replied, 'Certainly not!'

"His wife then arose and led her husband into the bedroom where the two boys lay, dead, and said, 'God wanted his jewels back.'. . .

"For the bereaved parent, functioning is somewhat like jumping aboard an already moving bus. You are out of breath, somewhat disheveled, but in motion nonetheless.

"The first rule in trying to function is not to bite off more than you can chew. Start small. Begin with essential everyday tasks. Work, cook, shop, pay your bills. Those things must be done. Make sure you complete your projects. It is very easy to become distracted when grieving. Then, gradually, add a few chores that can be—and have been—put off. Balance your checkbook, file all those office letters you have let pile up, clean out that ridiculously overstuffed closet. . . .

"It may come as a surprise that once you have taken the first step, others will follow. Of course, there will be times you falter and seem to go backward. But, as time goes on, the setbacks become smaller and fewer while the momentum of living propels you forward."

MOTHERHOOD AND MOURNING:
Perinatal Death
by Larry Peppers and Ronald Knapp
1980, 164 pages

from
Praeger Publishers
Div. of CBS, Inc.
521 Fifth Avenue
New York, NY 10017
$21.95 hd.

One may wonder immediately how two men came to write a book on mourning in motherhood. They answer that question themselves in the introduction; while teaching a college course on death, one of their wives (who had miscarried 15 years earlier) brought up the subject of miscarriage and stillbirth. Peppers and Knapp, who had considered themselves very learned on the subject of death, realized then that they had overlooked an obvious fact: Babies die. And parents grieve. Both Peppers and Knapp have doctorates in sociology, a background which is reflected in the book's style. It is completely footnoted and documented, with many referrals to other studies throughout. To my surprise, however, the book is not dry or emotionally restrained; it is warm, sensitive and sometimes very dramatic.

Motherhood and Mourning is an excellent exploration of the elements involved in a child's death—be it before birth, at birth, or in the year or two that follows. By using actual quotations throughout. Peppers and Knapp shed light on such issues as the hospital experience, breakdowns in communication between doctor and mother, lack of community support for her extended grief, communication and sexual difficulties with husbands, and decisions about autopsies, burials, etc. They also discuss how differences in bonding are reflected in how one grieves, and that frequently parents live in a state of 'shadow grief' for many, many years. One of the largest problems, they conclude, is that grieving parents lack *listeners*, and they highly recommend lay support groups such as AMEND, SHARE, or Compassionate Friends (see index). How to start such a group is covered in the last chapter.

Also included is a very interesting and unusual chapter which discusses and analyzes how we offer our sympathies to grieving parents. (PM)

"It is difficult for a friend or even a relative to grieve for the death of a child whom they have never known. This lack of an established social circle around the infant can certainly account for the inability of most people to grieve with the mother for the child. It is because of this that fortunately, or perhaps unfortunately, Americans have adopted the practice of sending sympathy cards as a symbolic acknowledgement of death. This is fortunate because the cards say to the mother that the sender recognizes the loss, and unfortunate because the cards serve to isolate the mother, deny the importance of the death, and offer an easy way to avoid the grieving mother. . . ."

ON THE DEATH OF A NEWBORN CHILD

The flowers in bud on the trees
Are pure like this dead child.
The East wind will not let them last.
It will blow them into blossom,
and at last to the earth.
It is the same with this beautiful life
Which was so dear to me.
While his mother is weeping tears of blood,
Her breasts are still filling with milk.

by Mei Yoo Ch'en

from *One Hundred Poems from the Chinese*, translated by Kenneth Rexroth, New Directions.

SUPPORT GROUPS

COMPASSIONATE FRIENDS
P.O. Box 1347
Oak Brook, IL 60521
312/323-5010

Compassionate Friends is a non-profit, self-help organization. Its purpose is to offer friendship and understanding to parents who have experienced the death of a child, and to facilitate the positive resolution of their grief. "Joining" the organization is accomplished through affiliation with a local chapter, each of which develops its own resources, newsletters, libraries, and community of caring people. Some chapters have also established professional advisory committees (made up of local doctors, nurses, clergy, social workers, psychologists, funeral directors, and others) who are available as resources to the chapter members and who may present educational programs to the parent groups. There are now over 200 local chapters in the U.S.

An individual or family who contacts the national headquarters office will receive the name, address and phone number of the closest local chapter leader. They will also receive a list of recommended books, an order form for relevant booklets, and several pages of advice for grieving parents, their friends, and medical personnel. These suggestions clearly have been developed by wise, gentle and compassionate people who have experienced first hand the loss of a child. The Compassionate

Friends are not at all academic or theoretical in approach; their communication is directly heart to heart. I truly felt a lot of love coming through in just a few pages of literature. (PM)

"Normal grieving, with many ups and downs, lasts far longer than society in general recognizes. Be patient with yourself.

— Crying is a very acceptable and healthy expression of grief for both mothers and fathers which releases built-up tension; cry freely as you feel the need.
— Whenever possible, put off major decisions (changing residence, job, etc.) for at least a year.
— Because the 'bonding' between mother and child begins long before birth, a father should expect the mother to have more intense feelings for a longer time; mourn with her and be supportive.
— The anniversaries of a baby's birth and death can be a most stressful time for parents—be good to yourself and allow yourself some emotional space and special time for grieving.
— When considering another pregnancy, give yourself time to mourn and recover physical and emotional strength.
— When you do have a new pregnancy, choose new names; each child is unique and does not deserve to be a surrogate."

HAND
3311 Richmond Ave. Suite 330
Houston, TX 77077
713/493-6792

Hope's Aid in Neonatal Death (HAND) is a support group of another organization called HOPE (Houston Organization for Parent Education). HOPE is an independent, educational group which presents information on all aspects of prenatal care, childbirth, and family education. Included in the organization are three support groups designed for parents who have experienced deliveries with unexpected outcomes: prematurity, cesarean, and stillbirth. This is where HAND comes in; it is for parents whose babies have died anytime from the moment of conception through late infancy. Although both groups are more or less specifically for the Houston area, they jointly publish a newsletter and a very excellent bibliography which is helpful to anyone concerned, regardless of where they live. The bibliography includes almost 200 separate listings of articles, books, films, and pamphlets. Of special interest are the books written especially for children to aid in their understanding of death. Write to HAND at the above address to request their *Parent and Perinatal Death*

Bibliography. To receive the newsletter, write to:
Karen Riley, Editor
14207 Locke Lane
Houston, TX 77077
(PM)

"Aims of HAND
"Provide understanding and mutual support to parents who have experienced an infant death. We hope by sharing experiences and providing educational programs at monthly meetings, as well as circulation of a bi-monthly newsletter, we will be able to reach parents who want to understand their grief.

"Improve communications, share feelings and ideas with the community in regard to newborn loss. The unique grief as well as specific needs parents have when a baby dies is not always understood by family, friends, or the medical community. In-service education is available to the medical profession, social workers, clergy, funeral directors, crisis centers, and counseling agencies to aid further understanding."

SHARE
c/o Sister Jane Marie Lamo
St. John's Hospital
800 East Carpenter St.
Springfield, IL 62702
(217) 544-6464 x-4500

Source of Help in Airing and Resolving Experiences (SHARE) is a self-help and support organization for parents who have experienced a miscarriage, stillbirth or the loss of a newborn baby. Most of SHARE's chapters are in Illinois; however, new chapters are springing up in many other states including California, Wisconsin, and New York. SHARE headquarters will put you in contact with the SHARE chapter closest to you or with another similar organization if it is closer. SHARE publishes a newsletter that frequently includes poetry and birth announcements of "special children" (those children born after the death of another).
(PM)

"As the result of SHARE, we contacted the coroner and he reluctantly made photos available to a mother. Where there was once fear and terror, a sense of peace and calm now remain for this parent. Additionally, the coroner has agreed from this point on to take footprints should he be called in on an infant."

Miscarriage/Stillbirth/ Infant Death — State and Local Organizations

In addition to the national organizations dedicated to parents' support, there are also local organizations in almost every state in the country. The most complete state-by-state listing is in the appendix of *When Pregnancy Fails,* by Borg and Lasker (see index). The authors note that new groups are formed all the time, so even this list may not be complete. Contacting a local hospital's Social Service Department, or local Childbirth Education Association may be helpful if there is no listing in your area. (PM)

STILLBIRTH
by Barbara Crooker

She said, "Your daughters
are so beautiful.
One's a copper penny,
the other's a chestnut colt."
But what about my first
    daughter,
stillborn
at term,
cause unknown?

Ten years later
and I sift the ground
for clues: what was
it I did?
Guilt is part
of my patchwork;
grief folds me up
like an envelope.

In the hospital,
the doctors turned
their eyes, told me
not to leave
my room.
But I heard them,
those babies in the night,
saw women from Lamaze
in the corridor.
They would be wheeled home
with blossoms & blankets,
while I bled the same,
tore the same,
and came home, alone.

Later, women showered me
with stories
of babies lost:
to crib death,
    abortion,
    miscarriage;
lost:
    the baby
    that my best friend
    gave up
    at fourteen.

They wouldn't let me hold her:
all I saw were fragments:
    a dark head,
    a doll's foot,
    skin like a bruise.
They wouldn't let me name her,
        or bury her,
        or mourn her.

Ten years later
and I do not have
the distance:
I carry her death
like an egg in my pocket.

Copyright©1981 by Barbara Crooker
"Stillbirth" appeared first in *Childbirth Alternatives Quarterly.*

THIS IS WHAT I DO WITH KERIN
by Marion Cohen
1980, 3 pages

from
Mothering Publications, Inc.
P.O. Box 2208
Albuquerque, NM 87103
request reprint No. 17-2
$.75 each

Marion Cohen is well known to those of us who read *Mothering Magazine* as the author of sensitive, moving poems regarding the death of her child. Her daughter, Kerin, who died two days after birth, is still very much a part of Marion's life. Marion has kept Kerin "alive" by exploring her sorrow, and sharing it with those who care. This reprint is Marion's story of the birth and death of her daughter and her experience with grief. Because it is so painful, so difficult, and yet so hopeful and loving, reading her story is really like sharing that part of her life with her.

Marion did get involved with an organization called UNITE (see index) and found it to be *wonderful*. To be sharing her grief with others who were there just for that purpose was the salve she needed for her pain. She later found it to be a way to help others, too. By staying involved with

UNITE, she found a way to actively keep Kerin's memory alive. "I go to be with Kerin. This is what I do with Kerin."

For parents who have experienced the loss of a child, reading this reprint might give them solace and support. It is as if Marion is hugging them and saying, "I know."
(Editor's Note: Marion is also working on an anthology of poems relating to child death, to be published soon. PM)

"I found myself looking forward to the next meeting with an urgency bordering on hunger. For the first time since it happened, I was actually looking forward to something. And this is the way I continue to feel, over the weeks, over the months (until I got pregnant again). And over the years, as I continue to attend meetings (as a "survivor" and UNITE graduate), over and over again, newly bereaved parents express the same feelings. 'I live from meeting to meeting,' they say, and 'the only people I'm interested in getting together with are UNITE people.' We laugh—no funny ha ha, but familiar funny. It's so true; as my mother pointed out, meetings are where we can talk about what we really want to talk about."

WHEN PREGNANCY ENDS WITH THE BABY'S DEATH: A Resource Book for Parents
by Laurie Randall and Nancy Johns
1980, 12 pages (booklet)

from
Booth Maternity Center
6051 Overbrook Ave.
Philadelphia, Penn. 19131
$3.00

When Pregnancy Ends With The Baby's Death is a small booklet prepared by the staff of Booth Maternity Center. It is simple, concise, and offers information pertinent to a parent *immediately* after a stillbirth or miscarriage, such as: Should an autopsy be done? Should we name the baby? Can we hold the baby? Photos? Baptism? What to do with the baby's body? Because much of the information is specific to Booth Hospital and the Philadelphia area, it is not the best general information book. However, it is an *excellent* example of something *every* hospital should prepare for grieving parents.   (PM)
"Too many decisions too soon: what are my options?
"Unfortunately, when death occurs, many decisions need to be made within a very short period of time. This is often hard to do because your hurt is so new and overpowering all you may want to do is be left alone, or even leave Booth (Hospital) as soon as possible. However there are laws we must adhere to following the death of the infant, and there are papers that must be signed. It was important for you to be 'in charge' of your pregnan-

cy. We now want you, as much as possible, to be in charge of arrangements for you and your baby. Therefore, by putting your options into writing (this booklet), we hope you will better understand what they are and, thus, be more equipped to make decisions appropriate to *you* and *your* family."

Bibiographies

In addition to these books and organizations, articles written in professional journals are another source of information—usually of an academic or research-oriented nature. It is not possible for us to list each article; however, annotated bibliographies are available. One very good one is in *BIRTH* (formerly *Birth and the Family Journal*), Summer, 1981. The bibliography was prepared by members of the Perinatal Mortality Counseling Program at . Shands Teaching Hospital in Gainsville, Florida. Back issues of the Journal are available for $4.00. Write to:
BIRTH
110 El Camino Real
Berkeley, CA 94705
request vol. 8, no. 2, Summer '81
Another excellent bibliography is available from HAND, an organization based in Houston, TX. See listing in this section.   (PM)

More Resources

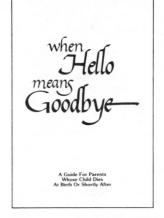

when Hello means Goodbye

A Guide For Parents
Whose Child Dies
At Birth Or Shortly After

WHEN HELLO MEANS GOODBYE

A booklet dealing with the psychological responses to the death of a child.

from
OB/GYN Professors
University of Oregon
Health Sciences Center
3181 Sam Jackson Road
Portland, OR 97201
$1.50

* * *

TELL ME, PAPA

A booklet written for kids, to answer their questions about death, funerals, etc.
$3.75, 16 pages

CHILDREN DIE, TOO

A sensitive booklet about the grief process for parents who have experienced the death of a newborn or older child.
by S. & J. Johson
$2.50, 14 pages

from
Creative Marketing
P.O. Box 2423
Springfield, IL 62705

SWIMMER IN A SECRET SEA
by W. Kotzwinkle
1979
Avon Books

A novel about a young couple's experience when their newborn dies within minutes of birth.

DEATH OF AN INFANT

THE CHILD IS DYING: WHO HELPS THE FAMILY

ANNIE IS ALONE: THE BEREAVED CHILD

These articles appeared in the *American Journal of Maternal-Child Nursing*, July/August 1981. Reprints are available: minimum order is 100. For single copies, order the back issue, $5.00

from
MCN Magazine
Editorial Services Division
555 W. 57th Street
New York, NY 10019

* * *

THE FROGS HAVE A BABY, A VERY SMALL BABY

THE FROG FAMILY'S BABY DIES

These coloring books give kids a chance to express painful emotions and offer parents an opportunity to deal with the anxieties and frustrations caused by grief and fear. These books are free.

from
Ms. Oehler
MCN Magazine
555 W. 57th Street
New York, NY 10019

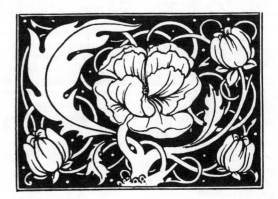

SUDDEN INFANT DEATH SYNDROME

Sudden Infant Death Syndrome (SIDS) is the largest single cause of death of infants between one week and one year of age, accounting for one third of all deaths that occur during that period. Its peak incidence is during the third and fourth month of a baby's life; during that period SIDS accounts for half the total deaths. Annually, SIDS claims the lives of 7,500-10,000 babies.

In a typical case, an apparently healthy infant, usually between the ages of four weeks and seven months, is put to bed without any suspicion that something is out of the ordinary. Some time later, the baby is found dead. There is no evidence of a struggle having taken place, although the baby may have changed position at the time of death. An autopsy may reveal, at most, some inflammation of the respiratory tract, but nothing serious enough to have caused death. Usually the autopsy reveals no evidence of illness.

Parents may feel tremendous guilt, or may place blame on a family member or baby sitter who was present, or on a doctor who pronounced the infant healthy shortly before it died. The truth is, however, that SIDS *cannot be predicted*, and *cannot be prevented*, according to our present limited knowledge of the syndrome.

For parents who have experienced the death of their baby to SIDS, there are now many fine organizations and publications that offer education and support. (PM)

FACTS ABOUT SIDS
by Public Information Office
Department of Health and Human Services
1972, 12 pages

from
Superintendent of Documents
U.S. Government Printing Office
Washington, DC 20402
(request DHEW pub. no. (NIH)72-225)
single copy, 10 cents

Using a question and answer format, this brochure covers much information regarding SIDS. It is thorough, clearly written, and very worthwhile. It also includes other sources of help and information and a short list of available publications.

The brochure was prepared by the Sudden Infant Death Research Team of Children's Orthopedic Hospital and Medical Center of Seattle, Washington. An almost identical brochure is distributed by the National Foundation for Sudden Infant Death, using the same title, *Facts About SIDS*. (PM)

"SOME BASIC FACTS ABOUT SIDS

— SIDS is a definite medical entity and is a major cause of death in infants after the first month of life.
— SIDS cannot be predicted or prevented, even by a physician.
— Research to date indicates that the cause of SIDS is not suffocation, aspiration or regurgitation.
— A minor illness such as a common cold may be present, but many victims are entirely healthy prior to death.
— There appears to be no suffering; death occurs very rapidly, usually during sleep.
— SIDS is not contagious in the usual sense. Although a viral infection may be involved, it is not a "killer virus" that threatens other family members or neighbors. SIDS rarely occurs after seven months of age.
— SIDS is not hereditary; there is no greater chance for it to occur in one family than in another.
— The baby is not the victim of a "freakish disease." As many as 10,000 babies die as a result of the sudden infant death syndrome every year (up to three per 1,000 live births).
— SIDS is at least as old as the Old Testament and seems to have been at least as frequent in the 18th and 19th centuries as it is now. This demonstrates that new environmental agents, such as birth control pills, fluoride in the water supply and smoking, do not cause SIDS."

SIDS COUNSELING AND INFORMATION PROGRAM/NATIONAL CLEARINGHOUSE FOR SIDS

from
SIDS Program Office
Bureau of Community Health Services
Room 7-36
5600 Fishers Lane
Rockville, MD 20857

On April 22, 1974, President Ford signed the Sudden Infant Death Syndrome Act (P.L. 93-270), which authorized the Secretary of Health, Education and Welfare to make grants for projects which include the collection, analysis and furnishing of information relating to the syndrome, and for the counseling of family survivors. The law also authorizes that public information and professional educational materials be developed and distributed to health care providers, public safety officials, and to the general public. An amendment enacted in December of 1979 (P.L. 96-142) required the extension of counseling and information services to all 50 states, District of Columbia, all territories and possessions by 1981.

SIDS Projects have been created and funded all across the country to achieve the program's goals. (PM)

"OBJECTIVES

—autopsies in all sudden, unexpected deaths of children up to 1 year of age
— certification of SIDS on the death certificate.
— prompt notification of the parents about the cause of death, preferably within a 24-48 hour period.
— educational programs for health care providers, safety officials, and the public.
— counseling for families affected by a SIDS loss.
— timely transfer of research findings into health care delivery services, including new diagnostic and treatment methods.
— early identification of vulnerable infants and provision of services which may prevent SIDS deaths."

SUDDEN INFANT DEATH SYNDROME
Bibliography
prepared by Charlotte Kenton
1981, 395 citations

from
National Library of Medicine
8600 Rockville Pike
Bethesda, MD 20209
(request literature search No. 81-6, SIDS)

This bibliography is part of the National Library of Medicine's Literature Search Series. It contains 395 citations, all of which are from professional journals. (PM)

SUDDEN UNEXPLAINED INFANT DEATH; 1970-1975: An Evolution in Understanding
by Marie Valdes-Dapena, MD
1977, 29 pages
(reprinted from *Pathology Annual*, part 1, Vol. 12, 1977)
Appleton-Century-Crofts)

from
U.S. Department of HSS
Public Health Service
Bureau of Community Health Services
Rockville, MD 20857
(request DHEW pub. no. (HSA) 80-5255)

This booklet, which is a reprint from a scientific journal, is very technical and detailed. It contains the first information that I came across indicating that perhaps SIDS babies, as a group, are *not* normal and healthy. By referring to study after study, the author points out interesting features that are characteristic in general of babies who die of SIDS; slow growth and weight gain, abnormally heavy right ventricles, lower Apgar scores, required resuscitation at birth, less intense responses to stimuli, and cries of unusual pitches —to name a few. She emphasizes, however, that "there is not yet a single one of these differences that can be employed, before or after the death, as a predictive or diagnostic criterion."

Other discussions cover the incidence of SIDS, socio-economic factors relating to the mother, factors relating to the baby, and environmental factors. The author also discusses the results of recent research and studies-in-progress.

This is a very technical, sophisticated and informative booklet, unusual in its content. (PM)

"Ideally, physicians should be able to identify the infant at risk for the sudden infant death syndrome before the fact. However, despite recent developments in our knowledge concerning the potential victim and his various characteristics, no one can yet single him out. We do know that he is more likely than not to be a male from a minority group, of low socio-economic origin, and to have been born of a young mother either prematurely or of low birth weight. There are apt to have been problems with establishment of his respiration initially. He was probably rather quiet with a relatively poor or peculiar cry, or poor capacity to suck. There will be a history that he did not develop or gain weight adequately, etc. Yet even these features are so non-specific and so common that they are actually insufficient to yield a high-risk population for purposes of investigation."

THE NATIONAL FOUNDATION FOR SUDDEN INFANT DEATH
1501 Broadway
New York, NY 10036
212/563-4630

The National Foundation for Sudden Infant Death (NFSID) is a national organization with chapters in many areas. The purpose of the organization is to assist parents, educate the community about SIDS, and promote SIDS research. NFSID offers factual, supportive literature for parents; material for medical and welfare organizations; information for newspapers and other media; a speakers bureau; guidance to established chapters and to those in formation; and a semi-annual newsletter.

The main concern of the chapters is to help the family struck by SIDS. All chapter leaders are themselves SIDS parents, and are dedicated to helping other parents cope with the death of their child.

The NFSID version of *Facts About Sudden Infant Death* contains the following suggestions regarding misinformation in the media: (PM)

"A great deal of misleading information and erroneous interpretation about sudden infant death finds its way into print. . . .

"If you read . . . obvious errors in the press, *you can help correct them.* Clip the statement or article out of the newspaper or magazine; identify the publication, date the appearance and page number; and mail to the National Foundation for Sudden Infant Death, 1501 Broadway, New York, NY 10036. It is extremely cruel and confusing for these statements to keep reappearing in print. If you feel qualified, you might write the publication yourself, *particularly* when articles suggest accidental causes. . . Your note should state that SIDS is *not accidental*, but a definite disease entity which is, at this time, *not preventable.* Refer them to the National Foundation for further information and strongly urge them to print a correcting statement as soon as possible."

SUDDEN INFANT DEATH SYNDROME REGIONAL CENTER
Health Sciences Center
SUNY at Stony Brook
Health Sciences Center
Level 2, Room 099
Stony Brook, NY 11794
516/246-2582 (24-hour answering service)

The SIDS Regional Center at Stony Brook University serves as the central agency for co-ordination of research on Long Island. It is included here as an example of how hospitals and/or university centers can serve the public in relation to SIDS.

The basis of the project is the family assistance program. Each family receives the guidance, support and medical services of the Center's associates without regard to racial, social, or residential requirements. Upon notification from the Medical Examiner of a "possible SIDS" death, the center offers prompt autopsy, immediate notification of results, concise medical information, and voluntary counseling and grief therapy through both lay organizations and Public Health nurse teams. In addition, the center contacts pediatricians, funeral directors, clergy,

other professionals, volunteer SIDS families and extended family members to facilitate a network of support for SIDS families. There is also a 24 hour hotline.

Besides offering services for families, the center offers training programs for health professionals and emergency care personnel, including police. (PM)

"The death of a child is an excruciatingly painful experience—one of the most traumatic events in a person's life. When a child dies, the parents' life is altered, their future affected, their hopes and dreams shattered and their family system strained. This pain is compounded by endless, self-searching questions and feelings of helplessness, shock, anger and guilt. While that pain seems unfathomable and endless, it may help when others are there—to care; to assure them they are not alone with their loss; that it was not their fault; that SIDS is not now preventable; that it is expected that they will need to mourn and talk about their child; that they may have reactions which to them are new and troubling; that turning to others for help is alright and, perhaps, advisable."

SUDDEN INFANT DEATH SYNDROME: Special Report for Fiscal Year 1982
1982, 18 pages, free

from
National Institute of Child Health and Human Development
Center for Research for Mothers and Children
Clinical Nutrition and Early Development Branch
Bethesda, MD 20014

The NICHD of the National Institutes of Health has the primary federal responsibility for research on SIDS. This document outlines some recent research accomplishments, as well as activities of many other projects relating to the syndrome.

The report seems somewhat disorganized, but clearly reflects the extensive involvement and interaction of many government agencies regarding SIDS. (PM)

INTERNATIONAL GUILD FOR INFANT SURVIVAL, INC.
6822 Brompton Road
Baltimore, MD 21207
301/944-2502

Founded in 1964, the Guild for Infant Survival (the "international" came later) is a non-profit, non-sectarian, charitable and educational organization. At the time of its charter, little was known about SIDS; it was not even considered a medical entity. Therefore, gathering up-to-date information became important in order to offer comfort to parents. It is now composed primarily of SIDS parents and provides service and information to bereaved families.

supports scientific research activities, and brings the scope and seriousness of the syndrome to the attention of the public. (PM)

"Because death comes so suddenly and silently, and because these innocent babies have had little time to become known outside their own family, the general public is unaware that this dilemma even exists. Nor do these infants linger in a handicapped or suffering condition to enlist society's sympathy and help. Yet for every victim, death is final. And all that remain are empty cribs, tiny graves, and broken hearts—mute evidence of the total destruction by this killer in our midst."

More Information

Some other sources of information on SIDS are:

Scientific:
SUMMARY OF PROCEEDINGS, SECOND INTERNATIONAL CONFERENCE ON CAUSES OF SUDDEN DEATH IN INFANTS (1971)

from
Superintendent of Documents
U.S. Government Printing Office
Washington, DC 20402
45 cents

PROCEEDINGS OF SECOND INTERNATIONAL CONFERENCE ON CAUSES OF SUDDEN DEATH IN INFANTS (1970)

from
University of Washington Press
Seattle, WA 98105
$10.00

General:
NATIONAL SUDDEN INFANT DEATH SYNDROME FOUNDATION
310 South Michigan Avenue
Chicago, IL 60604
312/663-0650

Request the publication price list and order form.

MENTAL HEALTH ISSUES IN GRIEF COUNSELING
by Stanley Weinstein, ed.
1979, 133 pages

from
U.S. Department of HSS
Public Health Service
Health Services Administration
Bureau of Community Health Services
Rockville, MD 20857
(request DHEW pub. no. (HSA) 79-5264)

"The question of what we mean by helping the family to adjust will be answered differently by different people. Do we mean the family should get on to new investments, another baby, another interest as soon as possible? Do we mean that the family should be able to put it in the past and forget it? Or do we mean that the family needs to be able to absorb it, have time for mourning, be informed in ways that relieve unrealistic guilt feelings, and integrate it into their lives as part of the sadness along with the gladness of life?"

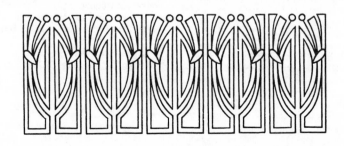

SOME OBSERVATIONS ABOUT BIRTH AND DEATH

by Theo Dawson

"In the past nine months I have assisted two sets of parents with stillbirths in the same hospital environment. Both couples were planning home births and were being seen regularly by both midwife (myself) and physician. Contact with both couples was frequent for six weeks after their births and intermittent into the sixth month.

"The first birth was not, legally, a stillbirth; it was a miscarriage according to dates and weight of the baby. The mother was twenty-one weeks pregnant when she woke one morning and felt for her cervix vaginally. This was a common practice for this woman since she had been using natural birth control and had gotten used to checking her cervix daily. What she felt this time was nothing like the cervix she was used to at all. When I arrived, a vaginal exam revealed that she was totally effaced. I could not feel dilation clearly because of my reluctance to explore too deeply into the vagina. We felt certain that she was going to miscarry, talked about where to give birth at some length and consulted with her doctor. It was decided that if we had the dates all wrong and the baby turned out to be viable none of us would feel good about doing the birth at home.

"We called our back-up obstetrician and arranged to go to the hospital. When we arrived, the nurses received us very graciously and were supportive of the parent's decision to birth the baby naturally and to hold their baby following delivery. The obstetrician seemed a little surprised at their desire to hold the baby but supported their decision. The labour was mild and the parents worked closely together throughout.

"When she was dilated, the doctor asked the mother to push. The tiny baby was born feet-first and there was a pause before the head was born. His tiny feet kicked wildly as the doctor hastened the birth of the after-coming head. I thought at the time that he was rushing the birth to make it easier for the mother. Yet it was hard to see this dying little person tugged on—it must have been frightening for him.

"He was only about 400 grams and perfect. The parents were given the baby after a delay of five minutes or so; I wanted to grab him and cradle him . . . he looked so cold and alone on the sterile green towel. Jordan (as the parents named the baby) was held in his mother's arms for about 45 minutes before they asked that he be taken away. As she was handed her child the mother wept quite openly, as did her husband, then both parents got down to the important business of looking the baby over. I have witnessed this many times with live

babies but the procedure had new significance when it was a non-living baby who was being examined. They counted toes and fingers, checked his eyes, ears, miniscule buttocks until they had covered every visible part. Then they asked questions. 'Why is the skin so transparent?' 'Where is the vernix?' 'Is the head too big?' 'Why does the skin looked bruised?' It was good to be there to help them with their questions; the hospital staff were unable to take the time because of the other women in their care and because they just didn't seem to know how to react.

"The parents decided to hold a funeral. There was much weeping, a tender parting, a final goodbye. Their family was very much there to offer support and help in the next weeks. A decision was made to postpone another pregnancy for at least six months to give the hurt time to heal. I received many calls over the next weeks and months— some sad, some lonely, some hopeful. And some angry. The anger was directed at the obstetrician, because he could not tell them *exactly* why the baby had been lost. Anger is a common feeling in the mourning process; this time anger was expressed over frustration at not being able to get *answers*. My job was to help them to see that the obstetrician, a warm, compassionate and skilled specialist was nevertheless not omniscient, that the absence of answers was something they needed to accept, as hard as that was. I was relieved again that midwives have not yet begun to teeter on the pedestal of omniscience.

"It is now over five months since this birth/death and we are working together again. The new baby is due in September. There is much excitement and joy; and there is a touch of fear that it could happen again. The parents are prepared to take this pregnancy one step at a time. They feel that their mourning is just about completed, or as completed as it can be and that they are embarking on this second pregnancy completely open to the new baby and a new experience.

"A second hospital birth/death experience held many lessons about medicine, love and people in crisis.

"We discovered on Friday that Jenny had an anencephalic baby growing inside her. She had had an ultrasound because of her polyhydramnios the week before and there was virtually no skull on her baby past the eye sockets. We were going

to tell her on her next prenatal visit if it seemed right at the time, but on Monday her water broke. As I left the office with my apprentice the doctor asked me what I would tell her and her husband, Bob. I did not know. I would have to feel the right time and way.

"We arrived, and as soon as I saw Jenny's face I knew we had to tell her right away. I held her hand as I told her—looked into her eyes explaining in as much detail as I could. Bob had a hand on her shoulder and together, we all wept. The questions followed, more than we had answers to and then they began to decide how they would like to do this birth.

"We would have stayed at home if all had gone as it ought, but labour never began. Twenty four hours later she developed a fever and we decided to go to the hospital. Labour was started with an oxytocin drip. The contractions and emotional shock caused Jenny to shiver uncontrollably as her husband and my apprentice held her. She did not want to see her baby, did not want to feel it being born. Later she said that she could see as far as the birth and no farther, she was unable to choose any more trauma even though she felt she was betraying herself and the baby.

"The doctors and the nurses all obviously felt that she should not see the baby. I felt that it would have been easier for her if she saw him—but mine is the long view—the hospital's role is over so soon. (I confess here that I was motivated, in part, by my desire to have an easier time with Jenny and Bob postpartum.)

"The doctor looked away as the baby was being born, covered its little head with a towel so no one would have to look. My heart pounded. The mother and father burst into tears as my apprentice bundled up the baby and took him out of the room, and I followed for a moment to look at this child and touch him. We saw his funny anencephalic face, tiny sculpted nose and wide mouth. We looked at his head, felt sad about the missing part, touched it so that its strangeness would lose its power, examined his little legs and arms which were longer than usual but still all there. Odd how the baby stopped looking ugly after we loved him a little.

"The parents exhibited strengths that they did not know they had. They wept fully and openly and faced each new feeling as it arose with great courage.

"We saw them often in the following days and weeks. Each visit saw Jenny in particular with new insights. Some visits were packed with torrents of tears, some, and these were as powerful, with talk of all the the growth happening inside. Guilt was an occasional feeling, awe, helplessness, denial, frustration, bargaining all appeared at various times. Jenny wondered what her baby looked like and we told her in detail what we had seen. She was unhappy about accepting the epidural, and doubted her future ability to handle labour. The worst weeks were in the second month, and then, slowly, the pieces began to fit together again and life began to be something more joyful.

"Six months after the birth we had a long talk. Jenny and Bob were looking forward to the next pregnancy. Jenny had decided *not* to have the test for an anencephalic baby, routinely given to women who have had one anencephalic child. She felt that she would be unable to terminate the pregnancy in any case. She wanted some reassurance that we would be available for the next birth (we wouldn't miss it!!). And she described a feeling that she had had during the delivery . . . 'A pleasant, warm sensation as the baby was born, it was so nice, something positive in the middle of so much hurt.'

"We did not learn the things from these births that we expected to learn. What follows is a short list of our discoveries.

"Not seeing their baby did not prevent Jenny and Bob from recovering from the loss of their child.

"Tears were not the only product of mourning—there were moments of discovery and much growth in everyone.

"The funeral ceremonies seemed very helpful to both sets of parents in saying their goodbyes.

"Turning away from a feeling was appropriate at times, and did not prevent facing that feeling at another time.

"Fathers needed other men around to help them to sort out their feelings.

"Some of the people in hospitals are terrified of death and need our support in a birth/death situation.

"Support and trust in the ability of people to deal with the pain of death are clearly the major roles of the midwife when birth is also death."

Reprinted by permission of Theo Dawson. This article first appeared in *Issue*, the newsletter of the Ontario Association of Midwives, P.O. Box 85, Postal Station C, Toronto, Ontario, Canada M6J 3M7.

Medical Reference

Medical reference books are an excellent source of information for parents on the anatomy and physiology of pregnancy, labor, and birth. There's no reason not to go right to the source, since many medical text books are written in language which lay people can understand. The books reviewed here were chosen as especially useful for parents planning a home birth and for student midwives and childbirth educators. Most are available at local public libraries, college libraries, or through your inter-library loan system.

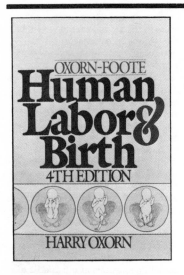

HUMAN LABOR AND BIRTH
(Fourth Edition)
by Harry Oxorn
1980, 726 pages, Illus.

from
Appleton-Century-Crofts
292 Madison Avenue
New York, NY 10017
$18.95 pap.

This is an excellent "first book" for learning about how labor and delivery work. Each of the 48 chapters treats a single subject in clear simple language with a minimum of technical jargon. The book covers pelvic anatomy, presentation and position of the fetus, normal labor and birth, malpresentations, abnormalities of labor and birth, obstetric operations and drugs, hemorrhage, episiotomy and repair, prenatal testing, prematurity, dystocia, cesarean section, the newborn and more. Material is presented in outline form with clearly marked headings, subheadings and numbered points, so it's easy to scan each page for the information you need. There are many clear line drawings throughout. The author states in his preface that he is biased in favor of a non-interventive approach to birth and this attitude is evident throughout his book.

"One of the key problems in obstetrics is to keep advances in perspective. It is tempting, but frequently not wise, to utilize a new procedure simply because it is new. However, a non-invasive, non-surgical ap-

proach often can be as safe and efficacious as an aggressive one. In such cases, we freely opt for the conservative approach, and this attitude is reflected in the presentation of material in this edition.

"A valid general principle is that, as long as the boundaries of medical safety are observed, every woman has the right to give birth to her baby in the manner she chooses. Only when a difficulty arises is interference justified . . . .

> "One of the key problems in obstetrics is to keep advances in perspective. It is tempting, but frequently not wise, to utilize a new procedure simply because it is new. . . . A non-invasive, non-surgical approach often can be as safe and efficacious as an aggressive one."

"So aggressive, impatient, and apprehensive have many North American obstetricians become, that it seems, sometimes, that the doctor is having the baby rather than the woman. Unless the baby falls out of the pelvis, cesarean section is performed. It is our opinion that, barring serious complications, vaginal birth is safer for both mother and child . . . .

"LIE Relationship of the long axis of the fetus to the long axis of the mother.
PRESENTATION The part of the fetus that lies over the inlet. The three main presentations are cephalic (head first), breech (pelvis first), and shoulder.
PRESENTING PART The most dependent part of the fetus, lying nearest the cervix. During vaginal or rectal examination it is the area with which the finger makes contact first.
ATTITUDE Relation of fetal parts to each other. The basic attitudes are flexion and extension. The fetal head is in flexion when the chin approaches

the chest and in extension when the occiput nears the back. The typical fetal attitude in the uterus is flexion, with the head bent in front of the chest, the arms and legs folded in front of the body, and the back curved forward slightly.
DENOMINATOR An arbitrarily chosen point on the presenting part of the fetus used in describing position. Each presentation has its own denominator.
POSITION Relationship of the denominator to the front, back, or sides of the maternal pelvis.

"With each contraction the head advances and then recedes as the uterus relaxes. Each time a little ground is gained. The introitus becomes an anteroposterior slit, then an oval, and finally a circular opening (Figs. 4A-C). The pressure of the head thins out the perineum. Feces may be forced out of the rectum. As the anus opens, the anterior wall of the rectum bulges through. With descent the occiput comes to lie under the pubic symphysis. The head continues to advance and recede with the contractions, until a

strong one forces the largest diameter of the head through the vulva (crowning), as seen in Figure 4D. Once this has occurred there is no going back, and by a process of extension (Fig. 4E) the head is born, as the bregma, forehead, nose, mouth, and chin appear over the perineum (Fig. 4F). At the stage where the

> "With each contraction the head advances and then recedes as the uterus relaxes. Each time a little ground is gained."

head is passing through the introitus, the patient has the sensation of being torn apart. Laceration of the vulva sometimes occurs.

"The head then falls back toward the anus. Once it is out of the vagina it restitutes (Fig. 4G) as the neck untwists. After a few moments, external rotation takes place (Fig. 4H) as the shoulders move from the oblique to the anteroposterior diameter of the pelvis."

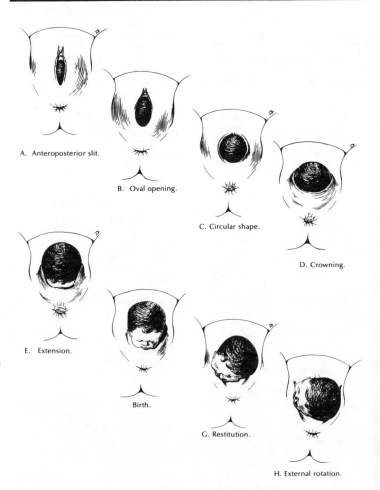

A. Anteroposterior slit.

B. Oval opening.

C. Circular shape.

D. Crowning.

E. Extension.

Birth.

G. Restitution.

H. External rotation.

Dilatation of the introitus and birth of the head.

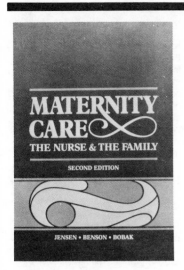

MATERNITY CARE, THE NURSE AND THE FAMILY (Second Edition)
by Margaret Jensen, Ralph Benson and Irene Bobak
1981, 1013 pages, Illus.

from
C.V. Mosby
11830 Westline Industrial Drive
St. Louis, MO 63141
$29.95 hd.

This textbook was written by two nurses and a doctor and while perhaps most useful to nurses and childbirth educators, it contains pertinent information about pregnancy and birth which non-medical persons will also find very useful. The glossary, illustrations and examples come in handy for those unfamiliar with medical terms. Besides informative chapters on biology, contraception, genetics, nutrition, pregnancy, labor and birth, special chapters to note are those on

fathers, alternative settings for childbirth, and a well-illustrated chapter on the normal newborn. The section on home delivery has "down-to-earth" instructions including a note to bake a medium-sized potato in the home oven when linen for the birth is being sterilized; if there is no oven thermometer or temperature setting—when the potato is done, the linens are sterilized! Complications in pregnancy, labor, and birth and newborn complications are discussed after each section, which outlines the normal and expected events. Appendices include the Pregnant Patient's Bill of Rights, the United Nations Declaration of the Rights of the Child, fetal positions and presentations (illustrated), standard lab values for the newborn, growth charts, immunization schedules, and a listing of community resources.

"Home birth has always been popular in certain advanced countries, such as Great Britain, Sweden, and the Netherlands. It is rapidly gaining popularity in the United States and Canada. In developing countries, hospitals or adequate lying-in-facilities often are unavailable to most pregnant women, and home birth is a necessity.

"Selective home birth in uncomplicated pregnancies is feasible, provided those women at high risk can be identified during the prenatal period and referred for hospital delivery and assuming that a transport system is available for transfer of suddenly complicated labors to a nearby adequate medical facility. Another acceptable plan provides for specialist care to be brought to the home by means of a so-called flying squad ser-

vice, which is utilized in Great Britain, for example. . . .

"One advantage of home birth is that delivery may be more natural or

> "One advantage of home birth is that delivery may be more natural or physiological in familiar surroundings. . . . Serious infection may be less likely, assuming strict aseptic principles are followed. Persons generally are relatively immune to their own home bacteria."

physiologic in familiar surroundings. The mother may be more relaxed and less tense than she might be in the impersonal, sterile environment of a hospital. The family can assist in and be a part of the happy event, and mother-father-infant (and sibling-infant) contact is sustained and immediate.

"In addition, home birth may be less expensive than a hospital confinement.

"Finally, serious infection may be less likely, assuming strict aseptic principles are followed. Persons generally are relatively immune to their own home bacteria.". . .

The following excerpt is from the instructions for emergency birth by a nurse.

"6. The perineum thins and distends. As the head begins to crown, the birth attendant should do the following:
 a. Tear the amniotic membrane

(caul) if it is still intact.
 b. Instruct woman to pant or pant-blow, thus avoiding the urge to push.
 c. Place the flat of the hand on the exposed fetal head and apply *gentle* pressure toward the vagina to prevent the head from 'popping out.' The mother may participate by placing her hand under yours on the emerging head. (NOTE: Rapid delivery of the fetal head must be prevented because (1) it is followed by a rapid change of pressure within the molded fetal skull, which may result in dural or subdural tears, and (2) it may cause vaginal or perineal lacerations.)

7. Instruct the mother to pant or pant-blow as you check for an umbilical cord. If the cord is around the neck, try to slip it up over the baby's head or pull *gently* to get some slack so that it can slip down over the shoulders.

8. Support fetal head as restitution (external rotation) occurs. After restitution, with one hand on each side of the baby's head, exert *gentle* pressure downward so that the anterior shoulder emerges under the symphysis pubis and acts as a fulcrum; then as *gentle* pressure is exerted in the opposite direction, the posterior shoulder, which has passed over the sacrum and coccyx, is delivered.

9. Be alert! Hold the baby securely because the rest of his body may deliver quickly. He will be slippery!"

Maternal progress in first stage of labor within normal limits.

from *Maternity Care, The Nurse and The Family*

Cervix			
Dilatation	0-3 cm	4-7 cm	8-10 cm
Effacement			
Duration	About 8-10 hours	About 3 hr	About 1-2 hr
Contractions			
Magnitude	Mild	Moderate	Strong to expulsive
Rhythm	Irregular	More regular	Regular
Frequency	5-30 min apart	3-5 min apart	2-3 min apart
Duration	10-30 sec	30-45 sec	45-60 sec (few to 90 sec)
Descent			
Station of presenting part	Nulliparous: 0 Multiparous: 0 to -2 cm	About +1 to +2 cm About +1 to +2 cm	+2 to +3 cm +2 to +3 cm
Show			
Color	Brownish discharge, mucous plug or pale, pink mucus	Pink to bloody mucus	Bloody mucus
Amount	Scant	Scant to moderate	Copious
Behavior and appearance	Excited; thoughts center on self, labor, and baby; may be talkative or mute, calm or tense; some apprehension; pain controlled fairly well; alert, follows directions readily; open to instructions	Becoming more serious, doubtful of control of pain, more apprehensive; desires companionship and encouragement; attention more inner directed; fatigue evidenced; malar flush; has some difficulty following directions	Pain described as severe, backache common; feelings of frustration, fear of loss of control, and irritability surface; vague in communications; amnesia between contractions; writhing with contractions; nausea and vomiting, especially if hyperventilating; hyperesthesia; circumoral pallor; perspiration on forehead and upper lip; shaking, tremor of thighs; feeling of need to defecate, pressure on anus

WILLIAMS OBSTETRICS
(Sixteenth Edition)
by Jack A. Pritchard and
Paul C. MacDonald
1980, 1179 pages, Illus

from
Appleton-Century-Crofts
292 Madison Avenue
New York, NY 10017
$52.00 hd

Williams Obstetrics was first written by J. Whitridge Williams in 1902 and has been continuously revised and expanded since then as obstetrical knowledge and practice have changed. The book is used as a standard text in medical education and may also be of use to midwives and interested parents.

Williams begins with a great deal of technical material on female anatomy, endocrinology, and physiology, including the ovarian cycle, menstruation, conception, the development of the placenta, fetal development, and maternal adaption to pregnancy. The chapters which will be of use in the management of pregnancy concern the diagnosis of pregnancy, pelvic anatomy, position of the fetus, and prenatal care. The 16th edition includes a new chapter on "Technics to Evaluate Fetal Health" which describes the controversial new tests and technologies which are being used more and more in obstetrics (amniocentesis, ultrasound, stress and non-stress tests, electronic fetal monitoring). Six fairly brief chapters (116 pages) cover the physiology, mechanism and conduct of normal labor, birth, labor drugs, the puerperium, and the newborn. The next 616 pages, more or less, are devoted to abnormalities including hemorrhage, ectopic pregnancy, twins, toxemia, illness during pregnancy, dystocia, injuries to the birth canal, puerperal infection, prematurity, newborn diseases and birth defects, forceps, breech extraction, and cesarean section. Each chapter includes listings of medical references and many good line drawings and photographs. The use of a new two-column format and bold headings has made the text easier to scan and read. (A word of warning: *Williams Obstetrics* contains many photographs of maternal, fetal, and infant abnormalities which are **very grim.** In fact, even the photos of normal processes appear to have been chosen by someone who doesn't think well of the female body. I was startled and frightened by some of these pictures during my first pregnancy and still will not leaf casually through this book.)

"If the patient is to be delivered at home, the room to be used for the confinement, should be inspected in advance and suggestions made as to its arrangement. The obstetrician should also inquire as to the number of wash-basins which are available; for with the increasing perfection of plumbing the portable wash-basin has become replaced by permanent washstands, so that in many modern homes it is difficult to find a sufficient number for disinfecting the hands and cleansing the patient. Four basins will be needed: three for the use of the physician and one for the nurse; and if so many are not already in the house a sufficient number, made of plain agateware and measuring 10 inches across the top should be procured." (from the 1931 edition)

"ATTENDANCE IN LABOR."

Ideally, the person who performs these measurements [in monitoring labor] is able to remain with the mother throughout labor to provide psychological support as well as discern promptly any fetal or maternal abnormalities. Haverkamp and co-workers (1976, 1979) have demonstrated that an equally satisfactory outcome for the fetus can be achieved without continuous electronic monitoring of the fetal heart rate, continuous intrauterine pressure recording, and fetal scalp blood pH measurement if the mother and fetus are closely attended by appropriately trained labor room personnel. Given a choice, many women would probably prefer the reassurance of the nearly continuous presence of the obstetrician or of a compassionate well-trained obstetric associate to that of a metal cabinet and its wires and tubes that invade her and her fetus." (from the 1980 edition)

HANDBOOK OF OBSTETRICS AND GYNECOLOGY (Seventh Ed.)
by Ralph C. Benson
1980, 808 pages, Illus.

from
Lange Medical Publications
795 Altos Oaks Drive
Los Altos, CA 94022
$10.00

Ralph Benson is one of the co-authors of *Maternity Care, the Nurse and the Family* which we have praised highly (see index). His handbook can be used as an introduction to labor and birth for parents and midwifery students and can also be easily carried to births in the medical kit (it's like a small bible with flexible binding, rounded page corners, and small print). Benson provides clear descriptions of the basics of normal and abnormal birth and many good line drawings and charts are included. His recommendations for the "Management" of birth are fairly interventive (shave the perineum completely, use anesthesia for second stage, always do an episiotomy) but his presentation of normal physiology is sound.

"There are 3 stages of labor: (1) The period from the onset of labor to full dilatation of the cervix; (2) The period from full dilatation of the cervix to the delivery of the fetus; and (3) The period from delivery to the recovery of the placenta. The hour immediately after the birth of the placenta, during which time the danger of postpartal hemorrhage is great, is often referred to as the 4th stage of labor; it will be considered here as part of the third stage.

"The onset of the first stage begins with demonstrable, progressive dilatation and effacement of the cervix (see Figs. 5-1 and 5-2). It is often difficult to determine the exact time of onset since the cervix may change very slowly or rapidly.

"The *first stage* of labor ends with complete (10 cm) dilatation of the cervix. This stage is by far the longest. The average duration of the first stage is about 13 hours for the primigravida and about 8 hours for the multipara. However, the first stage of labor may be less than 1 hour or more than 24 hours depending upon (1) parity of the patient, (2) the frequency, intensity, and duration of uterine contractions, (3) the ability of the cervix to dilate and efface, (4) fetopelvic diameters, and (5) the presentation, position, and size of the fetus.

"The *second stage* of labor begins when the cervix becomes fully dilated and ends with the complete birth of the baby. The second stage varies from a few minutes to several hours, depending upon (1) fetal presentation and position, (2) fetopelvic relationships, (3) resistance of maternal pelvic soft parts, (4) the frequency, intensity, duration, and regularity of uterine contractions, and (5) the efficiency of maternal voluntary expulsive efforts.

"The *third or placental stage* of labor is the period from the birth of the infant to one hour after delivery of the placenta. The rapidity of separation and means of recovery of the placenta determine the duration of the third stage." (from the Sixth Edition)

16: MECHANISM OF NORMAL LABOR IN OCCIPUT PRESENTATION

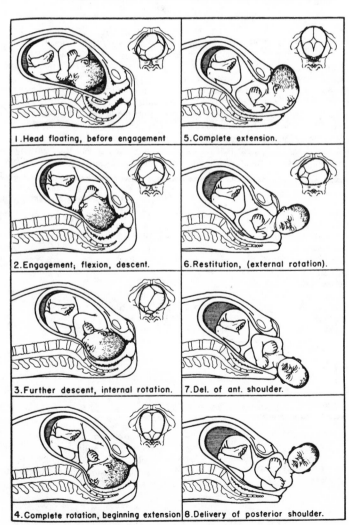

1. Head floating, before engagement
2. Engagement; flexion, descent.
3. Further descent, internal rotation.
4. Complete rotation, beginning extension
5. Complete extension.
6. Restitution, (external rotation).
7. Del. of ant. shoulder.
8. Delivery of posterior shoulder.

Fig. 16-1. Principal movements in the mechanism of labor and delivery, left occiput anterior position.

AN INTRODUCTION TO MID-WIFERY
by Maureen A. Hickman
1978, 501 pages, Illus.

from
Blackwell Scientific Publications
publisher
Blackwell Mosby Book Distributors
11830 Westline Industrial Drive
St. Louis, MO 63141
$19.95 pap.

This English midwifery text is divided quite simply into four main sections: normal pregnancy, labour and puerperium; abnormal pregnancy, labor and puerperium; the fetus and neonate; and health and social services (the last section is applicable only to services in Great Britain but provides an interesting contrast to the relative lack of social services for childbearing and rearing in the U.S.). Within each section, material is organized in outline form with many clear illustrations. Though first published in 1978 (that is, fairly recently), this book reflects a much less intervention-oriented approach to midwifery than recent editions of Myles (see index). Hickman has written a good general text which is informative on technical points *and* sensitive to the needs of women in labor.

"If arrangements are made for a home confinement or early transfer home following delivery, a home assessment is undertaken before the arrangements are finalised.

"Suitability of the home for early transfer includes:
a. Adequate standard of cleanliness.

b. Adequate accommodation with no overcrowding.
c. Indoor bathroom and toilet.
d. Hot and cold running water.
e. Adequate heating day and night.
f. Help available until the tenth postnatal day to undertake household chores and shopping.
g. Household pets under control.
"In addition to the items mentioned above the following would be noted when assessing the home for a home confinement.
a. Adequate lighting as the delivery may take place at night.
b. Telephone in case of an emergency.
c. Toilet and bathroom on same floor as mother's room.
d. Working surface for delivery pack.
e. Access for ambulance, summer and winter . . . .

"The mechanism of labour describes the changes in the attitude and position of the fetus in its descent through the birth canal. Because these movements are necessary for the fetus to adapt to the shape and size of the mother's pelvis it is logical to describe the mechanism of labour in relation to the maternal pelvis and fetal skull although it must also be considered in association with the physiology and management of labour.

"At the commencement of labour the fetus lies longitudinally in the uterus in an attitude of flexion. In the primigravida the head is normally already engaged in the pelvis; in a multigravida, owing to greater laxity of the uterine and abdominal wall muscles, flexion may be less complete

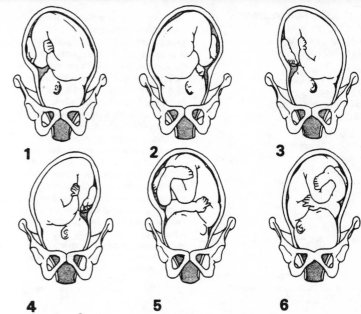

Fig. 4-3 Positions of the vertex: 1. left occipitoanterior; 2. right occipito-anterior; 3. left occipitolateral; 4. right occipitolateral; 5. left occipitoposterior; 6. right occipitoposterior.

and engagement does not usually take place until labour has already started.

"As labour progresses the fetus descends through the birth canal and there is increased flexion. The occiput meets the resistance of the pelvic floor and internally rotates forward through 45° (Fig. 3.64). When the occiput escapes under the pubic arch and the biparietal diameter is level with the ischial tuberosities, exten-

sion of the head takes place (Fig. 3.65). Because internal rotation of the head is not accompanied by rotation of the shoulders, a twisting of the neck occurs (Fig. 3.66). This is released (restitution) as soon as the head is born. Following restitution of the head, the shoulders rotate and descend causing the occiput to externally rotate a further 45° following the direction of restitution (Fig. 3.67)."

MIDWIFERY
by Jean L. Hallum
1972, 152 pages, Illus.

from
Arco Publishing Company Inc.
219 Park Avenue South
New York, NY 10003
request price information

The best way to describe this book is to quote the synopsis which appears on the front of the cover:

"This clear, accurate text written for obstetric nurses, midwives in training and all those who view Childbirth as a natural phenomenon, reviews the anatomy of the female genital organs and the physiological changes associ-

ated with childbirth. Patient care, the management of normal pregnancy and labour as well as postpartum care and care of the newborn are explained. While the complications of pregnancy and labour are considered, the emphasis throughout is on childbirth as a natural phenomenon, with unnecessary interference in the process to be avoided."

The book lives up to its description: it is a useful handbook, brief, comprehensive, and well-illustrated.

"Labour is defined as the process by which a viable foetus (28 weeks gestation) is expelled from the uterus. The whole process is due to *retraction* of the involuntary muscles in the upper uterine segment and passive stretching of the lower uterine segment and cervix. Midwives should understand retraction. When a muscle contracts, muscle fibres shorten: with relaxation their length is restored. This action occurs in the upper uterine segment throughout pregnancy. Retraction means that after a contraction, the muscle fibres fail to relax completely and gradually become shorter and shorter. In this way the length of the upper uterine segment diminishes. Consequently there is

progressively less room for the foetus in its bag of membranes, and pressure is exerted on the lower uterine segment and cervix. The internal cervical os dilates with slight separation of the chorion from the lower segment of the uterus. The cervical canal is drawn up and disappears. Pressure on the external cervical os causes dilation and the complete drawing up of the cervix. The period from the commencement of retraction until full dilatation of the cervix is known as the *first stage of labour.* In a primigravida the maximum time should not exceed 24 hours. A multiparous cervix, which has previously dilated, stretches more rapidly and the first stage should not exceed 12 hours. Frequently the time is less . . . .

"*The relief of pain.* With modern drugs a midwife should not allow a patient to become distressed with pain during labour. However, a relaxed patient, provided labour is normal, may not wish to have analgesics (pain relieving drugs) and none should be forced on her. All analgesics are potentially dangerous to the foetus, especially if the baby is born with a low birth weight. . . ."

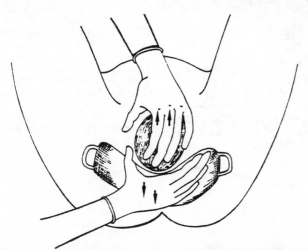

Fig. 10.16 Guarding the perineum

TEXTBOOK FOR MIDWIVES
(Ninth Edition)
by Margaret Myles
1981, 890 pages, Illus.

from
Churchill Livingstone, Inc.
19 West 44th Street
New York, NY 10036
$29.75

For many years, midwives and parents interested in alternative childbirth have looked to England as a model of better maternity care, since the English health system has involved the widespread use of professional midwives for normal births and the availability of services for home birth ("domicilliary confinement.") Unfortunately, this is changing as England becomes more "Americanized" and the new edition of Myles' midwifery text continues the trend away from non-interventive birth. The midwife is described as a member of the "obstetrical team" and the front cover photographs show her, in every case, using a machine to provide care to mother or baby. The already small section on home confinements has been reduced from six to four pages, the use of drugs rather than psychological support for pain relief is promoted, induction of labor and electronic fetal monitoring are praised without mention of adverse effects, etc. The sections on normal labor and birth are still well-illustrated with drawings and photographs which clearly show concepts, techniques, and especially, materials and methods for midwifery teaching. But the overall tone and direction of Myles is ultimately disappointing and saddening. Quite ironically, this new edition of *Textbook for Midwives* is more "conservative," dogmatic, technological in approach, and disapproving of consumer input than is the new edition of *Williams Obstetrics.*

"Pregnant women are inadvisedly exhorted by certain groups to demand "natural childbirth" and to refuse any interference. But when left to nature, labour can be long, painful, exhausting to the mother and lethal to both mother and child. Women today are not aware of the disastrous results of 'natural childbirth' at the beginning of this century and in some underdeveloped countries today.

"*Childbirth has been made safer, shorter, and easier by the very scientific procedures some misinformed women object to.* Reverting to primitive methods is a retrograde step which has no justification and should not be condoned . . . .

"To the expectant mother, labour is a very personal experience which engenders the presumption that she ought to participate in professional decisions and dictate regarding her obstetric care. But she may have little understanding of the tremendous amount of knowledge and years of experience needed in the practice of competent obstetrics. If she knew more she would realise the wisdom of having faith in professional experts and allowing them to make decisions regarding her own and her baby's wellbeing and safety throughout labour . . . .

"Drugs are more efficacious when the woman has been educationally conditioned to approach labour with equanimity based on confidence. Midwives should prepare expectant mothers to cope with such stresses as may occur using suggestion and distraction to heighten the pain threshold. Trust in the hospital staff, who will care for her, is a valuable aid. Complete reliance on the psychological method of pain relief is a subordinate feature in the management of labour today: prolonged labour is no longer permitted; it intensifies the perception of pain which becomes unbearable as the woman's stamina wanes. New drugs and epidural analgesia are now preferred to psychoprophylaxis."

EMERGENCY CHILDBIRTH

EMERGENCY CHILDBIRTH
by Gregory J. White
1958, 64 pages, Illus.

from
Police Training Foundation
3412 Ruby Street
Franklin Park, IL 60131
$4.95

Gregory White is a home birth physician and has been active in the alternative childbirth movement. His wife, Mary White, is one of the founding mothers of La Leche League. This manual was originally written to teach police, fire, and other emergency workers how to deliver a baby without a doctor. But it has also become a classic in the home birth movement, appearing on many "required reading" lists and helping many parents give birth at home without medical assistance. This is one of the clearest guides to "non-interventive" management of normal labor and birth. The first section, describing the basics, can be read at leisure, but there's also a back section of "Condensed Instructions for Emergency Use" which gives an easy-to-use outline, printed in large letters, to keep at your bedside during labor. Extensive details on complications in birth are not presented; nor are the fine points of birth technology and technique. The overall tone, however, conveys a strong sense of, and confidence in, birth as a normal process.

"Generally speaking, mechanical assistance is rarely needed, but psychological or emotional support to the mother is almost always in order. This is usually given by means of a calm and confident manner and the frequent assurance that all is going well. Such moral support is given to the mother not just because she is a fellow human being undergoing a trying experience, worthy as that reason is, but because calmness on her part and confidence in nature, in herself, and in her attendant make it possible for her to do her part of the job better. Giving birth, at its best, is something a mother *does,* not merely something which happens to her . . . .

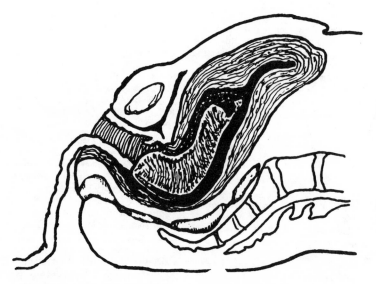

The placenta, or afterbirth, has loosened and is sliding out of the uterus. The mother is on her back. Do NOT pull on the cord.

"The afterbirth will follow the baby, usually in a few minutes, sometimes after many hours. If the woman is not bleeding, no effort should be made to hasten the delivery of the afterbirth. If there is some bleeding, or if the mother begins to feel severe cramps, the uterus should be felt through the belly wall. If soft, it should be massaged until it becomes very hard, and gentle downward pressure within the limits of the mother's comfort will usually deliver the afterbirth at this point. NEVER pull on the cord to deliver the afterbirth. Too vigorous massage—enough to cause the mother considerable pain—may deliver only part of the afterbirth and increase rather than diminish the blood loss. The entire afterbirth, all solid matter passed, should be saved (on ice if necessary) so that the doctor can inspect it for completeness when he comes. If the woman is to be taken to the hospital, the afterbirth should be taken with her.

"The afterbirth on the side detached from the womb resembles raw liver; the side toward the baby is covered by the shiny bag of waters and large blood vessels radiating out from the cord."

EMERGENCY CHILDBIRTH HANDBOOK
by Barbara Anderson and Pamela Shapiro
1979, 204 pages, Illus.

from
Delmar Publishers, Publisher
Van Nostrand Reinhold, Distributor
135 West 50th Street
New York, NY 10020
$8.20 paper

This manual was written by an obstetrical nurse and an ICEA-affiliated childbirth educator. It provides a more detailed presentation of birth than White's *Emergency Childbirth,* including fairly extensive chapters on the male and female reproductive systems and fetal development as well as on normal and abnormal labor, birth, and postpartum. The book is illustrated with very nice drawings and excellent photographs supplied by police and fire departments in Hawaii. A very useful set of appendices provides a list of emergency supplies, Lamaze techniques for use in emergency birth, instructions on how to hold an infant, a glossary of terms, and a self-test with answers.

Though the manual is intended for emergency personnel, it is so thorough and comprehensive that it would make good all-purpose reading for childbirth education classes whether or not an unattended birth is anticipated.

"The delivery of breech positioned babies is usually spontaneous and the outcome is generally good. However, it does involve more risk to the infant than a head presentation. The danger comes from the trauma of delivery and the chance of a prolapsed cord. Also, labor is usually longer for a breech delivery. Therefore, more time is available to get the woman to a hospital. This should be done if at all possible. If, however, the birth is happening rapidly, delivery usually is not difficult. This is because a rapid breech delivery usually means the baby is small, the contractions are strong and forceful, and

there is ample room in the birth canal. The baby will probably deliver spontaneously with little need of assistance.

"Preparation for Breech Delivery

"When the presenting part can be seen at the vaginal opening and immediate delivery of the baby is inevitable, prepare the expectant mother as you would for any delivery. Details were given in the preceding chapter. Briefly, they include these considerations:
Provide privacy
Explain what you plan to do
Position the woman (firm surface, knees bent, legs apart, head raised)
Drape her properly
Scrub your hands and arms thoroughly
Comfort and reassure the expectant mother
When delivering a baby in breech position, focus your attention on: (1) guiding and supporting the emerging infant, (2) helping the baby breathe, (3) handling it with care, (4) preventing infection in the mother and child and (5) reassuring the mother.

IF THE HEAD DOES NOT DELIVER WITHIN 3 MINUTES

"Rest the baby on the palm of your hand, with its legs stradling your forearm.

"Insert two fingers in the vagina and place them gently in the baby's mouth. With the fingertips, gently bend the baby's chin down on its chest. This places the head in a position where it can be more easily expelled. DO NOT PULL or use force. Sterile gloves should be used when available.

"Apply firm downward pressure on the mother's abdomen to help expel the head. *Caution:* Do not pull the baby. Pulling may permanently damage the baby's spinal cord, nerves, and/or breathing organs.

IF THE HEAD STILL DOES NOT DELIVER

"Create and maintain an air passage to the baby's nose so the infant will not suffocate.
Move the two fingers towards the baby's face.
Press the wall of the vagina away

from the baby's face with the back of your fingers.
"Form a 'V' by placing your fingers at each side of the baby's nose. The baby can breathe with this assistance until the head is delivered, or until medical help arrives."

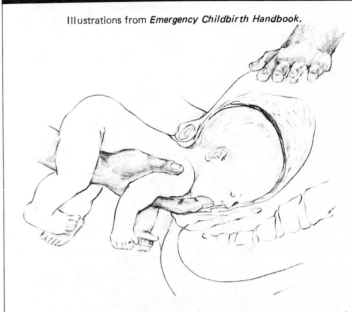

Illustrations from *Emergency Childbirth Handbook.*

Fig. 8-7 If the head does not deliver after the baby has rotated and is facing the mother's back, two fingers may be inserted to pull the lower jaw down and so bend the head; at the same time firm downward pressure is applied to the woman's abdomen. DO NOT PULL the baby out.

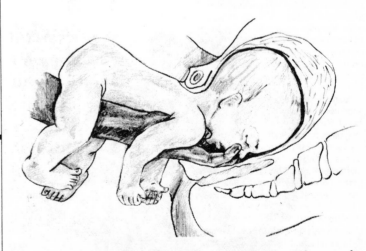

Fig. 8-8 If the head will still not deliver, make an air passage. With two fingers, form a "V" around the baby's nose. Press the back of the fingers against the vaginal wall so there is room for the baby to breathe until medical help arrives.

EMERGENCY CHILDBIRTH
by Rosemary Romberg Wiener
2 pages

from
Rosemary Romberg Wiener
6294 Mission Road
Everson, WA 98247
$.10 plus self-addressed, stamped envelope

This fact sheet provides basic instructions and points to remember for delivering a baby in an emergency.

"If the choice is between getting in the car and making a mad frantic dash to the hospital or birth center, versus having the baby at home by yourself, your safest choice is to stay at home. (If you as the mother are at

home with no other adult present, this is your *only* choice! Please don't be foolish enough to try to drive while you are in labor!!) The number of people killed or injured in traffic accidents, especially with a speeding, emotionally frantic driver, vastly outnumbers any dangers of medically unattended birth. Also, you are running the risk that the baby will be born in the car before you reach your destination. If this happens, the husband or other accompanying person will be busy driving and won't be able to help with the birth. The mother will not be very comfortable giving birth in a moving vehicle, and during the colder part of the year, the baby will be exposed to a greater possibility of getting chilled."

BIRTH ATLAS
Set of 19 charts in easel-back book
14" x 20", black and white
$25.00

RELATION OF GROWING UTERUS TO OTHER ORGANS
Set of 5 charts, 17" x 28"
black and white
$6.00

both from
Maternity Center Association
48 East 92nd Street
New York, NY 10028

The Birth Atlas uses photographs (life size) of the Dickinson-Belskie medical sculptures to illustrate in detail fertilization, development of the embryo and fetus, labor, and birth. The sequence showing cervical dilation and the movement of the baby through the birth canal is excellent. *Relation of Growing Uterus to Other Organs* uses drawings by Eva Schucardt to show how the mother's body adapts to the growing baby.

Both the Dickinson-Belskie sculptures and the Schucardt charts are reproduced in a smaller format (8½ x 11") in *A Baby Is Born* (see index).

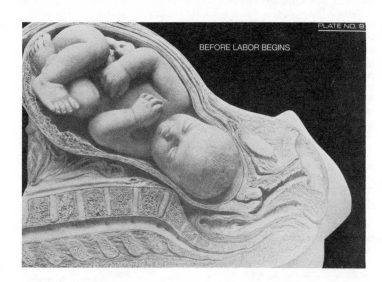

PLATE NO. 9

BEFORE LABOR BEGINS

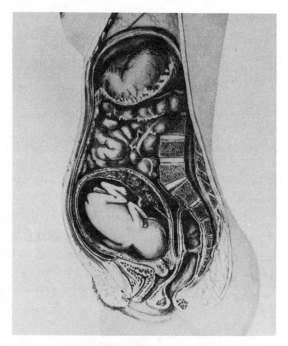

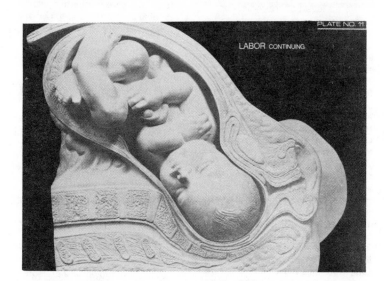

PLATE NO. 11

LABOR CONTINUING

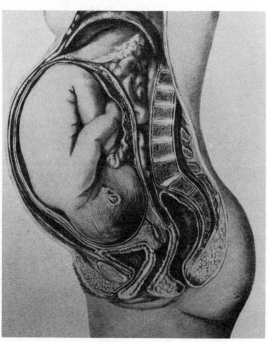

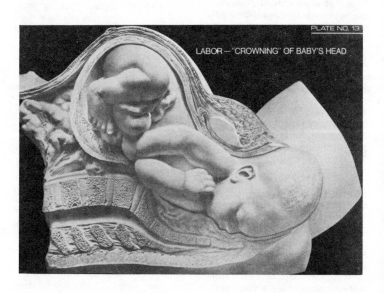

PLATE NO. 13

LABOR — "CROWNING" OF BABY'S HEAD

DILATION OF THE CERVIX

During labor the cervix or "neck" of the uterus enlarges from an opening of just a few millimeters wide to an opening large enough to permit the passage of the baby. Cervical dilation is most commonly measured in centimeters and a diameter of 10 centimeters is considered to be full or complete dilation. During labor the birth attendant may do an internal examination to determine the state of dilation. This helps to determine how labor is progressing. Student midwives and others who are learning how to feel for cervical dilation sometimes find it handy to cut circles of several diameters up to 10 centimeters out of cardboard. Running your finger around the edge of the circle helps teach the hand how to measure cervical dilation.

APGAR SCORE

The Apgar scoring system was devised by renowned neonatologist Virginia Apgar (see index for review of her book for parents, *Is My Baby All Right?*). The Apgar score is used to assess the condition of the newborn immediately after birth, to determine the possible need for resuscitation, and to provide a diagnostic tool for predicting the health of the baby in the first weeks of life. The scoring can be done by a birth attendant usually without interrupting any other care the baby may be receiving, and while the baby is being held by its parents.

The "signs" listed in the chart appear in order of their importance, from top to bottom. Heart rate is most important and is checked by observing pulsation of the umbilical cord or by using a stethoscope on the baby's chest. "Respiratory effort" means how well the baby is breathing. Vigorous crying is common if a healthy newborn is handled roughly at delivery, but crying as a sign of good respiration may not be so reliable when the baby is born more gently. A baby with good muscle tone will keep her arms and legs well flexed and resist efforts to extend them. Again, the poking and prodding which define the response of reflex irritability may not be necessary if the more important signs are good. Color is the least important sign. One to three minutes may go by before the baby's entire body is pink. The hands and feet will be the last to change color.

The Apgar score is usually done at 1, 5, and 15 minutes after birth. A score of 7 to 10 indicates a healthy baby, probably requiring no treatment. A score of 4 to 6 probably indicates a need for resuscitation. A score of 0 to 3 means the baby is severely depressed and must be resuscitated immediately.

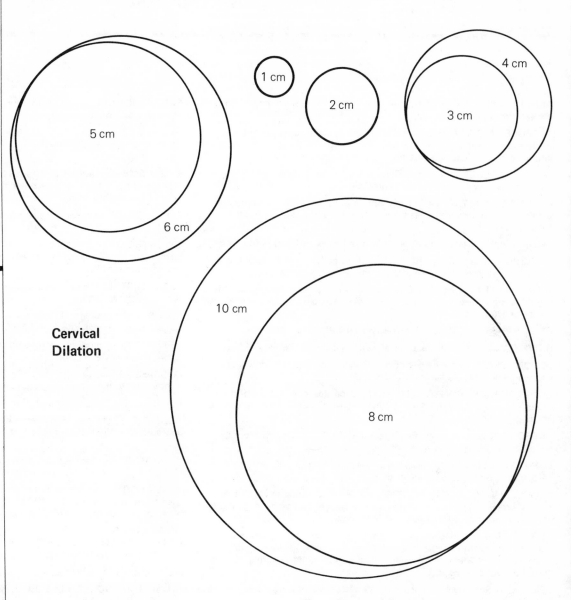

Cervical Dilation

Apgar Score

Sign	0	1	2
Heart Rate	Not detectable	Slow (below 100)	Over 100
Respiratory effort	Absent	Slow, irregular	Good, crying
Muscle tone	Flaccid	Some flexion of extremities	Active motion
Reflex Irritability 1. Response to slap on sole of foot.	No response	Grimace	Cry
2. Response to catheter in nostril.	No response	Grimace	Cough or sneeze
Color	Blue, pale	Body pink, extremities blue	Completely pink

GLOSSARY OF TERMS

ABRUPTIO PLACENTA Premature separation of a normally implanted placenta from the uterine wall.

AMNIOCENTESIS A procedure done to test for fetal abnormalities, maturity and sex. Done by inserting a needle through the abdomen and uterus into the amniotic fluid and withdrawing a sample for analysis.

AMNIOTIC FLUID The watery fluid within the amniotic sac, which surrounds the embryo and fetus during pregnancy.

AMNIOTIC SAC The "bag" of membranes which lines the uterus and contains the fetus before birth. Made up of two layers, the chorion and the amnion.

AMNIOTOMY Artificial rupture of the membranes during or before labor.

ANTERIOR The front or belly surface of the body. In an anterior position of the fetus, its back lies toward its mother's belly (see posterior).

AUSCULTATION Listening to sounds in the chest and abdomen. Specifically, listening through the uterus to the fetal heart beat, usually with a stethoscope or fetoscope.

BAG OF WATERS The amniotic sac and amniotic fluid within it.

BIRTH CANAL The vagina, especially during labor and delivery.

BLOODY SHOW A discharge of blood-tinged mucus from the cervix as it begins to dilate in early labor (see mucous plug).

BRAXTON-HICKS CONTRACTIONS Mild, painless contractions of the uterus which occur intermittently during pregnancy before the onset of true labor.

BREECH PRESENTATION Presentation at the cervix of the buttocks, knees, or feet of the fetus. (see presentation)

CAPUT SUCCEDANEUM Swelling of the presenting part of the baby's head, caused by pressure during labor.

CEPHALOPELVIC DISPROPORTION (CPD) A condition in which the head or presenting part of the fetus cannot engage or pass through the mother's pelvis, either because of shape, size, or position.

CERVIX The narrow lower end or "neck" of the uterus, which extends from the body of the uterus into the vagina. The cervix is closed during pregnancy and dilates to a diameter of about 10 centimeters during labor to permit passage of the baby.

CESAREAN SECTION Surgical delivery of a baby by lifting it out through an incision made through the abdominal wall and uterus.

COLOSTRUM Yellowish fluid which precedes breast milk and which is rich in antibodies and nutrients.

CONTRACTION The rhythmic shortening (contraction) and thickening (retraction) of the uterus during labor which work to efface and dilate the cervix and expel the fetus.

CROWNING That stage of delivery when the largest diameter of the baby's head is encircled by the vaginal opening.

DILATION (sometimes Dilatation) Enlargement of the opening of the cervix caused by the contractions of the uterus during labor.

DYSTOCIA Long or difficult labor or delivery caused by various mechanical or muscular factors.

EDEMA Retention of water in the tissues, often causing swelling of the ankles and legs. Severe edema may be a sign of toxemia.

EFFACEMENT Thinning of the cervix as it is drawn up into the body of the uterus by labor contractions.

EMBRYO The developing human being from the second or third week after conception to about the eighth week. A period of fundamental tissue and organ development.

ENGAGEMENT Descent of the fetal head or presenting part down into the pelvis, past the pelvic inlet. Usually occurs just prior to labor (in a primapara) or just after the beginning of labor (in a multipara).

EPISIOSTOMY A surgical incision of the perineum to enlarge the vaginal opening.

EXPECTED DATE OF CONFINEMENT (EDC) Estimated date of the baby's birth; "due date"; calculated as 40 weeks after the first day of the last menstrual period (LMP).

FETAL DISTRESS Poor condition of the fetus during labor, indicated by slow or irregular fetal heart rate.

FETUS A developing child in the uterus from about the eighth week after conception until birth; distinguished from embryo.

FETOSCOPE A modified stethoscope used to listen to fetal heart tones during pregnancy and labor.

FORCEPS An instrument made of two spoon-like, curved blades which is inserted into the vagina and used to extract the fetal head during delivery.

FUNDUS The large, upper end of the uterus.

GESTATION The period of pregnancy, usually lasting about 38 weeks from conception or 40 weeks from the first day of the last menstrual period.

GRAVIDA A pregnant woman
    PRIMAGRAVIDA A woman pregnant for the first time
    MULTIGRAVIDA A woman pregnant for the second or subsequent time.

HEMATOCRIT A measure of the percentage of red blood cells in the blood, used to test for anemia. Normal hematocrit levels range from 38% to 45% in non-pregnant women and may be normally lower (to 34%) in pregnant women.

HEMORRHAGE Heavy bleeding
    INTRAPARTUM HEMORRHAGE Bleeding during labor.
    POSTPARTUM HEMORRHAGE Excessive bleeding after delivery.

HYPERTENSION High blood pressure.

INDUCTION, INDUCED LABOR Labor started artificially by prematurely rupturing the bag of membranes or by giving an oxytocic drug or both.

I.V. Abbreviation for "intravenous." Injection of continuous "drip" of drugs or fluids into a vein.

LABOR The process of uterine contractions which dilate the cervix and expel the fetus and placenta. Usually divided into three stages.
    FIRST STAGE: The period of effacement and dilation of the cervix. Begins with the onset of regular contractions and ends with complete dilation of the cervix.
    SECOND STAGE: The period of expulsion of the baby through the birth canal. Begins with complete dilation and ends with the birth of the baby.
    THIRD STAGE: The period of expulsion of the afterbirth or placenta. Begins with the birth of the baby and ends with the delivery of the placenta.
    (Also see "Transition")

LITHOTOMY A conventional position for delivery in which the woman lies flat on her back with her knees bent and legs spread wide apart with stirrups.

GLOSSARY OF TERMS

LOCHIA   The discharge of mucus and blood from the uterus after childbirth. Usually lasts about six weeks.

LAST MENSTRUAL PERIOD (LMP)   The length of pregnancy is usually calculated from the first day of the last menstrual period because the actual date of conception or ovulation is often not known. Therefore, a woman who is 16 weeks pregnant LMP, for instance, is in fact 14 weeks pregnant.

MASTITIS   Breast infection.

MECONIUM   A dark, greenish brown substance which accumulates in the bowel of the fetus and is usually discharged right after birth. Passage of meconium during labor (causing staining of the amniotic fluid) may be a sign of fetal distress.

MOLDING   Change in shape of the fetal head as it passes through the birth canal.

MUCOUS PLUG   A mass of mucus and blood which plugs the cervix during pregnancy and may be discharged from the vagina as labor begins.

NEONATAL   The period immediately after the baby is born.

OCCIPUT   The back part or "crown" of the head which usually leads and emerges first during passage through the birth canal.

OXYTOCIN   A postpituitary hormone responsible for mediating many of the processes of reproduction, including orgasm, labor contractions, and the milk ejection or "let-down" reflex.

PALPATION   Examination of the body by touching; specifically, feeling through the abdomen and uterus to determine the size and position of the fetus.

PARITY   The state of having carried a pregnancy to the stage of viability of the fetus.
   NULLIPARA   A woman who has not been pregnant or carried a pregnancy to viability.
   PRIMAPARA   A woman who has carried one pregnancy to viability, usually used to describe a woman pregnant for the first time.
   MULTIPARA   A woman who has carried two or more pregnancies to viability, used to describe a woman pregnant for the second or subsequent time.

PELVIC FLOOR   The muscular structures stretching across the bottom of the pelvis which support the pelvic organs. The urethra, vagina, and rectum pass through the pelvic floor.

PELVIS   Bony structure which cradles the pelvic organs.
   FALSE PELVIS   Upper portion, which varies considerably in size and does not affect childbearing capacity
   TRUE PELVIS   Lower portion, through which the fetus actually passes to be born. Small or irregular diameters of the true pelvis, combined with the size of the fetal head, may produce cephalo-pelvic disproportion.

PERINATAL   The period immediately before, during, and after birth.

PERINEUM   The triangular area of tissue between the anus and the back of the vaginal opening. This is the site of the episiotomy incision or of perineal lacerations or tears resulting from birth.

PITOCIN   The trade name of a synthetic form of oxytocin. Used to induce labor or augment labor contractions.

PLACENTA   The bloody organ which makes possible the exchange of nutrients and waste materials between the fetus and the mother. Attached to the fetus by the umbilical cord.

PLACENTA PREVIA   A condition in which the placenta develops low in the uterus and partially or completely covers the cervical opening.

POSITION   The position of the fetus in the uterus, described as the relationship between the fetal back and the front (anterior), back (posterior) or sides of the mother's pelvis. Thus, a fetus lying with its back toward the left, front side of its mother's body is described as being in a left anterior position (this is the most common position).

POSTERIOR POSITION   Position in which the back of the fetus is toward the back of the mother. Usually results in a longer, more difficult labor because the fetal head is not in the best position to move through the birth canal.

POSTMATURE LABOR   Labor beginning more than two weeks after the expected date of birth.

POSTPARTUM   The period after birth, usually lasting for about six weeks.

PREMATURITY   Birth of a baby before reaching a gestational age of 37 weeks LMP, or about three weeks or more before the estimated date of birth.

PREMATURE RUPTURE OF MEMBRANES   Spontaneous rupture of the bag of waters before the onset of labor. (see amniotomy)

PRENATAL   Before birth.

PRESENTATION   The part of the fetus which "presents" or appears first at the pelvic outlet. May be a vertex presentation (head first), breech, arm (indicating a transverse lie), or face.

PROLAPSED CORD   A condition in which the umbilical cord falls below or in front of the presenting part of the fetus.

PUERPERIUM   The postpartum period of about three to six weeks after birth, or specifically, the period until the uterus has returned to its nonpregnant size.

TERM   The complete period of gestation, about 38 to 42 weeks LMP.

TOXEMIA   A metabolic disorder of pregnancy also known as:
   PRE-ECLAMPSIA   A toxemia of pregnancy characterized by increasing blood pressure, edema, and protein in the urine.
   ECLAMPSIA   A severe form of toxemia characterized by convulsions and coma in addition to the symptoms of pre-eclampsia.

TRANSITION   The last phase of first stage labor in which the cervix dilates from about 8 to 10 centimeters.

TRIMESTER   A period of three months, used to divide pregnancy into three trimesters.

UMBILICAL CORD   The cord which connects the fetus with the placenta.

UTERUS   The hollow, muscular organ in which the fetus and placenta develop and which contracts to expel these "products of conception."

VERNIX   A white, creamy substance which covers and protects the skin of the fetus and newborn baby at birth.

Mail-order Books and Supplies

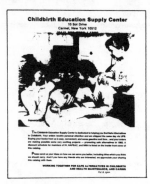

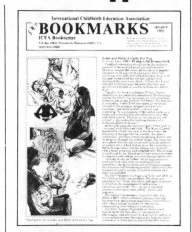

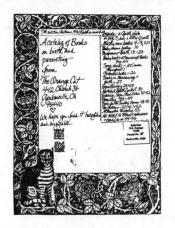

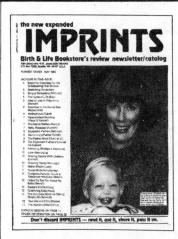

CHILDBIRTH EDUCATION SUPPLY CENTER
10 Sol Drive
Carmel, NY 10512
914/225-7763 and 4809
free catalog

Childbirth Education Supply Center (CESC) is operated by John Crockett and Pat Way. John teaches Informed Homebirth classes and has been active in alternative childbirth since 1976. CESC stocks almost 150 books on pregnancy and birth, midwifery, medical reference, nutrition, breastfeeding, parenting, books about birth for children, personal growth, and related subjects. CESC also carries anatomical charts and a selection of birth supplies. As a special feature CESC includes a library card and pocket (for childbirth educators' lending libraries) with each book ordered and also encloses "Tru-Breast" and "No Smoking-Fetal Growth in Progress" posters with each shipment. CESC offers a discount to current members of NAPSAC, the National Midwives Association, and Informed Homebirth.

CESC is also gathering information for the National Resource Referral Service for Safe Alternatives in Childbirth, a computer database which will help parents locate birth resources in their area. A data sheet is included in the CESC catalog.

ICEA BOOKCENTER
P.O. Box 20048
Minneapolis, MN 55420
612/854-8660
free catalog

ICEA Bookcenter has been a service of the International Childbirth Education Association since 1964. ICEA members receive a 10% discount on prepaid orders of $30. or more and all proceeds from the sale of books go to further the work of ICEA. The Bookcenter publishes a biannual newsletter/catalog, *Bookmarks,* which includes news and reviews of new books and the complete annotated book list of over 400 titles in childbirth preparation, pregnancy and birth, cesarean birth, midwifery, teenage pregnancy, breastfeeding, parenthood, infant/child development and care, fathers, women, health and family planning, grief, nutrition, for children, for childbirth educators and groups, professional books, and poetry and humor. The Bookcenter is the main source for all ICEA publications (over 30 books and pamphlets) and bulk rates are available for most of these. Service on all orders is very prompt.

THE ORANGE CAT (GOES TO MARKET)
442 Church Street
Garberville, CA 95440
707/923-9960
free catalog

The Orange Cat is a mail-order book business offering books on birth and parenting. Owner Kathy Epling produces a delightfully personal catalog which includes book listings with her own reviews, many lively illustrations from old manuscripts, and personal notes on the growth of young son Garth (whose birth motivated his mother's entry into the book-selling business). Book categories include pregnancy and birth, medical reference, miscarriage and death, breastfeeding, natural birth control, exercise, yoga, meditation, and parenting. She also lists books for the creative woman, for children, alternative education, and note cards.

"I had imagined birthing my child in my home, harmoniously reclining in John's arms, surrounded no doubt by candles and flowers and love. I had a very long (but very supported—I still get tears in my eyes thinking of the intense and continued loving energy poured out to me by my birth attendants) labor at home, but ended up going into the hospital, where Garth was born. John did support me at the moment of birth and it was undrugged and miraculous. But there were no flowers and candles, silver nitrate was used in Garth's eyes. It wasn't THE PERFECT HOME BIRTH. But love was there, and a great affirmation (and much much learning—I learned more of myself from those long hours of labor than from many years of my life). Perhaps what I am trying to say is—yes, plan your perfect dream birth. Do everything to make it so. But then remember *any* birth is a miracle, *any* labor an affirmation of your own strength and self and being—and love is present wherever you may be."

BIRTH AND LIFE BOOKSTORE
P.O. Box 70625
Seattle, WA 98107
206/789-4444

For many years Lynn Moen operated the ICEA book service from Seattle, and when ICEA consolidated its operations in Minneapolis in 1980, Lynn Moen continued on her own with Birth and Life Bookstore. She stocks over 400 titles in childbirth preparation, pregnancy and birth, alternatives and home birth, books for childbirth educators and groups, cesarean birth, medical texts and references, family planning, teenage pregnancy, women and health issues, food and nutrition, breastfeeding, humor, parenthood, grief and loss, the human condition, child care and books for children. She also carries pamphlets and recordings. Her newsletter/catalog *Imprints* includes reviews and listings of new books, advertisements, and the complete annotated mail-order listing. Service is very prompt.

COLLIN'S FAMILY-BIRTH BOOKSTORE
4940 SW West Hills Road
Corvallis, OR 97333
503/758-1435
free catalog

This family business features books on pregnancy and childbirth, medical reference, family planning, parenting, breastfeeding, health care, nutrition, and humor plus ovulation thermometers, birthing dolls, and other special items.

NOAH'S ARK BOOKS
P.O. Box 463
South Sutton, NH 03273
603/927-4237
free catalog

Noah's Ark offers an extensive selection of books on alternative life styles and self-sufficiency, including about 45 titles on birth, children, and parenting.

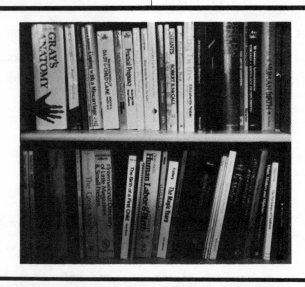

BIRTH SUPPLIES

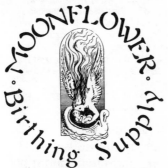

MOONFLOWER BIRTHING SUPPLY
8593 Highway 172
Ignacio, CO 81137
303/259-3129

Patricia Pedigo and Christopher Junkin of Moonflower describe their business this way:

"Moonflower Birthing Supply is a home business that supplies medical equipment for midwives and parents interested in homebirths, a full range of pertinent books including over 25 titles of technical books and a wide variety of natural baby paraphernalia, bumper stickers and T-shirts for homebirth supporters all in one handy catalog. We keep a large inventory and are usually able to fill your order within 2 business days. Almost all the items were chosen from personal experience and have been tested in birth situations many times. Our satisfied customers from all over the U.S. and various other parts of the world feel well-served. There is a 10% discount available to current members of Informed Homebirth on most items if the order totals more than $10.00. Call or write for a free brochure."

Moonflower sells a parent's Basic Birthing Kit (13 items) for about $16. and a Basic Midwifery Kit (9 items) for from $100. to $135. Other birth supplies available separately include wooden and metal fetoscopes, hemostats, speculums, surgical scissors, infant scales, portable oxygen units, sterile barrier towels and underpads, bulb syringes, gauze pads, sterile gloves, betadine scrub, cord clamps, urine test strips, and much more. These items are all available to "lay" people. Moonflower also stocks some "controlled" items which are available only to medical professionals. These include sutures and needles, mucus traps, and a stainless steel amniotome.

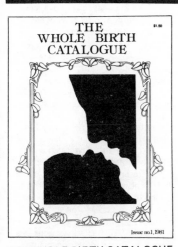

THE WHOLE BIRTH CATALOGUE
20 London Road West
Guelph, Ontario
N1H 2B5, Canada
519/837-2796
$1.50 per catalog

The Whole Birth Catalogue is a mail-order business sponsored by the Ontario Midwives Association. The *Catalogue* features maternity and nursing clothing in ethnic styles, breastfeeding aids, notecards, lambskins, herbs, vitamins, cassette tapes and records, a complete line of birth supplies (including FDA-restricted items which are not restricted to lay people in Canada), and an extensive list of books (almost 250 titles) on sex education, pregnancy and birth, exercise, nutrition, breastfeeding, family planning, health consciousness, self-healing, death, parenting, medical reference, and much more. Nice photographs and a list of Canadian and U.S. resource organizations is included.

"Many specific herbs have been used throughout the centuries by pregnant and lactating women. A popular herb for pregnancy, red raspberry leaf tea is believed in many cultures to facilitate labour and delivery by toning the uterus. Chinese women have used this tea 3 times daily in the last 3 months of pregnancy. In other cultures it has been used daily throughout pregnancy and lactation with the belief that the tea prepares the female organs to get them ready for childbirth. Others feel that it is the psychological benefits of sipping tea while meditating on the child within that is most beneficial to the pregnant woman. After all, the attitude a woman has towards herself and her baby make all the difference in the birthing experience . . . ."

SUGGESTED SUPPLIES FOR PRENATAL CARE AND HOME BIRTH

Fetoscope (to hear baby's heartbeat)	$ 30.00
Blood pressure cuff	30.00
Urine text sticks (100 per bottle)	20.00
Sterile gloves (for internal vaginal exams), 1 dozen	6.00
Sterile underpads (to absorb birth fluids, create "sterile field" in birth area), 1 dozen	3.00
Sterile 4" x 4" gauze pads (for perineal support, misc.), 1 box	4.00
Betadine scrub (to wash hands), 1 bottle	4.00
Fingernail brush (to clean under fingernails)	1.00
Isopropyl Alcohol (to cover sterile instruments, care of umbilical cord stump), 1 pint	1.00
K-Y sterile lubricant or olive oil (for perineal massage)	2.00
Scissors (to cut umbilical cord)	10.00
Umbilical clamps, or cord tape, or sterile shoelaces (to tie off cord before cutting)	1.00
Bulb ear syringe (to suction mucus from baby)	2.00
Plastic squeeze bottles (to apply oil for perineal massage and for perineal care after birth)	1.00
Maternity-size sanitary napkins and belt (to absorb after birth flow of lochia), 1 dozen	2.00
Large cook pot (to boil instruments)	10.00
Large bowls (to catch placenta, misc.)	10.00
Hot water bottle or heating pad (for labor comfort)	10.00
Large plastic sheet (to protect mattress or floor from birth fluids)	5.00
Thermometer	3.00
Flashlight	2.00
Disposable Diapers (to absorb mother's "drips" during labor and to diaper newborn)	3.00
List of emergency phone numbers	
Approximate Total Cost	170.00
Plus estimated midwife's fee	500.00
total	$670.00

(Estimated cost for hospital delivery and stay / $3,000.00)

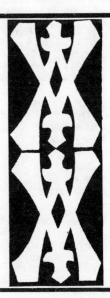

CASCADE BIRTHING SUPPLIES CENTER
P.O. Box 1300
Philomath, OR 97370
503/754-6184
free catalog

Donna and Paul Ruscher of Cascade Birthing Supplies offer a complete line of home birth kits and midwifery supplies. Unusual items include umbilical cord tape, stainless steel reuseable cord clamps, a cord bander, pelvimeters, instrument trays, instrument "milk," bed pans, sterilization wrap and tape, and unrestricted medical dopplers.

Childbearing in Perspective

Psychology and Sociology of Childbirth

How does childbirth affect the mind of the individual and of society? Since childbirth has been defined as a medical event in our society, people often do not place enough importance on the effects of thought and feeling on birth. But many experienced midwives feel that the psychological state of the mother is the single most important factor in determining the progress of labor, more important than the particular physical factors involved. Women come to childbirth with a complex set of expectations and mental skills and with specific psychological "tasks" to accomplish. A woman's own personality and also the "personality" of her culture and surroundings affect how she prepares for birth and how she responds to the stresses of labor. A woman who has a good, positive birth experience, in which she feels she has achieved something and done the best she can for her baby and herself, will feel good about herself and her baby and be a stronger person. A woman whose important needs and desires are frustrated in birth will carry that scar and re-live that bad experience for the rest of her life, very often with negative consequences for the baby and the family.

Some doctors feel that a woman's desire for a "good birth experience" should not take precedence over medical safety. But childbirth advocates know that these two interests are rarely incompatible. What's good for a woman's mind and self-esteem is also good for her body and for the baby. Good birth experiences are a source of great power and competence for women as well as the source of healthy babies. The way we experience birth affects our health and growth as women and as mothers, affects the health of our children, and ultimately makes its mark upon the well-being of our society.

THE PSYCHOLOGY OF CHILDBIRTH
by Aidan Macfarlane
1977, 140 pages, Illus.

from
Harvard University Press
79 Garden Street
Cambridge, MA 02138
$3.95 pap.

Two developments of recent decades—the reevaluation of women's role in society and the control of birth by male medical specialists—have spurred increased interest in examining the complex psychological aspects of childbearing, especially as medical control and sex role models effect physical outcomes in childbirth. In his prologue to *The Psychology of Childbirth,* author Aidan Macfarlane says, "Mothers now having babies are considered 'patients in hospitals' rather than human beings who go through normal physiological and psychological developments. To a certain extent we seem to have reached a point of diminishing returns: increasing interference provides less and less in terms of improved outcome. In spite of lip service paid to the idea that psychological and physiological changes are so linked that changes in one area do not occur without changes in the other, little use is made of the connection. Nevertheless, psychological factors can be used both to predict where trouble may occur in pregnancy and birth and to improve the quality of the experience." With the aims of prediction and improvement in mind, Macfarlane looks at birth and the constellation of events which surround it, briefly presenting what current studies and literature have to say about the baby's intrauterine experience, the effects of labor induction and hospitalization for birth, methods of pain relief in labor, the significance of the first minutes after birth, what the baby is able to perceive at birth, the effects of early mother/infant separation, and events in the early weeks at home. While recognizing the contribution of some medical advances in lowering mortality, Macfarlane feels that birth care is best provided in a context which acknowledges and provides for the psychological needs and functioning of mothers and babies.

"A healthy woman who delivers spontaneously performs a job that cannot be improved upon."

"In all discussions of home versus hospital delivery, the childbirth practices in The Netherlands inevitably come up. Holland has a lower death rate among babies than either the United States or England, and yet a very substantial number of the deliveries are carried out at home.
"G.J. Kloosterman, Professor of Obstetrics at the University of Amsterdam, has summarized the philosophy on which the organization of obstetrics in The Netherlands has been based since the beginning of this century. 'Childbirth in itself is a natural phenomenon and in the large majority of cases needs no interference whatsoever—only close observation, moral support, and protection against human meddling.' A healthy woman who delivers spontaneously performs a job that cannot be improved upon. This job can be done in the best way if the woman is self-confident and stays in surroundings where she is the real center (as in her own home). . . .
"The philosophy in Great Britain and the United States is quite different. It operates on the basis that it is impossible to predict which women will be 'at risk,' so that all women having babies must be treated as if they were high risks and hospitals are the places to deal with them. Therefore, if a mother has her baby at home, she is increasing the risks not only to her own health but to that of the baby. Again a question of values is involved. Each time a pregnant woman crosses a street she is increasing the risk of death for herself and her unborn baby, but no one would question her right to cross the street."

THE PEOPLE PLACE
1465 Massachusetts Avenue
Arlington, MA 02174
617/643-8630

"The People Place is a Family Counseling Service founded in 1974 and involved in Childbirth Counseling since 1978. We strongly believe that supportive family living is the only antidote to our present economic stress, skyrocketing divorce rates and increasing alienation and conflict. We now know that childbirth experiences and their accompanying adjustments greatly influence the future effectiveness of each family system.

"Our Childbirth Counseling Program is aimed primarily at producing emotionally positive birth experiences for all family members, regardless of where or how parents choose to birth. We believe parents deserve the highest support for choosing the birth experiences most suited to their needs, as well as those of their unborn children, without guilt or self-recrimination.

"In order for each birth to be emotionally welcomed with the freshness and newness parents and children deserve, it may be necessary to clear parents of previous painful birth-related events. Through a process of awareness and release, the body, mind and spirit can be relaxed and opened for a positive birthing.

"Over the past four years, we have developed some special and unique techniques for couples seeking VBAC (Vaginal Birth After Cesarean). Through the use of visualization, guided fantasy and yoga breathing, parents (especially women) can regain faith in the functioning of their physical bodies and experience the emotional relaxation and self-confidence necessary to produce effective labor and vaginal birth.

"We have also developed a program for 'Parents-in-Grief'—those parents/grandparents who have lost their children through miscarriage, still-birth and infant death. Effective grieving is necessary for all family members so that the profound sorrow and loss can be healed without prolonged suffering, guilt and blame."

Publications available from the People Place include:

THE EMOTIONAL UPS AND DOWNS OF CHILDBIRTH: A Healing Handbook
by Claudia S. Panuthos and Barbara Bierkoe-Peer
$8.00 plus $1.00 postage

ENLIGHTENED PARENTHOOD
by Claudia S. Panuthos
$10.00 plus $1.00 postage

EIGHT STEPS TO POSITIVE BIRTHING
by Johanna M. Silva
$2.00 plus $.25 postage

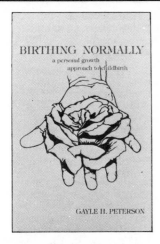

BIRTHING NORMALLY: A Personal Growth Approach to Childbirth
by Gayle H. Peterson
1981, 203 pages

from
Mindbody Press
1749 Vine Street
Berkeley, CA 94703
$10.95

While psychologists and sociologists study and speculate about the relationship between mind and body in childbirth, Gayle Peterson and her collaborator Lewis Mehl have developed a practical program for putting the relevant concepts to work. The aim appears to be twofold: first, to help birth attendants identify those women who are "at risk" psychologically, and secondly, to help women and their care givers optimize the birth experience through awareness of the effects of emotional factors. Peterson describes her theory of "holistic" childbirth preparation, explaining the importance of attitudes and beliefs in affecting the course of pregnancy and birth. She provides a detailed outline of a series of prenatal classes which can help women become more aware of their feelings about birth and which teach "psychophysiological" methods for coping with labor pain and stress. Peterson draws upon many of the techniques of the "human potential movement" (relaxation, use of mental imagery, touch and massage, breathing patterns, creative trance states, hypnosis, etc.) to create a prenatal program which aims to integrate mind/body functioning. Her presentation will be useful for parents but is particularly geared toward childbirth educators and others who may be teaching prenatal classes. Examples are given of how birth attendants can use "psychological intervention" to facilitate the progress of labor. Two sections also provide detailed descriptions of "holistic screening for obstetrical risk" (by Lewis Mehl) and "psychophysiological risk screening." In all, birth is seen as an expression of a woman's total being and personality, calling into play her unique configuration of hopes, fears, memories,

beliefs, and habitual ways of coping. The more a woman understands these facets of herself, and the more her attendant understands and appreciates the mother's emotional background, the better birth will proceed for all concerned.

"Use of the toilet. As mentioned in an earlier case history, the bathroom is a place in which most of us have repeatedly experienced letting go of the sphincter muscles in the urethra and anus. Because of this physical association, which may perhaps even constitute a conditioned reflex, it can be advantageous for a woman to sit on the toilet during contractions. When used as an intervention, sitting on the toilet has increased the strength and hardness of contractions for some women. If the woman is sexually inhibited during labor, or romantically inclined, and experiencing uterine inertia, the environment of the bathroom and the act of sitting on the toilet may break the romantic atmosphere, precipitating hard contractions. Sitting on the toilet, particularly if labor is stopped at 7-10 cms. or in second stage, may increase pressure on the rectum, bladder, and vagina, which further reinforces the conditioned response to let go of the sphincter muscles themselves. The desire to push may also be enhanced, and effectiveness of pushing may greatly increase on the toilet when no other position has yielded any progress."

PSYCHOPHYSIOLOGICAL ASSOCIATES
1749 Vine Street
Berkeley, CA 94703
415/843-2766

Gayle Peterson, MSW and Lewis Mehl, MD, PhD, are codirectors of Psychophysiological Associates. They travel extensively throughout the country providing a series of workshops on Holistic Prenatal Care and Risk Screening, based on concepts discussed in their book *Birthing Normally.* The workshops present the Mind/Body approach for assessing risk and improving birth outcome and are designed for midwives, nurses, physicians, childbirth educators, and psychotherapists. The three-day series costs about $55. and is offered once a month in a different city. Write for a calendar schedule.

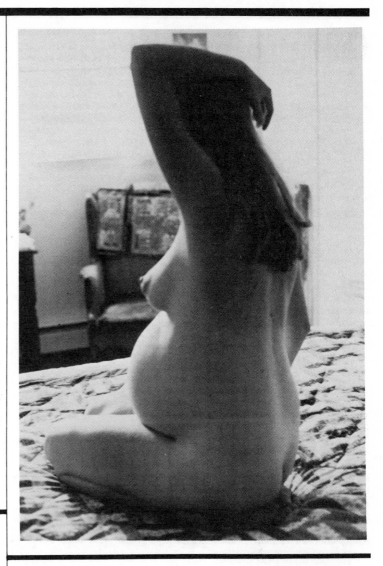

ASSOCIATION FOR BIRTH PSYCHOLOGY
444 East 82nd Street
New York, NY 10028
212/988-6617

The Association for Birth Psychology was founded in 1978 by Leslie Feher, who has trained in psychoanalysis and hypnosis. The goal of the Association is to promote the establishment of birth psychology as "a relevant and autonomous science of human behavior." The discipline of birth psychology is defined as follows:
1. The study of the psychological, sociological and ethical attitudes towards birth.
2. The study of embryology, neurology and physiology preceding, during and after birth as they interact and affect adult emotional patterns.
3. The study of the effects of medical practices on the psychological reactions of mother, child, doctor, father and family.
  A. Prenatal care
  B. Medical procedures and technology
  C. Attitudes and interactions of obstetrician with mother, child and family
  D. Pediatrician's interaction with mother, child and family.
4. The implications for future research in medicine, psychology and psychotherapy.

The Association publishes a biannual journal, *Birth Psychology Bulletin,* which is available to nonmembers for $8.00. The Association also sponsors an annual conference on birth psychology. Membership is $25. per year, which includes free admission to the annual conference, free subscription to *Birth Psychology Bulletin* and discounts on publications and workshops. Membership is available to all professionals and paraprofessionals who deal with psychological aspects of birth, such as obstetricians, psychiatrists, psychologists, midwives, counselors, nurses, sociologists, pediatricians, etc. Student memberships are available at $15. per year.

PSYCHOLOGICAL ASPECTS OF PREGNANCY, BIRTHING, AND BONDING
by Barbara L. Blum, Ph.D., ed.
1980, 380 pages
(Vol. IV in *New Directions in Psychotherapy Series,* an official publication of the National Institute for the Psychotherapies)

from
Human Sciences Press
72 Fifth Avenue
New York, NY 10011
$25.95 hd.

Changes in medical science, public health, and public life (industrialization, changes in women's status, improvements in infant mortality rates, prenatal diagnosis, use of contraceptives and abortion) have changed the way we experience pregnancy and childbirth. So we try to adapt our attitudes and values to keep pace with the changes possible in our behavior. That's the premise of this book, a collection of papers written by professionals (psychologists, social workers, doctors, nurses, educators) for professionals who may have to deal with the psychological adjustments of their pregnant clients. The book is laced with psychology jargon ("Object relationships," "countertransference") and assumes a familiarity with and acceptance of Freud's theories, including concepts like "penis envy" and the "oedipal conflict." The contributers provide many useful or at least thought-provoking ideas but there is a tendency to view mothers' psychological prob-

lems as arising more from their own internal ego structures than from external forces, such as the low social status of mothers, or the lack of adequate services. The result is that therapists are encouraged to "intervene" in the individual problem pregnancy by providing psychotherapy, without much thought to working for change in the social context of childbearing. And mothers may feel that seeking out an "expert" to help them solve their personal problems would be more effective than banding together with their peers to change their situation. I find these ideas disturbing, mainly because they tend to "blame the victim" and direct remediation toward her, rather than her oppressors, so to speak. However, three of the papers would be particularly useful to parents: Patsy Turrini's "Psychological Crises in Normal Pregnancy," based in part on her work with the Model Mother's Center in Hicksville, Long Island; "A Psychohistorical View of 19th and 20th Century Birth Practices" by Alice Eichholt; and "The Prevention of Birth Trauma and Injury Through Education for Childbearing" by Doris Haire.

"Pregnancy and childbirth, as other life transitions, have always been times when conflicts and feelings regarding one's adequacy, fears, hopes, and relationships to past generations arise. Pregnancy, childbirth, and parenting involve major life changes in the woman's body, in interpersonal relationships, in the dy-

namics of the family, and in social status. Childbirth implies the birth of a life-style as well as of a child; new roles are taken on, old roles are discarded, and social patterns may change. People's ability to cope with the stresses of major life transitions, which is dependent upon their available ego resources as well as upon the sociocultural milieu, results either in psychological growth or in disturbance. In the past, culture and religion provided men and women with elaborate ceremonies, rites, and rituals to mark and to help them cope with the anxieties and conflicts of life transitions . . . . In our postindustrialized society, while some religious ceremonies remain (e.g., circumcision, baptism), most cultural rituals regarding conception, pregnancy, and childbirth have been discarded. Yet, much of the anxiety persists. In fact, new anxieties and new stresses, resulting from medical, cultural, and technological changes have emerged.

"Some people elect to leave decisions and choices regarding pregnancy and childbirth to authority figures (e.g., doctors, clergy) and remain passive and dependent. Others question procedures, attitudes and methods, and become active participants in the choices made. The control exerted over pregnancy and childbirth choices probably is representative of the manner in which these persons handle other important life decisions."

—from the Introduction

PSYCHOLOGICAL EFFECTS OF MOTHERHOOD: A Study of First Pregnancy
by Myra Leifer
1980, 291 pages

from
Praeger Publishers
521 Fifth Avenue
New York, Ny 10017
$22.95 hd., $8.95 pap.

Leifer's study of the psychology of pregnant women closely parallels that of Breen (see *Birth of a First Child,* listed in index) and their conclusions are quite similar; basically, that pregnancy is a time of rapid and active psychological change and adjustment. This book is well-organized and discusses the emotional changes of pregnancy, development of maternal feelings, attitudes toward breastfeeding, responses to the experience of birth itself, and conflicts between "the dream and the reality" of American motherhood. Dr. Leifer provides a feminist analysis of the many questions raised and outlines her recommendations for improving the social context for childbearing. I found the chapter on childbirth to be especially interesting and saddening because it shows how often the important psychological tasks of motherhood are undermined by insensitive handling during labor and delivery.

"Most medical personnel rely on technology to help the laboring women, and few provided practical assistance, such as suggesting a change in position or a simple breathing technique, or giving a back massage. Aside from routine and perfunctory comments, genuine emotional reassurance, support, and encouragement were usually absent. It was touching and rather saddening to see how extraordinarily grateful women were for any sign of personal interest, consideration, or respect from the staff. One woman spoke warmly about a medical student who (in contrast with other physicians who left abruptly after their examinations, without explaining what they had done or found) took the time to discuss with her how her labor was progressing. 'It really made a big difference to me,' she recalled, 'though it was such a small thing. It was as though he was the first person to treat me as an intelligent adult and not as a body to be examined.' . . . The few incidents like this that occurred had powerful effects on the women and were long remembered, indicating that even a relatively simple humane response from the medical staff can do much to provide reassurance to laboring women."

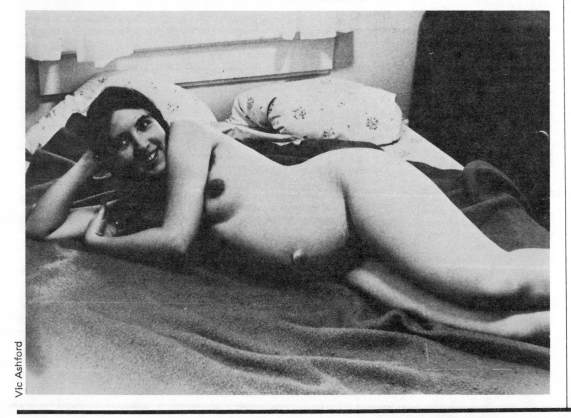

Vic Ashford

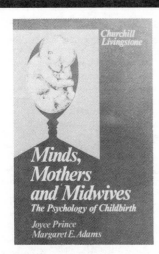

MINDS, MOTHERS AND
MIDWIVES: The Psychology of
Childbirth
by Joyce Prince and Margaret E.
Adams
1978, 179 pages, Illus.

from

Churchill Livingstone Inc.
19 West 44th Street
New York, NY 10036
$13.95 pap.

This book was written to introduce English midwives and midwifery students to concepts in psychology which affect childbirth. A wide range of topics is discussed, including recent changes in medicine and society which affect birth (contraception, the status of women, neonatal technology, etc.), sex preferences for offspring, feeding practices, "neonatal abilities," theories in child development, birth defects, psychological factors in pregnancy, cultural and medical management of labor, postnatal events, and family structure.

". . . Until fairly recently midwife and psychologist have had neither interest nor concept and language in common, and they have therefore had little occasion for communication with each other. Since the 1960's there have been some remarkable developments in the practice of midwifery and obstetrics. Discoveries about the abilities and perceptions of young babies have coincided with these changes. It is becoming increasingly clear that the areas of interest of the midwife and the psychologist are interlocked. Premature delivery, feeding difficulties, the non-thriving baby and non-accidental injury to infants, to take only a few examples, are recognized as being affected by psychosocial as well as physiological factors.

"Psychologists are interested in behaviour and experience while midwives concern themselves mainly with normal (meaning physiologically normal) pregnancy, labour and puerperium. Physical and mental events cannot be separated rigidly for they affect one another intimately . . . .

"Another area of conflict which has emerged in this century is the association of pregnancy with medical care and hence with illness. The first antenatal hospital bed was provided in Edinburgh in 1902 (Donald, 1972) From an obstetric point of view, the developments which followed were highly desirable and no one would want to return to the high maternal and infant mortality rates of the past. The fact that a considerable amount of antenatal care is provided in a hospital setting, however, inadvertently reinforces the view that pregnancy is pathological. Rosengren (1961) found that women who regarded pregnancy as an illness have significantly longer labours. This can be interpreted as showing that the illness role carries with it expectations of behaviour which the subject endorses. Margaret Mead (1950) in her anthropological studies has found that in some cultures morning sickness is expected for primiparae only, in some it is always expected, and in others it is regarded as abnormal. The numbers of women experiencing morning sickness varies with social expectations. Recent developments in obstetrics can only strengthen the association between pregnancy and illness. Pregnancy is *diagnosed,* there may be some discussion about a *therapeutic* abortion, an amniocentesis to make a *diagnosis* of the condition of the fetus, ultrasound cephalometry which involves some medico-technical procedures, and finally delivery itself has become mystified in medical technology. Pregnancy, which in some societies is seen as the peak of female vigour, health and good fortune, is in the advanced societies a confusion of low status, illness, pleasurable anticipation and fulfillment . . . .

"The progress of labour may be normal and natural and the patient free to walk around until late first or second stage of labour. When the labour is induced, accelerated, and monitored, movement is often restricted by the infusion and cardiotocograph. Some women in antenatal classes express their apprehension at the idea of being attached to machinery and being unable to get off the bed. There is a number of possible reasons for this. The control of bowel and bladder movement is very deeply ingrained by early training, as is a strong reticence about their activity. Complaints about not being able to get up to go to the lavatory must be one of the most common in all hospital patients. The return to infancy implied by soiling, or dependence on someone else to deal with these primitive needs, is a trauma not to be lightly dismissed. In addition many women in normal labour find walking about of some comfort.

Physiologically it is a better position for facilitating childbirth than being flat on a bed. . . .

"A patient who is immobile because she is attached to apparatus is bound to feel passive rather than active. Her movements, behaviour, progress in labour, her bodily sensations are constrained or initiated at the behest of someone else. She is passively expected to react to management by others, to follow instructions rather than determine the course of events for herself. This becomes more markedly the case for patients who have epidural analgesia. An increase in epidurals seems to be associated with an increase in instrumental delivery. The enormous motive power from within is reduced to a less efficient level. One woman we know had all her four healthy children at home. On every occasion she refused to call the midwife until the very last moment because 'I didn't want anyone to come and fiddle about with me.' Dana Breen (1975) found that the women 'who went through the experience of having a child with least difficulties, were those women who were able to feel themselves to be active, not only after the birth of the baby but also during pregnancy. Such a sense of initiation and activity is one which has often been denied women in our culture.' (Breen 1975) It is denied to too large a number of women who are managed during their labour. The midwife does need to use considerable tact and skill to help a woman in normal labour to retain her initiative and active integrity."

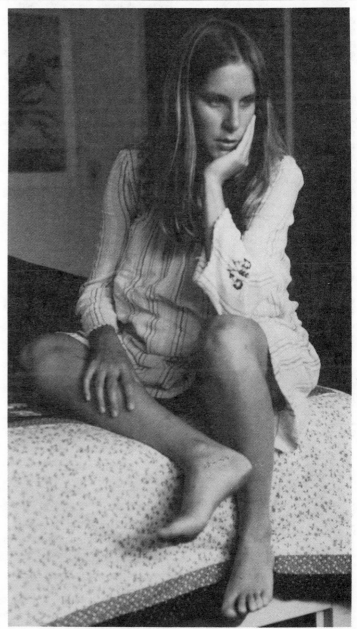

J.I.A.

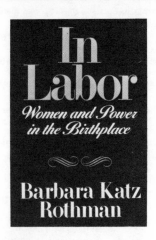

**IN LABOR: Women and Power
in the Birthplace**
by Barbara Katz Rothman
1982, 320 pages

from
W.W. Norton
500 Fifth Avenue
New York, NY 10110
$14.95 hd.

This book is being called "the first systematic feminist analysis" of childbirth in the U.S. and it is indeed a very exciting and insightful new work. Barbara Katz Rothman is a sociologist and gave birth to her own two children at home, the first in New York City in 1973, a time and place when not many women were having home births. I am personally very pleased that Katz Rothman has written this book because it provides the kind of very useful, sociological, feminist analysis of the home birth movement which has been lacking until now, and puts home birth firmly back in the context of the struggle for women's rights.

Katz Rothman begins by discussing the politics of maternity care, that is, who controls birth, how and why. She describes the "medical model" of childbirth, in which pregnancy is seen as a deviation from the (male) norm and contrasts it with the "midwifery model," her term for those ways of birth in which childbirth is an integrated experience and in which women learn to give birth with confidence in their own bodies. She outlines the history of childbirth, tracing the transition to total hospitalization for birth. Her discussion of the inherent difficulties in the "nurse-midwife" role is especially interesting. Katz Rothman then describes the history and present status of consumer movements in maternity care, providing a critical look at the deficiencies of male theories of "natural childbirth." She also provides an excellent discussion of conflicts within the childbirth movement which until now have been known only to "insiders": the cooption of ASPO-Lamaze by the hospital system, the split between pro- and anti-abortion forces in the home

birth movement and the role of men in childbirth (are fathers "in charge" at home births or is it basically a woman's event?). This material is must reading for women who want to confirm home birth and midwifery as proper concerns of feminism.

In Part II, Katz Rothman looks at how the medical and midwifery models work in practice, showing how the two approaches affect the experiences of infertility, pregnancy, giving birth, breastfeeding and maternal bonding. In the final section, she looks specifically at the nurse-midwives who are involved in home birth and birth centers, describing their work in detail and documenting their growing "radicalization" as home birth practice affects and reshapes their "medical" thinking.

Being able to "take off your cultural glasses" and really *see* your own society is one of the most important skills we can cultivate and *In Labor* is one of the rare books which helps us do this. It is an enlarging, stimulating, *vital* book. For women who are involved in the movement to regain control of birth, *In Labor* may be the most important book reviewed in this *Catalog*. For women who are considering giving birth in a hospital, *In Labor* should be considered essential first reading.

"It may be that 'nurse-midwife' is a contradiction in terms, with an inherent dilemma. Nurses, in our medical system, are defined by their relationship to doctors, and midwives are, in the meaning of the term derived from Old English, 'with the woman.' Nurse-midwives operating in the medical establishment, paid by that medical establishment, have a hard time as 'advocates of the childbearing couple.' The essential elements of cooption—job, prestige, professional recognition—are all right there. As has been demonstrated with lawyers, clients come and go, but the institution and the people working for the institution, D.A. or M.D., remain. For a midwife to stand firm as an advocate of the right of any given client to birth in her own way would jeopardize her relationship with physicians, nurses, and hospital administrators. Ultimately, it would cost her her job . . . .

"ASPO [the American Society for Psychoprophylaxis in Obstetrics, which teaches the "Lamaze" method] has not supported childbirth outside of the hospital, and home-birth advocates have been denied acceptance into ASPO teacher-training programs. The hospital is unchallenged as the location for birth, and the training the pregnant woman receives usually does not teach her to understand and manipulate the hospital environment. For the most part, rather than teaching in detail about hospital facilities and personnel, the childbirth-educa-

tion classes instruct the woman in ways to avoid dealing with external events. The laboring woman is taught to take a 'focal point'—a picture or flower she brings from home, or simply a spot on the wall—and focus on that alone, blocking out all other happenings during a contraction. Rather than being alerted to which hospital procedures are arbitrary or might be unnecessary in her case, the woman is taught instead how to ignore—'breathing through'—enemas, perineal shaves, repeated examinations, transfer from bed to stretcher, and so on. The focusing technique is thus one for dealing with the hospital, and may not be directly related to the birth experience itself . . . .

"In the medical model, responsibility is something shouldered by the doctor. This is of course not unique to obstetrics, but has long been a part of the traditional clinical mind. In the medical model the practitioner is expected to see himself as responsible for the outcome of treatment, and since pregnancy is a disease-like state, its care comes under the treatment model. The physician 'manages' the pregnancy, attempting constant, usually minor, adjustments in order to bring the physiological picture of the woman back to 'normal.' In the midwifery model the mother herself holds the responsibility for her pregnancy and makes her own decisions. The midwife is a teacher and a guide for the pregnant woman and her family during the experience.

"Thus, where a physician might spend ten to fifteen minutes at each prenatal visit (or even less, if ancillary staff does part of the work), a routine midwifery prenatal visit takes thirty minutes, an hour, or even more. Essentially the same physical screening procedures are performed (frequently by the mother herself), but the socio-emotional context of the pregnancy is also evaluated and discussed. One might make the argument that the physicians' prenatal visits are limited to just a few minutes based on purely economic motives. While I do not doubt that efficiency and financial gain are important considerations, from the point of view of the medical practitioner the essential business of the visit takes only a few minutes. The machinery of the body is what matters. If the woman's signs are good, then she needs no further treatment until the next visit. If her signs are not good, then the appropriate treatment is prescribed. The job of the physician is to diagnose and to treat, and in the relatively straight-forward work of pregnancy management, these routines are handled quickly. But creating a 'milieu' that is safe and supportive in which individuals can discover for themselves what it means to give birth is a more time-consuming goal. Getting to know women and their families, educating and sharing information, all take time and involve the

midwife in the lives of her clients to a greater extent than does checking blood pressure . . . .

"Giving birth at home changes things. It reshapes the experience of birthing women and their families. It lessens the monopoly that hospitals have had on childbirth in this country. And it deeply affects the nurse-midwives.

"For a nurse-midwife with standard hospital-based training, doing home births is a radicalizing experience. It makes her think hard about her work and its meaning. In this new setting she has to question many of the taken-for-granted assumptions of the medical setting and the medical model. And she finds herself constructing a new model, a new way of explaining what she sees. This is the process of *reconceptualization*, taking something you've confronted maybe a hundred times, and suddenly seeing it anew, seeing it as something else entirely . . . .

"For a nurse-midwife with standard hospital-based training, doing home births is a radicalizing experience. It makes her think hard about her work and its meaning. In this new setting she has to question many of the taken-for-granted assumptions of the medical setting and the medical model."

"Maybe, by accident, things will get better. Careful planning is bringing us regionalization of maternity care (the sorting and matching of women and hospitals in risk categories), more and fancier technology, and a well-thought-out attempt to coopt midwives and the home-birth movement. Maybe they will just put flowered sheets on the beds, hang a plant on the IV pole, and go on about business as usual. But maybe it will backfire. Maybe the attempt to coopt those seeking alternatives will end by creating change in the medical institutions, as doctors and nurses work in the new settings. Maybe obstetrics will go through some changes too."

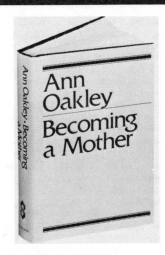

BECOMING A MOTHER
by Ann Oakley
1979, 328 pages
$18.95 hd.

WOMEN CONFINED: Towards A Sociology of Childbirth
by Ann Oakley
1980, 334 pages
$12.95 hd.

both from
Schocken Books
200 Madison Avenue
New York, NY 10016

Ann Oakley is concerned with how women respond emotionally to the childbirth experience and particularly with how medical maternity care affects their feelings about becoming mothers. In 1974 she began a research project which involved extensive interviews with sixty-six women who were expecting their first babies. In *Becoming a Mother*, Oakley discusses the institution of motherhood, the harmful effects of the medicalization of birth, the short-comings of "natural childbirth," and the limitations of feminist alternatives. She then presents the experiences of the women who were her research subjects, for the most part using the women's own words. The book is a powerful rendering of the reality of motherhood in our culture, an experience for which many if not most women are inadequately prepared. Oakley says, "It is the moment when she becomes a mother that a woman first confronts the full reality of what it means to be a woman in our society."

Women Confined is based on the same research but presents Oakley's conclusions more in the form of a sociological treatise. In this book Oakley is particularly concerned with pointing out the psychological constructs which surround birth and the problems caused by sexist bias in sociology and science in general. Taken together, these books are extremely stimulating and thought provoking and will be of interest to people who are working to achieve the twin goals of making childbirth care more humane and bringing women to full humanity.

"I am a feminist, an academic sociologist, and a woman with children. I was not a feminist until I had children, and I became a sociologist as an escape from the problems of having children . . . .

"In the past and still in many cultures today women have babies without any medical help. Their attendants are other women, usually those who have had babies themselves. Babies are born in the home, in a family setting, and birth proceeds as the woman's body dictates it should; there is little or no intervention in the natural process. None of this holds in industrialised societies where childbirth 'is medicalised.' Attendants at childbirth are professional deliverers (for women are no longer their own deliverers in birth, they are delivered 'by' someone); hospital is the proper place for having a baby, which has become an occasion on which the family is split up, not united; trust in nature has been replaced by trust in technology, as tests and machines and instruments become the necessary paraphernalia of birth. This colonisation of birth by medicine is a thread in the fabric of cultural dependence on professional health care. People are not responsible for their own health, their own illness, their own births and deaths: doctors are saviours, miracle-workers, mechanics, culture-heroes. From being necessary to the cure or treatment of a probably quite small number of illnesses, they have been given responsibility for *all* illness, and anything to which, like birth, the label of illness can be attached . . . .

"Many feminists have been distinctly anti-natalist. The concerns of organised feminism since the 1960's have been with *freeing* women from their child-bearing and child-rearing roles (more abortion and contraception, more state child care) to increased participation in the non-domestic world (equal pay for equal work, equal opportunities and education, legal and financial independence from men). A major theme has been the redefinition of sexuality, its liberation from the constraints of the patriarchal stereotype. Thus feminism has unconsciously echoed the patriarchal view of women; women as sexual objects condemned by their biology to motherhood. The pain of childbirth has been seen as unnecessary suffering—the heritage of the Judeo-Christian condemnation of women to a punishment from God. The ability of women to grow and breastfeed babies and give birth to them in pain but with satisfaction is only now beginning to be seen by feminists as a valid and valuable aspect of being a woman, a resource to be drawn on rather than a burden to be disposed of . . . .

"I felt more exhausted. But it was labelled postnatal depression.

The sister, and everyone else picked it up, and said yes, that's postnatal depression. I said to the sister, Piccadilly Circus is more restful than this place. Oh it was so bad, I had one hour's sleep for three nights running, and no sleep during the day. I recognized that I might have broken down.

"I think with the loss of the blood and the manual removal of the placenta which was pretty ghastly really, although I was knocked out for it, I felt terrible just after the birth. Finally I got in such a state that I rang my mother (a GP) at four o'clock in the morning which I've *never* done . . . because I was having problems with the doctors and sisters, not getting the rest, and someone who's lost a lot of blood has got to have a lot of rest and a high protein diet, neither of which I was getting. The diet was appalling and the rest was non-existent. Routine was what mattered. If you'd fed the baby at five in the morning, you still had to get up at six to join the band. I just wasn't sleeping, and I thought you've just got to get out of this place or you'll go mad. I thought if I have to go one more night in this place, I'll go crazy. I'm feeling I'm crazy anyway. My mother realized this and she said well I'll ring the doctor in the morning. So she rang, she got hold of the registrar and he said I was obviously having a postnatal depression . . . .

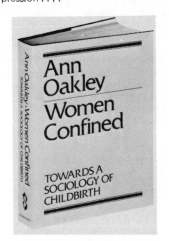

"The trouble with childbirth (sociologically speaking) is that it only happens to women. But this does not mean that women's reactions to it can be explained in terms of their womanhood, their adherence to certain standards of feminine personality and behaviour. The trouble with women is that they are also people, and it is this status that is so easily forgotten in both sexist and anti-sexist types of analysis. It has long been clear that the task of a feminist consciousness in social science is not only the exposition of sexism but its correction, and in the pursuit of this end it is essential to develop fresh modes of thinking about women, a new conceptual apparatus. The trouble with sociology (as with many other academic subjects) is that it is not merely sexist on the surface but deeply and pervasively so. Bias against women as people equal in stature to men cannot therefore be expunged piecemeal; a fundamental process of revision must be engaged in . . . .

"The third way in which psychoanalytic ideology has particularly handicapped the psychology of reproduction is through the view that individual psychodynamics are the main determinant of responses to reproduction. The dominant orientation is towards 'blaming the victim.' Problems in pregnancy, birth and the postpartum period are interpreted as arising from personal failure or personality 'defect,' a methodological feature that follows from the *en masse* treatment of women as residing in a psychology of their own. For, by implication, problems with motherhood cannot be traced to the *human* condition and must therefore be located in the feminine psyche. . . .

"Veiled by the mystiques of feminine psychology and deterministic biology, mothers' reactions to motherhood have been regarded by medical and social science as in a class of their own: a female secret negotiated by, and on behalf of, hidden personality factors. But because women's biological reproductivity has a social function—the reproduction of a society—any difficulties women have with motherhood constitute a 'social problem.' Science, responding to an agenda of basically social concerns, has provided the label 'postnatal depression' as a pseudo-scientific tag for the description and ideological transformation of maternal discontent. Thus labelled, maternal difficulties remain impervious to male scientific understanding, as we have seen in this book; it is only the alternative approach of considering responses to childbirth as a species of a larger genus, human reactions to life events, that their intrinsic character can be mapped out."

Anthropology and History of Childbirth

Our society is often accused of having a very short memory. We tend to forget events even of the recent past, thinking that current ways and ideas have no background or precedent. We also tend to be quite insular, regarding our own culture as the highest and describing others as "primitive" or under-developed. This historical and cultural isolation can be damaging for those who are struggling to understand the controversies in childbirth today. We need to be able to see our present concerns in their historical and cross-cultural context, for an understanding of how childbirth has been regarded in other times and places can help us to "see" and understand our own "ways of birth."

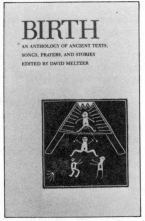

BIRTH: An Anthology of Ancient Texts, Songs, Prayers, and Stories
edited by David Meltzer
1981, 248 pages, Illus.

from
North Point Press
850 Talbot Avenue
Berkeley, CA 94706
$8.50 pap.

Many people in the alternative childbirth movement are consciously seeking to reincorporate ritual and spiritual significance into their birthing practice. The literature and artwork of "pre-industrial" peoples and past cultures is often used as a source of symbols and ideas. This book presents a wide range of cultural material, gathered from many ethnographic and historical sources. The emphasis is on how people throughout time have responded to the awe-inspiring nature of birth which is so closely linked with death in the life cycle. Included are creation myths and accounts of "fabulous births," conception lore, charms and spells to provide magical protection for mother and baby, accounts of pregnancy and birth, and ritual events after the birth. In addition to a complete bibliography, Meltzer also includes an interesting listing of books which "help to further define the feminine aspect in history and culture."

"The romavali's thick stem supports
a pair of lotuses, her high and close-set breasts,
on which sit bees, the darkening nipples.
These flowers tell of treasure
hidden in my darling's belly."

Translated by Daniel H.H. Ingalls, from *Sanskrit Poetry from Vidyakara's "Treasury"* (Daniel H.H. Ingalls, editor and translator; Harvard University Press, 1968).

Slowly the unborn babe distends life's pathway,
   torn by the child's head;
Now the living child
   long cherished by the mother beneath her heart,
Fills the gateway of life.
There is no room to pass safely through; —
   The child slips downward,
   It becomes visible
   It bursts forth into the light of day, —
The waters of childbirth flow away."

Translated by Willard Trask, from *Songs and Tales of the Sea Kings: Interpretations of the Oral Literature of Polynesia* (J. Frank Stimson, editor; The Peabody Museum (Salem), 1957).

BIRTH IN FOUR CULTURES: A Crosscultural Investigation of Childbirth in Yucatan, Holland, Sweden and the United States
by Brigitte Jordon
1980, 109 pages, Illus.

from
Eden Press Women's Publications
245 Victoria Avenue, No. 12
Montreal, Quebec
H3Z 2M6 Canada
$6.95 pap.

Because birth is defined as a medical event in Western culture, there has been little study of the social aspects of Western birth practices. Brigitte Jordon did original work in studying and recording the birth practices of Indians in Yucatan. She contrasts their system with that of the U.S. and with Holland and Sweden, the countries with the lowest infant mortality rates in the world. Her crosscultural comparison shows "the tremendous range of variation in the organization of birthing systems." An important idea introduced by Jordan is that cultural systems of birthing are justified from the "inside out" which means that "the judged provide the criteria for judging." She shows how the medical definition of birth in the U.S. has forced all discussions of birth alternatives to begin with a statement on their "safety" even though medical safety may not be the most important factor in evaluating birth practices or in contributing to good birth outcomes.

"The sense of *moral* requiredness figures in the expression of disbelief and outrage that properly socialized participants frequently show vis-a-vis the practices of other systems. To illustrate: since it was known in each particular fieldwork situation that I had participated in births in other cultures, a standard and instructive type of interaction with local birth personnel consisted of their asking me questions about other systems' practices. While eliciting information, these questions typically at the same time expressed disbelief that anybody could engage in what appeared, from the local point of view, as obviously unnecessary, ridiculous, chancy, stupid, barbaric, etc. Thus Dutch midwives asked me, (in a tone that said: Tell me I'm wrong), 'Do they *really* do episiotomies on all women in the United States?'; Swedish midwives wanted to know why American obstetricians still use outmoded forceps when, in their view, vacuum extractors are much safer; and an eminent Swedish obstetrician considered differential care depending on ability to pay "an obscenity." American doctors often questioned me about the "backward" practices of the Indians, while the Indians, in turn, spoke only with moral indignation of such standard hospital procedures as vaginal examinations ('They put their hands inside of you'), episiotomies ('They cut you') and the feet-in-stirrups position ('They expose you.').

"In the United States, we find a pervasive, unspoken assumption, shared by medical practitioners and their clients alike, that our practices are, in fact, scientifically grounded, even though a given medical practitioner, at any one time, may not just then have the data at hand which support his conviction. He *knows* that they exist and can be found in the biomedical research literature. It may come as a surprise, then, that on examination the evidence on which this conviction is based is sometimes nonexistent, and if it does exist, is frequently far from clear-cut."

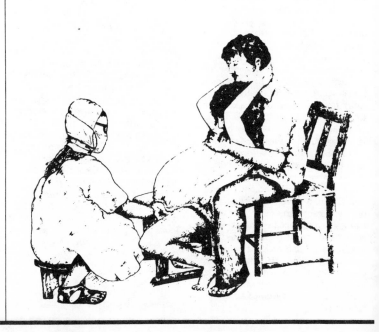

ANTHROPOLOGY OF HUMAN BIRTH
by Margarita Artschwager Kay
1982, 445 pages

from
F.A. Davis Company
1915 Arch Street
Philadelphia, PA 19103
$25.00

People in every culture are accustomed to thinking that their own way of doing things is the only or the best way. This is true for the intimate events of life like sex, birth, and death and also true for systems of medicine and science. But, as Margarita Kay says in her preface to this book, "Women's health care in every society is a reflection of the total culture. Each childbearing system relates to the social organization, the political system, and the religious system as much as it does to the medical system of a particular society . . . The values, sentiments and beliefs of each group are reflected in the practices they maintain."

In a time when America's way of birth is subject to such intense scrutiny and criticism, people are especially interested in learning how others perceive and manage pregnancy, labor and birth. *Anthropology of Human Birth* is a collection of articles by many ethnographers which provides a fascinating glimpse into the birth practices of other cultures (Malaysia, Japan, Taiwan, Egypt, Nigeria, Benin, India, Mexico, Guatemala, St. Kitts, Ireland) as well as sub-cultures in our own country (Mexican-American, home birth, the Ashram, lesbian mothers, Mormons, American Indians).

Margarita Kay explains that her book was written to fill the needs of her own teaching work. "Scientific obstetrics, or biomedicine, also represents the culture from which it is derived. In an attempt to help health care providers realize their own ethnocentrism, I introduced a course in the anthropology of childbirth." She points out that each of the contributors to this book is a woman, an important asset in studying cultures which limit men's access to childbirth. This book will be of great value in helping health care providers and parents to "see through" the veils and trappings of their own culture.

"Labor is feared to a certain extent by all people. The proud Bariba woman attempts to deliver alone to conquer this fear. In most other societies, the husband is expected to be a major source of encouragement, and scientific childbirth culture now permits his presence, or that of someone else referred to in the latest jargon as the 'significant other.' The traditional American Indian prefers the support of her mother or some other female to that of her husband, and the Japanese woman is "too

ashamed" for her spouse to see her. The Lesbian woman wants her lover to be welcomed as her husband would be. Women who give birth at home may choose to do so because their children can participate in the entire process. Mexican women prefer giving birth in the hospital for exactly the opposite reason, because they do not want their children to see what is going on. Navajo women are helped by their older daughters . . . .

"Culturally sensitive observers have urged policymakers and program planners to undertake studies of regional and local birthing customs and related cultural institutions prior to introducing integrated maternal and child health and family planning programs. . . . According to this scheme, harmful practices, such as severe dietary restrictions placed on pregnant and lactating women, and septic treatment of the umbilical stump, are to be discouraged in favor of scientifically approved practices. Beneficial practices, such as breastfeeding, are to be encouraged. Neutral or harmless practices, such as the performance of birth rituals, may be tolerated because they are medically innocuous, or to be encouraged for their positive psychological benefits. Uncertain practices, such as the administration of herbal teas during labor, may be allowed until medical research determines their safety . . . .

"The Mayan midwife (*iyom* or *ilonel* in Quiche and *comadrona* in Spanish) is regarded as having a supernatural calling. This destiny or *mandado* is revealed in various ways, such as birth signs (being born with a veil or on a certain day), repetitive dreams, finding strange objects (shells, scissors, mirrors, special shaped stones), and serious illness. These are considered messages sent by God or the spirits, and are interpreted by a shaman as indicating the midwife's calling. If she does not follow her destiny, she shall be subject to supernatural sanctions which may take the form of worse illness or death for herself or members of her family. Even the midwives who do not subscribe to the belief of supernatural or divine recruitment, such as the Latino midwives, believe they receive divine assistance from God, the spirits of dead midwives (*comadronas invisibles*), Mary, and Santa Ana (patroness of childbirth). During the birth, they are accompanied by these spirits, who tell them if the birth is normal or not, how to massage, what to do if the baby is in an incorrect position, and what herbs and medicines to use. . . .

"Though Grantly Dick-Read is known for his natural childbirth approach, even his landmark book *Childbirth Without Fear* begins with

a championing of the technological view: 'Goaded on by the humiliation of woman's helplessness in distress, man hunted through the armory of science to find some weapon he could wield in her protection and defense. The natural reaction of the male to such a situation is anger, destruction, obliteration and annihilation of the aggressor.' In this view, the course of pregnancy and delivery is the province of male physicians and is best conceptualized in terms of aggressive technological measures. While his language leaves one with the impression that overkill is a distinct possibility, he seems unaware that all of the weight attached to 'destruction,' 'obliteration,' and 'annihilation'—even if it is of distress—may ultimately have a harmful effect on the woman. One prospective father put his finger on the more ludicrous aspects of the technological view when he said, 'Are we going to the moon, or is my wife having a baby?' "

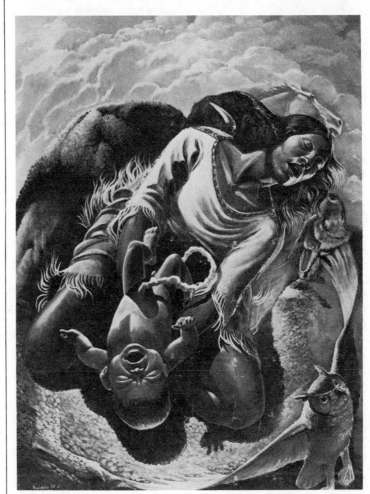

GIVING LIFE
by Parker Boyiddle
poster reproduction, 24" x 36"
$25.00 postpaid

from
Boyiddle-Bahti
1708 E. Speedway
Tucson, AZ 85719

This signed and numbered reproduction of an original acrylic painting by Kiowa artist, Parker Boyiddle, was produced in a limited edition of 1000.

"[the painting] powerfully depicts the life cycle of a man in the traditional world of the Kiowa People. Born beneath the night skies of the Universe and on the Earth, one sees to the left of the child the form of a buffalo rising from the earth as they did in the Kiowa Creation Legend. The buffalo will provide him and his family with food, clothing, shelter and tools. The horse will carry him on hunting trips and into battle. The coyote—Sayn-day—will, through the many stories he will hear from his elder, teach him of the Kiowa legendary past and what it means to be a Kiowa. Finally there is the owl, who will call when his death approaches and he is returned to the earth from which the owl's wing flows in this remarkable painting."

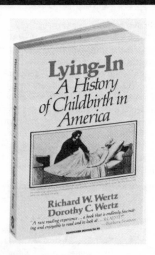

LYING-IN: A History of Childbirth in America
by Richard W. Wertz and Dorothy C. Wertz
1979, 260 pages, Illus.

from
Schocken Books
200 Madison Avenue
New York, NY 10016
$5.95 pap.

Dorothy Wertz has a doctorate in religion and society and Richard Wertz has taught in the humanities. Together they have written an excellent introduction to the history of childbirth in America, showing not only how practices and personnel have changed over the years (home to hospital, midwife to doctor, "social" to "technological") but also how the American experience has been different from that in Europe, where midwives were not suppressed and still manage the majority of normal births. They discuss many important topics in the development of American birth practices including the concept of "social childbirth" in colonial days, the influence of 19th century scientific medicine on midwifery, the rise of the male medical profession in America, how American women came to accept male doctors as birth attendants, the effects of Victorian ideas of female morality and modesty, the transition from home to hospital birth, the acceptance of anesthesia, social characteristics of the "natural childbirth" movement, and government involvement in maternity care.

Lying-In is written in a very accessible, popular style and is liberally illustrated with fascinating historical drawings. It will be of great interest to childbirth educators, midwives, and parents who want to better understand the roles they play and the social forces which act upon them as they participate in childbirth in America.

"Midwifery itself paid less than other types of practice, for many doctors spent long hours in attending laboring women and later had trouble collecting their fees. Yet midwifery was a guaranteed income, even if small, and it opened the way to family practice and sometimes to consultations involving many doctors and shared fees. The family and female friends who had seen a doctor 'perform' successfully were likely to call him again. Doctors worried that, if midwives were allowed to deliver the upper classes, women would turn to them for treatment of other illness and male doctors would lose half their clientele. As a prominent Boston doctor wrote in 1820, 'If female midwifery is again introduced among the rich and influential, it will become fashionable and it will be considered indelicate to employ a physician.' *Doctors had to eliminate midwives in order to protect the gateway to their whole practice.*

"In recent years some social historians have been examining the character of Victorian separate-sex culture, the reasons for it, its extent, and its consequences. That culture expected women to be primarily wives and mothers, homebound, pious, and dependent upon husbands and other males, and it seems that some women were content in this arrangement. Doctors as a group helped both to define and to enforce the boundary between what men and women were expected to do. Thus, arguing that women could not and should not be midwives or doctoresses, male doctors were expressing a cultural judgment as well as protecting their own professional and economic interests. At the same time, they were also, of course, saying what men could and should sometimes do. Sex-linked attributes and prerogatives in birth became a central cultural event, a ritualistic definition of sexual place. *In the most simple sense, it became unthinkable that a woman could both give birth and attend birth.* Giving birth was the quintessential feminine act; attending birth was a fundamental expression of the controlling and performing actions suitable only for men. . . .

"One [19th century] medical writer indicated that the touch, far from being an affront, had such near-magical significance that it might be the occasion for a bit of flim-flam. He instructed doctors to act as if they caused all that happened in birth, even if they were not present:

'A Patient, after the waters are discharged, requires a little management. It is not just to stay with her at this time; and yet it is necessary, if we leave her, to leave her in confidence. Therefore we may give her the idea of making provision for whatever may happen in our absence; we may pass our finger up the vagina or opening of the womb, and make a moderate degree of pressure, for a few seconds, on any part of it so that she may just feel it; after which we may say to her, "there ma'am, I have done something that will be of great use to your labor." This she trusts to: and if, when she sends for us, we get there in time, it is well; if later than we should be, we easily satisfy her. "Yes! You know I told you I did something which would be of great use to your labor!" If the placenta is not yet come away—"Oh, I am quite in time for the after-birth, and that, you know, is of the greatest consequence in labor!" And if the whole has come away—"We are glad that the after-birth is all come away in consequence of what we did before we last left, and the labor terminated just as we intended it should." '

"Here is an excellent example of symptomatic treatment that gave the doctor credit for birth's success, even though it was usually an inherently successful natural process. . . .

"Technical routines to control natural processes compounded with social procedures to process the patient no longer seemed warranted by the danger of birth but seemed instead to stand in the way of a humane and meaningful delivery.

"[By the 1950's] Hospital delivery had become for many a time of alienation—from the body, from family and friends, from the community, and even from life itself. The safe efficiencies had become a kind of industrial production far removed from the comforts of social childbirth or the sympathies of the proverbial doctor-patient relation. A woman was powerless in the experience of birth and unable to find meaning in it, for her participation in it and even her consciousness of it were minimal. She was isolated during birth from family and friends, and even from other women having the same experiences. She had to think of herself instrumentally, not as a woman feeling love and fear or sharing in a creative event, but as a body-machine being manipulated by others for her ultimate welfare. She played a social role of passive dependence and obedience.

"Hospital birth became a regime against which many women began a critical struggle, questioning the need for such extensive manipulation, questioning the safety of the procedures, and demanding that birth be an experience that permitted them a sense of self-fulfillment. They set out to regain possession of their bodies and of the life they had lost. . . .

"That the husband was until recently the only outsider allowed to be present during labor or birth bears witness to the early relationship between natural childbirth and the Feminine Mystique. 'Togetherness' was for husband and wife only; it did not include female friends and relatives, not even the woman's mother, who had traditionally helped in birth. The presence of an unmarried father was unthinkable. Natural childbirth was thus a means of strengthening the middle-class marriage.

"Other cultural conditions also made the Read method attractive to postwar middle-class women. One was the religious revival of the 1940s and 1950s, which raised church attendance and interest in theology.

"In the 1950s, when Christian ethics were interpreted mostly as personal or family ethics, in tune with the 'privatization of life' described by Friedan, natural childbirth, which avoided potential damage to the baby's brain by anesthesia, appeared to some women as a 'heroic' Christian act. In the days before the civil-rights movement made social action a viable choice for Christians, having a natural birth was perhaps the only ethical action, Christian or otherwise, that many women could take. . . .

"Because the Lamaze method stressed autonomy, a psychoanalyst argued that only the 'dissatisfied woman . . . wants it to complete her drive for masculine powers,' for she believes that 'the wound of womanhood, of not having been a boy, will be healed by giving birth, and she wishes to consciously establish her psychic virility.' The Lamaze method was clearly not in tune with psychoanalysis or the feminine mystique. . . .

By the 1970s many doctors were prepared to offer a more natural childbirth. Most often, however, it was a peculiarly American 'natural birth' they provided, for they drew routinely upon the arts of medicine. Episiotomy, outlet forceps, Demerol, and even epidural anesthesia were combined with the Lamaze method. Doctors were satisfied with Lamaze only if they could adjust it to keep birth from being overly time-consuming and to permit them enough activity to justify their professional presence and fees. *Anesthetists accepted Lamaze so long as enough drugs were given to require their presence or the hospital ruled that even a nonanesthetized mother must pay for their services.* Many women accepted the assurance that they had had a natural delivery when, in fact, many interventions were made. Probably only a Caesarean section or Twilight Sleep would not have qualified for natural birth in American practice."

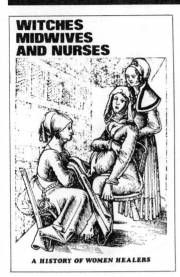

WITCHES MIDWIVES AND NURSES

A HISTORY OF WOMEN HEALERS

WITCHES, MIDWIVES AND NURSES: A History of Women Healers
by Barbara Ehrenreich and Deirdre English
1973, 48 pages, Illus.

from
The Feminist Press
Box 334
Old Westbury, NY 11568
$2.95 plus .50 postage

This pamphlet is an early classic of the women's health movement of the 1970's. Written in 1973, it traces the history of women healers and their persecution from the witch hunts of the middle ages through to the outlawing of midwives in America at the turn of the century. Ehren-reich and English provide a political framework for the suppression of women in medicine and help us see that political action, not personal adaptation, is the solution. Their description of the Popular Health Movement of the 1830's and 1840's will be particularly poignant and galvanizing for women's health activists of today. Since writing this pamphlet Barbara Ehrenreich has continued working as a political activist and writer and Deirdre English has become editor of *Mother Jones* magazine. Under her leadership, *Mother Jones* has reported on many important issues of interest to women, including the cesarean epidemic (see index) and the Bendectin controversy (see index). Ehrenreich and English are also the authors of *For Her Own Good: 150 Years of the Experts' Advice to Women,* published by Doubleday in 1978.

"Women have always been healers. They were the unlicensed doctors and anatomists of western history. They were abortionists, nurses and counsellors. They were pharmacists, cultivating healing herbs and exchanging the secrets of their uses. They were midwives, travelling from home to home and village to village. For centuries women were doctors without degrees, barred from books and lectures, learning from each other, and passing on experience from neighbor to neighbor

and mother to daughter. They were called 'wise women' by the people, witches or charlatans by the authorities. Medicine is part of our heritage as women, our history, our birthright. . . .

"American obstetricians had no real commitment to improved obstetrical care. In fact, a study by a Johns Hopkins professor in 1912 indicated that most American doctors were *less* competent than the midwives. Not only were the doctors themselves unreliable about preventing sepsis and ophthalmia but they also tended to be too ready to use surgical techniques which endangered mother or child. If anyone, then, deserved a legal monopoly on obstetrical care, it was the midwives, not the MD's. But the doctors had power, the midwives didn't. Under intense pressure from the medical profession, state after state passed laws outlawing midwifery and restricting the practice of obstetrics to doctors. For poor and working class women, this actually meant worse—or no—obstetrical care. (For instance, a study of infant mortality rates in Washington showed an increase in infant mortality in the years immediately following the passage of the law forbidding midwifery.) For the new, male medical profession, the ban on midwives meant one less source of competition. Women had been routed from their last foothold as independent practitioners. . . .

"Women have always been healers. . . . Medicine is part of our heritage as women, our history, our birthright."

"Professionalism in medicine is nothing more than the institutionalization of a male upper class monopoly. We must never confuse professionalism with expertise. Expertise is something to work for and to share, professionalism is—by definition—elitist and exclusive, sexist, racist and classist. In the American past, women who sought formal medical training were too ready to accept the professionalism that went with it. They made *their* gains in status—but only on the backs of their less privileged sisters—midwives, nurses and lay healers. Our goal today should never be to open up the exclusive medical profession to women, but to open up medicine—to all women."

FOR MORE READING

The following books contain chapters or sections on childbirth which illuminate the social and cultural nature of childbirth practices.

THE HORRORS OF THE HALF-KNOWN LIFE: Male Attitudes Toward Women and Sexuality in Nineteenth Century America
by G. J. Barker-Benfield
1976, 352 pages

from
Harper and Row
10 East 53rd Street
New York, NY 10022
out of print

Contains a very interesting 60-page account of the suppression of midwives in America and the rise of the male obstetrician/gynecologist.

WOMEN AS MOTHERS
by Sheila Kitzinger
1979, 240 pages

from
Random House
201 East 50th Street
New York, NY 10022
$8.95

Kitzinger's book on motherhood contains two chapters on childbirth and the use of "ritual and technology" in the hospital.

OF WOMAN BORN: Motherhood as Experience and Institution
by Adrienne Rich
1976, 328 pages

from
W.W. Norton
500 Fifth Avenue
New York, NY 10036
$12.95

Rich's powerful book on the institution of motherhood contains two chilling chapters on the suppression of midwives ("Hands of Flesh, Hands of Iron") and on hospital birth ("Alienated Labor").

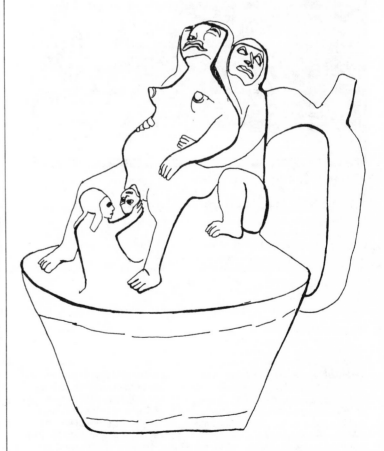

An example of "maternity pottery" of the Moochila period (500 A.D.), on display in the Herrer Museum in Lima, Peru. Two women are shown assisting the mother in labor. Sketched by Betty LaDuke (see index for another sample of her work).
© 1983 Betty LaDuke

CHILDBIRTH IN HISTORICAL ILLUSTRATION

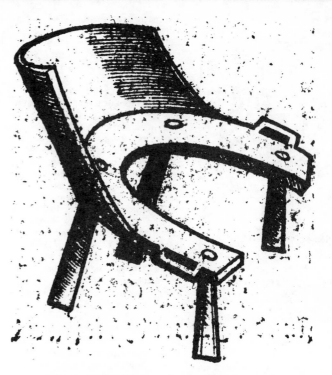

BIRTH STOOL. Woodcut illustration from (Roeslin, E.). Der Swangern Frauwen und Hebammen Rosegarten. (Strassburg, 1513) Courtesy of the National Library of Medicine.

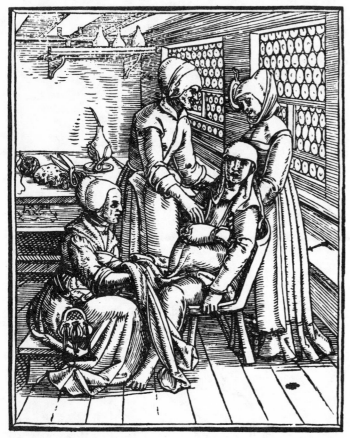

WOMAN IN LABOR, on birth chair, assisted by three women (midwives?). Woodcut illustration from J. Ruff. Ein schon lustig Trostbuchle. Zurich, 1554. Courtesy of the National Library of Medicine.

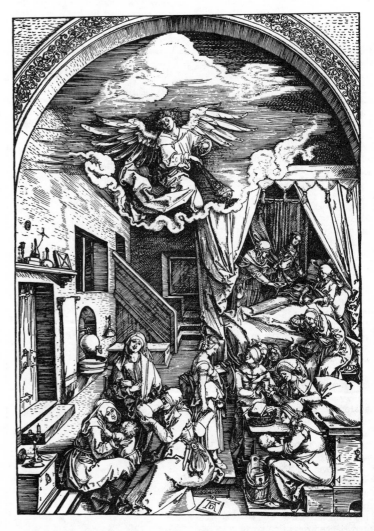

THE BIRTH OF THE VIRGIN. Woodcut designed by Albrecht Durer (German, 1471-1528), Nuremburg, 1505. "One of the most famous and charming delineations of birth in the history of the graphic arts. It was more or less traditional to conceive of the nativity of Christ in terms of fantasy and imagination, but to treat the birth of the Virgin as a genre piece with a wealth of realistic detail. In this picture the actual accouchement has just taken place, and we see the exhausted mother receiving nourishment, the tired midwife sitting nearby, and a jolly company of housewives busied with various occupations, such as bathing the child, preparing the cradle, and generally having a good time." Reproduced from *Medicine and the Artist (Ars Medica)* by permission of the Philadelphia Museum of Art. Published by Dover Publications, Inc., 1970, Carl Zigrosser, editor.

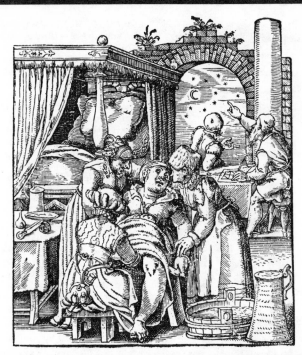

CHILDBIRTH. "This woodcut by Jost Amman (Swiss-German, 1539-1591) appeared in Rueff's *De Generatione Hominis,* Frankfurt, 1580, a famous and widely used handbook for midwives. An astrologer is seen in the background, casting a horoscope of the newly born." Reproduced from *Medicine and the Artist (Ars Medica)* by permission of the Philadelphia Museum of Art.

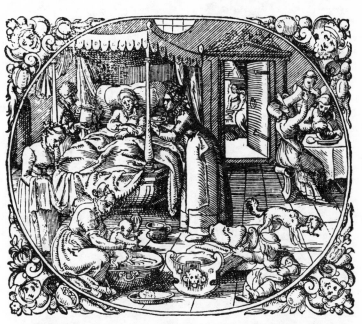

MATERNITY BEDROOM SCENE; new mother is attended by two women and two others bathe the baby; another child plays on the floor. Woodcut illustration from J. Ruff. De conceptu et generatione hominis. Frankfurt, 1580. Courtesy of the National Library of Medicine.

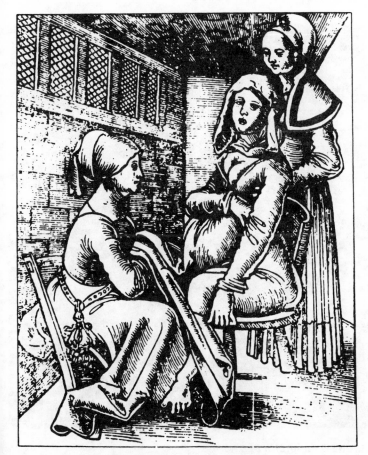

A GERMAN MIDWIFE assisting at the delivery of a woman on a birth stool. Detail of a 16th century woodcut, source unknown.

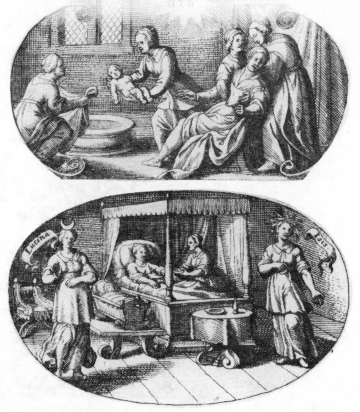

DETAIL FROM FIVE VIGNETTES, some with mystical figures, including a woman on a birth chair, with four attendants, one handing baby to another, and a bedroom scene with mother in bed and baby in cradle. Engraved title page. Louise (Bourgeois) Boursier. Hebammen Buch. . . Hanau, 1644-52. Courtesy of the National Library of Medicine.

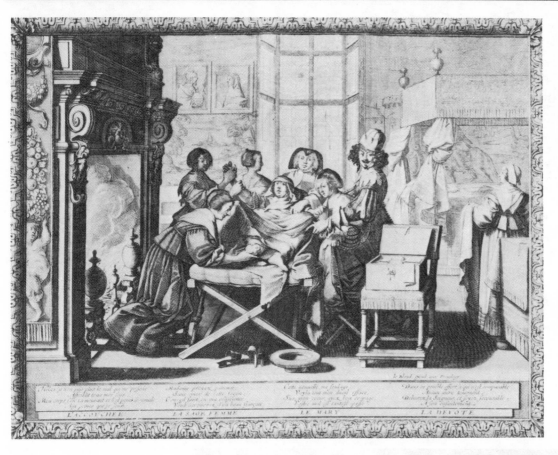

L'ACCOUCHEE   *LA SAGE FEMME*   *LE MARY*   *LA DEVOTE*

L'ACCOUCHMENT. "An etching by Abraham Bosse (French, 1602-1676) made in 1633 at Paris. The *dramatis personae* of the tableau include the mother, the midwife, the friend of the family (Devout Woman) and the husband. Each recites, as it were, a quatrain, engraved below the picture and translated as follows. The Mother: 'Alas, I can no more; the pain possesses me, enfeebling all my senses; my body is dying, and there is no remedy for the pangs I feel.' The Midwife: 'Madame, have patience; do not cry out so; it's all over, by my faith, you are delivered of a fine son.' The husband: 'That news comforts me; all my grief has vanished; keep on, dear heart, take courage, your pain will soon be over.' The Devout Woman: 'From this painful effort, so unlike any other torment, deliver her, oh Lord, and be of help in her childbirth.' "*

* Reproduced from *Medicine and the Artist* (Ars Medica) by permission of the Philadelphia Museum of Art.

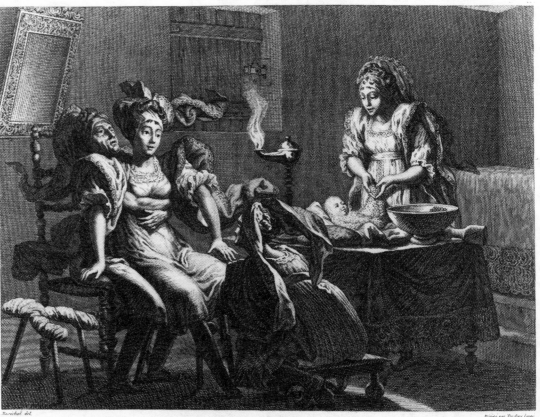

ACCOUCHEMENT D'UNE FEMME GREQUE DE L'ARCHIPELE. One midwife holds the mother as another removes the afterbirth; another attendant puts a powder substance over the baby. Engraving after Marechal, published by Tardieu l'aine, 18-- . Courtesy of the National Library of Medicine.

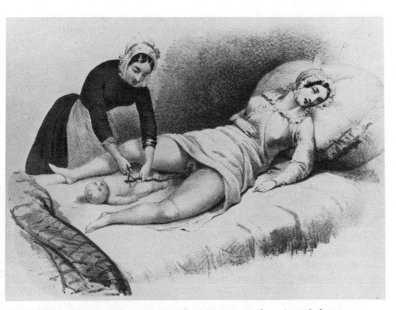

NEONATAL SCENE with nurse-midwife cutting cord of newborn infant, lying between legs of mother on bed. Lithographic illustration, colored. W. Beach, *Improved System of Midwifery.* New York, 1850. Courtesy of the National Library of Medicine.

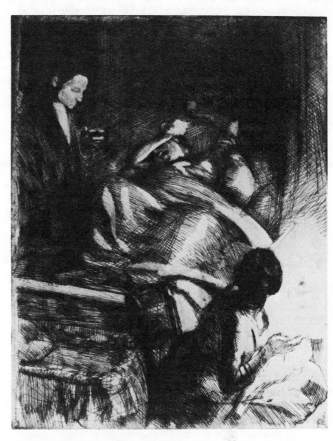

INTERIOR OF BEDROOM, with woman in labor on bed, attended by another woman and a doctor. Drypoint by Paul Albert Besnard, 19- - Courtesy of the National Library of Medicine.

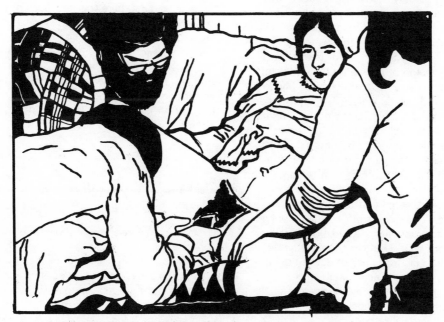

HOME BIRTH IN ILLINOIS, 1976. The mother rests between labor contractions, as the father supports the baby's crowning head. Two friends give comfort and support. Ink drawing from a photograph, Janet Isaacs Ashford, 1980.

CHILDBIRTH IN MY FAMILY

A few years ago, in preparation for a book on home birth, I asked my two grandmothers and my mother to tell me about their experiences in giving birth. The answers I received were quite strikingly varied and show something of how birth has been conducted in our country over the past 65 years.

The first story is that of my father's mother, Jean Chisholm Isaacs, who was born in Pittsburgh in 1888. She was about twenty-six at the time of the birth of her first child, my Uncle Jim. The second story is that of my mother's mother, Florence Scriven Munro, who was born in Philadelphia in 1886. She was about thirty-five at the time of the birth of her first surviving child, my mother, in 1921, in Los Angeles. Twenty-eight years later, my mother, Alice Munro Isaacs, gave birth to me in Los Angeles, as she describes in the third story. My own daughter, Florence Jean, is named for her two great-grandmothers, who were each about ninety years old when they recorded these stories. Florence Jean's birth is recorded in pictures in the section on home birth in this *Catalog*.   (JIA)

February 26, 1978

"Dear Janet,

You asked sometime ago if I could tell you about my three pregnancies in case there was something of value you could use in the book you are writing about your experiences

"Of course, my first one was pretty serious and both the baby (Jim) and I came very close to not 'making it' because of uremic poisoning developing early in the seventh month. That situation doesn't seem to be prevalent today, but then in 1915 it was something doctors were constantly on the lookout for.

"My mother's youngest sister, who was expecting in December 1915, sometime, died in September after my experience. She was 35, a graduate of Vassar. She had a woman obstetrician who allowed the condition to continue too long before taking steps to end the pregnancy and clean out the uterus. She finally did take the baby (girl), who weighed two pounds, but Aunt Mabel went into convulsions and died. The baby lived five days.

"I was dead set against going to a hospital to have my baby. There had been several cases in the news about that time in which nurses were accused of being careless about handling the infants and the mothers were never sure they had the right baby. But my family doctor convinced my husband and my parents I must go to the Magee Hospital and have the pregnancy terminated for I was so full of poison that if I had *one* convulsion that would be fatal. He did not tell me this but persuaded me to go for treatment.

"We had figured the baby would be due about the middle of April. I entered the hospital the afternoon of March 3. My doctor took me and mother in his Ford (touring car). My feet, legs, hands, face were badly swollen. I had to wear my grandmother's underwear and old-fashioned shoes (garters) with elastic in the sides.

"This Magee Hospital was the first maternity hospital in Pittsburgh. At the time I was there it was housed in a very large mansion belonging to some wealthy Pittsburgh brothers named Magee, who gave the building plus several acres of ground and money for the new building then in progress, in memory of their mother who had died in childbirth with the last of a large family. As soon as I got to the hospital the head doctor examined me and did not tell me what he was doing or why, but by inserting instruments began dilation about 5 p.m. I went into labor about 7 or 8, but I did not know what was happening. As far as I knew I was just getting "treatment," but by 9 p.m. they took me down stairs to a small room and then I lay on a hard cart with a nurse who kept taking my blood pressure. I had a severe backache.

"The doctor came in about 10 p.m. and I asked him what was going on. He said, 'Jean, don't you know you are in labor?' I cried very hard. I said, 'Doctor, I can't have this baby now, I haven't

been married nine months till the 16th of March. People in the church are going to talk about us.' He said, 'Well, there's nothing can be done about it now. Just send the people to me. Anyhow you are allowed two weeks with the first.'

"In the meantime the hospital had called John and my parents and my doctor. They got there about 11 p.m. The nurses told me they were outside the delivery room but were not allowed in. My doctor was, but he was not permitted to have any participation.

"For two hours I suffered Hades. Because of the high content of uremic acid and my high blood pressure the doctors said I couldn't have enough ether to put me out, only little whiffs. Jim's head was visible, but he was wedged sideways and face forward. Finally I heard my doctor say, '*Hurry*. She's getting too weak. Never mind the baby, *save* her!' So the obstetrician used instruments and grabbed the baby *wherever* he could and *pulled*. You can well imagine I was badly lacerated.

"I could just barely see the doctor hand the baby to the nurses who began to walk away with him, but I was alert enough to know the baby did not cry. I cried out, 'Something's wrong. That baby didn't cry. Do something.' The doctors said something to the nurses and my doctor moved over beside me and took my hand. He said, 'It's all right, Jeanie.' I was aware of some activity in the corner where the nurses had gone and then after a bit I heard a faint cry and I said, 'Oh, Jimmy, your mother's awful sick!' The doctor said, 'How did you know it was Jimmy?' I said, 'He's always been Jimmy.' My doctor told me the doctor thought the baby was dead. He was nearly black and did not seem to breathe, and after the way he was simply pulled out they thought he could not be alive. If I hadn't called out, the nurses were just putting him in a small basket and doing nothing. Jim has a large scar up the front of his skull and another just behind an ear just at the base of the brain where the instruments had grabbed.

"The doctors knew I was badly torn but my blood pressure was still so high they decided I'd have to have repairs later. When Jim was two years old I went to another hospital and had it done. The surgeon told me there was not much of the neck of the uterus left and I had fifteen stitches in the vagina and hemorrhoid repair also. He said he didn't see how I could carry another baby, but two years later almost to the week I was back in the hospital, and your Dad was born with no complications. He was small-boned and plump. Bob was born at home with my mother and my family doctor. No anesthetic with either one.

"I don't know how this will be of any value to you. Obstetrics has greatly improved since 1915.

Love,
Grandma Jean"

(From a taped conversation between my mother and my grandmother Florence.

"Your Dad and I talked it over and we decided it would be nice if we had a baby. I was told nothing about childbirth by my mother or by my older sisters. Neither of them were married, of course. They did check for pregnancy in those days, but I didn't have any checking done, I just knew when I was pregnant. My sister-in-law Hazel was there with me the first time and she told me everything about things because she had had children. My first baby was born back East and it was a very large baby and broke its shoulder in delivery, so it passed on. You were born here in California and I had had such a hard time with that first baby and all that I was almost afraid to have anything. Then my mother talked to a woman that told her about Dr. Shafer and that she was a very good person for bringing in the babies or anything like that. So I went up and saw her and I took her course. I went every Tuesday, or maybe every other Tuesday and I got everything from Dr. Shafer. She had some sort of liquid stuff that she got from China and this was supposed to help your whole insides work very smoothly so you wouldn't have very many hard labor pains. She was a homeopathic doctor. She said to eat plenty of greens and I got the herbs from her. I felt pretty fair during the pregnancy.

"Your dad, Jimmy, had bought a car and we went for a ride and when we got back I wasn't feeling too good so I decided to go up and see how I was getting along. So in the afternoon the next day we went up to Dr. Shafer's office and she told me to stay there because she said, 'You're almost ready for labor pains.' Your dad was with me. Dr. Shafer had a nurse. We were at her home up in the mountains, up in the hills somewhere. She and the nurse both went to bed. Your dad said he'd stay with me and Dr. Shafer said she'd just be in the next room and the nurse was going to be in the other room. So your dad stayed there with me and then I told him I was beginning to feel some pains. And then I said, 'Jimmy, you'd better get her right here because the baby's coming!' I knew it was coming myself. But you came before the doctor and the nurse got there. But of course, they were right there in the house and your dad was right there. They fixed your dad on a cot bed so he could stay all night, a few nights. He stayed right there. The nurse took care of the baby. But I got a terrific headache, something terrible. So they were afraid the milk wouldn't be good for the baby. But I gave the baby some and I guess I did all right. They had you in another room and I said, 'You take that baby out of that room because I saw a mouse coming out of that room.' I said, 'You put that baby right in here with me.' So they put you in with me. Then your dad had to go back to work, so my sister Emmy got a cab and came up and got me and the baby and brought us home to 58th street. She'd never done anything like that before in her life. She wasn't that brave. I wanted to nurse you but I didn't have enough milk so I wasn't able to. Dr. Shafer gave me something for you that was very good. I wasn't able to get it for Arthur [my mother's younger brother] but at the end of 57th street there was a family that had a goat and I got goat's milk for the baby."

"After we had been married for two years, I made an arrangement with your dad that on our second anniversary we would stop using contraceptives because I wanted to have children. He was not so keen about it, he liked things just the way they were but he went along with it. I had been told very little about childbirth by anyone. When I was a child I was told nothing. I believed that babies actually came down in a special room in the hospital directly from heaven. So it was quite a shock to me when I found out it just wasn't that way and it turned me into an atheist for some period of time when I realized there was no direct connection between heaven and earth.

"I knew I was pregnant when I missed the first period, because I was so regular. So when it came around to the second period and I didn't have one, I went to the doctor and had a test done and sure enough I was pregnant. In the beginning I went for prenatal visits once a month, then twice a month, then once a week. I generally saw the same doctor. She was a woman. However, she was not married and she had no children. It was a medical clinic that I went to and they really charged us a tremendous amount, because at that time in the state of California, a medical clinic could have its own pharmacy. So when I went to the doctor they always gave me all the vitamins and the calcium pills and so on and so forth right there. And none of it was billed until you were born and then it was a tremendous shock when we got the bill. For the most part it was just vitamin pills except that in the beginning I was quite sick at my stomach and so I had to go up once a week and have a shot in the arm for the nausea. As for diet, they just kept telling me to not eat too much. I started getting cramps in my legs about the third or fourth month and then they told me to start taking calcium. After I got over those first three months I felt fine. I did have some constipation and so I had to take something for that regularly.

"With you I had a saddle block, which was a new kind of thing at that time (1949) and they considered this to be the best thing to do and so that's what I said I wanted to do. You were two weeks overdue. There were no pains at the beginning—the water broke. I was at Grandma and Grandpa's because your Dad was up at USC going to school. My dad and mother took me up to the hospital. I walked up the front steps, quite a few steps up into the hospital, and told them at the admissions desk what had happened and they immediately sent a wheelchair down and got me in it and told me not to get up again. Afterwards they told me that there is danger after the water breaks of having the cord come down first and strangling the baby.

"I was in a little room and the labor pains were not too bad. My Dad went over to USC and got Jack and they brought him over. He came up and stayed with me for a little while. It was in a private labor room. It was around six or six-thirty in the evening. It wasn't very long after your dad came that they came in and said they were going to give me something that would either make me go ahead and have the baby or make me go to sleep, it would do one or the other. At least, that's what I understood them to say. And so I did just simply go to sleep and then I remember they came in, woke me up and they said, 'You know you have to do some work if you're going to have a baby, you're going to have to do some pushing.' And I didn't want to be bothered, but they kept telling me 'You've got to work on this. You're going to have to push now.' So then I did push because they annoyed me so. They took me in, gave me the saddle block, and you were born, at about eight or nine in the morning. Most of the night, the whole thing, is just a blank as far as I'm concerned. Whatever they gave me just wiped it out. I do remember I did have the episiotomy and I remember that the doctor had apparently an intern or a resident watching her and she kept saying, 'Now feel this. Feel how smooth this is. It has to be just this smooth,' when she was stitching me up. She was instructing this person in how to do it as she was doing me. It was a man she was instructing.

"I felt no pain during the delivery. I was not fearful. I felt okay. I really wasn't worried about it, I don't know why. With both you and your brother forceps were used. Of course, with the saddle block you're not aware of any feeling at all, so after the episiotomy she used the forceps and took you. When you were very first born she said 'Oh, it's a little boy,' and then she said, 'No it's not, it's a little girl.' I didn't get a very good look at you. They didn't bring you up and show you to me. I know you cried immediately because I was listening to hear that. I wasn't allowed to touch you in the delivery room. They took me to my room and your dad came up to see me after he saw you in the nursery. I was able to see you pretty soon after, I think, and I was not only allowed to undress you but I was asked to undress you and look you over and make sure everything was okay. And I remember they pointed out the fact that they had used forceps and that those marks on either side of your forehead would go away."

Women's Birth Art

At the time I became pregnant with my first child in 1976, I was working as a printmaker, making silk-screened political posters (see index). I had hoped to sell enough posters to sustain a small home business, but unfortunately my pregnancy cut short my printmaking activities. Silkscreen ink contains several harmful chemicals and even though I normally used a chemical filter mask while working, I felt I could not take even a small chance of harming the fetus with noxious fumes. So I stopped making prints, but my interest in art continued. I began to think about the possibility of incorporating images of pregnancy and birth into my art work. I asked my husband to photograph me during pregnancy and arranged for someone to take pictures of the birth. I wanted to have lots of graphic material available for future art work.

During my pregnancy an article by feminist art critic Lucy Lippard appeared in an art magazine ("The Pains and Pleasures of Rebirth: Women's Body Art," by Lucy Lippard, *Art in America,* May/June 1976). Lippard noted that while formerly taboo subjects like menstruation, aging, and sex had appeared in women's art, women artists were not using pregnancy and childbirth as major images in their work. She speculated about why this might be (women artists don't have children? women artists want to recognize intellectual, not biological creation? the pregnant figure is considered unattractive?) and called procreativity in art "the next taboo to be tackled." I vowed to start making "birth art" as soon as my baby was born. I wanted to create strong, powerful images of women giving birth—images which would convey the sense of personal power which women can achieve (and are often denied) in childbirth.

After my baby was born, though, the demands of breastfeeding and baby care kept me from resuming either printmaking or painting, both of which require large chunks of uninterrupted work time (the ink dries in the screen; the paint dries on the canvas). I took up writing instead, which can be done in half hour bits throughout the day whenever the baby naps. By the time my son was old enough to permit a change in my schedule, I had become too deeply involved in writing about birth to turn back. Way led on to way until I found myself editing the *Whole Birth Catalog.*

I have yet to create my body of "birth art." Just one painting is done so far. But others are working in this area. While researching this *Catalog,* I wrote to the editor of *Women Artists' News* and she published my call for birth art for the *Catalog.* I received a selection of excellent submissions from women artists around the country, many of which are reproduced here. I asked the artists to write a brief explanation of how and why they came to make their birth art and their words are also included here. One of my projects for the future is to research and mount an exhibition and catalog of contemporary women's birth art and to include more examples in future editions of the *Catalog.* If you know of anyone or are yourself producing art work with pregnancy, childbirth, or breastfeeding as central themes, please contact me, as described in "Contributing to Future Editions" in this *Catalog.*

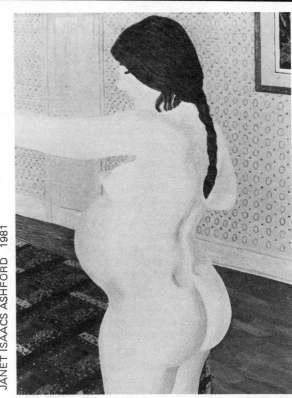

SELF-PORTRAIT AS A PREGNANT WOMAN   Acrylic on canvas, 30" x 24"
JANET ISAACS ASHFORD   1981

MARIA IN EXILE
Mixed media, 41 3/8" x 29 1/2"
1981

by
Josely Carvalho
216 E. 18th St.
New York, NY 10003

Josely Carvalho is a Brazilian artist who now lives in New York City. She has exhibited extensively in Brazil, Washington D.C., and New York since 1974 and is currently director of The Silkscreen Project at St. Marks Church-in-the-Bowery in New York. *Maria in Exile* was shown as part of an exhibit "A Diary of Images: Women 1980/81" at Central Hall Artists in New York City in 1982. Each image was accompanied by poetic documentation, which "Intensifies the total impact of the works."

Smell of fish.
I, you, we,
all
women that fish,
that sew, that farm,
that nourish, that fight,
that cry, that lose,
that dream, that ignore,
you, lost women in an unknown
    world.
you, failed women by the jails of
    our daily life.
You, mummy-bride,
Why do you marry?

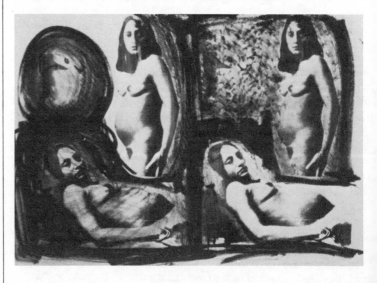

ENTRANCE
Oil on canvas, 24″ x 48″
1978

PANGS OF GREEN
Oil on canvas, 40″ x 48″
1979
by
Francia
c/o Westbeth Artists Community
463 West Street
New York, NY 10014

Francia studied at the Art Student's League and the Brooklyn Museum Art School and has been widely exhibited in New York City and Kentucky (where she was an artist in residence). She has received a grant from the National Endowment for the the Arts and is listed in the *World Who's Who of Women.* Francia is represented by the Martha White Gallery, Louisville, Kentucky, and Virginia Miller Galleries, Coral Gables, Florida.

"It was the birth of my son Sascha that lead to the paintings and drawings I call my *Birth Series.* On July 30, 1977, Sascha was born; my husband Bruce and midwife Sandy Woods were at my side during the entire labor. Although the birth took place in Roosevelt Hospital in New York City my experience had none of the typical qualities of a hospital delivery. Bruce and Sandy's responsiveness made my birth a very positive and exhilarating one from beginning to end. It left an indelible visual stamp on my brain and I felt a strong need to translate what I experienced into a visual language.

"I have for some time been interested in forms of organic imagery which express the qualities related to being a woman. My work has represented the coming together of my conscious and unconscious into the creation of an organic fantasy world. The primary inspiration is nature: the key sources are rock, land and quarry formations, clouds and the human figure. These elements have become abstracted by my transforming nature, sensations and feelings into my own visual language.

"In the *Birth Series,* which began in September, 1977 and lasted until March, 1979, I was involved in depicting the life force. I continued to examine the contours, crevices, and mounds of organic forms through color contrasts, volume, luminosity and the tension that arises between the forms. Both the internal and external of the human body pulsate and have a sensuality that I continue to explore on each canvas. In these paintings my use of dark against light creates a third dimension to the forms. The luminosity in each work can be seen as brilliant light edges against dark ones which represent the spiritual glow of giving birth at the end of a dark tunnel. The placenta appeared as a beautiful crimson red ameoba-like form with the delivery room lights creating a sparkling turquoise backdrop. The thin smooth layers of oil paint mold the forms into breathing matter: massive areas against smaller ones and muted tones against luminous ones. The paintings generally try to express the sensation of pushing down and opening up or flowering in parallel to the process of giving birth. In the piece *Entrance* I see the top form as the beginning of the engagement process when the uterus is ready to open up. *Pangs of Green* shows the stage of pushing and pulling, the gusts of force that are the labor process. That same push and pull relationship exists between the colors and forms of each canvas."

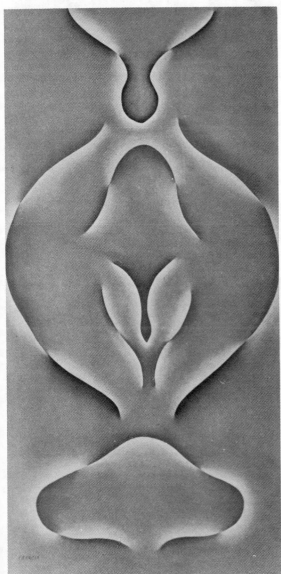

Entrance

Pangs of Green

CHILDBIRTH DREAM
360° Internal Hologram
1978-1980

from
Box GZ-12
Cal Arts
McBean Parkway
Valencia, CA 91355
signed, limited edition
about $1200. with rotating display

Postcard with an image from *Childbirth Dream* by Alexis Krasilovsky

"A new art form was born a few decades ago, and everybody is still waiting to find out what it will look like when it grows up. Essentially like three-dimensional photography, holography grabbed my attention around the same time I was beginning to re-examine my life and artistic capabilities in feminist terms. Here was a form that could address inner as well as outer space, and an industry in which women could participate from the ground floor up.

"For me, exploring childbirth through art was a ritual which brought my body, my thoughts and my emotions into balance for the first time. But I was aware that I was denying myself the life experience and the joy which my mother had had in giving birth to me, even though completely anesthetized and divided from herself. Ironically, I would have made more money as a welfare mother than as an artist supported by grants. But my hands were tied to 1,632 drawings of a

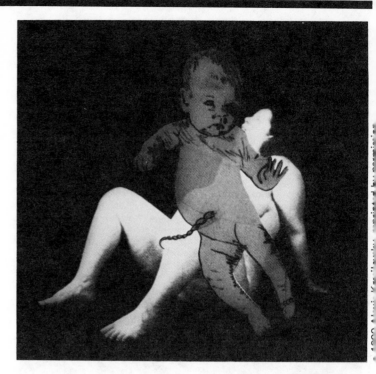

pregnant mother and a newborn baby, while my womb was begging the rest of me to give it a baby right there on the animation table, if necessary!

"I found a source of strength in the repetitive task of drawing hundreds of 3-D umbilical cords as they turn in space, but I also found myself questioning over and over again the extent of my rights and freedom to choose this kind of labor. I know, because I've had the time to think about it, that I could not have made my hologram if I had gotten pregnant, and I battled—sometimes physically—for the right to choose my art over another life, in order to fulfill this aspect of my own.

"I am particularly happy that the hologram will be shown in a women's context. *Childbirth Dream* is a pro-Choice hologram, meant to encourage women to ask themselves, 'How do I feel about this experience?' 'Is it a beautiful dream?' The men who postponed the printing of it at the Holographic Film Company for many months called it a nightmare. As it turns in space, how many times is a baby born? How many times satisfies us? How many babies do we want? Is this modern work of art a fertility symbol, or a reminder of our choices?

"Some men have objected to the fact that *Childbirth Dream* does not present the typical, blonde, slim-though-pregnant Hollywood stereotype, nor is the hologram a "Madon-

na and Son," but rather, a real mother dreaming about her daughter's birth.

"Holography is still young enough not to be treated just like any old technology. At the same time as we work to improve holographic techniques, we can insist on hours that allow us to raise another generation while we work for a world

in which it can grow. We can insist on imagery that raises us out of the sexual degradation and violence of mass media. We can create a new mythology in the fourth dimension that sustains us through difficult times ahead. We can honor the creative impulse in women and men without which life has little meaning."

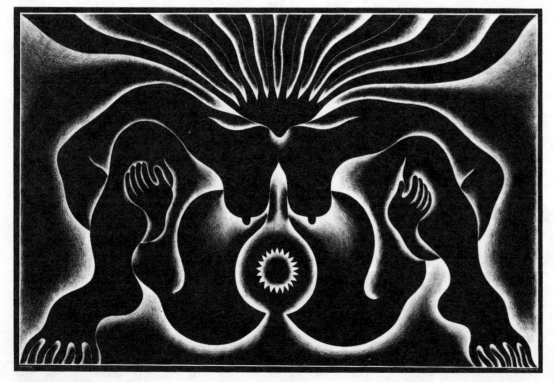

THE CROWNING
by Judy Chicago
poster, 25" x 38"

from
JC/WIN
1728 Bissonnet
Houston, TX 77005
$10.00 unsigned
$20.00 signed
plus $3.00 shipping

This poster is one of the images from feminist artist Judy Chicago's new *Birth Project* (her last project was The Dinner Party). The *Birth Project* is being funded by Through the Flower Corporation, a nonprofit organization founded by Chicago and colleagues to help produce and distribute women's art. The poster is being distributed through the Judy Chicago Word & Image Network (JC/WIN). The JC/WIN catalog states "Judy Chicago became aware that the subject of birth is scarcely recorded in Western art despite its central importance in women's lives. Addressing the imbalance caused by omitting this universal human experience from our culture's store of symbols, Judy Chicago has been designing a series of images related to birth and the birth process to be executed under her supervision in a wide range of needlework techniques by people around the country."

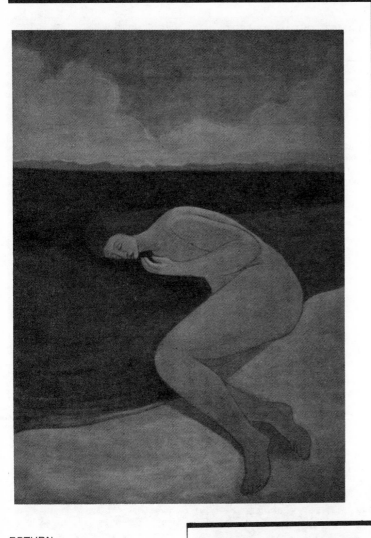

BIRTH PAINTING
Acrylic on canvas, 66" x 72"
1982

Cindy Pink
c/o 64 Grand Street
New York, NY 10013

Cindy Pink studied painting at Columbia University and at the New York Studio School. Her drawings have been shown in various group shows and her collaborations have been shown at ABC NO RIO and Fashion Moda in New York City.

Cindy and I met when we were invited to attend the home birth of a mutual friend.

"I felt enthusiastic when I started the birth painting because I knew it would be shown in a good context. It was to be part of a larger piece on home birth which I was preparing for "Carnival Knowledge," a continually evolving traveling show on the subject of reproductive rights. Most of the contributing artists and performers were women. I was also spurred on by having recently witnessed a birth at home. The experience had served as a wonderful antidote to my own two children's births—both in hospitals and both experiences leaving me emotionally frustrated. The surprise came as I got into working on the painting. The figures came alive for me and were not just models. They started to move of their own accord, to vibrate, and create their own gestures. This was something I had never experienced in drawing "the figure"— an academic conception. First I drew the baby crowning, which is such a beautiful form to see. But the figures all seemed to move and the baby just came forward. I literally felt I had to stop the time sequence or I would have had to draw the baby fully emerged and I knew I wanted that strange moment when it's still 'stuck' in order to get the pictorial imagery I wanted.

"Doing the painting was far more of a catharsis than I expected. Each figure had become connected to someone I knew. The subject matter of birth had worked its magic. This heightened the emotional intensity to such a degree that at one point I broke down and started to sob. At times I identified with each figure in the painting, with the mother and with the helpers. My indentification with the baby was less conscious. At one point a vibrant image of my mother as she was when I was seven or eight came to me. I yearned with the desire that my children would find such immediate vitality in me.

"This painting led to a rebirth and new integration for me in my work. Right afterward I began work on a series of oil pastel drawings of the human face done from imagination."

RETURN
Oil on canvas, 76" x 48"
1977

Frances E. Lyshak
57 East 4th Street, Apt. 5B
New York, NY 10003

Frances Lyshak was educated at the Center for Creative Studies and Wayne State University in Detroit and at Pratt Institute in New York. Her work has been exhibited in a variety of galleries and shows since 1976.

"*Return* is an outgrowth of an inner image. The inner image surfaced, no doubt, in response to a deep need for simplicity, repose and the tender caressing feeling that immersion in quiet water provides.

"When I paint, the process of bringing the image to fruition in the painting becomes like an extended meditation. The image is a visual metaphor which I must paint in order to fully unearth its significance; and, thereby, I begin to resolve this particular outcry from my unconscious."

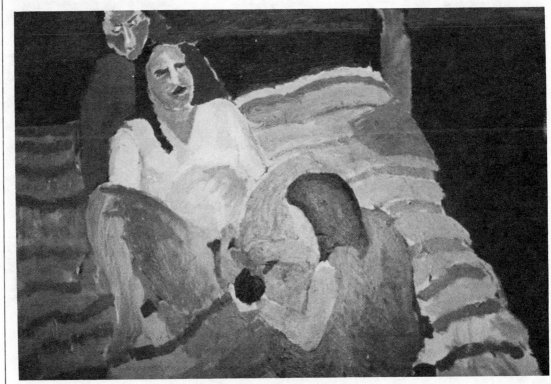

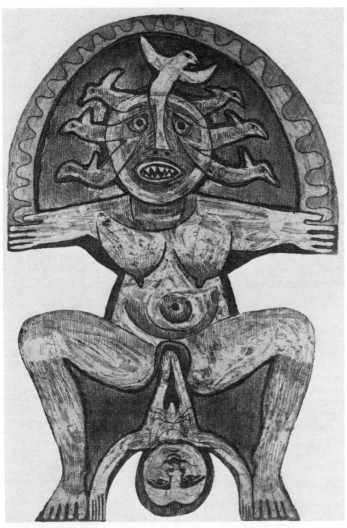

Rites of Passage

BIRTHING IMAGES
A series of four etchings reproduced in color, 11" x 14" each
Print titles:
Birth Rite
Cassowary's Baby
Rites of Passage
Cormorant Lady

Betty LaDuke
610 Long Way
Ashland, OR 97520
$12.00 per set of four

Betty LaDuke is a professor of art at Southern Oregon State University, and has been exhibiting her work since 1953. She has traveled extensively in South America and Asia, and draws much of her inspiration from the art of third world cultures. *Birthing Images* is based on fertility myths and folk tales of Papua New Guinea. She has also created work based on totems, creation myths, and "feminine mythical views" of landscape. Contact Betty LaDuke for information on traveling exhibitions, slide presentations, and lectures on these subjects.

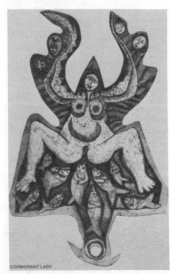

Cormorant Lady

LAMAZE CHILDBIRTH POT
clay, 14" high, 9½" wide

Susan Grabel
c/o The Prince Street Gallery
121 Wooster Street
New York, NY 10012

"I had been making large covered jars with figures on them at the time of my first pregnancy. My husband and I went through the Lamaze course and had our child using the Lamaze method of childbirth. The experience was so profound and exhilarating that it spurred me on to taking the pots a step further.

"I began to use the figures in a narrative context rather than as decorative elements. And the first story I told was the story of the birth of our child.

"On top is a woman giving birth and around the sides are relief figures depicting the Lamaze exercises: front, simulated contraction with man timing it; back, tension/relaxation; sides under handles, stretching exercises."

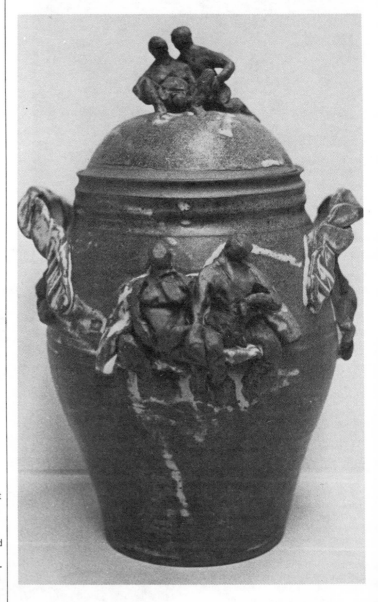

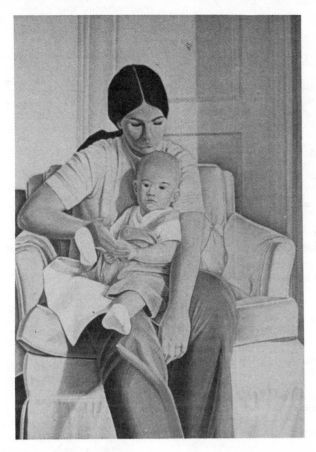

FIGURES IN AN UPHOLSTERED CHAIR
Oil on masonite, 6" x 8½"
1974

Laura Schechter
c/o Forum Gallery
1018 Madison Avenue
New York, NY 10003

Laura Schechter was born in Brooklyn in 1944 and studied art at Brooklyn College. She has exhibited her work extensively in one-person and group shows since 1971. Her work is part of the permanent collections of the Boston Museum of Fine Art, the Brooklyn Museum, the Museum of Art of the Carnegie Institute and other institutions. She has worked as an artist-in-residence at colleges in Baltimore, Boston, Arizona, New York City, and Long Island. See other work by Laura Schechter on page 49.

"I want women to know that you can continue doing your work after your baby is born, but you have to know that you will have to give up other things and you will have to be resolute in devoting yourself to your work and to child care. My son was born by cesarean section, so my recovery was longer. But when my son was ten or eleven days old, I started painting again, at first for just an hour a day and I worked up to painting four or five hours a day until he was about three years old, even though I was totally responsible for his care during that time. I learned that I must paint when I could. Whenever he was asleep I would paint and I found that the experience of painting for an hour here and an hour there built up my tolerance and discipline so that now that he is in school I paint all day long, eight to nine hours a day.

"I developed what I call the 'washerwoman theory' of childrearing. I see an image of the washerwoman, with ten or eleven kids all around her and she's in the midst of them, washing clothes for a living, and she has to keep working all the time even though she has these kids all around her. I figured that if my child saw me painting all the time, from the minute he was born, he would accept it. When he was a toddler, and going to sleep late, I would start painting around seven in the evening and he would be there in the studio. I would be taking care of him; changing his diapers, giving him a bottle, whatever, but I would keep on painting all evening. This is how I survived as an artist/mother. But in order to do this I had to be very single-minded and strong. When my son was a baby I had to give up everything else—reading, friends, socializing. All I did was take care of the baby and paint. The trouble with being a modern working mother is that you can be totally isolated. I used to see women in the park who were totally into motherhood as their sole occupation and as the definition of their self. But I couldn't do that. I had to keep painting and I did."

UNTITLED
Acrylic on canvas 72" x 50"
1977

Mary H. Nash
8536 Aponi Road
Vienna, VA 22180

Mary Nash was born in Washington, DC in 1951 of creative parents who had worked as entertainers in vaudeville for many years. Because of her parents' creative inclinations, Mary became interested in pursuing a career in art. She earned B.A. and M.F.A. degrees in 1973 and 1976 and has since pursued a life of painting in the studio full-time. Her work has been previously influenced by American folk art, but has increasingly displayed her own individual reaction to her life, herself, and her ideas. The work of Mary Nash is owned by seven public collections and has been exhibited in shows across the United States. Mary Nash has been listed in *Who's Who in American Art, Personalities of the South,* and *Who's Who Among Students in American Colleges and Universities.* Mary makes her home in the suburbs of Washington, DC, where she lives and works with her husband, Richard.

"The painting, *Untitled,* 1977, is an examination of a young woman who is ready to commence a journey to hike up a hill to a building which represents the unknown. Her infant child is very wise as the woman is herself. The terrain consists primarily of plowed fields which will be farmed soon. The woman and the child are in an area where there is a concern for natural food and surroundings. As they hike towards the unknown, they hope to experience spiritual development, and so they are both dressed in white. The unknown building is like a temple; it too is white, but no one really knows what will happen there. This painting on another level represents the journey of life and mind—a form of becoming. I chose to make this painting because at the time that I made it, these were all issues of concern to me. The woman is somewhat Egyptian in appearance, especially her hair, because for a time I was especially interested in the stylistic concerns of Egyptian Art."

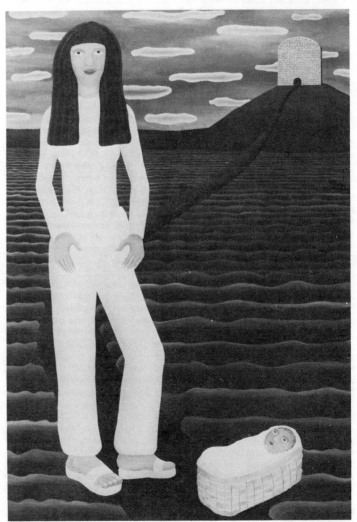

Mary H. Nash, *Untitled* (photo by Joel Breger), © 1980 Mary H. Nash. Reprinted by permission.

Childbirth in Literature

Childbirth has not often been depicted in literature, in part because many of the fine women writers of the past were able to write only because they were childless and thus unencumbered. Women make up half the world and our collective experience of childbirth should have provided us with a tremendously rich heritage of writing on this most important of life events. But all this has been lost. Women's voices and uniquely female experiences have been feared and suppressed for a long time and only recently have writers, who are also mothers, begun to bring their experience into the realm of literature. Some of these voices are presented here.

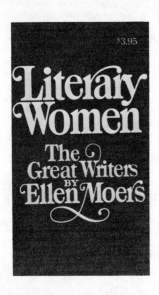

LITERARY WOMEN: The Great Writers
by Ellen Moers
1977, 496 pages, Illus.

from
Anchor/Doubleday
245 Park Avenue
New York, NY 10017
$3.95 pap.

This fascinating and inspiring book by the late Ellen Moers is about "the major women writers" and the effect their sex had upon their lives and literary production. Most interesting in the context of childbirth is the chapter on "Female Gothic" in which Moers discusses Mary Shelley's *Frankenstein* as, in effect, a fantasy based on her childbearing experiences. In an inspired introduction, Dr. Moers compares a passage from *Frankenstein* (quote follows) with Dr. Spock's descriptions of the appearance of a newborn baby in *Baby and Child Care* (see page 5 of the 1976 Pocket Books edition).

(This book made me so excited about women's literature that I went out to a used book store and bought a whole stack of novels by the Brontes, Jane Austen, George Sand, George Eliot, etc., and had a wonderful time reading them.)

"Mary Shelley was a unique case, in literature as in life. She brought birth to fiction not as realism but as Gothic fantasy, and thus contributed to Romanticism a myth of genuine originality: the mad scientist who locks himself in his laboratory and secretly, guiltily works at creating human life, only to find that he has made a monster.

'It was on a dreary night of November, that I beheld the accomplishment of my toils. With an anxiety that almost mounted to agony, I collected the instruments of life around me, that I might infuse a spark of being into the lifeless thing that lay at my feet. . . . The rain pattered dismally against the panes, and my candle was nearly burnt out when, by the glimmer of the half-extinguished light, I saw the dull yellow eye of the creature open; it breathed hard, and a convulsive motion agitated its limbs. . . . His yellow skin scarcely covered the work of muscles and arteries beneath; his hair was of a lustrous black, and flowing . . . but these luxuriances only formed a more horrid contrast with his watery eyes, that seemed almost of the same color as the dun white sockets in which they were set, his shrivelled complexion and straight black lips.'

"That is very good horror, but what follows is more horrid still: Frankenstein, the scientist, runs away and abandons the newborn monster, who is and remains nameless. Here, I think, is where Mary Shelley's book is most interesting, most powerful, and most feminine: in the motif of revulsion against newborn life, and the drama of guilt, dread, and flight surrounding birth and its consequences. Most of the novel, roughly two of its three volumes, can be said to deal with the retribution visited upon monster and creator for deficient infant care. *Frankenstein* seems to be distinctly a *woman's* mythmaking on the subject of birth precisely because its emphasis is not upon what precedes birth, not upon birth itself, but upon what follows birth: the trauma of the afterbirth."

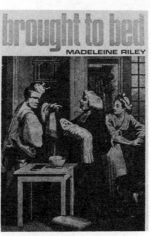

BROUGHT TO BED
by Madeleine Riley
1968, 138 pages, Illus.

from
A.A. Barnes and Co.
Cranbury, NJ 08512
out of print

This unusual book is apparently out of print. I found my copy by chance through a sale of remaindered books, but readers may be able to find it in a used book shop or a library. Madeleine Riley, an Englishwoman, has collected together references to childbirth in English literature since the 18th century, and provides many excerpts along with her comments. Topics include the preference for sons, illegitimate births, abortion, infanticide, the rivalry between doctors and midwives, women's behavior in labor, superstitions and dreams, how husbands behave, and changes in childbirth in the last century. Much of the writing is by men (Tolstoi, Dickens, Fielding, Galsworthy, etc.) but there are excellent excerpts from Doris Lessing, Enid Bagnold and others, and some discussion of why women writers may have avoided childbirth in their work. Also included are several fine historical illustrations.

"The eighteenth century regarded childbirth, it seems, as a natural, frequent event involving all the community in which the mother lived. They recognized that it was an event which was likely to include death, which would require humour, endurance and good luck. In the childbirth scenes in these novels there are many characters, some giving advice and assisting at the birth, some coming in to chat, eat and drink; the atmosphere is convivial, busy and easy going. The women in labour are, for the most part, brave and practical. The husbands are well looked after; they reserve their love and any anxiety for their wives and mistresses and show little concern for the child. The doctors and midwives, with their free enterprise methods and their rivalry, have a bracing attitude to

childbirth and, though the need for concealment and courage is not minimized, the most carefree illegitimate births come from this period.

"In nineteenth-century novels childbirth is treated quite differently. These novels have the most unhappy, bleak confinements: deaths abound and are less casually treated than formerly. The impression is that childbirth is a difficult, secret, exclusively feminine affair. Anxieties have increased—fear of death, money worries, the health, itself, of the women before and after childbirth, is more delicate and precarious. In this era illegitimate births are tragedies; prostitutes who give birth easily and comfortably have disappeared to be replaced by pure young girls who are seduced with frightful consequences. A wife who is about 'to cry out' has become a 'virtuous mother in the sacred pangs of childbirth.'

"By the middle of the twentieth century childbirth is no longer sacred. The 'virtuous mother' is now being described as 'lying almost naked, her tight knotted belly sticking up in a purple lump, watching with fascination how it contracted and strained.' The traditional womanly modesty is disappearing and documentary descriptions are being written. In these accounts the doctors and midwives have been cleaned up and become antiseptic, respectable professionals. It is hard to imagine Mrs. Gamp or Dr. Bangham as their predecessors. The baby has become much more important both in embryo and at birth. It arouses passionately strong paternal feelings in the sensitive husbands of the twentieth century. There are fewer people involved in the birth, which is now a more important and exclusive event in the lives of both fictional parents."

"The eighteenth century regarded childbirth, it seems, as a natural, frequent event involving all the community in which the mother lived. . . . The atmosphere is convivial, busy and easy going. The women in labour are, for the most part, brave and practical."

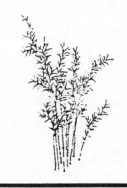

THE DOOR OF LIFE
by Enid Bagnold
1938

William Morrow and Co.
out of print
(published in England as *The Squire*, by Wm. Heinemann, 1938).

Enid Bagnold (author of *National Velvet*) describes the birth at home of a seventh child to an upper-class English woman who feels confident about her birth attendants and her ability to give birth. She is an early adherent of "natural childbirth" and cooperates with her doctor and midwife, whom she calls the "monk" and the "nun."

"The monk and the nun were about her bed, acutely directed on her, tuned to her every manifestation. With eyes fast shut she lent herself to their quiet directions, clinging to the memory of her resolve that when the river began to pull she would swim down with it, clutching at no banks. With a touch of anaesthetics from a gauze mask to help her she went forward. Her mind went down and lived in her body, ran out of her brain and lived in her flesh. . . . Now the first twisting spate of pain began. Swim then, swim with it, for your life. If you resist, horror and impediment. If you swim, not pain but sensation! Who knows the heart of pain, the silver, whistling hub of pain, the central bellows of childbirth which expels one being from another. None know it who, in disbelief and dread has drawn back to the periphery, contracting the will of pain,

braking against inexorable movements. Keep abreast of it, rush together, you and the violence which is also you! Wild movements, hallucinated swimming. Other things exist than pain.

"It is hard to gauge pain. By her movements, by her exclamations she would have struck horror into anyone but her monk and nun. She would have seemed tortured, tossing, crying, muttering, grunting. She was not unconscious but she had left external life. She was blind and deaf to world surface. Every sense she had was down in Earth to which she belonged, fighting to maintain a hold on pain, to keep her pace with it, not to take an ounce of will from her assent to its passage. It was as though the dark river rushed her to a glossy arch. A little more, a little longer. She was not in torture, she was in labour; and she had been thus before and knew her way. The corkscrew swirl swept her shuddering until she swam into a tunnel—the first seconds of anaesthesia.

"Now the shocked and vigorous cry of the born rang through the room. From its atavistic dim cradle, from a passage like death, crying with rage, resenting birth, came the freed and furious cave child coated in mystery, the heavy-heeled, vulnerable young, the triumph of the animal world, the triumph of life.

"Now out of her river the mother was drawn upwards, she became the welcomed, the applauded, the humoured. Faces smiled over her.

" 'What is it?' Nine months of wondering in one second solved.

" 'A boy, a beauty.' "

A PROPER MARRIAGE
by Doris Lessing
1970

from
New American Library
1301 Avenue of the Americas
New York, NY 10021
$3.95 pap.

This novel is part of Doris Lessing's series, *Children of Violence*. Her heroine, Martha Quest, labors alone in a maternity home and is determined to maintain her control over the pain of her labor.

"For some time she lay stiff on the narrow slope of the table and waited. In this position it seemed that the pains were worse. Or rather that she could not command herself as well. She climbed down and walked up and down the deserted room. Now it was every four minutes; and she was doubled up with them, shutting her teeth against a desire to groan, cautiously unfolding herself again. . . . Tight, stiff, cautious, she felt the baby knot and propel itself down; it recoiled and slackened and she with it. The pain had changed. She could mark the point at which, just as it abruptly changed its quality a couple of hours before in the bath, so now it ground into a new gear, as it were. It gripped first her back, then her stomach, then it was as if she and the baby were being wrung out together by a pair of enormous steel hands. But still she kept the small place in her brain alive and watchful. She would not give in . . . The small lit place in her brain was dimming most alarm-

ingly with the pains . . . she entered a place where there was no time at all. An agony so unbelievable gripped her that her astounded and protesting mind cried out that it was impossible such pain should be. It was a pain so violent that it was no longer a pain but a condition of being. Every particle of flesh shrieked out, while the wave spurted like an electric current from somewhere in her backbone and went through her shock after shock. The wave receded, however, just as she had decided she would disintegrate under it; and then she felt the fist that gripped her slowly loosen. Through the sweat in her eyes she saw that ten seconds had passed; she went limp in a state of perfect painlessness, an exquisite exhaustion, in which the mere idea of pain seemed impossible —it was impossible that it could recur again. And as soon as the slow flush of sensation began, the condition of painlessness seemed as impossible as the pain had seemed only a few moments before. They were two states of being, utterly disconnected, without a bridge, and Martha found herself in a condition of anxious but exasperated anger that she could not remember the agony fifteen seconds after it had ended. . . .

"Later, Martha heard the bright voice calling, 'Yes, doctor, she's ripe!' The room was full of people again. She was sucking in chloroform like an addict, and no longer remembered that she had been determined to see the child born. . . .

"When her eyes cleared, she caught a glimpse of Dr. Stern holding up a naked pallid infant, its dark hair plastered wet in streaks to its head, mouthing frustratedly at the air. Martha momentarily lost consciousness again and emerged, feeling it must be years later, to Dr. Stern in the same position, still holding the white baby, which looked rather like a forked parsnip and was making strangled grumbling gasps. Two nurses were watching him. This humanity comforted Martha. She heard someone say, 'A lovely little girl, isn't she?' Then the pink nurse bent over her and began lifting handfuls of Martha's now slack stomach and squeezing it like oranges. Martha shrieked, with the intention of being heard. 'Oh, drat it,' said the nurse: and the dome of white chloroform came down again over Martha's face."

THE DIARY OF ANAIS NIN, 1931-1934 (from a 7-volume set)
1978

from
Harcourt Brace Jovanovich
757 Third Avenue
New York, NY 10017
$22.50 set

In this excerpt from her diary of 1934, Anais Nin describes her miscarriage of a baby girl at six months of pregnancy. Her labor is induced in a maternity clinic, after the doctor fails to detect a fetal heart beat.

"August, 1934 . . .

"I lie back so quietly. I hear the ticking. Softly I drum, drum, drum. I feel my womb stirring, dilating. My hands are so weary, they will fall off. They will fall off, and I will lie there in darkness. The womb is stirring and dilating. Drum drum drum drum drum. 'I am ready!' The nurse puts her knee on my stomach. There is blood in my eyes. A tunnel. I push into this tunnel. I bite my lips and push. There is fire, flesh ripping and no air. Out of the tunnel! All my blood is spilling out. 'Push! Push! It is coming! It is coming!' I feel the slipperiness, the sudden de-

liverance, the weight is gone. Darkness.

"I hear voices. I open my eyes. I hear them saying, 'It was a little girl. Better not show it to her.' All my strength is coming back. I sit up. The doctor shouts, 'For God's sake, don't sit up, don't move!'

'Show me the child,' I say.

'Don't show it,' says the nurse, 'it will be bad for her.'

"The nurses try to make me lie down. My heart is beating so loudly I can hardly hear myself repeating, 'Show it to me!' The doctor holds it up. It looks dark, and small, like a diminutive man. But it is a little girl. It has long eyelashes on its closed eyes, it is perfectly made, and all glistening with the waters of the womb. It was like a doll, or like a miniature Indian, about one foot long, skin on bones, no flesh. But completely formed. The doctor told me afterwards that it had hands and feet exactly like mine. The head was bigger than average. As I looked at the dead child, for a moment I hated it for all the pain it had caused me, and it was only later that this flare of anger turned into great sadness.

"Regrets, long dreams of what this little girl might have been. A dead creation, my first dead creation. The deep pain caused by any death and any destruction. The failure of my motherhood, or at least the embodiment of it; all my hopes of real human, simple, direct motherhood are lying dead, and the only one left to me, Lawrence's symbolic motherhood, bringing more hope into the world. But the simple human flowering denied to me.

"Perhaps I was designed for other forms of creation."

"There is blood in my eyes. A tunnel. I push into this tunnel. I bite my lips and push. There is fire, flesh ripping and no air. Out of the tunnel! All my blood is spilling out."

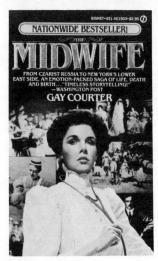

THE MIDWIFE
by Gay Courter
1982, 521 pages

from
New American Library/Signet
1633 Broadway
New York, NY 10019
$3.95 pap.

Gay Courter makes films on child-birth and childbirth preparation (Parenting Pictures, 121 NW Crystal St., Crystal River, FL 32629). She has drawn upon this background, her own midwifery training, and much research to produce this wonderful historical novel about Hannah Blau, a Russian Jewish immigrant midwife who struggles to gain recognition for herself and her profession in New York at the turn of the century. Each chapter centers around the birth of a baby (three in Russia, two "between" two worlds and three in America) and Courter provides excellent detail on the management of these births as a midwife like Hannah may have conducted them. The connecting characters and plot are very compelling and filled with insight into the problems of anti-Semitism, Jewish immigrant life, politics and the class system, marriage relationships, women's status in society, and the medical profession. Courter's treatment of all these subjects is exemplary from the point of view of the women's health and alternative childbirth movements and it is heartening to see that this book, with its strong advocacy of midwifery, has become a best-seller.

"Lazar was interrupted as one of the ship's officers came toward them. 'That's the one who helped arrange a larger food allotment in exchange for our section requiring fewer services from the crew,' he said in Hannah's ear.

" 'Mr. Sokolovsky,' First Officer Braden said, touching his hand to the brim of his stiff cap.

" 'Yes, sir!' Lazar responded in German, clicking his heels together with mock respect.

" 'Do you have any doctors among your group?'

" 'What kind of a doctor do you require?'

" 'In second class we have a couple, a Jewish couple, and the woman is going to have her baby. Upon boarding she advised us it was not expected until November, but now she thinks otherwise.'

"Hannah tugged at Lazar's sleeve. 'A baby! My wife is a doctor, a doctor of midwifery. She studied in Moscow. I am certain she could attend the case.'

" 'How fortunate! Is this your wife, then?'

" 'Hannah, will you go with him?'

" 'Of course,' Hannah replied quietly, not wanting to reveal her excitement.

" 'Do you need anything?'

" 'My medical bag. Mama knows where everything is better than I do. Have her bring it to me and I'll go with the officer.'

"Turning to him, she spoke slowly in Yiddish, knowing he would understand since some of the words were almost identical with German. 'Has she been in labor a long time?'

" 'They just wanted a doctor. That is all I know, ma'am.'

"Hannah followed him up the outside stairway near the forward smoke-stack and down the narrow passage-way, which, in that part of the ship, was carpeted with a ruby wool that looked like a long tongue reaching down into an endless mouth. They made three confusing turns before reaching cabin B-56.

"She knocked and the door opened immediately. Hannah stared at the strikingly handsome man who stood before her.

" 'I'm, I'm Mrs. Sokolovsky.'

" 'We asked for a doctor.'

"Hannah spoke quickly to try to impress him with her credentials. 'I'm a midwife; I've studied medicine at the Imperial College in Moscow.'

" 'But you look so . . . young.' The man almost apologized for his doubts.

" 'I have much experience in both Gentile and Jewish births. I have even delivered noble ladies in Moscow,' she added, sensing he was a man who wanted the best for his wife.

"A tired woman, her thick wavy hair pulled back into braids, lay on a lower bunk, her face partially covered by the floral-patterned curtain that hung above the berth on a shining brass track. 'What did you expect on this ship? A professor?' she asked her husband."

REVELATIONS: Diaries of Women
edited by Mary Jane Moffat and
Charlotte Painter
1975, 411 pages
$4.95 pap.
from
Vintage/Random House
201 East 50th Street
New York, NY 10022

Revelations is a wonderful collection of excerpts from diaries written by famous and less well-known women from the early 1800's to the present. The excerpts are arranged to cover the life span from childhood to old age and included are three excerpts concerning childbirth. Evelyn Scott (1893-1963) describes the birth of her first child in Rio de Janeiro just before World War I. "In the portion of her diary we have excerpted," say the editors, "she reflects the sweet pleasures of carrying her lover's child and the way that joy is undercut by a doctor who treats her as an object and by the humiliation of being poor." Frances Karlen Santamaria writes of the first postpartum days after her son's birth, including his Jewish circumcision ritual. But the most extraordinary account is from the obscure diary of Martha Martin, who delivered her own baby while stranded for the winter in a cabin in Alaska in the early 1950's. Martha gained such strength and sense of independence from her experience that she was almost reluctant to leave her small domain when finally rescued by Eskimos.

"I made a birth cloth today from one of Don's union suits. It is all wool and should serve nicely to wrap a newborn child in. . . .

"I plan to use string raveled from a flour sack to tie the cord. I boiled a piece to make sure it is clean. . . .

"I've worked again on the fur, and I'm pleased with the result. I used a different system—pulled it back and forth around the bunk pole. I admire the fur more and more, and I want so much to get it soft enough to use for my baby. . . .

"Since the baby came down to live in the lower part of my abdomen, I have been constipated, and I don't like it. I think it's the cause of my swollen ankles. I had absolutely nothing here to correct it, so I looked around to see what the wilderness might provide, and hit on the idea of eating seaweed. Certainly it can be called roughage . . . I went along the beach and gathered a mess . . . I picked it over well, washed it thoroughly, and ate quite a lot—ate it raw. It wasn't too awful, but I certainly don't like the stuff. It was very effective, almost more effective than I desired it to be. I was busy all day with the honey bucket . . . "

THE GARDEN OF EROS
by Dorothy Bryant
1979, 170 pages

from
Ata Books, publisher
The Crossing Press, distributor
P.O. Box 640
Trumansburg, NY 14886
$6.00 plus $1.00 postage

Dorothy Bryant is the author of the much-celebrated novel, *The Kin of Ata are Waiting for You* (Ata Books, 1976). In *The Garden of Eros* Bryant tells the remarkable story of a young blind woman who labors and gives birth alone, stranded by a rain storm, in a small house in the hills near Berkeley. Her first person account of the labor is mingled with the mother's reflections on her life: the accident which caused her blindness, her feelings for the baby's father, and her struggle to become strong and independent.

". . . Nothing real but the pain. It's the world. The pain is the universe. It takes, swallows everything. The pain wants all my strength, my sweat, my grunting and straining. It wants me to help it tear me open, tear out the life that is in me, then tear out my own life. And when I see this, when I know it . . . then it creeps away and hides. Quiet. Nothing. Nowhere. Where is it? How can it—it knows my mind will say, Impossible! Shocked, stunned, my mind, not able to believe it was here.

Then it will come back, it will fill the whole universe. Dizzy, my poor mind is spinning off, away, ready to leave me, leave . . . it almost did the last time, at the top of the last pain. And if it spins away, will it come back with the pain? Or will it . . .

"No! Coming back, starting again. Oh, Friend, help me. Help me get away. I can't do it. Grab legs. Slippery; I can't! Breathe. Can't! Help me! I'm a coward, can't do this. Push! No, I've got to get away. Escape! Someone. Friend, help me get away! Push! No, not me, not my mind. I'm running away, I'm escaping. Leave this body—pushing—pushing—no, I won't come back! Let me go. Going! Help! Coward. Giving up. A coward. Go where? I can't go. It's going. Pain going for now. But not me. I can't go anywhere. I can admit I'm a coward but I can't go. Not like the soldier. He can desert when the test comes. Turn and run. Disgrace, guilt, shame, but safety. Not me. I have no choice. Coward or not, I have to do it. No medals. No one caring about whether or not I was brave. Don't tell about it, not like the man in battle. No one wants to hear. Old wives' tales. Disgusting. Women talking about childbirth, disgusting. Men talking about killing, exciting. Giving life is messy. No glory, no dignity, no heroism. Just bare-assed grunting and pushing. No one wants to hear about it. . . . "

THREE WOMEN: A Poem for
Three Voices (in *Winter Trees*)
by Sylvia Plath
1972

from
Harper and Row
10 East 53rd Street
New York, NY 10022
$8.95

Sylvia Plath gave birth to her two
children at home in England. A description of the births is included in

Letters Home, edited by Sylvia
Plath's mother. *Three Women* was
produced as a radio play by the BBC.
Three women in a maternity ward
describe their experiences: the first
is giving birth to a wanted baby, the
second is suffering an unwanted miscarriage, and the third intends to
give up her unplanned baby for adoption. *Winter Trees* contains other
poems on birth and children.

SELECTED POEMS, 1942-1970
by Judith Wright
1971

from
Angus and Robertson
102 Glover
Cremorne , New South Wales
Australia

These two poems are from the
work of Australian poet, Judith

Wright, born in 1915. The poems
show a progression from the ambivalence of early pregnancy, in which
the fetus is described as "the eyeless
labourer" to the strong maternal feeling which comes after the birth and
recasts the imagery which describes
the pregnancy ("O node and focus
of the world").

First Voice:

Who is he, this blue, furious boy,
Shiny and strange, as if he had hurtled from a star?
He is looking so angrily!
He flew into the room, a shriek at his heel.
The blue color pales. He is human after all.
A red lotus opens in its bowl of blood;
They are stitching me up with silk, as if I were a material.

What did my fingers do before they held him?
What did my heart do, with its love?
I have never seen a thing so clear.
His lids are like the lilac-flower
And soft as a moth, his breath.
I shall not let go.
There is no guile or warp in him. May he keep so.

Second Voice:

It is a world of snow now. I am not at home.
How white these sheets are. The faces have no features.
They are bald and impossible, like the faces of my children,
Those little sick ones that elude my arms.
Other children do not touch me; they are terrible.
They have too many colors, too much life. They are not quiet,
Quiet, like the little emptiness I carry.

I have had my chances. I have tried and tried.
I have stitched life into me like a rare organ,
And walked carefully, precariously, like something rare.
I have tried not to think too hard. I have tried to be natural.
I have tried to be blind in love, like other women.
Blind in my bed, with my dear blind sweet one,
Not looking, through the thick dark, for the face of another.

I did not look. But still the face was there.
The face of the unborn one that loved its perfections,
The face of the dead one that could only be perfect
In its easy peace, could only keep holy so...."

Third Voice:

I am a mountain now, among mountainy women.
The doctors move among us as if our bigness
Frightened the mind. They smile like fools.
They are to blame for what I am, and they know it.
They hug their flatness like a kind of health.
And what if they found themselves surprised, as I did?
They would go mad with it.

And what if two lives leaked between my thighs?
I have seen the white clean chamber with its instruments.
It is a place of shrieks. It is not happy.
'This is where you will come when you are ready.'
The night lights are flat red moons. They are dull with blood.
I am not ready for anything to happen.
I should have murdered this, that murders me."

WOMAN TO MAN

The eyeless labourer in the night,
the selfless, shapeless seed I hold,
builds for its resurrection day—
silent and swift and deep from sight
foresees the unimagined light.

This is no child with a child's face;
this has no name to name it by;
yet you and I have known it well.
This is our hunter and our chase,
the third who lay in our embrace.

This is the strength that your arm knows,
the arc of flesh that is my breast,
the precise crystals of our eyes.
This is the blood's wild tree that grows
the intricate and folded rose.

This is the maker and the made;
this is the question and reply;
the blind head butting at the dark,
the blaze of light along the blade.
Oh hold me, for I am afraid.

WOMAN TO CHILD

You who were darkness warmed my flesh
where out of darkness rose the seed.
Then all a world I made in me;
all the world you hear and see
hung upon my dreaming blood.

There moved the multitudinous stars,
and coloured birds and fishes moved.
There swam the sliding continents.
All time lay rolled in me, and sense,
and love that knew not its beloved.

O node and focus of the world;
I hold you deep within that well
you shall escape and not escape—
that mirrors still your sleeping shape;
that nurtures still your crescent cell.

I wither and you break from me;
yet though you dance in living light
I am the earth, I am the root,
I am the stem that fed the fruit,
the link that joins you to the night.

Living in Family

The process of childbearing doesn't end when the baby is born, as all new parents quickly learn. After the stresses and excitement of being pregnant and giving birth, comes the reality of living as a family. There are still many decisions to be made and things to be learned. Hopefully, the consumer skills we gained in pregnancy will continue to serve us well as parents. This section of the *Catalog* will review resources for parents in postpartum adjustment, breastfeeding, baby and child care, parenting, and family planning.

The Postpartum Period

Caring for a newborn baby is one of the most demanding jobs in the world and many new parents are shocked to discover how much time and effort it can take. Particularly if your baby cries a lot and/ or doesn't sleep much, you will be living under conditions of near-constant stress and sleep-deprivation. If your childbirth experience was very strong and positive, the confidence you gained will help you in the postpartum period. But if your birth experience was not what you had hoped for, your reaction to it, combined with the normal stress of the postpartum period, may lead to feelings of depression. Remember that this difficult period *will pass* and that there are resources available to help you. Some of these are listed in this section.

MOTHER CARE: Helping Yourself through the Emotional and Physical Transitions of New Motherhood
by Lyn DelliQuandri and Kati Breckenridge
1978, 206 pages

from
St. Martin's Press
175 Fifth Avenue
New York, NY 10010
$7.95 hd.

Many new mothers are dismayed to learn just how demanding, tiring and "un-romantic" it can be to care for a new baby. This book acknowledges the stressful realities of new motherhood and helps mothers see the challenges as opportunities for change and growth. Written by a psychiatric social worker and a clinical psychologist (both are mothers), *Mother Care* describes relaxation techniques for coping with stress and gives advice on the "myth" of maternal instinct, nutrition and exercise for the postpartum period, and on changing relationships with the father. The authors stress that learning to care for ourselves as mothers is never selfish because an emotionally and physically healthy mother provides a foundation of health for her family.

"After the birth of your baby, life will never be the same. For the person called 'mother,' the physical and psychological changes are always ex-traordinary, sometimes disturbing, and rarely easy. . . .

"The early months of motherhood often bring an overwhelming sense of isolation and confinement. If you were working before the birth of your baby, you may feel the loss of companionship and stimulation, even if you didn't especially like your job. Your husband may be gone ten hours of every day. Your family may be far away. Your nonparent friends will have a very different schedule from yours. And of those friends who have babies, you may not want them to know you feel less than adequate in your new role. As a mother you are often the target for invidious remarks about 'housewives' and even discrimination by employers."

LIVING WITH YOUR NEW BABY:
A Postpartum Guide for Mothers and Fathers
by Elly Rakowitz and Gloria S. Rubin
1978, 272 pages

from
Franklin Watts
730 Fifth Avenue
New York, NY 10019
$8.95 hd.

Berkley
200 Madison Avenue
New York, NY 10016
$2.95 pap.

During pregnancy most of our planning and preparation is geared toward the crucial hours of labor and delivery. But what happens after the baby is born? Parents are often shocked by the amount of time and energy required by new baby care and mothers are often left to cope in relative isolation. *Living With Your New Baby* is a book to read before the baby is born. The authors feel that "Preparing for postpartum can help you and your mate face the realities of this period so that stress, frustration, guilt, worry, and resentment can be reduced." Elly Rakowitz is a childbirth educator in the Lamaze method. Gloria Rubin is one of her students who was not prepared for the emotional turmoil of her postpartum period. Together they provide advice on preparing for postpartum (avoiding isolation, finding a pediatrician, breast vs. bottle), changes to expect after the birth (physiological changes, medical exams and procedures for mother and baby, what newborns are like, fathers' feelings, postpartum blues, postpartum rap groups, the special concerns of post-cesarean parents), and how to cope with typical problems in the postpartum period (feeding, body image, sex, birth control, getting out, babysitters, advice, crying baby, the working mother, the single mother, and more). There is lots of good advice here to help parents cope with the nitty-gritty details of living with a new baby.

"Seriously consider breastfeeding your baby. Besides the many other advantages nursing has for mother and child, it is less work than bottle-feeding—no formula to prepare, no bottles to wash and/or sterilize and take along with you when you go out. At 2 A.M. you will not have to stagger to the kitchen half asleep to warm a bottle. Also, nursing forces you to sit down, put your feet up, and relax. If you bottlefeed, you might be tempted to prop a bottle—which is dangerous because the baby may gag and choke—and go about your chores. This defeats your efforts to relax. You can't prop a breast. As you nurse, a hormone is released that will give you a warm, relaxed feeling conducive to sleeping. Take advantage of this feeling and go to sleep when the baby dozes off at the end of the meal, night or day. . .

"If your baby cries a lot, your feelings of concern and sympathy can lessen as your stress tolerance level is reached. It is well known today that continual noise pollution from airplanes, electronically amplified rock music, loud motors, etc., is bad for our ears and entire organisms. It can affect our state of mind and our digestive processes. Crying is noise; incessant crying is constant noise and a constant source of stress to those present, including parents. If, in addition, there are other causes of stress occurring at the same time—a dog barking, the telephone ringing, the TV blaring, other children crying, yelling, whining, talking, demanding attention—the recipient is unquestionably under a lot of stress. Since stress tolerance levels vary, each individual reacts differently to a given situation. But a woman who has just undergone childbirth and whose hormones are out of balance, who is fatigued from the birth process and lack of sleep, who may be overwhelmed by being responsible for a new human being and possibly is shocked by the dramatic changes in her lifestyle, who is perhaps unsure of her abilities to cope, who is possibly being pressured by relatives to do things their way, whose bottom is sore and back is achey, and whose body image is not what she'd like, may not have a high level of resistance to the stress of noise. . . .

"Some mothers complain, 'How can I set aside a specific time for chores or getting out of the house when the baby has no specific time for crying? I may have to hold him all during my 'choretime' or 'reading time!'

"If you are the type who needs a specific hour-by-hour schedule, perhaps you can plan your choretime to coincide with your child's fussytime and take him or her with you from room to room as you work. Some chores can be done while the baby is happily strapped to your back or chest, papoose-style (ironing, mending, cooking, laundry, billpaying). Keeping the baby with you and close to you may be soothing in itself (as well as more interesting than lying unoccupied and alone in a crib) and may afford you the time to accomplish what you'd like."

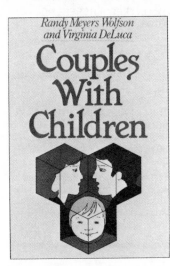

COUPLES WITH CHILDREN
by Randy Meyers Wolfson and
Virginia DeLuca
1981, 190 pages

Red Dembner Enterprises, publisher
W.W. Norton, distributor
500 Fifth Avenue
New York, NY 10110
$12.95 hd.

Randy Wolfson and Virginia DeLuca are both past officers of COPE (Coping with the Overall Pregnancy Experience, see index), an organization which offers counselling to expectant and new parents. When they began leading support groups for new parents they expected questions about the details of new baby care but soon found their clients were most interested in the impact of childrearing on couple relationships. *Couples with Children* discusses many of the issues which COPE parents found important, including pressures to be a "perfect" parent, coping with the first few months, changes in social life, sex after childbirth, working outside the home, sharing child and house care responsibilities, and working for change in childrearing patterns. Many personal anecdotes from parents enhance the authors' discussions. The emphasis is on helping parents integrate children into a couple relationship in a time when men's and women's roles and expectations are changing.

"Many men feel guilty for not spending more time with their children, and when they try to remedy that, are left feeling anxious about their standing at work. There is not much support given a man caught in this conflict. If he makes it known that his family needs come first, his boss questions his commitment to the job. If he makes it known that his work comes first, his wife questions his commitment to the family. It's understandable how many men see themselves in a no-win situation; they either risk failure in terms of their job, or risk failure in terms of their marriage."

"All of us are constantly encouraged to try and keep up the image of eternal youth, and after having children we feel even more vulnerable to this pressure. We're disappointed and even devastated when no amount of dieting, running, or swimming brings back pre-pregnant bodies. We may look great and feel great; but our bodies have changed. A woman who feels she can only be sexually attractive when her stretch marks disappear or her breasts miraculously uplift, will have a hard time enjoying, or wanting to make love. . . .

"In the effort to balance each other's attitude toward limits and boundaries, couples often exaggerate their natural tendencies. One parent becomes locked into the role of the 'heavy,' while the other becomes the 'nice guy.' When you think your partner is too strict, you may overlook as much as you can to balance the situation. Then the parent who feels the need for tighter controls, may increase them to offset what they perceive as too much benign neglect. And you're off in a vicious cycle.

'Cynthia is just too hard on the kids,' said Jon. 'She's always telling them—don't do this, play outside, and so on. It makes me furious sometimes, when she yells at them to keep the noise down, when all they're doing is playing normally.'

"What may be background noise to one parent, may be an intolerable assault on the ears of the other. It's important to discuss what behavior is really bothering us and to explain why. Often we label each other as too permissive or too strict without ever discussing the issue at hand. . . .

"The pressure on families to be havens, where adults and children are nurtured, totally removed from work, friends, education, and other social commitments, is unrealistic and often results in friction between family members. When our institutions, schools, medical services, social services, work places and media images ignore or inadequately reflect the needs of parents and children we end up feeling terribly alone in our struggles. What parents today are trying to do is integrate family life into the center of the community, and make families a place where nurturance and warmth can mesh with the other needs, desires, and commitments that make up our lives."

HI MOM! HI DAD!: 101 Cartoons
for New Parents
by Lynn Johnston
1981, 107 pages, Illus.

from
Meadowbrook Press
18318 Minnetonka Blvd.
Deephaven, MN 55391
$3.75 postpaid

These cartoons are funny! They take us from birth to the baby's first birthday, illuminating all the silly situations in between. Lynn Johnston is a mother of two and draws the "For Better or Worse" comic strip which appears in many newspapers. She helps us laugh at our struggles as parents and know that we're not alone.

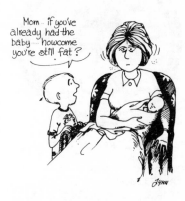

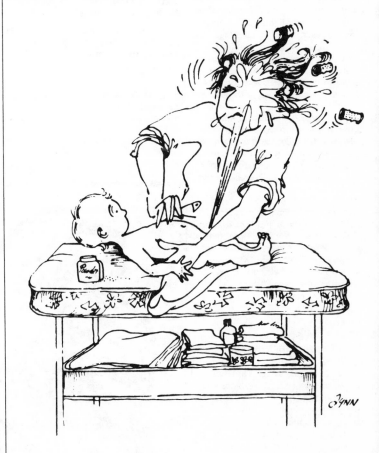

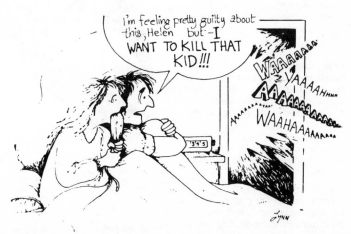

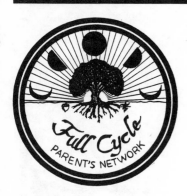

FULL CYCLE PARENTS NETWORK
P.O. Box 685
Capitola, CA 95010
408/475-6866

"Full Cycle Parent's Network is a group organized to help families after the birth of their babies with household chores, marketing, cooking nutritious meals, nurturing the family as a whole. We also offer information regarding the years of childrearing, referrals to professionals, groups, classes, friends, networking with people in similar situations and emotional support. We provide instruction to ladies interested in working for us to help sensitize them to go into a newly birthed home. In addition we provide workshops focusing on postpartum and parenting skills, sponsor seminars emphasizing nurturing at home and abroad and compile information and make it available to mothers and their families through our newsletter and pamphlets. We have been in existence over four years and have helped over 400 families with the transitions a new baby brings. We currently have a network of 38 groups in 21 states which Full Cycle has helped begin."
—Laura Peduto, founder and director

This sounds like a great idea and a much needed service. The usual home health care services are more geared to the needs of the elderly and the handicapped and nurse's aides are not really necessary for a mother who simply needs more time to be with her baby. Groups like Full Cycle can provide parents with really useful homemaking services, performed by people who are sensitive to their needs as a postpartum family. Hopefully Full Cycle will serve as a model for similar groups around the country. Send a SASE for a copy of Full Cycle's descriptive brochure. Services include Postpartum Care ($4. an hour), Standard housecleaning ($5.50 an hour), and Special cleaning ($8.00). Scholarships are available.

"Here is an example of a mother's helper 3 hour stay for a newly postpartum family.

½ hour arrival and emotional support for mom and dad or discussing things that are happening right at the moment (breastfeeding, sleep patterns

or needs for additional services from Full Cycle)

½ hour childcare while mother bathes

1 hour house tidying

½ hour nurturing mom while nursing by answering phones, bringing a snack and drink to mom, then straightening mother's bed area giving her and the baby a nice place to retreat for a nap

½ hour mother and baby nap while mother's helper cleans kitchen and/or prepares lunch to be eaten later or perhaps prepares dinner to be enjoyed by the whole family that evening."

FULL CYCLE
by Sally Nesmith
1981, 36 pages, Illus.
$3.00 plus .50 postage

A collection of poetry and pictures "celebrating life's montage." Proceeds go to further the work of Full Cycle.

SEASONS: A POSTPARTUM PRESS
Quarterly Newsletter
$3.00 a year

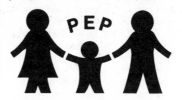

POSTPARTUM EDUCATION FOR PARENTS (PEP)
c/o Jane Honikman
927 N. Kellogg Avenue
Santa Barbara, CA 93111

PEP is a California group which provides local services for postpartum support: a "warm line," parent discussion groups, baby basics classes, presentations for childbirth preparation classes, etc. PEP has also developed publications to help people around the country establish a similar service in their own community.

A GUIDE FOR ESTABLISHING A PARENT SUPPORT PROGRAM IN YOUR COMMUNITY
116 pages
$10.00

Describes how PEP began and provides a detailed explanation of PEP's services, volunteers, structure, finances, and community relations.

VOLUNTEER'S REFERENCE GUIDE
70 pages
$6.00

Provides background information to help volunteers deal with the common concerns of new parents.

A LEADER'S GUIDE FOR TRAINING VOLUNTEERS IN PARENT SUPPORT SERVICES
139 pages
$10.00

Describes PEP's volunteer training program in depth. Includes outlines, a reading unit, handouts, and suggestions for role playing.

MORE RESOURCES FOR THE POSTPARTUM PERIOD

C.O.P.E.
(Coping with the Overall Pregnancy/Parenting Experience)
37 Clarendon Street
Boston, MA 02116
617/357-5588

COPE provides individual counseling and support groups for parents in Massachusetts and can provide information to those who wish to set up similar services in their own area. See index for a complete listing.

THE MOTHERS' CENTER
c/o United Methodist Church
Old Country Road and Nelson Ave.
Hicksville, New York 11801
516/822-4539

The Mothers' Center provides support groups led by trained peer-support mothers. The Center is the first of its kind in the nation and can provide information on setting up a Mother's Center and a list of other Mother's Centers currently in operation. See index for complete listing.

THE PEOPLE PLACE
1465 Massachusetts Avenue
Arlington, MA 02174
617/643-8630

The People Place provides postpartum counseling for individuals and groups. (See index for complete listing.)

". . . we work with the birth process to heal painful birth experiences. Some of these might be considered 'normal' medical deliveries, while others are complicated by Cesarean or breech delivery."
—Claudia S. Panuthos, director

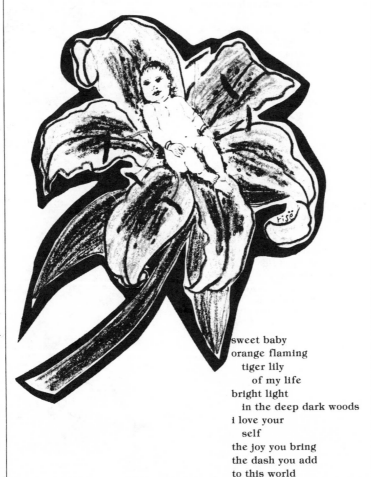

sweet baby
orange flaming
  tiger lily
    of my life
bright light
  in the deep dark woods
i love your
    self
the joy you bring
the dash you add
to this world

—from *Full Cycle* by Sally Nesmith

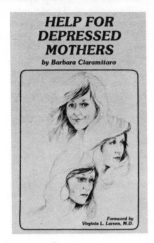

HELP FOR DEPRESSED MOTHERS
by Barbara Ciaramitaro
1982, 153 pages

from
The Chas. Franklin Press
18409 90th Avenue West
Edmonds, WA 98020
$7.95

This book is for women who are seriously depressed after the birth of a baby, written by a woman who had this experience and brought herself back to recovery. Barbara Ciaramitaro begins with a "self-help workbook for depressed mothers" which describes specific strategies for coping with depression, including getting enough rest, eating well, exercising, consulting professionals, and meeting needs for love. Part II presents "case histories": letters from "formerly-depressed" mothers which illustrate the range of circumstances and ways that women have helped themselves. Part III provides information on what is currently known about the causes of postpartum depression, through medical and psychological literature. Ciaramitaro's approach is very woman-centered and caring—she doesn't blame women or point her finger at their deep psychological "problems." She recognizes the many social and environmental factors which contribute to postpartum depression and offers useful tools for recovering.

"Being depressed is like stepping unexpectedly into quicksand. You feel yourself being sucked down, quickly and helplessly. Your impulse is to panic and struggle against the grip of these gloomy feelings. But fearing the way you feel and trying to fight off your depression will only weaken you all the more.

"Quicksand is mostly water. The way to keep it from sucking you under is to lay out flat on your back on its surface as though you were floating in a pool. In the same way, to keep on top of your depression, you must learn to relax in the face of it—to accept it as normal under the circumstances, to realize that you can and will get better as your body recovers its strength.

"Being depressed is like stepping unexpectedly into quicksand. You feel yourself being sucked down quickly and helplessly. Your impulse is to panic and struggle against the grip of these gloomy feelings. . . . The way to keep it from sucking you under is to lay out flat on your back on its surface as though you were floating in a pool."

"Every depressed mother feels a need for the kind of acceptance, love and reassurance that we call mothering. If your mother is able to give you this love, by all means tell her of your need for her special attention. However, you can also learn to mother yourself, even if no one else has ever mothered you much.

"The first thing to remember is that love is a physical thing—it must be felt. Here are some ways you can make yourself feel loved:
a. allow yourself to express your angry and sad feelings as well as your happy ones,
b. wrap your arms or a warm blanket around yourself and ask others to hold you,
c. care for your body's needs,
d. get help with jobs that are too difficult to do alone,
e. avoid people who make you feel badly,
f. praise your own accomplishments to yourself and take other's compliments deep into yourself, and
g. find direct ways to do what you want to do and to have what you want.

"The more love you give yourself, the more love you will have to give to your baby."

"You can give love to your baby by allowing him or her to express anger and grief as well as pleasure, by holding him or her often in a relaxed way, by caring for his or her physical needs, by helping him or her do the things he or she wants to do, by allowing him or her to avoid people who upset him or her, and by praising his or her accomplishments.

"The more love you give yourself, the more love you will have to give to your baby. . . .

"While no woman can consider herself totally immune to postpartum depression, it is true that some women run a higher risk than others. Much more research is needed before we will be able to predict with certainty which women will suffer a postpartum depression. However, doctors and researchers have noted a number of factors which indicate a higher than normal risk.

HIGH RISK FACTORS

1. a postpartum depression after a previous birth
2. a previous manic-depressive or schizophrenic episode
3. parents or siblings who have had manic, depressive or schizophrenic episode
4. an alcoholic or aggressively anti-social father
5. the loss of a parent through death or divorce during childhood
6. an unhappy childhood due to a cold or abusive parent
7. a neurotic personality structure
8. an unwanted pregnancy
9. a long or difficult labor or complicated birth
10. having a premature, ill or defective baby

A woman who is aware of having more than one of these high risk factors in her background should certainly consider the possibility of not having a child (or more children). Should she get pregnant unexpectedly she should certainly consider an abortion. If she decides to have a child she should be particularly careful to receive adequate nutrition and rest during the pregnancy, the best medical care, and household help and emotional support during the first year after giving birth."

POSTPARTUM DEPRESSION
edited by Rosemary Cogan
1980, 8 pages

from
ICEA Bookcenter
P.O. Box 20048
Minneapolis, MN 55420
$1.00 plus 60 cents postage

This very useful issue of *ICEA Review* (August, 1980) provides an introduction to the characteristics of postpartum "blues," postpartum depression, and postpartum psychosis, pointing out that social and environmental factors appear to be more important than physiology in affecting our emotions after childbirth. Included are abstracts of 12 journal articles and an axcellent commentary by Niles Newton, author of *Maternal Emotions.*

"Topics included in the Prenatal Instruction of Gordon and Gordon

1. The responsibilities of being a mother (and not a martyr) are learned, hence get help and advice.
2. Make friends of other couples who are experienced with young children.
3. Don't overload yourself with extra, less important tasks.
4. Don't move soon after the baby arrives.
5. Don't be too concerned with appearances when other things are more important.
6. Get plenty of rest and sleep.
7. Don't be a nurse to elderly relatives at this period.
8. Confer and consult with husband, family, and experienced friends and discuss your plans and worries.
9. Don't give up your outside interests, but cut down the responsibilities and rearrange your schedules.
10. Arrange for babysitters in advance.
11. Learn to drive a car.

Changes Made by Women Who Did Well During the Postpartum Period

1. *They made more friends of couples with young children.*
2. They gave less emphasis to tidiness in the home.
3. They obtained more experienced help with the baby.
4. The husband became more available in the home, and reduced his outside activities.
5. The couple continued to socialize outside the home, but *less* frequently.
6. The wife continued with her outside interests, but *limited* her responsibilities."

"Social factors in prevention of postpartum emotional problems. Gordon, RE and Gordon, KK. *Obstet Gynecol* 15, 433-438, 1960."

"Perhaps the very best thing a mother can do is to feel 'low' enough so that she will rest and stay near her baby."

". . . we should not pathologize ordinary blues that occur transiently in some women after birth, which may be triggered both by hormonal changes and environmental stresses.

"We could even look at mild changes leading to inactivity as having biological value. Perhaps the very best thing a mother can do is to feel 'low' enough so that she will rest and stay near her baby. Many other mammals have periods of quietly staying very close to their infants immediately after birth. When a mother rat does this we simply describe her behavior as 'normal.' When a human mother recedes to similar inactivity, we are tempted to rate her as slightly depressed."
By Niles Newton, Ph.D.

SEX AFTER THE BABY COMES
by Sheila Kitzinger
1980, 4 pages

from
the pennypress
1100 23rd Avenue East
Seattle, WA 98112
50 cents single copies
$20.00 per 100

Sheila Kitzinger discusses several of the factors which can affect sex after childbirth including "concepts of pollution" (cultural taboos), tiredness, depression, pain (from episiotomy stitches, etc.), breastfeeding, fear of getting pregnant, and interruptions. She also discusses in detail the importance of building strength in the pelvic floor muscles.

"Perhaps the important thing to realize is that there is a wide range of feelings and that goal-oriented sex, feeling under pressure to have an orgasm because you cannot be a 'complete woman' (or he isn't a 'complete man') unless you have a climax every time, destroys any potential for spontaneous pleasure. If you are finding that intercourse is not very exciting and it is your first baby, it is understandable that you may get anxious that things have changed forever and that you will never be able to enjoy sex in the same way again. But all the evidence goes to show that women who have reduced libido, less intercourse and fewer orgasms while breastfeeding, find their sex drive returns in full force when

the baby is weaned. If you enjoyed sex before, you will enjoy it again, in your, and the baby's own good time. . . .

"If you enjoyed sex before, you will enjoy it again, in your, and the baby's own good time."

"Get ready for going to bed and create the atmosphere you like well before the late feed so that you have ample time to spend with the baby first. Then put the baby in another room close by, or behind a screen, where you cannot hear every little sniffle and grunt. Turn on the radio or TV low, or leave a loudly ticking clock next to the baby. Babies sleep better with a regular background of repetitive sound than in total silence. If you put the record player or tape recorder outside your door, both you and the baby hear it, and you may find that a background of sound allows you to draw into yourself and focus on feelings in a way you cannot otherwise. Even the whirr of a fan heater can help you concentrate on your body instead of being distracted by the baby's movements, breathing and little noises."

POSTPARTUM INFORMATION
by Rosemary Romberg Wiener
1981, 3 pages

from
Rosemary Romberg Wiener
6294 Mission Road
Everson, WA 98247
15 cents plus SASE

This fact sheet provides advice on dealing with the postpartum flow of lochia, on getting enough rest, postpartum "blues," regaining your figure, exercise, and breastfeeding.

"'Lochia' refers to the normal vaginal bleeding that occurs during the first few weeks after the birth of a baby. As a rule most women bleed fresh red blood for about 1-2 weeks following delivery. This gradually tapers off and becomes whitish or brownish for about 1-2 more weeks. The type and amount of bleeding varies considerably from woman to woman, and some women bleed very little following birth. The amount and length of lochia can depend on many things. Generally women tend to have less postpartum bleeding if they are breastfeeding. This is because the suckling of the infant stimulates the uterus to contract. The opportunity to nurse the baby shortly after birth and often during the first couple of days also contributes to less postpartum bleeding. Sometimes women who have been heavily medicated during labor and birth tend to bleed more. Also, problems with 'third stage' (expul-

sion of the placenta), for example, if the placenta did not come out in one piece, often results in heavier bleeding. Finally, if the mother does a lot of 'running around,' doing too much physical exertion within the first few weeks after birth, this can cause an increase in bleeding. This is one of the reasons that it is very important to relax and not do too much during the postpartum period.

Shopping List for the Post Partum Period: . . .

1. Two boxes of 40 each, 'super-size' sanitary napkins. You may not need this many, but this is a good amount to have on hand. (Save your husband an embarrassing trip to the store!) Some stores sell 'obstetrical' pads which are larger and thicker than ordinary pads and are regularly used in hospital maternity departments. You may wish to purchase this kind also, especially if you will be giving birth at home, in a birth center, or leaving the hospital shortly after birth. If you will be staying in the hospital for a few days following birth, they will provide them while you are there and you will probably not need that kind once you get home. You may wish to purchase the type of pads that attach to your underpants with an adhesive strip. These eliminate the need for a belt. This type is especially helpful if you have a Caesarian birth, as the belt tends to irritate the incision."

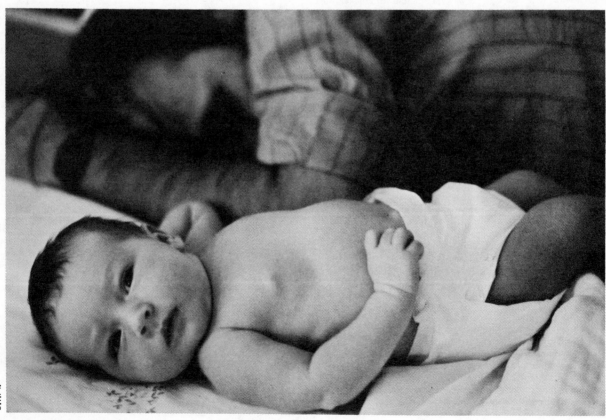
J.I.A.

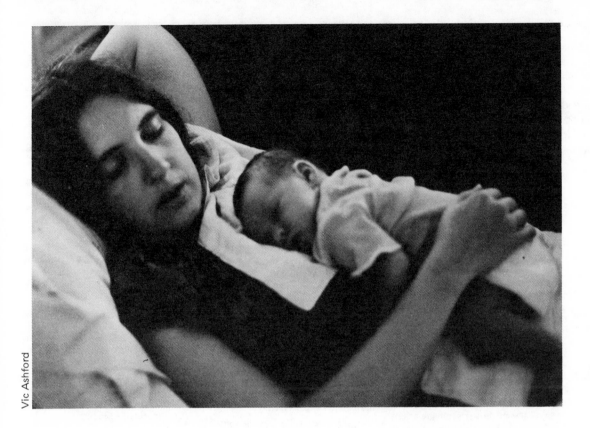

Vic Ashford

roller coaster

in the short weeks after birth
woman's roller coaster of emotions
and reverb perceptions
and deep flowing hormones
go from a faraway place
it took nine months
and a slow motion implosion of body birth
to come to
and which it will take a slight six weeks
in some corners of her borders
to return to
while the rest of her will continue to change
faraway
as she follows the nurseling at her breast

we must take care of her
she is wide open and spinning away
she is the caretaker of an angel

by Karen Hope Ehrlich

from *Birth Song,* reviewed on page 104

© 1979 Karen Hope Ehrlich. Reprinted by permission.

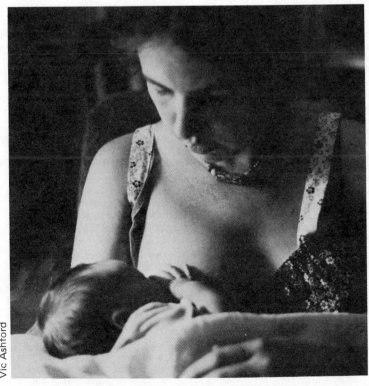

Vic Ashford

Breastfeeding

Breastfeeding *is* best, both physically and emotionally, for mother and baby. Breast milk is uniquely suited to the nutritional needs of the baby and provides immunologic protection. Because of the many special properties of breast milk, bottle-feeding with formula or cow's milk is not a totally adequate substitute. In addition to its physical benefits, nursing develops love and closeness between mother and baby and teaches us, from the earliest moments of life, that people and not things are the source of nurturance and satisfaction. Please consider breastfeeding your baby, for as long or as short a time as you are able. Encourage your friends and acquaintances to breastfeed, support breastfeeding women in your community, and work to make breastfeeding easier for women who work outside the home.

LA LECHE LEAGUE
INTERNATIONAL
9616 Minneapolis Avenue
Franklin Park, IL 60131
312/455-7730

La Leche League, an organization composed entirely of volunteers, has done more to promote the return to breastfeeding in our country than any other single force. The League stands not only as a symbol of breastfeeding and the special nurturing of babies it involves, but also as a model of success for consumer health organizations. The League has provided sound, scientific information and warm, personal support for breastfeeding in a time when the medical profession has, for the most part, provided neither.

La Leche League was founded in 1956 in Franklin Park, Illinois, by a group of seven mothers, all of whom still serve on the League's board of directors. The "founding mothers" all had experienced difficulties in learning to breastfeed their children and felt the need for an organization which could provide "mother-to-mother" encouragement and advice on breastfeeding to women in their own communities. After 25 years, there are now about 14,000 League leaders around the world who conduct the regular monthly series of four meetings in their homes. Pregnant women and new mothers with their babies come to learn about the benefits and techniques of breastfeeding and to offer advice and support to each other. Group leaders share their special experience and also provide telephone counseling, all on a voluteer basis. The League's main office now has a staff of over 50 to answer the many thousands of letters and telephone calls received each year. A Professional Advisory Board of over 40 medical professionals provides the League with expert information and review of all League publications. The founding mothers and all the League leaders and members who came after have succeeded admirably in their goal—to help women relearn the "womanly art" of breastfeeding and to convince everyone that breastfeeding is best for mother, baby, and the family.

What the La Leche League Believes. . .

"1. Mothering through breastfeeding is the most natural and effective way

LA LECHE LEAGUE

of understanding and satisfying the needs of the baby.
2. Mother and baby need to be together early and often to establish a satisfying relationship and an adequate milk supply.
3. In the early years the baby has an intense need to be with his mother which is as basic as his need for food.
4. Breast milk is the superior infant food.
5. For the healthy, full-term baby breast milk is the only food necessary until baby shows signs of needing solids, about the middle of the first year after birth.
6. Ideally the breastfeeding relationship will continue until the baby outgrows the need.
7. Alert and active participation by the mother in childbirth is a help in getting breastfeeding off to a good start.
8. The father's role in the breastfeeding relationship is one of provider, protector, helpmate, and companion to the mother; by thus supporting her he enables her to mother the baby more completely.
9. Good nutrition means eating a well-balanced and varied diet of foods in as close to their natural state as possible.
10. Ideally, discipline is based on loving guidance."

La Leche League Meetings

All League meeings are held "in the relaxed atmosphere of a member's home." The series of four monthly meetings is given regularly throughout the year by local League leaders and includes the following:

1. Advantages of Breastfeeding to Mother and Baby.
2. The Art of Breastfeeding and Overcoming Difficulties.
3. Baby Arrives; The Family and the Breastfed Baby.
4. Nutrition and Weaning.

To find a group in your area, the League suggests that you consult the calendar section of your local newspaper, the white pages of your phone book (under La Leche League), or ask among your friends, neighbors and local childbirth educators, doc-

tors, and hospital maternity wards. If you have difficulty, contact LLL directly for the name of the League leader nearest you. There is no charge for League meetings or services, but mothers are encouraged to become League members.

Membership

Regular (includes one year of *La Leche League News*) $12
Supporting (includes one year of *La Leche League News* and calendar) $25

La Leche League News

La Leche League News is a 20-page bimonthly newsletter which is included in all categories of League membership. Issues include news of League conferences and activities and letters from mothers sharing their breastfeeding experiences. A four-page state insert is included for each of the fifty states, compiled by each state coordinator, to provide more local news and contacts.

Publications

The League's publication service produces and/or sells almost 150 different flyers, brochures, books and other materials on breastfeeding, childbirth, child care and nutrition for parents and professionals, along with gift items, packets, and visual aids. A selection of League-produced publications is listed below. These are available through local League leaders or by mail-order. Write for a complete catalog.

Breastfeeding and Working?—75 cents
Twins—30 cents
Breastfeeding After a Cesarean Birth—25 cents
Losing Your Milk?—15 cents
Does Your Baby Need a Pacifier?—15 cents
Thoughts About Weaning—15 cents
Mother-Baby Togetherness—15 cents
The Biological Specificity of Milk—30 cents
Environmental Contaminants in Mother's Milk—15 cents
Successful Lactation and Women's Sexuality—15 cents

Books

Gerald the Third $3.95
by Faye Early Young
Tale of a family welcoming a new baby (through the eyes of a 6-year-old). 32 pages.

Especially for You $11.95
by Kaye Lowman and Kay Kaszonyi
A "baby record book"—complete with references to breastfeeding and weaning the baby. 88 pages.

The LL Love Story $5.95
by Kaye Lowman
The story of La Leche League with photos and anecdotes from the early days to present. 92 pages.

Mother's in the Kitchen $4.95
by Roberta Johnson
Tasty and easy recipes submitted by LLL mothers. 228 pages.

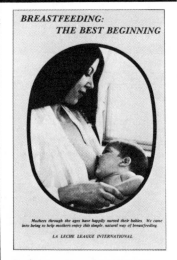

BREASTFEEDING:
THE BEST BEGINNING

Mothers through the ages have happily nursed their babies. We came into being to help mothers enjoy this simple, natural way of breastfeeding.

LA LECHE LEAGUE INTERNATIONAL

BREASTFEEDING: THE BEST BEGINNING
1981, 12 pages, Illus.
free, in single copies or in bulk

This brochure is illustrated with lovely photographs of nursing "couples" and families and provides an introduction to breastfeeding, including the many advantages of nursing, basic "how-to" tips, common concerns, a description of the League and its work, and an order form for selected League publications and other products. This brochure is available in bulk and is perfect for use in clinics, doctor's offices, hospitals, childbirth classes, and parents' information packets.

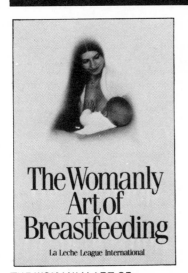

The Womanly Art of Breastfeeding

La Leche League International

THE WOMANLY ART OF
BREASTFEEDING
by La Leche League, Int'l
1981, 368 pages, Illus.
$12.95 hd
(order from La Leche League,
opposite page)

The 1963 edition of this classic book on breastfeeding was a bestseller for 18 years, with over one million copies in print. The new, third edition has been completely revised and updated and is based not only on the seven authors' experiences but also on the accumulated wisdom of 25 years' worth of League work. The new edition is twice as long as the previous one and includes, for the first time, many lovely photographs.

The basic components of the LLL approach to breastfeeding are still the same and are presented here along with much detailed advice on the day-to-day experience of breastfeeding and mothering and with personal comments from many parents. These basics include: the advantages of breastfeeding, planning for your baby (including becoming a parent, planning the birth, preparing your nipples, etc.), the first days with your new baby (coping with hospital routines, when the milk comes in), at home with your baby (day-to-day feeding concerns, care of the nursing mother, sex and breastfeeding), the "manly art of fathering," advice on weaning, nutritional know-how, and breastfeeding in special circumstances (including after cesarean, when the baby is premature, twins, birth defects, sore nipples, illness, handicapped mothers). These chapters are the real "how-to" *gold* which can help mothers cope with virtually any nursing difficulty.

Several of the LLL founding mothers gave birth at home and while the League does not officially promote home birth, it is clear that the opportunities for early suckling and bonding which home birth provides are important in establishing a successful nursing relationship. The new edition provides an expanded section on planning your baby's birth, explaining how natural childbirth, family-centered care, birth centers, and home birth can contribute to breastfeeding and a strong parent-child tie.

New to this edition is a chapter for working mothers. While recognizing the change in women's working patterns over the years, the League makes a strong argument for the advantages of staying at home with your baby for a while. The authors discuss other ways in which financial needs might be met and suggest part-time or at-home work as compromises. But they do provide a special section on how to really manage breastfeeding when the mother is working full-time outside the home.

Also new to this edition is a section on the new scientific evidence on the advantages of breastfeeding and breast milk and an overview of world trends in breastfeeding.

"The sooner you put your baby to the breast, the better. Most babies are ready and even eager to nurse at some time within the first hour after birth. The sucking reflex of a full-term healthy newborn is usually at a peak about twenty to thirty minutes after he is born, provided he is not drowsy from drugs or anesthesia used during labor and delivery. If this prime time to begin nursing is missed, the baby's sucking reflex may be less acute for about a day and a half.

"Early nursing is mutually beneficial to mother and baby. Aside from getting breastfeeding off to a good start, your newborn's immediate nursing hastens the delivery of the placenta. You will have less blood loss than you would have without this help from your little friend. For the baby, being so close to his mother is comforting, and the first milk, the colostrum, is priceless as a source of protective immunities against disease. . . .

"Hospitals want what is best for the patients, but often their size and bureaucracy come between their good intentions and the kind of care you need. Be prepared to speak up for what you want. Often, getting what you want is simply a matter of dogged persistence. One mother said that whenever she was told 'I'm sorry, we can't do that' in answer to a request, she would say that she did not want anyone to go against hospital policy, but that she would like to talk to someone who had the authority to alter the policy. Carrying her appeal up the line did at times result in a happy resolution of the problem."

NURSING YOUR BABY
by Karen Pryor
1973, 289 pages, Illus.

from
Pocket Books
1230 Avenue of the Americas
New York, NY 10020
$2.75 pap.

Karen Pryor's book is an excellent guide to breastfeeding, describing the social, emotional, and physical components of nursing along with the "how-to" techniques. Pryor defines the mother and baby as a "nursing couple" and explains the wonderfully complex bond which joins them both emotionally and physiologically. She gives particular attention to pointing out the many social factors which can discourage women from breastfeeding (uncooperative doctors, hospital routines, social prejudice) and gives advice on overcoming them. Her discussion of cultural versus biological femininity and of "milk emotionalism" are especially enlightening.

The "how-to" section is very good, defining the first six weeks as "the learning period" and the time after two months as "the reward period." A selection of historical illustrations are included, which show how the "classic nursing pose" has not changed since the days of early Egypt.

"When the baby nurses, he does not actually remove milk by suction. Such suction as he exerts is merely sufficient to keep the nipple in place in the back of his mouth. Then with tongue and jaws he compresses the areola and the large milk sinuses beneath, and presses the milk that is in the sinuses into the mouth. In this way he milks the breast; and this is the way all mammals (except of course, the platypus) get their milk. When the baby starts to nurse, he usually empties the milk sinuses fairly quickly. Meanwhile, the tactile sensations received by the mother from the highly sensitive nipple trigger the release of the hormone that causes the basket cells to contract. The milk lets down. The sinuses refill immediately, as fast as the baby can empty them. He need hardly make the effort to milk the breast; the milk comes pouring into his throat of its own accord. Even a very tiny or weak baby can thus get plenty of milk, almost effortlessly. In fact a newborn baby can be quite overcome by the sudden abundance from a strong let-down reflex. He may choke, gasp, sputter, get milk up his nose, and have to let go and catch his breath while the milk goes to waste, spraying all over the bedclothes and his face. Fortunately, most babies are excited rather than upset by this misadventure, and come back to the breast with avid greed. . . .

"The let-down reflex is a simple physical response to a physical stimulus. It is supposed to work like clockwork. Why then is failure of the let-down reflex the basic cause of almost every breastfeeding failure? Because this reflex is greatly affected by the mother's emotions. Any disturbance, particularly in the early days of lactation, can cause inhibition of the let-down reflex. Such stress as embarrassment, irritation, or anxiety actually prevent the pituitary from secreting oxytocin. Thus the woman who dislikes breastfeeding or is very much afraid she will fail may actually give less milk than the mother who is interested and hopeful of success. A strong disturbance, such as real anger or fear, sends adrenalin through the system, which causes the small blood vessels to contract, so that oxytocin, even if released, does not reach the basket cells which make the milk let down. . . .

"Margaret Mead has stated that undue admiration for milk is one of the most harmful ideas that we Westerners give to other societies, not only because it encourages women in primitive environments to abandon breastfeeding in favor of artificial feeding, but because it suggests that the only purpose of breastfeeding is the giving of milk. The non-Western mother gives the breast without reservation. She doesn't worry about when the baby ate last, or whether the breast seems full or empty. She isn't nursing to get milk into the child, anyway; she's nursing to keep him comfortable and happy. If he cries, she offers the breast; if he gets hiccups, or bumps his head, or feels shy of a stranger, she offers the breast. In the process, the baby gets all the milk he needs, but the milk is incidental.

"However, when the giving of milk becomes paramount, then the mother feels free to withhold the breast if she supposes that the baby has had enough, or is not hungry. From the baby's point of view, the comfort of the breast is lost. It becomes the mother, not the baby, who makes the decision as to whether the baby needs the breast, and when he gets it. This is a profound change from the normal pattern of most cultures; it makes a visible difference in the personality development of the babies, and hence eventually in the culture itself."

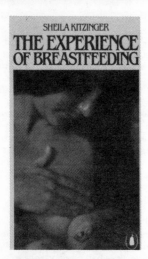

THE EXPERIENCE OF BREAST-FEEDING
by Sheila Kitzinger
1980, 255 pages

from
Penguin Books
625 Madison Avenue
New York, NY 10022
$3.50 pap.

In this book Sheila Kitzinger extends her "psychosexual" approach to pregnancy and childbirth (see pages 1 and 41) into breastfeeding and directs her discussion as much to men as to women. "In my own experience," she says, "I have found that over and over again a man's support for his wife during the time she is starting to feed their baby, his confidence in her and the basic knowledge he has of how lactation works, are decisive factors in her ability to breastfeed happily." Kitzinger begins by explaining the ways in which human mother's milk is uniquely suited to the needs of human babies. She considers the arguments against breastfeeding (my breasts are too small, my husband doesn't like it, I'll lose my figure, etc.) and tries to dispel myths that can get in the way. She describes in detail the importance of close contact in the early minutes after birth, the early days of nursing, dealing with the hospital environment, individual differences among babies and nursing difficulties. Also included are coping with the transition to parenthood, the effects of drugs and pollution on breast milk, nutrition, family communication and relationships, sexuality in breastfeeding, weaning, and social attitudes about breastfeeding. These subjects are discussed in many other books, but somehow Kitzinger brings a special warmth and *enlarging* social perspective to every topic she considers. She strives always to present breastfeeding as a dynamic, ever-changing process which exists within a framework of unique personal relationships and social influences. In fact, this book will be just as interesting to students of human behavior and

social anthropology as it will be to new parents.

"Birth is an intense and dramatic psychosexual experience, quite as much or even more so than lovemaking and intercourse. In the same way breastfeeding is psychosexual too, involving as it does a giving of the woman's body, release to let the milk flow, and relations between bodies, her own and the baby's. This is not to say that the feelings a woman has when giving the baby the breast are identical to or even similar to those she has when making love. They may be markedly different and are often quite distinct in her mind. Some women experience orgasms when breastfeeding. Probably most women do not. But orgasm is not the only pleasurable experience in sexuality. We know that goal-oriented sex which looks to orgasmic release as the only 'successful' kind of climax tends to be self-defeating and often in the end strangely unsatisfying. Sex is much more than that and is composed of far more varied and subtle themes. The sense of the completeness of her own body, her satisfaction in giving, her closeness to and union with the baby as she breastfeeds, are some of these other aspects of sex, which are no less to be valued because they do not lead to orgasm. . .

"There is one powerful argument for bottle feeding: that the mother herself prefers to do it that way. No other reasons for bottle feeding approach anywhere near the strength of such a statement and if a mother wishes to bottle feed it is her right to do so. She should be able to do this without being made to feel guilty. The choice is hers. Her breasts belong to her. . . .

"A babymoon is a holiday spent by the new parents with their baby which takes place for the most part in the bedroom. They get in food and drink in advance and make forays to the kitchen, but spend most of the time in bed with their baby. They do not receive visitors, and make it known beforehand that they will be otherwise occupied. They might even put up a notice on the door 'parents resting.' The only other person who is allowed in is the midwife who pays her daily visit and, if they are fortunate, a cleaning lady or a friend or relative willing to take on this role who washes the dishes and the nappies, but keeps out of their way. Couples in our society need babymoons even more, perhaps, than they need honeymoons. They need a space in their lives when they come to terms with the momentous event which has occurred and can begin to understand their baby's signals. Since the man will have to take time off work the babymoon may only last a few days, but even if it is that brief it can be an important contribution to the psychological well-being of the new family."

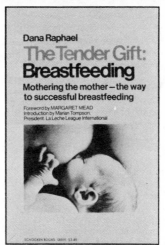

THE TENDER GIFT: BREAST-FEEDING
by Dana Raphael
1976, 200 pages, Illus.

from
Schocken Books, Inc.
200 Madison Avenue
New York, NY 10016
$4.50 pap.

The social isolation of young mothers in our culture is a common cause of breastfeeding failure. Dana Raphael is an anthropologist and has observed breastfeeding in many cultures. She is convinced that in order to breastfeed successfully, women need the support and encouragement of a friendly social network. The special contribution of Raphael's book is her introduction of the concept of the "doula," a supportive friend or companion who helps "mother the mother" so that she can breastfeed her baby.

Often a local La Leche League group can serve this purpose. Sometimes a woman's husband is her doula. Sometimes it's her own mother or a special friend. What does a doula do? Sometimes s/he moves in or visits regularly in the early weeks to help with housework, shopping, and cooking so that the mother can concentrate on her baby; the doula can take care of older children; sit with the baby so the parents or the mother can be alone for a while; she can entertain the baby's visitors, etc.

In essence, Raphael is saying that mothers need help in learning how to be mothers and that we can draw on the collective mothering experience of other cultures to recreate what has been lost in our own. (Raphael has also included a helpful chapter on breastfeeding the adopted baby.)

"In most countries, women usually decide what is right or wrong for infants. In America, we prefer to leave the responsibility to medical authorities, who are usually male and often uninformed about some simple, even critical aspects of breastfeeding. Their answers are sometimes medical prescriptions for problems that

are social and emotional. For instance, one doctor suggested that the mother consult an ear-nose-throat specialist for a baby described over the phone as choking at the breast. One quick glance at the nursing pair by someone who *knew* would have revealed that she was holding the baby in a smothering position. But these days, who ever sees a woman breastfeeding?

"At home and but a few days out of the hospital, the new mother comes to the awful realization that she and her hungry infant are going to have to make it alone. In such an isolated and nonsupportive environment, the breastfeeding mother is almost certainly condemned to an anxiety—milk-loss—failure syndrome. . .

"The common denominator for success in breastfeeding is the assurance of some degree of help from some specific person for a definite period of time after childbirth.

"I call this help 'mothering the mother.' Sometimes it takes the form of rituals and prohibitions. Sometimes it means doing chores like housekeeping or minding the baby so the mother can nap, but ultimately it permits the mother time to feel secure and to establish the essential rhythm of breastfeeding.

"In non-Western societies where this caretaking is prescribed, if the flow of the mother's milk is disrupted temporarily, several lactating women are usually around to keep the baby fed. Other experienced women are there to calm her, 'Be patient, all is well.' Reassured by their experience and presence, she relaxes and usually, in due course, adequately nurses her infant. The supportiveness of others has allowed her time to get the ejection reflex established.

"Once this rhythm of sucking and letting-down the milk is set in the first crucial weeks, fatigue and tension are less likely to disturb or prevent it. It also follows that the longer the mother is mothered by others, the more secure she becomes and the less prone she is to trouble with her milk supply.

"Many people think that the milk will just turn on. They expect that with a bit of good will the maternal instinct will take care of everything. We've discussed milk failure and shown that a major problem can be the establishment of the ejection reflex. And even maternal instincts often seem unable to withstand the social pressures of a world hostile to breastfeeding, nor can they pull the mother from the occasional doldrums brought on by this new and awesome event of childbirth when it must be experienced all alone.

"What is needed if a woman wants to breastfeed is someone, almost anyone, with a helping hand and a willing friendliness to make it possible."

BABIES, BREASTFEEDING AND BONDING
by Ina May Gaskin
1983, Illus.

from
The Book Publishing Company
156 Drakes Lane
Summertown, TN 38483
$8.95 pap.

"Breastfeeding is a natural and instinctive act. Today many mothers want to achieve this close, intimate interaction with their newborn. *Babies, Breastfeeding and Bonding* is a complete manual for the nursing mother; it is also a thorough discussion of the politics and sociology surrounding this experience.

"*Babies, Breastfeeding and Bonding* helps liberate women and babies from society's tendency towards depersonalization and regimentation. It encourages a loose, comfortable attitude towards breastfeeding, free of inhibitions and restrictions, to promote a rich, loving relationship that can last a lifetime. Written in a lively, humorous style, this book contains much practical advice for parents and for professionals who counsel them.

Chapters include:

* Attitudes toward Breastfeeding
* Bonding
* Nutrition of Mother's Milk
* Getting Off to a Good Start
* Common Problems
* Fathers and Breastfeeding
* Working Mothers
* Teenage Mothers
* Chemicals, Medications, and Drugs
* The Third World and Breastfeeding

"Ina May Gaskin is also the author of *Spiritual Midwifery,* which has sold over 130,000 copies and is currently translated into two languages. It has become a classic in the natural childbirth movement around the world. Ina May's team of midwives have delivered 1,350 babies since 1970 with better statistics than U.S. hospitals' national averages.

"Ina May is also senior editor of *The Practicing Midwife Journal*, which is published four times a year. Features include women's interest articles, book reviews, and international reports for midwives, parents and the medical community."
(from a pre-publication press release provided by The Book Publishing Company)

"People are the only mammals who have devised an alternate means to the glandular method of feeding our newborn young. In certain cases, this bottle technology can be helpful, but we are to be commended for this invention only if we, as a species, do not forget the skill of breastfeeding, which has kept us surviving for millions of years. . . .

"The first few minutes and hours following delivery are very special. This is the time when mother and baby really 'claim' each other, when their physical relationship enters a new, more active phase. The feelings of both mother and baby are subtle, yet strong, and impressions are made that last a lifetime. . . .

"Remember this: it is a feminist action to breastfeed your baby, if you are a female, or to make it possible, if you are a male. Our society will be much more liberated if we relearn and repopularize breastfeeding. To accomplish this, we need extensive cooperation among men as well as women. It represents a change in consciousness that is one of the most important projects for the 80's."

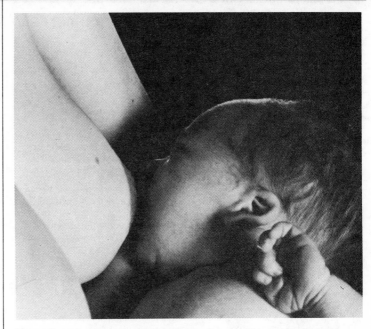

Illustration from *Breastfeeding: A Family Event,* a slide series with audio cassette. Available from BABES, c/o Deanna Sollid, 59 Berens Drive, Kentfield, CA 94904.

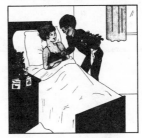

The Other Side Makes Chocolate

*This side makes vanilla...
the other side makes chocolate.*

A Look at the Humorous Side of Breastfeeding and Parenting

**Written and illustrated by
Joan McCartney**

THE OTHER SIDE MAKES CHOCOLATE
by Joan McCartney
1981, 88 pages, Illus.

from
Joan McCartney
475 West End Avenue, Suite S6
North Plainfield, NJ 07060
$2.50

Joan McCartney has put together an amusing book of cartoons which bring out some of the inherently humorous aspects of breastfeeding as well as some of the "funny" episodes caused by the clash between breastfeeding and public prejudice against it. McCartney's aim is to let women know they are not alone, despite the often harried and unappreciated life of the nursing mother.

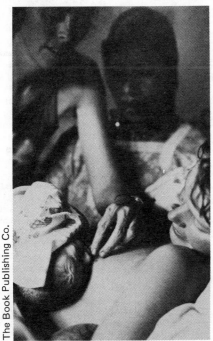

The Book Publishing Co.

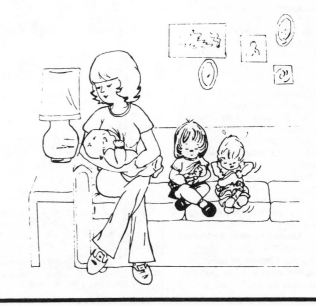

BREASTFEEDING PAMPHLETS

The pamphlets and flyers listed below are produced by consumer-oriented organizations and are excellent choices both for parents and for midwives, doctors, and childbirth educators who want inexpensive, responsible materials on breastfeeding to give to their clients.

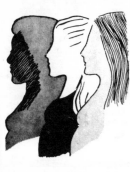

Prenatal Breast Care

Preparing
For Breastfeeding

PACKET OF BREASTFEEDING PAMPHLETS
$3.00

from
Health Education Associates
211 South Easten Road
Glenside, PA 19038

This organization provides teaching aids, speakers, seminars, and a series of twelve attractive illustrated pamphlets on breastfeeding. A sample packet includes one of each for $3.00 and bulk rates are available. The series titles include:

Nursing is Easy
Why Do Mothers Breastfeed?
Have You Thought About Breastfeeding?
Time Out for Breastfeeding Mothers
Fathers Ask: Questions About Breastfeeding
Breastfeeding: Those First Weeks at Home
Breastfeeding Your Twins
Adjusting to Parenthood: Making Love
Breast Massage and Hand Expression of Breast Milk
Weaning Your Breastfed Baby
Nursing and Weaning: The Older Baby and Toddler

BREASTFEEDING
by Rosemary Wiener
11 pages, pamphlet

from
Rosemary Romberg Wiener
6294 Mission Road
Everson, WA 98247
$.50 plus self-addressed, business size envelope with two stamps

In this pamphlet Rosemary Wiener introduces the work of La Leche League, discusses the benefits of breastfeeding for mother and baby, and provides a very informative question-and-answer survey of "common misconceptions" about breastfeeding.

" 'Only women with large breasts can nurse their babies.'

"All breasts of normally functioning adult women are equipped with the same basic milk producing glands and system. The varying sizes of different women's breasts is almost entirely due to fat cells. Therefore the size of one's breasts has nothing to do with the ability to produce milk. There are some women who have very little breast development *except* when they are pregnant or nursing their babies. Even women with silicone implants can nurse their babies."

BREASTFEEDING SAMPLER
by Doris Haire
1967-72, 5 pamphlets, Illus.

from
ICEA Bookcenter
P.O. Box 20048
Minneapolis, MN 55420
$.50 plus 60 cents postage
bulk rates available

Doris Haire has written five very clear and simple pamphlets to help mothers understand and enjoy breastfeeding. Titles include:

Have You Considered Breastfeeding?
How the Breast Functions
Instructions for Nursing Your Baby
Simple Instructions for Nursing Your Baby
Check List for Counseling Breastfeeding Mothers

"More and more women are becoming aware of the important advantages of breast-feeding to their babies and to themselves. Breast-feeding develops a special closeness between a mother and her baby that is beneficial to both. Your breast milk is the perfect food for your baby, ideally suited to his nutritional needs and bodily development. Breast-feeding benefits your baby by providing added protection against disease, infection, tooth decay and allergy."

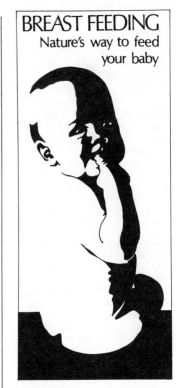

BREAST FEEDING
Nature's way to feed your baby

BREAST FEEDING: Nature's Way to Feed Your Baby
1978, brochure
25 cents single copy
bulk rates available

BREAST MILK IS BEST
color poster 18 x 24 inches
$6.00 laminated
$3.00 standard
bulk rates available

from
Center for Science in the Public Interest
1755 S. Street, NW
Washington, DC 20009

The Center for Science in the Public Interest is a non-profit organization which "provides the public with reliable, up-to-date information about the effects of science and technology on society." CSPI's special interest is in food and health, including breastfeeding. In addition to the brochure and poster listed above, CSPI produces an excellent monthly newsletter, Nutrition Action, and a variety of lively posters, T-shirts, books and brochures on nutrition. Write for their current publications catalog.

"A good diet is especially important if you plan to nurse you baby. You should eat more whole grains, low-fat dairy foods, poultry, vegetables, and fruit. You should eat less animal fat. Avoid liver and freshwater fish, which often contain pesticides and other unwanted pollutants."
(from *Breast Feeding: Nature's Way to Feed You Baby*)

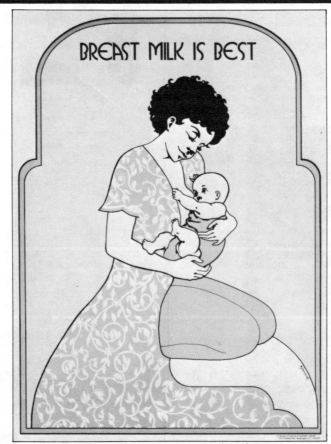

BREAST MILK IS BEST

from Center for Science in the Public Interest (right)

BREAST-FEEDING YOUR BABY
by Marsha Walker and Jeanne Watson Driscoll
1981, 60 pages, Illus.

from
Avery Publishing Group, Inc.
publisher

Order from
Boston Association for Childbirth Education
c/o Jan Crick
291 Woburn Street
Reading, MA 01867
$2.95 plus 75 cents mailing

This useful booklet was produced under the auspices of the Nursing Mothers' Council of the Boston Association for Childbirth Education (BACE) and is organized in workbook fashion with helpful hints, lists of suggestions, a question-and-answer series, and illustrations. Topics include how the breasts function, prenatal preparation, in the hospital, nursing after a cesarean, special situations, going home, the working mother, weaning, and getting support for breastfeeding. A set of appendices includes recommended reading, sources for breastfeeding aids (milk cups and breast pumps), support organizations, and a bibliography.

"As your baby and your own body adjust to nursing, you will notice that your let-down matures. This means that the milk will let down sooner after the baby begins each feeding, that it will do so regularly, and that milk will tend not to leak between feedings, especially when just thinking about the baby. Your breasts will seem softer and less engorged. This does not mean you have less milk. The following are guidelines for maintaining a good milk supply.

1. Frequent nursing: about ten times in twenty-four hours during the first two weeks or so.
2. Remember: Supply will increase to equal the demand.
3. Adequate fluid intake (two to two-and-one-half quarts per day).
4. Adequate rest: Nap when baby does, especially during the weeks with night feedings.
5. Good nutrition (refer to Table 6-1).
6. Relaxation during feedings to insure proper let-down (use relaxation breathing prior to nursing)."

WHY BREAST-FEED
by Ruth Levy Guyer and Margaret Wolf Freivogel
1981, 17 pages

from
Alliance for Perinatal Research and Services
P.O. Box 6358
Alexandria, VA 22306
$2.00 plus 25 cents postage

Ruth Guyer has a doctorate in immunology and she is especially interested in the unique properties of breast milk. In this booklet she discusses the ways in which human milk is different from cow's milk, how it affects the baby's health and development (particularly the effects on the growth of bacteria in the gut and the presence of antibodies), and health differences between breast and bottle-fed babies. She describes the problems associated with bottle-feeding (allergy, sudden infant death syndrome, obesity, faulty formula) and the problems associated with breastfeeding (environmental contamination and drugs in breast milk). The "pitfalls to successful breast-feeding" are also discussed.

"Throughout the nursing period, human milk changes to meet the needs of the maturing baby. Over time, some nutrients decrease while others increase in amount, and their specificities may also shift. For example, the concentration of antibodies is at first very high, then drops, and later may rise again. In addition, the mix of antibodies continuously changes as the mother's body responds to the diseases to which she is exposed. Even dog food manufacturers realize the changing needs of growing puppies and market 'cycle' dog food. In contrast, infant formula remains standard, with the result that the composition of any one formula is always the same. . . .

"Many women are working away from the home and very few employers have special arrangements for nursing mothers. This problem is an increasing one. Interestingly, it is not a problem everywhere because many countries are more enlightened than our own. In 1919, the the International Labor Organization, an autonomous unit associated with the United Nations, developed a list of recommendations (described in an article in *Environmental Child Health,* October 1975, Pp. 249-257) designed to make breast-feeding feasible for women who wished or needed to remain in the work force. Over the years, numerous countries have adopted the recommendations and have set up child care facilities for infants, have made arrangements for frequent short nursing breaks for employees, and so on. Because the United States has not adopted these recommendations, women must often choose between nursing and working, and the choice frequently reflects economic considerations rather then personal preferences. Now, more women are working than ever before, and more data show that breastfeeding is important. The time is right for enlightened federal policies to protect both the health and birthright of the infant and the right of every mother to both nurse her babies and work."

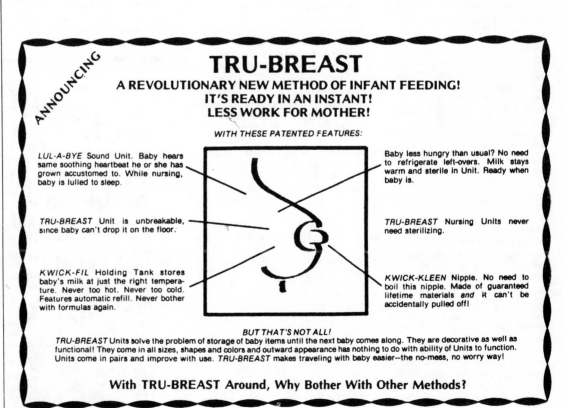

BREAST MILK AND ENVIRONMENTAL CONTAMINATION

BIRTHRIGHT DENIED: The Risks and Benefits of Breast-feeding
by Stephanie G. Harris and Joseph H. Highland
1977, 66 pages

from
Environmental Defense Fund
444 Park Avenue South
New York, NY 10016
$3.50 postpaid

The Environmental Defense Fund, founded in 1967, is a coalition of scientists, lawyers, and concerned citizens who work to protect environmental quality through legal action and public education. This publication looks at the possible "risks" of breastfeeding caused by environmental contamination of human breast milk with agricultural and industrial chimicals. These risks are balanced against the benefits to mother and baby of breastfeeding. The composition of infant formula is explained and common contaminants of formula are described. The report concludes by giving guidelines for making a decision and lists ways to minimize exposure to contaminants in the diet.

"From their first exposure *in utero* to their continued exposures in the early years of life, children have become the newest victims of our uncontrolled production, use and discharge of synthetic organic chemicals. Not only has the onset of exposure to these chemical hazards begun earlier but the extent of exposure has greatly increased over the past few years. Children today face an unprecedented situation; a world contaminated with chemicals, the exposure to which may not produce visible effects for decades to come.

"During the past ten years we have made significant progress in controlling our exposure to toxic chemicals. The use of several hazardous pesticides has been banned or greatly restricted, the discharge of many industrial chemicals into our air and water has begun to be regulated and a general awareness of the potential problems caused by carcinogens in our environment has developed. However, much remains to be done and until as a society we take the steps necessary to protect ourselves we will personally have to alter our own lifestyles in order to limit or prevent our exposure to these chemicals.

"While under normal circumstances EDF would support a parental decision to breast-feed a child, these are not normal times so this recommendation will have to be tempered. If our worst fears are realized a tragedy awaits us. If our strongest hopes prevail, our cautions today will have an enormous impact in the years to come. The decisions are ours. . . .

"Diet is probably the major source of PCBs and pesticide exposure for most people without an occupational exposure. It is relatively simple to outline a nutritious diet which minimizes these chemicals. As has been discussed on page 8, the major dietary source of PCBs is fish which have lived in fresh water for part or all of their lives. Therefore, this is one food which should be avoided. In particular, the fish to avoid are: bottom feeding estuarine fish (e.g. catfish, flounder, sole), Great Lakes fish (e.g. salmon, carp), and fatty fish (e.g. buffalofish and eels). Ocean fish (e.g. cod, haddock, halibut) are usually free from PCB residues.

"The major dietary source of chlorinated hydrocarbon pesticides is in foods of animal origin (meat, dairy products) and fish as the pesticide residues are bioaccumulated in the fat over the lifetime of the animals and fish. If meat is to be eaten, the fat should be removed and the drippings discarded. The better cooked the meat, in general, the lower its fat content. . . . the types of meat in which pesticide residues are most frequently found are: beef, veal, chicken, and turkey, while the animals in which residues are least frequently found are: sheep, goats, and swine. Also, grass-fed beef should have much lower residues than the usual grain-fed beef. If fish is to be eaten, only deep-sea fish should be chosen (e.g. cod and haddock).

"Only low-fat dairy products should be eaten (e.g., yogurt, skim milk, buttermilk, ice milk, uncreamed cottage cheese) and high-fat products (e.g., butter, cream, ice cream, high-fat cheese) avoided. Eggs have surprisingly low residues of most pesticides (with the exception of DDE) and can be eaten with relatively low risk."

PCBs AND BREAST MILK: Weighing the Risks
by Marcella R. Mosher and Greg Moyer
November 1980, 4 pages, Illus.
(Vol. 7, No. 11 of *Nutrition Action Magazine*)

from
Nutrition Action
Center for Science in the Public Interest
1755 S Street, NW
Washington, DC 20009
$1.25 for single back issue copy

See index for CSPI's other materials on breastfeeding. This article describes the extent of PCB contamination of breast milk, the risks associated with PCB exposure, and provides guidelines for reducing PCBs in the diet. PCB (polychlorinated biphenyl) is an industrial chemical which has seeped into the food chain and is present in virtually all samples of human breast milk tested.

"One person who has consistently focused on both the risks and benefits of breast-feeding is Stephanie Harris, a chemist by training, who worked on pesticide issues for Ralph Nader's Health Research Group . . . Due to a family history of allergies, she chose to nurse both her children, though she knows her milk contains some PCBs. . . .

"She offers women who may become pregnant these precautions for limiting an infant's exposure to PCBs:

* Eliminate from the diet freshwater fish, like salmon and carp, and bottom-feeding estuarine fish, like catfish, flounder, and sole. Eat more fresh vegetables, especially organic vegetables, and grain products since more PCBs are ingested through animal and dairy products. *Note:* don't expect diet to make a difference overnight. Studies show that PCBs remain in the body for years after the initial exposure. All that you can do is stop increasing the PCBs to your system.
* Lose weight *before* pregnancy to reduce the fatty tissue that keeps PCBs in the body. Once pregnant, maintain your weight. Weight reduction during pregnancy only releases more contaminants from the fat cells into the blood stream and eventually through the placenta.
* Avoid breast-feeding if you know you are exposed to unusually high levels of PCBs where you work or live.
* Consider breast-feeding one or two weeks to reap the known benefits of colostrum, the secretion preceding milk, then shift to bottle-feeding.
* Mix breast and bottle-feeding throughout the lactation period depending on the amount of PCBs you suspect yourself of carrying."

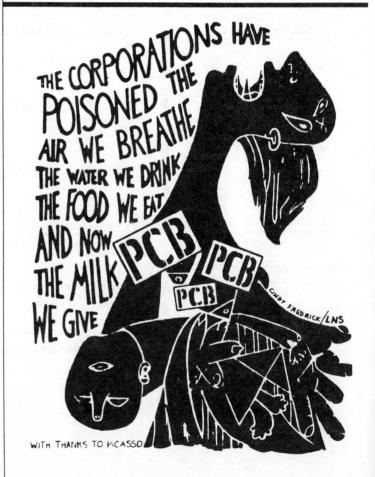

THE CORPORATIONS HAVE POISONED THE AIR WE BREATHE THE WATER WE DRINK THE FOOD WE EAT AND NOW THE MILK WE GIVE

PCB PCB PCB

CINDY FREDRICK/LNS

WITH THANKS TO PICASSO

DRUGS IN BREASTMILK

Before taking any drug, whether you are nursing a baby or not, it's a good idea to read the package insert provided with the drug (ask your doctor or pharmacist for a copy), or look up the same information in the *Physician's Desk Reference* at your local library. The package insert lists harmful side effects of the drug and may contain specific information concerning use by nursing mothers.

BREASTFEEDING AND DRUGS IN HUMAN MILK
by Gregory J. White, M.D., and Mary Kerwin White
1980, 44 pages

from
La Leche League
9616 Minneapolis Avenue
Franklin Park, IL 60131
$5.00

This booklet is in fact a supplement to Volume 22 of *Veterinary and Human Toxicology*, published by the American College of Veterinary Toxicologists at Kansas State University. It includes an introduction to the subject of drugs and breastfeeding, a list of drug brand names, and an extensive table of drugs listed by class or generic name, outlining their known effects on breastfeeding and keyed to a list of over 250 references. Particularly harmful drugs are highlighted in color. Authors Mary and Gregory White are a founding mother of La Leche League and a home birth physician, respectively.

"When prescribing a medication for a nursing mother, some physicians routinely insist on weaning as a precaution simply because they are not certain about the drug's possible effect on the nursing baby. Also, of late, a new rationale for weaning has

"If a drug prescribed for the mother is considered to pose some risk for the baby, it is usually possible to substitute another drug with lesser or no risk. . ."

appeared on the scene. With some drugs, even though they have not been found to affect the nursling, breastfeeding is being proscribed for 'medico-legal' reasons (Lipman, 1978). In other words, the doctor is afraid of being sued. Too often he does not realize the many benefits of which the baby is being deprived, nor the serious implications of weaning. . . .

"Abrupt weaning can be a traumatic experience for both mother and baby. Mother may develop painfully engorged breasts, risking a breast infection and compounding the problems for which she was advised to take the medication in the first place. The whole mother/baby relationship changes. Caring for the baby and keeping him content is difficult or impossible, the baby is often utterly inconsolable. . . .

"If a drug prescribed for the mother is considered to pose some risk for the baby, it is usually possible to substitute another drug with lesser or no risk. . . .

"The conclusion then can only be as Dr. Blake has observed: 'Breastfeeding has many benefits for mother and baby. Apart from a relatively few drugs and specific conditions, these beneficial effects easily outweigh the small risk attached to the presence of drugs in breast milk.' (Blake, 1980)"

DRUGS IN BREAST MILK: A Consumer's Guide
by Paula C. Rothermel and Myron M. Faber
1977, 12 pages

from
BIRTH Journal
110 El Camino Real
Berkeley, CA 94705
$1.50

This reprint provides an introduction to the mechanism of drug excretion in breast milk, discusses the effects of certain drugs on the baby, and describes problems in the study of drugs and breast milk. Included is an extensive table showing the effects on the nursling of over 50 different categories of drugs, referenced to a list of 32 research papers.

"Drug excretion in breastmilk is one of the most complex routes of drug action to follow experimentally. While not an important avenue of drug excretion, breastmilk has been found to harbor drugs in concentrations at or above those present in the mother's blood. Some drugs do not appear at all, while others are found in trace amounts only. . . .

"Effect on Nursling: Although only trace amounts of a drug may be found in breastmilk the cumulative effect over a 24 hour period of nursing may equal a full dose for an infant."

MEDICATIONS (IN THE USUAL DOSE) AND CHEMICALS PERMISSIBLE

ACTH
Antidiarrheal agent (nonabsorbable)
Antimalarial drugs
Barbiturates
Cephalosporins
Codeine
Digoxin
Epinephrine
Erythromycin
General Anesthetics (after mother has recovered)

Insulin
Laxatives (mineral oil, castor oil, methylcellulose, stool softeners, senna, saline)
Local anesthetics
Penicillins
Phenytoin
Thyroxin

MEDICATIONS (IN THE USUAL DOSE) AND CHEMICALS THAT SHOULD BE MONITORED

Acetylsalicylic Acid
Acetaminophen
Alcohol (one social drink only)
Antihistamines
Caffeine
Contraceptives (Hormonal only 1 month after birth)
Corticosteroids
Ethambutol
Isoniazid
Methadon
Methantheline (Banthine and Quaternary anticholinergics)
Naladixic Acid

Nicotine (smoking) (Only up to 10 cigarettes a day)
Nitrofuradantin
Opiates
Phenothiazines (Chlorpromazine)
Polybromated biphenyls
Polychlorinated biphenyls
Propranolol
Rifampin
Theophylline
Thiazides
Tricyclic antidepressants (Imipramine)

MEDICATIONS AND CHEMICALS TO AVOID

Amphetamines
Anticoagulants (oral coumarin types)
Antineoplastic drugs
Atropine (Tertiary anticholinergics)
Benzodiazepine (Diazepam)
Butazones
Bromides
Chloral Hydrate
Chloramphenicol
Demerol
Dihyrotachysterol
Ephedrine
Ergot
Heavy metal intoxication (lead and mercury)
Heroin
Hypoglycemics (oral)
Indomethacin

Iodides
Laxatives (Cascara, danthron, rhubarb, aloe)
Levodopa
Lindane (Kwell)
Lithium
Meprobamate
Mercurial Diuretics
Methyprylon (Noludar)
Mysoline
Metronidazole (Flagyl)
Novobiocin
Pseudoephedrine
Radioactive compounds
Reserpine
Streptomycin
Sulfonamides
Tetracycline
Thiouracil

Information provided by the Poison Control Center of the Nassau County Medical Center, 2201 Hempstead Turnpike, East Meadow, NY 11554.

ADVICE ON BREAST-FEEDING AND DRUGS
by Annabel Hecht
November, 1979, 2 pages

from
Food and Drug Administration
Office of Public Affairs
5600 Fishers Lane
Rockville, MD 20857
free

This reprint from the November, 1979, issue of FDA Consumer discusses the negative effects of some commonly used drugs on nursing babies. Included are tranquilizers, caffeine, lithium, antithyroid drugs, Flagl, radioactive iodine, Darvon, and some over-the-counter laxatives.

"Because of the possibility that her baby might be affected, it is a good idea for the nursing mother to ask her doctor about all the medications she is taking—both the prescription and the over-the-counter varieties. It may be that some drugs she is taking aren't really necessary, or that a substitute can be prescribed for a product that is known to affect the nursing infant. Whether she should stop nursing will depend on the importance of the drug to the mother's health."

THE HUMAN LACTATION CENTER
666 Sturges Highway
Westport, CT 06880
203/259-5995

"The Human Lactation Center, Ltd. is an unique institute whose major purposes are: research, teaching and publishing about breastfeeding. The Center's current activities include: research into the effects of lactation as a factor which inhibits fertility; consultation for national and international governments, industry and medical institutions on infant and maternal nutrition and feeding practices; design and management of conferences on lactation to encourage dialogue among professionals regarding lactation; cooperative meetings with groups in health and family planning; development of methodology for use by researchers in anthropology, nutrition and public health in field work on childbirth, breastfeeding and family planning; expansion of library and library notation system on human lactation; publication of *The Lactation Review*, a journal concerned with nutrition and feeding practices of women and children, occasional papers, proceedings, reprints and books; public education programs; tutorials for students and interns on research related to breastfeeding."

—Dana Raphael, director

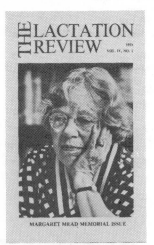

THE LACTATION REVIEW
Published and edited by Dana Raphael, director of the Human Lactation Center

Included with membership or available alone. Write for current rates.

"During another such visit, [Margaret Mead] picked out of our discussion three separate themes: Data which indicated (as did her early field observations) that mothers fed their infants a variety of foods besides breast milk soon after birth; demographic findings that suggested if the first two children of a couple live, the security they feel permits

them to have at least two fewer children; and, a universally accepted old wives' tale which suggests that breastfeeding prevents pregnancy (by inhibiting menstruation and ovulation).

"Immediately, she put these ideas into a broader context. She asked me to consider how they relate to population. Her train of thought went something like this: A baby's appetite and development outstrips the mother's milk supply sometime around three months of age. A hungry baby will whine or scream, and generally upset the mother. Unnerved, her milk supply dwindles, the infant cries more and she loses more milk. Now she becomes scared, afraid her baby will die. But, once she feeds the infant some additional foods, the baby is content. The mother calms down, her milk supply holds, breastfeeding continues and the child lives. By continuing to breastfeed, the mother's chances of becoming pregnant are reduced, the baby's chances of living are increased and the couple, feeling secure, parent fewer children."

(Editor's Note: In 1979 I wrote to the international headquarters of the Nestle company protesting their policy of promoting the use of artificial infant feeding in Third World countries. In reply I received a packet of materials which included a copy of an article by Dana Raphael in *The Lactation Review* on breastfeeding and weaning among the poor. I was disturbed to find a publication from a breastfeeding advocacy organization included in a packet from Nestle and confused by many of the issues raised in Raphael's article. I wrote to Dr. Raphael for clarification and she was very helpful in replying at length to my questions. Dr. Raphael maintains that the arguments behind the Nestle boycott are oversimplified and don't take into account the complex reality of breastfeeding in poverty. She feels that the breast/bottle controversy has been "politicized" to the detriment of mothers and babies, who are usually left out of policy-making. The questions raised are complex: is artificial feeding ever desirable, can women be forced to breastfeed, should supplemental foods be used during the first three months? These issues are discussed at length in many of the publications from the Human Lactation Center and concerned readers may find them helpful in stimulating their thinking about a difficult controversy. For more information on the Nestle boycott see index.)

BREASTFEEDING IN POST-INDUSTRIAL SOCIETY
BIRTH Journal, special issue
Winter 1981, Vol. 8, No. 4
81 pages, Illus.

from
BIRTH
110 El Camino Real
Berkeley, CA 94705
$4.00 for single back issues

The entire Winter, 1981 issue of *BIRTH Journal* (formerly *Birth and the Family Journal*) was devoted to breastfeeding. Following is the complete list of contents.

"Breastfeeding and Reproduction in Women in Western Australia," P.E. Hartmann, et. al.
"Special Properties of Human Milk," William B. Pittard.
"The Pharmacology of Human Milk," Joseph S. Bertino, Jr.
"Breastfeeding and Jaundice," M. Jeffrey Maisels.
"The Management of Breastfeeding," Edward R. Cerutti.
"The Romance and Power of Breastfeeding," Mayra Bloom.
"Dancing in the Dark, I: Romanticized Motherhood and the Breastfeeding Venture," Linda Blachman.
"Dancing in the Dark, II: Helping and Not-So-Helping Hands," Linda Blachman.
"Administrative Petition to Relieve the Health Hazards of Promotion of Infant Formulas in the United States," Angela Blackwell and Lois Salisbury.

"What becomes evident as we analyze the nature of assistance offered women as they decide to or attempt to breastfeed is that what is being supported is not a unique individual or personal relationship between a woman and a child, but rather a romantic ideal. What these authors and others who wish to assist mothers have yet to grasp is that it is the romanticized ideal that not only works to keep many women from breastfeeding, but keeps the nursing mother from getting the supports and recognition she needs.

"It may seem farfetched to find anything hazardous in others who, having had a positive if not euphoric nursing experience, wish to spread their joy around and help others to have similar pleasure. So many women who romanticize breastfeeding start off reaching out to assist other women authorities but end up sounding dangerously like the experts and authorities they eschew—patronizing, coercive, and having *the* answer. There are as many answers as there are women."

—from "Dancing in the Dark II: Helping and Not-So-Helping Hands," by Linda Blachman

BREASTFEEDING
by Audrey Palm Riker
1964, 18 pages, Illus.

from
Public Affairs Pamphlets
381 Park Avenue
New York, NY 10016
50 cents each
bulk rates available

In 1964 only two out of five women attempted to breastfeed their babies and many of those failed. The situation is quite a bit better today, but this pamphlet's discussion of cultural pressures against breastfeeding is still relevant.

"When approval and support are absent, a new mother may be confused and concerned by the attitude of discouragement or indifference she meets—even from doctors and nurses. In humorous exasperation, one woman categorized the kind of solicitous disapproval she met from 'that large and intolerant group who produce bottlefed progeny':

First six weeks: Are you going to *try* to nurse the baby?
Second six weeks: Are you still trying to nurse the baby?
Fourth month: My next-door neighbor nursed her baby fine for four months and then went completely dry just like that!
Fifth month: What do you do when the baby bites? (Her answer: Scream!)
Sixth month: Are you *still* nursing the baby?
Seventh month: Why are you still nursing the baby?
Eighth month: Won't it be inconvenient for her to interrupt kindergarten to come home and nurse?

"Clearly, the nursing mother can use a sense of humor and a touch of plucky independence. More important, perhaps, she needs an awareness of the considerable advantages of breastfeeding—to both mother and baby."

RESOURCES IN HUMAN NURTURING, INTERNATIONAL
3885 Forest Street
P.O. Box 6861
Denver, CO 80206
303/388-4600

Resources in Human Nurturing is a non-profit organization for professionals and parents concerned with promoting and protecting human nurturing through breastfeeding. The organization provides continuing education seminars, a clearinghouse service, and is the primary source for Lact-Aid breastfeeding supplies (see index). The organization also produces a variety of publications including *Keeping Abreast Journal* (back issues are available), a monograph series, and reprints. Topics include adoptive nursing, premature infants, and human milk banks. Write for a complete publications list.

YOU CAN BREASTFEED YOUR BABY: Even in Special Situations by Dorothy Patricia Brewster 1979, 624 pages, Illus.

from
Rodale Press
33 E. Minor Street
Emmaus, PA 18049
$12.95 pap.

This book has everything! The author covers virtually every problem which could interfere with establishing or continuing breastfeeding—Brewster provides clear descriptions of each situation or condition, offers advice on dealing with it, and adds personal comments from mothers who have had the experience described. Probably the best way to give an idea of the scope of this very useful book is simply to list the chapter titles. These are:

1. "What's Normal?"
2. "Nursing Techniques"
3. "Nutrition for Mother and Baby"
4. "Breast and Nipple Problems"
5. "Nursing after a Cesarean Childbirth"
6. "Nursing a Premature Baby"
7. "Newborn and Infant Problems"
8. "Malformation of Baby's Nose, Mouth, and Digestive Tract"
9. "Problems Related to Baby's Altered Body Chemistry"
10. "Nursing a Baby with Special Developmental Conditions"
11. "Dealing with Allergies"
12. "When Baby is Sick or Hospitalized"
13. "When Mother is Sick or Hospitalized"
14. "Working Together: Doctor, Hospital, Parents"
15. "Inducing or Reestablishing Your Milk Supply: For Natural Born or Adopted Baby"
16. "Nursing While Pregnant"
17. "Nursing Siblings"
18. "Nursing Twins"
19. "Nursing an Older Baby"
20. "Nursing Strikes and One-Sided Nursing"
21. "Nursing during Stressful Times"
22. "Mothers with Special Physical Problems"
23. "Nursing and Working"
24. "Traveling with a Nursing Baby"
25. "When You Go It Alone"

Dorothy Brewster has been a La Leche League leader for over 15 years and breastfed her four children. As a mother of twins, she knew the importance of advice and support for breastfeeding in special situations. In her book, she tries to provide that support for others. Much of the material in her book is based on the experience of other League mothers who responded to Brewster's call for personal stories on coping with unusual nursing situations. For women with any of the problems listed above, this book will be invaluable. Several of the chapters will also be useful to mothers in a normal nursing situation.

"The ability to easily hand express your milk is a technique that can be extremely helpful in certain situations, such as when your baby's suck is not yet well developed, when your baby is premature, when you are separated from your baby due to hospitalization, when you are inducing lactation for an adopted baby, or when you are nursing and working. The technique can also be used to give you relief if you are engorged (overly full with milk), or have extremely sore, cracked or bleeding nipples. If you want to increase your milk supply, expressing in addition to nursing will enable you to produce more milk. . . .

"Dr. John D. Michael, a pediatrician who has helped many mothers of premature babies learn to express their milk, suggests that the four steps of normal nursing just described be approximated in the following ways, in order to get maximum expression of available milk:
1. Apply warmth to your breasts: use a moist towel wrapped around a heating pad or hot water bottle, or any other method to *gently* warm the skin of your breasts, but not the nipple area itself. The heat may be applied several times during the day, ideally for half an hour prior to nursing. The warmth seems to increase the blood supply reaching the milk production cells.
2. Stimulate your nipples by physical rolling (like rolling a marble between your fingers), or any other gentle rhythmic stimulation, just prior to expression. (Be sure your hands are clean before touching nipple or areola area.)
3. Massage your breasts with your hands, starting back at the chest wall and moving down toward the areola. Smooth, strong, compressive strokes should be used, two or three times at each position. Rotate your hands so that you are massaging from different points all around the breast. The purpose is to compress the milk glands and to push milk down the ducts to the sinuses.
4. Next, place the tips of your thumb and first finger or fingers on opposite sides of the areola, then squeeze them rhythmically together. Rotate around the nipple, trying to empty all the sinuses which surround the nipple."

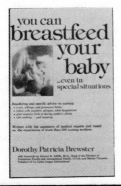

MILK BANKS

In 1980, New York became the first state to pass a law advocating the promotion of breastfeeding. The new law, an amendment to the public health statutes, (Section 2505), declares that human breast milk is "the preferred food for all infants" and states that breast milk should be made available to any infant who requires it through the establishment of human "milk banks." The law authorizes the commissioner of health to adopt regulations for such milk banks and to provide information on the availability of breast milk. Milk banks make breast milk available to infants who cannot tolerate formula. Priority is usually given to infants who are premature or of low birth weight or who are allergic to cow milk or formula. For these babies breast milk can literally be a lifesaver.

Following are excerpts from a Memorandum on the breast milk law, issued by the Governor of New York:

"It has been established that human breast milk is the preferred food for infants not only because it is uniquely suited to their nutritional needs, but also because it contains properties, lacking in other forms of infant nutrition, which afford protection against infections and necrotizing enterocolitis. Included among diseases preventable by breast-milk feeding are aminoacidemia in premature infants, acrodermatitis enteropathica, allergy, iron deficiency anemia, neonatal hypocalcemia, and pyrodoxine deficiency. Breast feeding also prevents dental disease ("nursing bottle syndrome") which occurs when bottle-fed babies drink milk, water or fruit juice sweetened with sugar, syrup or honey which

pools around their teeth resulting in bacterial growth causing rampant caries and which also results in the early development of a taste for sweets and consequent obesity. Breast feeding is beneficial to mother and child by creating a psychological bond between them and a sense of security in the child; it is convenient and eliminates the chore of preparing formula and cleansing nursing bottles; it assures proper nutrition for infants whose mothers are unable to prepare formula properly; and it has financial advantages over artificial feeding.

"Uniform, statewide standards and procedures are needed for screening breast milk donors to rule out those taking any medication or drug hazardous to infants or who are in ill-health or whose infants are in ill-health or whose infants are sick. In addition, uniform standards are needed for collecting breast milk; assuring that breast milk supplies are of appropriate types and proper quality; testing for bacteriological contamination; processing and storing breast milk in "banks" to assure an available supply when needed; and distributing the milk to the infants."

Groups of nursing mothers are forming around the country to donate milk on an informal basis for mothers and infants in their communities. If you are in need of human breast milk for your infant or would like to donate milk, contact the nearest regional milk bank or your local La Leche League leader (see index).

BREAST-FEEDING: A Commentary in Celebration of the International Year of the Child, 1979 by the Nutrition Committee of the Canadian Paediatric Society and the Committee on Nutrition of the American Academy of Pediatrics 1979, 11 pages

from
American Academy of Pediatrics Publications Department
P.O. Box 1034
Evanston, IL 60204
50 cents

The American Academy of Pediatrics (AAP) has recommended that all full-term newborn infants be breastfed. In this paper, the AAP Committee on nutrition looks at the nutritional and physiological properties of human milk, the epidemiology of breastfeeding, factors responsible for the decline of breastfeeding, and ways to increase breastfeeding. A list of 133 references is included.

"The routine in many hospitals makes breast-feeding difficult; therefore, efforts should be made to change obstetrical ward and neonatal unit practices to increase the opportunity for successful lactation. Changes may include the following:
1. Decrease the amount of sedation and/or anesthesia given to the mother during labor and delivery because large amounts can impair suckling in the infant.
2. Avoid separation of the mother from her infant during the first 24 hours.
3. Breast-feed infants on an 'on-demand' schedule rather than on a rigid three- to four-hour schedule, and discourage routine supplementary formula feedings.
4. Reappraise physical facilities to provide easy access of the mother to her infant. Rooming-in of mother and infant is important to successful lactation."

BREAST PUMPS

ORA'LAC PUMP
$30.00 complete
wholesale inquiries welcome

from
Ora'Lac Pump, Inc.
Box 137
Sitka, AK 99835
907/747-3434

This breast pump was designed by a nursing mother, Frances "Jill" Lunas and is slightly different from other manual breast pumps. The mother uses the sucking action of her mouth rather than a hand pumping action to pump the breast.

"My nick-name is Jill and like Jack, I am adept at many trades, and master of few. I designed the pump. I can also rebuild a gasoline engine, wire and plumb a house (according to code too!), carpenter, cook, clean a chicken, butcher a steer, can and freeze what we grow, be receptionist for my husband (an Internist—M.D.), am a labor coach (*not* Lamaze), a foster parent, a parent (4), am active in our organization against family violence (have housed many beaten wives), and most recently have been closely associated with the elderly and the dying (I am comfortable with both). In short, I love people and dealing with them.

"Two of the women who assemble and package the pump have marked physical handicaps—one cannot walk and the other is blind—which led me to design a jig to help solve their problems. Now my blind employee is probably my most consistent."

R & SS SALES
4924 Heatherdale Lane
Carmichael, CA 95608
916/487-2313

"My husband and I operate a small family-oriented business—mostly mail order, but including setting up other distributors across the nation.

"Our largest seller is breastpumps. We carry both the Marshall Comfort Plus Breastpump and the Nursing Mother Breastpump by Mary Jane. We feel they are the best two pumps on the market for the price. We discovered the Marshall Breastpump in 1979 while in Japan. I was desperate for an effective, efficient breastpump. We have been selling the pump ever since. The pump was like a miracle to me and countless women across the nation have found it to be No. 1! We have recently taken on the Nursing Mother Breastpump by Mary Jane, finding it to be a close second. Comfort Plus Breastpumps retail from us for $22., the Mary Jane for $18.

"Other products we sell include Breast Care Shields, a Natural Family Planning Kit, plus other home health care products including otoscopes, blood pressure units, stethoscopes, Family Black Bags, and Astrodents."

BREAST MILKING AND FEEDING UNIT
$23.95 plus $1.75 postage

from
Happy Family Products
12300 Venice Blvd.
Los Angeles, CA 90066
800/228-2028, ext. 34 (toll free)

Happy Family Products produces a manual breast pump which comes with a useful, 12-page booklet on *How to Manage Breast Milking and Breastfeeding.* Happy Family sells a variety of other products to aid breastfeeding mothers, including books, nursing bras, reusable bra pads, and hydrous lanolin. Write for their free catalog.

"Breastfeeding and Working. Many mothers today choose to give their babies the nutritional benefits of their breast milk even though they must be away. Breastfeeding your baby as often as possible helps to maintain your milk supply and keeps your special relationship growing. Allow time for the eye-to-eye communication that is so important to babies and mothers.

"Some mothers are able to be with baby during lunch hours. Others pump at that time, and refrigerate the breast milk for baby's lunch the following day. Some babies begin to wean to a bottle and refuse to suckle at the breast before you real-ize what is happening. Others are willing to bottle feed and breastfeed for many months (2-3 years). Some will sleep much more while you are away so they will be awake when you are home. A sitter who is supportive of your breastfeeding is worth the search.

"Taking baby to bed with you makes night feedings easier and full-time mothering on weekends helps."
—from *How to Manage Breast Milking and Breastfeeding.*

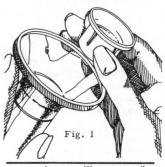

Fig. 1

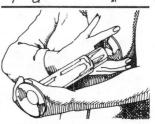

Fig. 2

EVENFLO BREAST FEEDING SET
Available in retail stores

from
Evenflo Products Company
Ravenna, OH 44266

Evenflo, a manufacturer of nursing bottles and nipples, also produces products to aid breastfeeding mothers. Their Breast Feeding Set includes a bulb-type manual breast pump, nursing pads, breast cream, and nipple shields. Request a copy of their free brochure, *The Joy of Nursing,* which describes the use of these products.

"More and more moms are bringing their babies with them when they go out to dinner, to the park, to visit friends. Nursing just makes it easier. If you carry a shawl or light baby blanket, it's easy to tuck the baby under your blouse, throw the shawl over your shoulder, and nurse inconspicuously.

"But what happens when you need or want to get out alone or with your husband for the evening? You don't want to take a chance that the baby will wake up hungry and no baby sitter wants to be left alone with a baby she can't feed. And what if you'd like your husband to take over one of the feedings—around suppertime, for instance, when you're tired and busy or you return to work part or full time.

"Breastfeeding mothers are advised against substituting formula or cows milk because their breasts need to be regularly stimulated in order to produce more milk.

"The Evenflo Breast Pump solves this problem. By expressing your own milk directly into a bottle, you are stimulating and emptying your breasts and continuing to give your baby 'the real thing' even when you go out. A breast pump is easy to use if you employ a gentle irregular pumping motion similar to baby sucking and place the horn off center of the nipple so that one side of the horn is pressing near the nipple."
—from *The Joy of Nursing.*

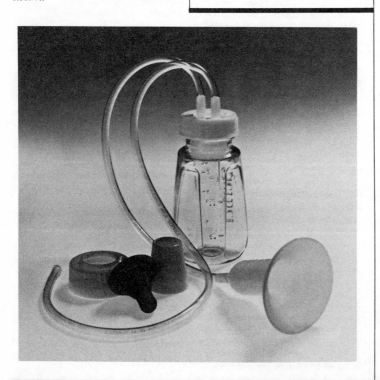

MILK CUPS

The milk cups listed below are all quite similar. They consist of a two-part, snap-together cup which fits over the nipple of the breast. The nipple pokes through a large hole in the center of the cup so that leaking milk falls into the cup. A small hole at the top permits air to flow through. Cups are made of light-weight, rigid, clear plastic.

CONFI-DRI MILK CUP
$5.30 plus 70 cents postage
set of one pair plus instructions
$2.50 plus 50 cents postage
single cups

from
CEA of Greater Philadelphia
814 Fayette Street
Conshohocken, PA 19428
215/828-0131

This cup is made to order for the Childbirth Education Association of Greater Philadelphia, which sells them by mail-order to mothers across the country.

"CEA Milk Cups are designed for women with flat or inverted nipples who plan to nurse. The cups are also very useful for women who are nursing and wish to collect leaking milk. The curved inner opening provides a smooth surface next to the breast. The cup gently applies pressure to the breast, encouraging the nipple to protrude. Separate parts permit easy cleaning. The CEA Milk Cup may be sterilized in your dishwasher or in boiling water, and reused many times."
—from CEA Confi-Dri brochure

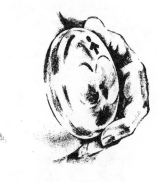

FREE AND DRY BREAST CARE SHIELDS
$5.95 plus 75 cents postage
set of one pair

from
Monterey Laboratories, Inc.
P.O. Box 15129
3301 W. Meade Avenue
Las Vegas, NV 89114
702/876-3888

Write for a free copy of this company's brochure, *Thoroughly Modern Mom*, which explains use of the breast shield.

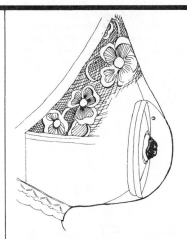

NETSY SWEDISH MILK CUP AND BREAST SHIELD
$8.95
set of one pair with instructions

from
The Netsy Company
34 Sunrise Avenue
Mill Valley, CA 94941-3398
415/388-3660

The Netsy milk cup is made in Sweden. Owner Marianne Alstrom says the goal of her business is "to help the new mother and newborn baby enjoy their new relationship and prolong the nursing experience."

"For the Nursing Mother
* No more wet clothes from milk leakage! This cup collects the excess and enables you to dispose of it discreetly.
* Helps to avoid or to treat sore or cracked nipples by holding your bra away from the nipples. This allows air to circulate around cracked areas and prevents the cracks from folding up into the nipples.
* Relieves painful engorgement as the continuous pressure exerted by the cup around the nipple helps evacuate excess milk. This pressure often helps to increase the milk supply when it is not sufficient."

NURSING THE ADOPTED BABY

RELACTATION: A Guide to Breast-feeding the Adopted Baby
by Elizabeth Hormann
1971, 21 pages

from
Birth and Life Bookstore
P.O. Box 70625
Seattle, WA 98107
$1.75 plus $1.00 postage

This booklet provides in-depth background and instructions for inducing lactation to breastfeed an adopted baby or a natural baby who has been weaned. A 1979 update is provided to address changes in the adoption scene.

"It may be that the permanent breast changes occurring in any pregnancy, put the mother who has borne a child at an advantage over the mother who has not, but our experience to date has not provided any substantial proof for this view. By and large, nulliparous adoptive mothers and mothers with no recent pregnancy or nursing expereince require roughly the same time to bring in their milk. Just as the sucking stimulus alone maintains milk supply by causing prolaction secretion, so, in the same way, can it start up a milk supply and enlarge the milk ducts to accomodate the milk. . . but it takes time. Breast changes in pregnancy take four to five months. This is not an unreasonable figure for accomplishing it outside a pregnancy either. Some women need less time (but hardly ever less than ten weeks for both tissue development and full milk supply) and some need more. Nearly all will have *some* milk . . . if only in drops . . . after two to six weeks of frequent stimulation."

LACT-AID NURSING TRAINER
Standard Nursing Trainer Kit
$24.50
Deluxe Kit
$36.50
Instructor Pack Kit
$34.50

from
Lact-Aid Service and Supplies Center
P.O. Box 6861
Denver, CO 80206

The Lact-Aid Nursing Trainer is a special device which enables mothers to start or increase lactation after an untimely weaning or separation or in order to nurse an adopted baby. The device consists of a clear plastic bag and nursing tube unit which attaches to the mother's bra and holds four ounces of formula, expressed breast milk or other liquid. A soft tube releases fluid into the baby's mouth as she suckles at the breast. In this way the mother's breast is stimulated in the natural way to produce more

NURSING AN ADOPTED BABY
1982, 8 pages

from
La Leche League
9616 Minneapolis Avenue
Franklin Park, IL 60131
30 cents

It is not easy but it is possible to induce lactation for an adopted baby, even if you have not been pregnant or had a baby before. Here is an excerpt from this La Leche League information publication.

"The way to proceed is to prepare formula just as if the baby were to be a completely formula-fed baby, but to put the baby to the breast to start with—and then to give the formula. Some mothers have inserted a dropper filled with formula into the corner of the baby's mouth while the baby is sucking at the breast to encourage the baby to continue sucking."

The following books contain chapters or sections on nursing an adopted baby. See the index of this *Catalog* for reviews.

The Womanly Art of Breastfeeding
by La Leche League

Nursing Your Baby
by Karen Pryor

The Tender Gift: Breastfeeding
by Dana Raphael

You Can Breastfeed Your Baby: Even in Special Situations
by Dorothy Patricia Brewster

milk, while the baby receives a supplement. As the mother's milk supply increases, less supplement is taken by the baby. The Lact-Aid Nursing Trainer is marketed exclusively by Resources in Human Nursing International (see index). Write for their free brochure.

SPECIAL NURSING TECHNIQUES
28221 Lomo Drive
Rancho Palos Verdes, CA 90274
50 cents

Dorothy Brewster, author of *You Can Breastfeed Your Baby: Even in Special Situations*, provides this updated listing of breast pumps, shields, and other products with manufacturers' addresses and current prices. Some items may also be ordered directly from her.

CLOTHING FOR BREASTFEEDING

Not only are more and more women breastfeeding, but more and more are coming "out of the closet" to nurse their babies in restaurants, stores, parks, and while visiting friends. Many of the books on breastfeeding include advice on how to handle nursing in public discreetly. Often all that's needed is to wear a blouse or sweater with pants or a skirt. If you pull your top up from the waist, your breast is completely covered by both your top and the baby and passers-by rarely notice that you're nursing.

Responding to the desire for attractive, convenient clothing for nursing mothers, many businesses have recently sprung up which supply patterns and ready-made clothing by mail-order. Many of these are home businesses run by women with breastfeeding experience. Some of these are listed below.

BABE TOO!
Route 1, Box 195
Assaria, KS 67416
$4.50 per pattern

RoJean Loucks has designed a very attractive collection of four basic dress patterns with concealed vertical openings over the bustline. Each pattern features a choice of dress and blouse lengths and several sleeve and neckline variations. Waistlines are loose or loosely gathered to provide postpartum comfort. Small (8-10), Medium (12-14), and Large (16-18) sizes are included in each pattern. Request a free descriptive brochure.

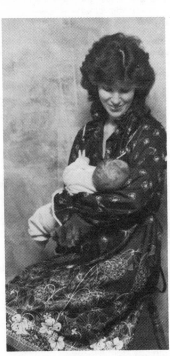

BABY LOVE
790 Griffith Way
Laguna Beach, CA 92651
714/494-6748
Nursing Tops about $16.
Nursing Dress about $27.

Baby Love sells two blouses and one dress design in a variety of cheerful calico, plaid, and print fabrics. Fabric swatches are available and vary with the seasons. Velcro strips are used in two of the styles (see heavy black lines in drawing) and side slits in the other. Specially designed turtlenecks are also available to be worn under blouses and dress. Request a free brochure.

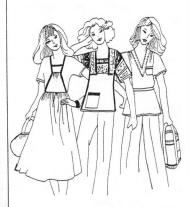

"For five years now we have been pleased to provide fun, yet practical clothes for the nursing mom at reasonable prices. We like to feel nursing moms are special and need to feel and look special."
—Marilyn Jones of Baby Love

MOM'S MATERNITY/NURSING GOWN PATTERN
c/o Cheryll Long
8704 Ralph
Rosemead, CA 91770
$3.25 per pattern

"I have designed a lovely nursing gown pattern which is super simple to to sew and pretty to wear. All sizes are included on each pattern. It requires 2¼ yards of fabric and uses only two pattern pieces. Two concealed slits make easy access to nursing. As a nursing mom I have worn and enjoyed this design for over a year."
—Cheryll Long of Mom's

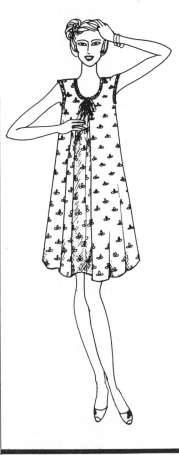

THE NURSING CONCERN
4305 Kensington Road
Baltimore, MD 21229
301/549-1248

The Nursing Concern features a line of blouses, jumpers, and dresses with invisible zippers. Prices range from $14. to $32. Request brochure.

"I make and sell clothing and accessories for nursing moms. My hope is that by making nursing more comfortable, fashionable and/or accessible more babies will be nursed more often and for longer periods of time to make happier, healthier children and future adults."
—Michele Belik of The Nursing Connection

CLOTHES FOR BREASTFEEDING
by Jacqueline McDonald
1981, 24 pages, Illus.
from
Jacqueline McDonald
Route 2, Box 338FF
San Marcos, TX 78666
512/392-6580
$2.50

Jacqueline McDonald offers many useful tips for choosing and adapting ready-made women's clothing and patterns for use in breastfeeding. Her booklet is especially geared to the needs of women who are "more conscious of modesty aspects," particularly those who want to nurse their babies in church.

"The most obvious and most convenient choice, at first, would seem to be a button-front dress or blouse worn with skirt, pants, or shorts . . . But instead of unbuttoning from the top, try unbuttoning from the bottom up (if a blouse). It is just not possible to nurse discreetly and undetected when the shirt or dress is opened from the neck down, unless nursing under some type of cover-up, such as a baby blanket or shawl."

HUGS & KISSES
P.O. Box 490
Crown Point, IN 46307

Hugs & Kisses offers a line of three ready-made blouses in a choice of red, blue, navy, and brown gingham, priced from $23. to $25.

"Each blouse comes complete with a white cord belt. Each blouse has a unique opening on each side that permits you to nurse discreetly. When not in use the opening closes in a way that is nearly invisible. Blouse openings can also be sewn shut after baby is weaned so the blouse can be worn continuously as a fashionable garment."

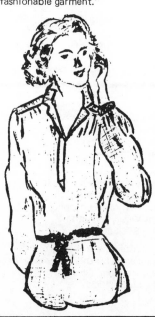

NURSING FASHIONS PACKET
$.50

from
La Leche League
9616 Minneapolis Avenue
Franklin Park, IL 60131

This packet contains many informative sheets, flyers, and brochures offering items for commercial sale and many that can be sewn yourself. Included are helpful hints on bras; ideas on adapting dresses for nursing; underfashions for expectant and breastfeeding mothers; nursing blouses, capes and dresses; numerous baby carriers, as well as the rebozo and the sling.

"Whether sewing your own or buying a ready-made dress, keep in mind that it's for you and baby. Milk stains and baby blanket lint don't show up so badly on prints or light colors. (Black and navy blue are the worst in this respect.) It goes without saying that you want machine-washable-and dryable fabrics. Consider wrinkling, too—a baby's going to be on your lap a lot."

MARY JANE COMPANY
5510 Cleon Avenue
North Hollywood, CA 91609
213/877-7166
$.20 brochure

The Mary Jane Company offers a complete line of maternity and nursing bras and other lingerie for pregnant and nursing mothers, including nightgowns, slips, panties, girdles and pantyhose. Several of their bras are available in cotton blends as well as in nylon and satin tricot. Bras range in price from about $4. to $12.

Mary Jane has also collaborated with La Leche League in producing two documentary, educational films on breastfeeding. Write for more information.

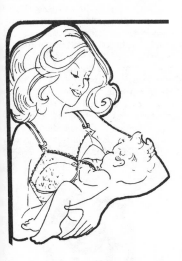

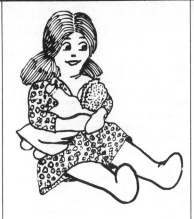

MILK AND HONEY
7345 Sichting Road
Martinsville, IN 46151
317/342-5093
Breastfeeding Dolls, set of handmade mother and baby, $24.00
Pattern, $3.00

"I hand make my patented breastfeeding dolls. I was sick of only finding baby dolls with plastic bottles for feeding them so I made these rag dolls for my daughter and went on to develop it as a business to help enforce breastfeeding through children's play. Also, I am a professional midwife and have helped establish the Indiana Midwives Association, same mailing address."

—Mary Edson of Milk and Honey

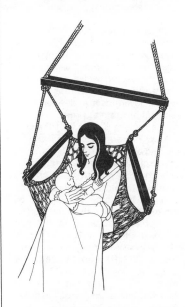

Global View—Auro International, an importer of handcrafted products, uses a nursing mother and baby to illustrate the comfort of their Hammock Chaise, made of cotton rope. The Hammock Chaise retails for about $59. Write or call for more information and a complete catalog of products. Global View—Auro International, Willow Gold, Route 3, Spring Green, Wisconsin 53588, 608/583-5311.

BREASTFEEDING AND WORKING

The issue of breastfeeding and working points up a basic dilemma experienced by mothers in our society. As a feminist, I recognize that women make an essential contribution to the economy and life of the greater community and nation and must be able to pursue their careers with equal access to job opportunities and pay. But as a mother, I know that breastfeeding and intimate care have made an invaluable contribution to the emotional and physical health of my children. I'm glad that I was financially able to stay home with them and provide the kind of care I felt was best. The problem is that our society does not truly value women in either of these roles and does not provide the kinds of programs and services which women need. We need paid parental leave; factories and offices with baby nurseries; flexible employment for parents; better child care services—so that nursing women can continue to work if they wish and so that fathers can spend more time in the day to day care of their children.

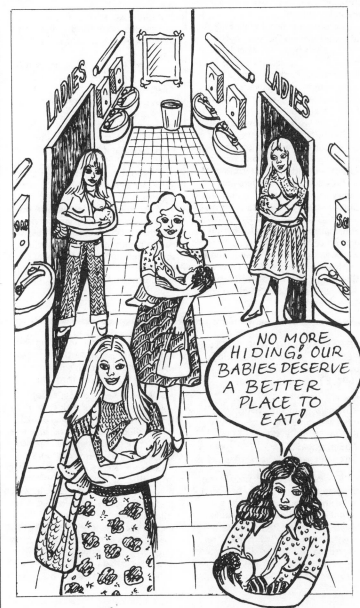

Illustration courtesy of *The Practicing Midwife,* see index.

Bottle Feeding

DOMESTIC FORMULA ABUSE

FORMULA
P.O. Box 39051
Washington, DC 20016

In 1978 the Syntex Corporation decided to stop adding salt (sodium chloride) to its two soy-based infant formulas. This resulted in a deficiency of an essential nutrient, chloride, which was not discovered until 1979 when the products were recalled from the market. An estimated 20,000 infants were fed the defective formula and many became seriously ill, requiring hospitalization, and bewere left with long-term developmental problems.

Carol Laskin and Lynne Pilot, two Washington, DC area mothers, were among those whose children became ill. As a result of their experience, they founded Formula, to make sure that defective formulas could never again reach the market. Both Laskin and Pilot and their husbands had worked in government and were familiar with the workings of the bureaucracy and of the Food and Drug Administration. As a result of this and their determined effort, Laskin and Pilot were able to achieve a major victory in one year's time—passage of the Infant Formula Act of 1980 (see below). Formula continues to provide information for concerned parents, particularly those whose infants may have used the defective formulas (Neo-Mull-Soy and Cho-Free). For more information send a self-addressed, stamped envelope to Formula.

INFANT FORMULA ACT OF 1980

Before the women of Formula began their campaign, the FDA did not set standards for nutrient content of infant formula and did not require routine testing to ensure that the formula matched its content labeling. The Infant Formula Act, which took effect on December 25, 1980, strengthens FDA's control over the safety and nutritional adequacy of infant formula. According to a report in the December 1980/January 1981 issue of *FDA Consumer,* the new law will:

* Set forth a list of nutrients to be provided in infant formulas, and permit FDA to revise the list as needed.

* Require manufacturers to follow effective quality control procedures, established by FDA regulations, to assure that safety and nutritional potency are built into the manufacturing process.

* Require manufacturers to notify FDA of significant changes in their infant formulations before they are made, and to notify FDA of the formulations before new products are marketed.

* Require manufacturers to notify FDA when they have knowledge that their products present a risk to human health, or otherwise violate the adulteration or misbranding provisions of the Federal Food, Drug, and Cosmetic Act.

PETITION TO ALLEVIATE DOMESTIC INFANT FORMULA MISUSE AND PROVIDE INFORMED INFANT FEEDING CHOICE
Prepared by Lois Salisbury and Angela Glover Blackwell on behalf of the petitioners
June, 1981

from
Public Advocates, Inc.
1535 Mission Street
San Francisco, CA 94103
415/431-7430
$7.00

An administrative petition to alleviate the misuse of infant formula in the United States and to promote informed choice in infant feeding, especially among our country's poor women, has been filed with federal agencies and is presently under formal consideration by the department of Health and Human Services and the Food and Drug Administration. The petition was prepared by Public Advocates, a San Francisco-based public interest law firm, which is dedicated to representing the rights of the underrepresented, typically racial minorities, women, the elderly, and children. The co-petitioners supporting the petition include ICEA, NAPSAC, INFACT, the National Women's Health Network, and many groups representing poor and minority women.

The petition documents the low incidence of breastfeeding among minority women, cites the many negative effects of formula feeding, and describes factors which discourage breastfeeding. The petition asks the federal government to develop a national program to promote breastfeeding and calls upon DHHS and FDA to perform specific actions, including banning formula giveaways by hospitals receiving federal funds, and requiring warning labels on infant formula containers. The complete 180-page petition, including over 500 references, was filed in June, 1981, and copies are available from Public Advocates for $7.00. Copies may also be available at no charge from Room 2323, Rayburn House Office Bldg., Washington DC 20500. The petition makes clear that abuse of infant formula is not a problem confined to poor, third world nations, but is adversely affecting the health of women and babies right here in the United States.

"Even with the new found popularity of breastfeeding among middle income women, the fact remains that today a substantial proportion of American women do not breastfeed and among those who do the duration of breastfeeding is severely limited. While the causes of the decline are complex, the important contributing factors are identifiable and include dominance of hospital-centered deliveries, attitudes and practices of medical professionals, and promotional practices of the infant formula industry. . . .

"The present practices in many United States hospitals severely obstruct lactation by interfering with this supply and demand process. These practices reduce the infant's ability or desire to suck and undermine the mother's confidence, thus negatively affecting her letdown reflex. According to the American Academy of Pediatrics Committee on Nutrition, 'Efforts should be made to change obstetrical ward and neonatal unit practices to increase the opportunity for successful lactation.' The practices which inhibit lactation include:
— sedation of the mother during delivery,
— use of lactation suppressants,
— routine separation of the infant and mother at birth,
— hospital layout,
— rigid hospital schedules which prevent demand feeding,
— supplemental feedings,
— distribution of discharge packages,
— general lack of breastfeeding information and support in the hospital setting. . . .

"Breastfeeding is a complex interaction between mother and infant that can be easily enhanced or inhibited by a wide range of social, psychological factors. Although it is a natural function, it is also learned behavior which must be taught to new mothers. . . . enlightened medical practice *can* substantially increase the prevalence and length of successful lactation. Providing information and support to expectant mothers, changes in hospital routines in the perinatal period, in-service professional education, and post partum advice, encouragement and support for lactating mothers have repeatedly been shown to dramatically increase the incidence and duration of breastfeeding in the populations studied. . . . this has been particularly true for low income Black, Hispanic, Asian and Native American women."

BREASTFEEDING AND BOTTLE-FEEDING: Some Considerations
by Rosemary Romberg Wiener
1981, 8 pages, Illus.

from
Rosemary Romberg Wiener
6294 Mission Road
Everson, WA 98247
$.35 plus SASE
bulk rates available

This pamphlet discusses some of the reasons women might not want or be able to breastfeed. For the parent who will be bottlefeeding, Wiener gives very useful advice on ways to make it a "warm, positive experience." She also discusses the use of infant formula and offers information on alternatives to the commercially made kind, including wet-nursing, expressing your own breast milk, milk banks, goat's milk, soy milk, and home made formula.

"When giving the bottle, hold your baby on different sides with different feedings. There is an eye disorder called 'amblyopia' or 'lazy eye' in which one eye does most of the seeing and the other is not working. This causes later reading and learning difficulties. Some cases of this have been linked to bottlefeeding, in which the infant was always held in one position so that one eye was busy looking and the other eye, pressed against the mother's or caretaker's body was not active. This does not happen with a breastfed baby since the mother nurses from both breasts."

THE NESTLE BOYCOTT

For the past several years, the Nestle boycott has focussed attention on the problem of infant formula feeding in the third world. Nestle Company was chosen as a target because it is one of the largest manufacturers of infant formula in the world. Though Nestle does not sell its infant formula in the U.S., the boycott has worked against the many Nestle products which are sold here (see list below).

The major organizer of the Nestle boycott is INFACT (Infant Formula Action Coalition). Throughout the campaign INFACT has made four demands of Nestle:

"An end to direct promotion to the consumer, including mass media promotion and direct promotion through posters, calendars, baby care literature, shows, wrist bands, and baby bottles.

"An end to the use of company milk nurses.

"An end to distribution of free samples and supplies to hospitals, clinics, and homes of newborns.

"An end to promotion to the health professions and through health care institutions."

All of these practices have contributed to what is called "bottle baby disease" in countries throughout Africa, Asia and South America. INFACT literature states:

"Most new mothers in poor countries . . . don't need, and can't afford, artificial baby formula products; their own breast milk is all their babies require in the first 4-6 months. Nevertheless, millions of mothers are abandoning breastfeeding for expensive powdered milks, encouraged by the aggressive promotion campaigns of a profit-hungry industry.

"Inappropriate use of these products—caused by poor sanitary conditions, contaminated water supplies, overdilution, and inability to read instructions for safe preparation—inflicts 'bottle baby disease' on millions of infants every year. Acute diarrhea, early infancy malnutrition, and even death result."

In 1979, the World Health Organization (WHO) and the United Nations Children's Fund (UNICEF) sponsored a meeting in Geneva, Switzerland, and developed guidelines for the marketing and sale of infant formula, which were adopted in 1981. The United Nations endorsed the voluntary code by a vote of 118 to 1, with the United States casting the only opposing vote. The code includes a ban on advertising of infant formula and on providing formula samples to mothers. In the Spring of 1982, Nestle Company announced that it would adhere to the WHO code and hired former Senator Edmund Muskie to head a Nestle-financed committee to monitor their compliance. However, INFACT will continue its boycott of Nestle products until it is satisfied that Nestle, through its actions as well as its words, adheres to the WHO code. Members of the International Nestle Boycott Committee, which support the boycott, include: the American College of Nurse-Midwives, the Childbirth Without Pain Association, the National Organization for Women, and the National Women's Health Network.

For more information on the Nestle boycott and other efforts to reduce the abuse of infant formula feeding in the U.S. and the world contact:

INFACT
(Infant Formula Action Coalition)
1701 University Avenue, SE
Minneapolis, MN 55414

Interfaith Center on Corporate Responsibility
475 Riverside Drive, Room 566
New York, NY 10027
212/870-2750

NESTLE BOYCOTT LIST

Chocolates
Nestle's CRUNCH; Toll House Chips; Nestle's Quik; Hot Cocoa Mix; Choco'lite; Choco-Bake; $100,000 Candy Bar; Price's Chocolates; Go Ahead Bar

Coffees and Teas
Taster's Choice; Nescafe; Nestea; Decaf; Sunrise; Pero

Wines
Beringer Brothers; Los Hermanos; Crosse and Blackwell

Cheeses
Swiss Knight; Wispride; Gerber Cheeses; Old Fort; Provalone Lacatelli; Cherry Hill; Roger's

Packaged Fruits, Soups, Etc.
Libby's; Stouffer frozen foods; Souptime; Maggi Soups; Crosse and Blackwell; Beech Nut Baby Foods

Hotels and Restaurants
Stouffer; Rusty Scupper

Miscellaneous
L'Oreal Cosmetics; Nestle Cookie Mixes; Deer Park Mountain Spring Water; Pine Hill Crystal Water; Kavli Crispbread; McVities; Keiller; James Keller & Son, Ltd.; Contique by Alcon; Ionax by Owen Labs; Lancome

This 18" x 22" poster is printed in black and red ink on brown paper. Copies are available for $2.00 each from the Interfaith Hunger Coalition, 813 S. Hope Street, Los Angeles, CA 90017. The five languages are Spanish, Korean, Vietnamese, Cambodian, and English.

First Decisions

The first important decisions about baby care have to be made in the first minutes and days after birth. These concern the use of silver nitrate in the baby's eyes, treatment of physiologic jaundice, and circumcision. It's a good idea to become familiar with the arguments for and against these procedures before your baby is born, so decisions don't have to be made at the last minute.

Silver Nitrate

Most states require that the eyes of all newborn babies be treated with medication to prevent infection or blindness which can result if the mother has gonorrhea at the time of the birth. Usually this medication is a one percent solution of silver nitrate (an irritant compound used in medicine as an antiseptic). However, silver nitrate can cause eye inflammation and cause the eyes to become puffy and swollen, interfering with parent-infant eye contact and bonding. In response to new questions about the safety and effectiveness of silver nitrate, several states, government agencies, and professional organizations have changed their recommendations to permit the use of alternative medications such as tetracycline or erythromycin eye preparations, which are less irritating to the baby. For more information consult the following resources.

AMERICAN ACADEMY OF PEDIATRICS
Publications Department
P.O. Box 1034
Evanston, IL 60204

The American Academy of Pediatrics has issued new recommendations, indicating that tetracycline or erythromycin are acceptable substitutes for silver nitrate, and also that instillation may be delayed up to one hour after birth to provide for parent-infant bonding. The new guidelines appeared in "Prophylaxis and treatment of neonatal gonococcal infections," *Pediatrics* 65:1047-1048, 1980.

PREVENTION AND TREATMENT OF OPHTHALMIA NEONATORUM
September, 1981, 4 pages

from
National Society to Prevent Blindness
79 Madison Avenue
New York, NY 10016
free

The National Society to Prevent Blindness has updated its statement on ophthalmia neonatorum to note that infectious conjunctivitis of the newborn can be caused by the mother's infection with chlamydia as well as gonorrhea and that silver nitrate does *not* prevent chlamydial infections, while both erythromycin and tetracycline are effective against chlamydia and gonorrhea.

THE SILVER NITRATE CHALLENGE
by Nancy Whittaker and Judy Strasser
1981, 4 pages

from
Mothering Reprints
P.O. Box 2208
Alburquerque, NM 87103
$.75

This reprint of an article in *Mothering Magazine* (Spring, 1981) describes one couple's successful effort to change the silver nitrate law in Wisconsin.

THE QUESTION OF SILVER NITRATE
by Rosemary Romberg Wiener
June 1981, 2 pages

from
Rosemary Romberg Wiener
6294 Mission Road
Everson, WA 98247
$.15 plus SASE

This useful fact sheet describes why silver nitrate is used, what the concerns are about its use, what the legal requirements are, and what alternatives are available.

"Most lay midwives attending home birth do not routinely administer silver nitrate. In practice it has been extremely rare for midwives to encounter any difficulty with babies' eyes because of this. However, occasionally it has happened that a mother did have gonorrhea, gave birth at home, and silver nitrate was not administered. In cases like this it has been learned that there is *time* to treat the baby's eyes before permanent damage takes place. Apparently the baby does not instantly go blind from the gonorrhea. Within the first day or two after birth the baby's eyes will ooze and become irritated, and if this happens it can be treated. If you are giving birth at home, if your birth attendant does not administer silver nitrate or other type of prophylactic ointment for the baby's eyes, and if there is any possibility that you may have gonorrhea, it is of utmost importance that you be alert to this, and get the baby to a doctor immediately to have his/her eyes treated if this should occur."

NEWBORN RIGHTS SOCIETY
Box 48
St. Peters, PA 19470-0048
215/323-6061

In addition to its work in circumcision education, the Newborn Rights Society provides information on the use of silver nitrate and alternatives.

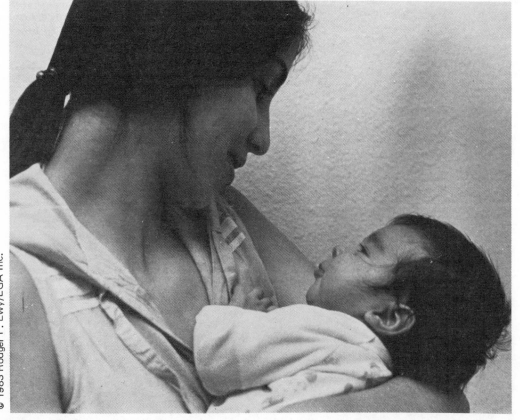

© 1983 Rodger F. Ewy/EGA Inc.

Jaundice

WHEN YOUR BABY HAS JAUNDICE
by Penny Simkin and Margot Edwards
1979, 4 pages

from
the pennypress
1100 23rd Avenue East
Seattle, WA 98112
$.50
bulk rates available

This pamphlet, written for parents, clearly explains what jaundice is, how bilirubin metabolism works, and what factors may be associated with jaundice. It describes the dangers of kernicterus (very high levels of unbound bilirubin) and the current methods of treatment. Advice is given on how to avoid jaundice and/or diminish possible harmful effects of treatment.

"Jaundice is a yellow discoloration of the skin and eyes due to an accumulation of yellow bile pigments (bilirubin) in the blood. In the adult it is caused by disease, malfunction or obstruction of the liver or intestine. In the newborn baby, it is almost always caused by immaturity in the system which metabolizes and excretes bilirubin, although disease or hereditary conditions do rarely cause jaundice in the newborn. Many babies need a week or two before they are able to handle bilirubin in the normal way. In the meantime they have jaundice. Noticeable jaundice is present in about half of full-term babies and about three-fourths or more of premature babies. In most of these babies, the jaundice is mild, lasts a few days and then subsides, without treatment. This type of jaundice is referred to as 'physiologic jaundice' of the newborn. . . .

"Drugs used during labor—some sedatives, tranquilizers, morphine, pitocin (used to induce or speed labor) and Vitamin K may also interfere with bilirubin metabolism. Of course, sometimes the need for the drug and the benefits to the mother are greater than the hazard of jaundice, but the possibility of jaundice in the baby should be considered when one contemplates using such drugs.

"The two main types of treatment are phototherapy and exchange transfusion, and their purpose is to prevent the accumulation of toxic bilirubin and Kernicterus. There is some disagreement among physicians on the need to treat physiologic jaundice.

PHYSIOLOGIC JAUNDICE OF THE NEWBORN
Edited by Susan McKay
1979, 12 pages

from
ICEA Bookcenter
P.O. Box 20048
Minneapolis, MN 55420
$1.00 plus .60 postage

This issue of *ICEA Review* (Spring, 1979) provides an excellent introduction to physiologic jaundice, including the psychological effects of treatment procedures which separate parents and infant. Included are abstracts from the medical literature, references, parent resources, and commentary covering causes of jaundice, how bilirubin is metabolized, "breast milk jaundice," what lab tests show, and different treatment regimens.

"Noticeably lacking in the literature . . . is information dealing with the psychological aspects of physiologic jaundice. Frequently, jaundice occurs at about the same time that the new mother is beginning to 'take

Many believe that phototherapy is safe and it is better to treat jaundice unnecessarily than to withhold treatment which might turn out later to have been necessary. Others believe that most jaundice is harmless and, after ruling out the possibility that the jaundice is anything but physiologic or breast milk jaundice, they watch the baby and check bilirubin levels without treating the baby. They might recommend placing the baby in the sunlight, giving extra fluids, and bringing the baby back to the doctor for checking the bilirubin level."

hold' as a parent, when her milk is just coming in, and when she is especially susceptible to postpartum blues. Knowledge that her baby has jaundice may exacerbate feelings of depression. Parents, who up to this time may have had extensive contact with their baby, are separated from the baby except for feeding periods. Few nurseries make provisions for the parents to spend time in the nursery stroking, comforting, and being near their affected baby while s/he is under the 'bili-light.' The mother may be dismissed from the hospital with empty arms while the baby remains an extra day for phototherapy treatment. . . .

"Even more difficult to evaluate are the psychological effects upon the baby. Sensory deprivation from having a mask over the eyes, sluggishness resulting from phenobarbital drug therapy, and the necessity of being naked under the phototherapy light with less frequent parental contact may cause sequelae of which health professionals are currently unaware."

"PHYSIOLOGIC" JAUNDICE OF THE NEWBORN
by Penny Simkin, Peter A. Simkin and Margot Edwards
1979, 18 pages, Illus.
(Spring, 1979 issue of *Birth and the Family Journal*)

from
BIRTH/Back Issues
110 El Camino Real
Berkeley, CA 94705
$4.00 single issue

This is a longer and more detailed analysis of jaundice and its treatment by the authors of *When Your Baby Has Jaundice* (this page). More detailed information is offered on the relationship between oxytocin during labor and later jaundice and the risks associated with phototherapy. A list of 61 references is included.

" 'Physiologic' jaundice is a time-consuming clinical problem. It is also a condition that exerts emotional stress upon the infant and family and may separate mother and child during the initial bonding period. While classical kernicterus is rare, the hazards associated with hyperbilirubinemia may warrant treatment of the many to save the few. However, new and more accurate tests may provide evidence to show that some cases of neonatal jaundice are indeed 'physiologic,' time-dependent and self-limiting, and that treatment is not necessary. . .

"Investigation is needed to determine the extent of normal 'physiologic' jaundice as opposed to jaundice secondary to iatrogenic factors. There is sufficient information on hand to suggest that certain drugs and obstetric practices are related to a rise in neonatal jaundice. A preventive approach might focus upon the relationship between drugs taken before conception, as well as drugs taken during pregnancy and intrapartum, and subsequent 'physiologic' jaundice. Utilizing a population of women with physiologic labors without any interventions or drugs may provide the basis for comparison that is difficult to find in current data. Surveys of clinical practice might determine whether environmental factors such as artificial versus natural lighting in the hospital nursery cause jaundice, and if continuous and frequent breastfeeding used in conjunction with phototherapy would increase or retard hyperbilirubinemia. A study of jaundiced infants discharged from the hospital with orders to nurse frequently and expose the infants to sunlight, would be valuable in determining whether or not simple treatment measures are efficacious."

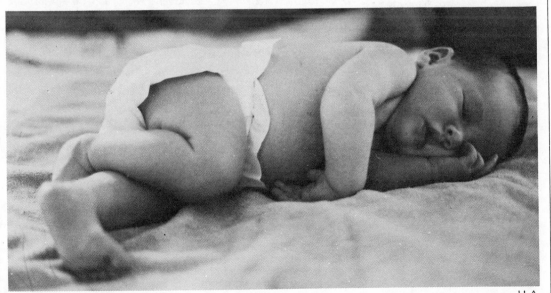

J.I.A.

Circumcision

INTACT EDUCATIONAL FOUNDATION
c/o Rosemary Romberg Wiener
6294 Mission Road
Everson, WA 98247
206/966-5582

The emotional trauma which followed the circumcision of Rosemary Wiener's first son led her to become involved in providing circumcision information to others. Through the INTACT Educational Foundation, she provides an excellent packet of 16 articles on circumcision, a circumcision slide series, and a medical information packet. Write for her complete catalog of informational material and teaching supplies.

INTACT SAMPLE PACKET
$4.00 postpaid

Each of the reprints included in this packet is also available in single copies and in bulk. Write for complete price information. Contents include:

Circumcision
    by Rosemary R. Wiener
The Circumcision Controversy
    by Jeffrey R. Wood
Care of the Uncircumcised Infant/What They Say
Circumcision in Social Perspective
    by Roger Saquet
INTACT Philosophy and Policy
    by Rosemary R. Wiener
Modern Ritualistic Surgery
    by Paul Zimmer
Quotes from *Circumcision: The Painful Dilemma*
    by Rosemary R. Wiener
A Nurse's View on Circumcision
    by Terry Schultz
Jesse's Circumcision
    by M. Pickard-Ginsberg
Guidelines and Suggestions for presenting INTACT Information
    by Rosemary R. Wiener
Why Not to Circumcise Your Baby Boy
    by Sylvia Topp
Circumcision Trauma/Circumcision Reconsidered
    by Rosemary R. Wiener
"The Circ Room" from *Labor and Delivery: An Observer's Diary*
    by Constance F. Bean
Whither the Foreskin?
    by Capt. Noel E. Preston
Should Your Baby Boy Be Circumcised?
    by Rosemary R. Wiener
Circumcision: My Own Story
    by Rosemary R. Weiner

MEDICAL INFORMATION PACKET
$15.00

A selection of 22 articles from the medical literature which support INTACT's position that routine infant circumcision is unnecessary.

CIRCUMCISION: THE PAINFUL DILEMMA
by Rosemary Romberg Wiener
unpublished manuscript

Rosemary Wiener has spent over three years writing an exhaustively researched book on infant circumcision which has already received very favorable comment from childbirth activists who have read it in draft form. Rosemary is now in the process of self-publishing her book. Write to her for more information.

> "We realize now that we made the wrong decision and our reasoning was ridiculous. Any other male children born to us will not be circumcised."

"My husband held the baby to the table while the doctor performed the operation. I found the screams unbearable and retreated to a chair in the waiting room. The doctor told my husband that at that age a baby's penis isn't really that sensitive and he was screaming out of fright and not pain. . . .' There is still a scar to remind me of the incident. We realize now that we made the wrong decision and our reasoning was ridiculous. Any other male children born to us will not be circumcised. . . .

"We decided not to subject our beautiful, whole newborn baby to mutilation and unnecessary pain. I asked a close friend why their son had been circumcised. She said, 'I thought you needed to! You mean you don't have to?!' "

—comments from parents included in *Circumcision: The Painful Dilemma*

—from *Should Your Baby Boy Be Circumcised?* by Rosemary Romberg Wiener, included in the INTACT Sample Packet.

Does Circumcision Hurt the Baby?

"Yes!

"This is what happens when a baby is circumcised. First his arms and legs are strapped down to a plastic board. Then the doctor takes an instrument and tightly pinches the end of his foreskin and cuts a slit in it to make a bigger opening. After that he tears the foreskin away from the glans. There are different ways that the foreskin can be cut off. Sometimes the foreskin is pulled up over the glans, smashed together with a metal device and then sliced off. By another method a small metal "bell" is placed under his foreskin and over his glans. Then a large metal clamp goes down over his penis and crushes his foreskin against the metal bell. After that it is cut off. There is yet another method in which a plastic "bell" is used. Instead of a clamp, a string is tied around the outside of his foreskin over the bell. Then part of the foreskin is trimmed away and the rest dries up and falls off with the piece of plastic in about a week.

"When skin is pinched, torn, clamped, and cut—this **HURTS!!** This hurts a person no matter how old he is! Babies are sensitive and aware of their surroundings. There is no truth to the idea that babies do not feel pain! People usually want to treat babies with a lot of love and gentleness. Cutting and pinching the baby's skin is not what most people want for their babies.

"Usually no anaesthesia is used when babies are circumcised. Most babies scream and cry when it is done. But some babies are so overcome with pain that they cannot cry! Often babies fall into a deep, "withdrawal" type of sleep after the operation.

"Many people believe that this traumatic operation can cause long lasting psychological damage to the child."

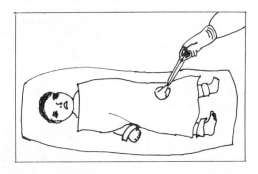

From *Should Your Baby Boy Be Circumcised?* by Rosemary Romberg Wiener, $.45 each from INTACT Educational Foundation, c/o Rosemary Romberg Wiener, see left.

INTACT EDUCATIONAL FOUNDATION
c/o Jeffrey R. Wood
P.O. Box 5
Wilbraham, MA 01095
413/596-8959

Jeffrey Wood is the founder and president of INTACT and has most INTACT reprints available in small quantities.

"INTACT stands for Infants Need to Avoid Circumcision Trauma—a conviction shared, in view of recent medical findings, by a growing number of people. Established in 1976 as a local resource, this grass-roots activity has attracted the devoted efforts of concerned individuals nationwide, achieving recognition by health care professionals and lay persons alike for its clear insight into what is rapidly becoming one of our society's more significant human rights issues. Unfettered by even the slightest trace of anti-Semitism, the scope of the Foundation's work encompasses the religious symbolism of both circumcision and non-circumcision, shedding critically needed light on an area of controversy too long enshrouded by ignorance and superstition."
        —Jeffrey Wood of INTACT

NEWBORN RIGHTS SOCIETY
Box 48
St. Peters, PA 19470-0048
215/323-6061

The Newborn Rights Society, headed by Paul Zimmer, provides information on "unnecessary medical procedures that are harmful and painful to the newborn," with an emphasis on circumcision but also covering the routine use of silver nitrate in the eyes of newborns.

"Surgical removal of a baby's foreskin (usually without anesthesia) offers no medical or social advantages for the child, but does cause unnecessary pain as well as the risk of permanent injury, bleeding, disfigurement and possible death. Beware that most health care providers have been taught to retract the foreskin of intact infants. This has been proven to be unnecessary and usually causes problems. DON'T LET THIS HAPPEN TO YOUR BABY.

"Silver nitrate drops are used in the eyes of the newborn to prevent gonorrhea-caused blindness and are useless and insulting to the 95% of babies whose mothers have been able to keep themselves free of gonorrhea. Silver nitrate itself causes chemical irritation to the eyes with possible temporary blindness and interference with bonding."
—from The Newborn Rights Society

The Society provides the following materials and others. Send a business-sized envelope with two stamps for a packet of information.

Modern Ritualistic Surgery
by Paul Zimmer
$.15 plus business-sized SASE
$10.00 per hundred

Circumcision "Nonessential" Pediatrics Academy is Told (from the *National Health Federation Bulletin*, January 1978)
$.10 plus SASE
$5.00 per hundred

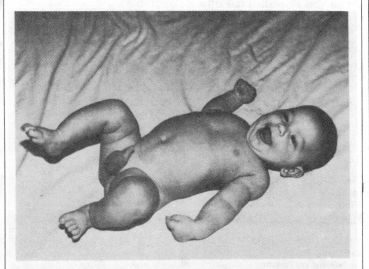

I was born perfect and fortunately my parents kept me that way.

Newborn Rights Society

REPORT OF THE AD HOC TASK FORCE ON CIRCUMCISION
Committee on Fetus and Newborn
American Academy of Pediatrics
1975

from
American Academy of Pediatrics
P.O. Box 1034
Evanston, IL 60204
free

Conclusions

There is no absolute medical indication for routine circumcision of the newborn. The physician should provide parents with information pertaining to the long-term medical effects of circumcision and noncircumcision, so that they make a thoughtful decision. It is recommended that this discussion take place before the birth of the infant, so the parental consent to the surgical procedure, if given, will be truly informed.

A program of education leading to continuing good personal hygiene would offer all the advantages of routine circumcision without the attendant surgical risk. Therefore, circumcision of the male neonate cannot be considered an essential component of adequate total health care.

AD HOC TASK FORCE ON CIRCUMCISION
Hugh C. Thompson, M.D., *Chairman*
Lowell R. King, M.D.
Eric Knox, M.D.
Sheldon B. Korones, M.D.

In 1971, the American Academy of Pediatrics stated that there are "no valid medical indications for circumcision in the neonatal period." Reviewing the question again in 1975, the Academy finds no basis for changing its statement.

OLYMPIC CIRCUMSTRAINT
promotional flyer

from
Olympic Medical
4400 Seventh South
Seattle, WA 98108
free

Olympic Medical manufactures a molded plastic restraining device with Velcro straps to keep infants immobilized during the circumcision procedure. Parents may want to see a copy of the flyer which shows this device in use, before deciding whether or not to have their newborn son circumcised.

"In less than 30 seconds, a nurse can immobilize the struggling infant securely in the correct position with Circumstraint. It works on a proven principle of positive 4-point restraint. Soft, wide Velcro straps encircle the infant's elbows and knees, depriving him of leverage. He's held safely and securely without danger of escape. Circumstraint's comfortable contoured shape positions the infant, hips elevated, perfectly presenting the genitalia. The platform between the infant's legs provides support for a circumcision clamp. Without pins, towels, plastic shells or the threat of strangulation, Circumstraint snugly and securely immobilizes the infant with his entire torso visible."

NON-CIRCUMCISION INFORMATION CENTER
P.O. Box 404
Ipswich, MA 01938

The Non-Circumcision Information Center, headed by Roger Saquet, works to discourage routine neonatal circumcision by distributing the following reprints free on request (please include a large, stamped envelope). The reprints are also available in bulk for the prices listed.

Whither the Foreskin?
by Noel Preston ($.10 each)
Circumcision in Social Perspective
by Roger Saquet ($.07½ each)
Penile Plunder
by William K.C. Morgan ($.07½ each)

OTHER RESOURCES

CHILDREN'S BETTER HEALTH INSTITUTE
1100 Waterway Blvd.
Box 567
Indianapolis, IN 46206

Provides a booklet with photographs of a baby being circumcised, available for $2.00. Other materials available.

CIRCUMCISION INFORMATION CENTER OF NEW YORK
Box 765, Times Square Station
New York, NY 10108-0765

Send $1.00 and a legal size SASE for packet of information on circumcision. (Mostly INTACT material)

CIRCUMCISION: An American
Health Fallacy
by Edward Wallerstein
1980, 281 pages, Illus.

from
Springer Publishing Company
200 Park Avenue South
New York, NY 10003
$12.95 pap.

Edward Wallerstein is a retired businessman and engineer who has worked in the application of telecommunications to the health field. Spurred by a personal curiosity and interest in the subject, Wallerstein has researched and written a comprehensive book on circumcision which covers the history of the procedure, why it is prevalent only in the U.S., and discusses the relation of circumcision to hygiene, venereal disease, cancer, premature ejaculation, and masturbation. He describes the pain and psychological trauma for the infant and the medical risks of the procedure. Also included are chapters on circumcision in the Jewish tradition and on female circumcision and genital mutilation.

"There appears to be a dilemma between medical theory and practice in regard to circumcision. Twenty-five years ago, it was rare to find an anti-circumcision article in the medical press. Since then, editors of medical journals have made impassioned pleas for objectivity and research. In the past decade, articles on the subject are more likely than not to be critical of one or all aspects of the practice; most express doubt and caution; few defend it outright. Yet the surgery continues with undiminished zeal. When tonsillectomy was questioned as often unnecessary, the incidence of its performance diminished; not so with circumcision. The reason for this dilemma will not be found in scientific rationale, but in the unique nature of circumcision. Unlike any other surgery, circumcision, in addition to being employed therapeutically and prophylactically, is heavily laden with sexual, religious, cultural, and social overtones. It is therefore difficult to obtain an objective analysis of the value of the practice. . . .

"Probably the most widely acclaimed circumcision benefit is that it simplifies penile hygiene. This is the key to all its other alleged advantages. The reasoning is as follows:

* The penis in its natural state is difficult to keep clean.
* Such lack of cleanliness provides a convenient place for smegma and dirt to accumulate and for germs to hide.
* The accumulated smegma, deposited on the cervix in coitus, causes cervical cancer, and the smegma infiltrating the urethra cause prostatic cancer.
* The subpreputial accumulations irritate (stimulate) the erogenous foreskin lining, causing masturbation.
* The very presence of the foreskin makes the glans excessively sensitive. This results in premature ejaculation.
* Over long periods, smegma can cause penile cancer.

The problems with the above statements is that, although they seem reasonable and logical, they are either patently false or at best unsubstantiated."

Summary: Care of the Uncircumcised Penis Before Retraction Takes Place:

1) Frequent bathing or sponge bathing of your baby is necessary.
2) Make sure all the folds and wrinkles of the genitals are cleansed after bowel movements and with diaper changes. The uncircumcised penis requires no extra cleaning—just wash, rinse, and dry it, along with the rest of the baby's bottom.
3) Wash away any smegma appearing on the outside of the penis, but don't try to wash or clean under the foreskin.
4) DO NOT retract (pull back) the foreskin over the glans of the penis. In a newborn, the foreskin is almost always attached to the glans. Forcing the foreskin back may damage the penis, causing pain, bleeding, possible scarring and adhesions, thus making circumcision necessary.
5) DO NOT let your pediatrician forcibly retract the foreskin of your newborn. Some pediatricians today remain uninformed on this matter, and believe that at birth the foreskin must be retractable. If it is not, they force it. As familiarity with the normal uncircumcised penis increases, there will be less of this improper care and improper advice.
6) Separation of the foreskin from the glans may take years.
7) To test whether or how much the foreskin has separated, either:
   a) observe an erection (all baby boys have them). If a full erection occurs, full retraction has also occured; or
   b) Hold the penile shaft with one hand and with the other hand, GENTLY push the foreskin back, only as far as it goes easily. STOP if the baby seems to be uncomfortable or if you feel resistance.
8) Test for retraction every few months.

After the Foreskin is Fully Retractable:

1) Until the child can bathe himself, an adult bathes him.
2) When washing the penis, retract the foreskin gently, wash the glans, rinse, and replace the foreskin, teaching the child that this is how the penis should be washed.
3) Sometimes, after the child takes over his own bathing, he is careless and the glans becomes red and sore. Washing the penis and applying a protective ointment will quickly clear up the problem.

—from *The Circumcision Decison*

THE CIRCUMCISION DECISION
by Edward Wallerstein
1980, 4 pages
50 cents each, bulk rates available

WHEN YOUR BABY BOY IS NOT
CIRCUMCISED
by Edward Wallerstein
1982, 4 pages
50 cents each, bulk rates available

from
the pennypress
1100 23rd Avenue East
Seattle, WA 98112

The pennypress provides two pamphlets on infant circumcision as part of the *Better Baby Series*. Both are written by Edward Wallerstein, author of *Circumcision: An American Health Fallacy*. *The Circumcision Decision* provides a summary of the pros and cons of infant circumcision and *When Your Baby Boy. . .* provides information for parents on caring for the uncircumcised penis.

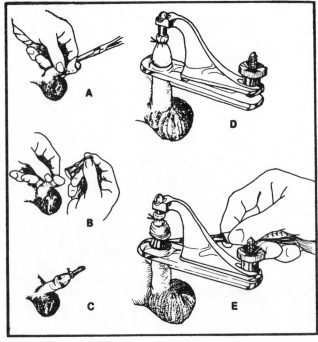

Circumcision with the Gomco Clamp.

CIRCUMCISION INFORMATION PAMPHLET
24 pages

from
Mothering Magazine
P.O. Box 2208
Albuquerque, NM 87103
$3.50

The pamphlet provides an anthology of articles which have appeared in *Mothering Magazine* on circumcision, including many letters from parents who regretted their decision to circumcise their sons.

Circumcision is a voluntary procedure. Though considered routine in many hospitals, a circumcision may not be performed without the consent of a parent.

"Even as I write now, two years later, the memory of those moments make it difficult to continue. I can still hear Jesse's crying. . . begging for someone to stop the pain . . . screaming of being violated. Elizabeth soaked a wash cloth in wine which he intermittently sucked; tears streaming down her face. His little hands clutched my thumb. Sharon's OMs occasionally drifted between screams—bless her. Steve was explaining that Jesse's foreskin was unusually tight; a dorsal slit was necessary. He asked how we were while holding the hemostat on Jesse's bloody penis after each cut. Hemorrhaging was important to avoid.

"Why didn't we stop him? Shock?

"He cut again. Pulling back the foreskin, Steve revealed the tip of Jesse's penis; the color of raw liver. This was circumcision? Finally, he put the bell clamp around the tip of Jesse's penis and clamped it. Jesse let out a scream we will never forget. It crescendoed up and up until his mouth hung open, face distorted, and no sound came out. Pure anguish.

"Twenty-five minutes had passed. A sacred boundary had been crossed. Never again will a son of mine be circumcised without medical reason.

"As was traditional, we said a few blessings and served cake and wine. To me this seemed barbaric. What had Jesse gained from this 'tradition'? What meaning could it have for him? How could Elizabeth and I justify violating this body? We couldn't and can't.

"I urge you to attend a circumcision if you are considering one for your son. Feel what he feels. How would you feel being tied down and cut? Foreskins are often tight and may take a few years (up to three sometimes) before they are fully retractable.

"Perhaps the circumcision shocked me into the reality of importance of the responsibility a parent bears for these delicate (though strong) souls we help bring into the world."
—from "Jesse's Circumcision" by M. Pickard-Ginsberg.

CIRCUMCISION
edited by Rosemary Cogan
1981, 8 pages

from
ICEA Bookcenter
P.O. Box 20048
Minneapolis, MN 55420
$1.00 plus 60 cents postage

This issue of *ICEA Review* (April, 1981) provides an introduction and abstracts of medical literature on circumcision, covering attitudes toward circumcision, effect on the neonate, complications, cancer of the penis, cervical cancer among women, and sensitivity of the penis. Included are line drawings and descriptions of the Plastibell and Gomco clamp circumcision techniques.

"Among some groups, circumcision has been carried out in adolescence and serves as a major part of a rite of passage from child to adult status. Among other groups, and most frequent in Western countries today, it is the neonate who is circumcised. Circumcision in the eighth day of life remains traditional among Jews; circumcision within the first two or three days of life is characteristic of other contemporary Western groups. The rate of circumcision has varied considerably at different times and places. Gairdner suggested that circumcision has become a common surgical procedure with the rise of modern surgery during the nineteenth century. In the United States, the circumcision rate increased from about 8% before 1870 to 20% from 1900 to 1910, 50% from 1930 to 1940, and about 80% during the 1950's. During the

> "The rate of circumcision has varied considerably at different times and places. Gairdner suggested that circumcision has become a common surgical procedure with the rise of modern surgery during the nineteenth century."

1970's, several large scale studies found that more than 90% of live born males in the United States were circumcised before they were discharged from the hospital at which they were born. Circumcision rates are considerably lower in other English-speaking countries such as Canada (50% circumcision rate), Australia ('45%), Newfoundland (30%) and England, where circumcision is rare."

circumcision

we have broken a child's spirit
he looked at me
before we began
and knew me for who i am
hey he said to me
in his gentle smile of recognition
hey you are the same as me
you must be who i am
and then i held down his legs
as we cut off his foreskin
infinitely sore tender life of orgasm
we rejected his life
force
power
he could not fight us off
despite the fact
that he fought with all his might
he gave up the fight
his legs lay beneath the ten ton fire
of my hands
and stayed there
with all his might drained
even after i had let him up

i cannot believe
that it does not harm so tender a life
to have his spirit broken
at this tender time of his life

at my hands
who has ushered in his life

from *Birth Song* by Karen Hope Ehrlich (see review and ordering information on page 104).

© 1979 Karen Hope Ehrlich. Reprinted by permission.

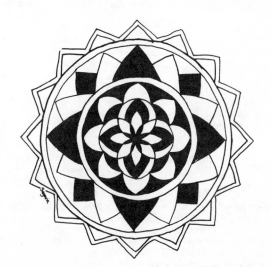

Baby and Child Care

Mary Scott, editor

There is so much information from all sorts of sources about how to care for babies that if any parent read all of it the babies would never be taken care of! Fortunately, most parents can sift through enough advice from friends, relatives, doctors, books, etc., to raise healthy, happy children. Your own baby is your best source of information. Either you will know intuitively or the little one will tell you of her/his wants and needs.

We include here some of the better pamphlets with basic information on baby care during the first year of life.

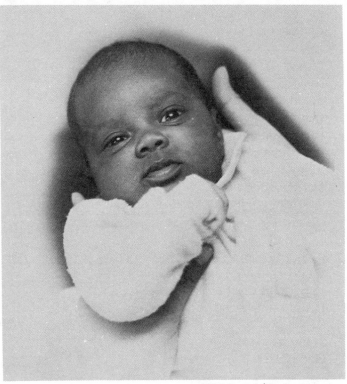

© 1983 Artemis/Harriette Hartigan

THE VERY NEW BABY: The First Days of Life
by June V. Schwartz and Emma R. Botts
1977, 28 pages (pamphlet No. 553)
50 cents

YOUR FIRST MONTHS WITH YOUR FIRST BABY
by Alicerose Barman
1979, 24 pages (pamphlet No. 478)
50 cents

from
Public Affairs Pamphlets
381 Park Avenue South
New York, NY 10018

The Very New Baby is a fairly complete layperson's guide to the first few days of life, discussing how the baby adjusts to its new environment and what signs to look for. In *Your First Months with Your First*

Baby, the author discusses the changes in lifestyle which a new baby brings, describing "the job and the joy" of first parenthood. Subjects include "sex education," "how life style changes," "a father's special role." Parental and child expectations of each other are discussed generally and in a friendly-advice style. (MS)

"Discipline should not be confused with punishment. A discipline is a body of knowledge; a disciple is a follower. Disciplining a child should really mean guiding him to learn what sorts of behavior will help him achieve socialization, learning, and pleasure for himself and make him acceptable to others."
—from *Your First Months with Your First Baby.*

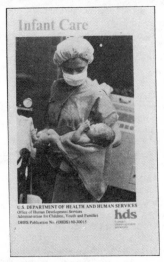

INFANT CARE
by A. Frederick North
1980, 67 pages

from
U.S. Department of Health and Human Services
Office of Human Development Services
Washington, DC 20201

This booklet has been continuously printed by the federal government since 1914 and was last updated in 1980. It provides clear and concise information which takes parents and children in complete stages from birth through the first year of life. Includes basics like feeding and bathing, but also goes into development and motor skills, common problems and worries, teething, laundering, and many more topics. A Safety Checklist is included for several sections, based on the baby's changing capabilities. Write for this booklet directly or ask your local Senator or Congressperson to get you a copy. (MS)

"Don't be surprised if one doctor doesn't give you the same advice as another, or even if they actually disagree with each other or with what you read in this book.

"For many problems, there are many successful treatments, and this book only mentions one. For some other problems, such as colds, each doctor may have a favorite medicine, none of which makes much difference. For still other problems (whether boys should be circumcised, for example) there are real differences of opinion. When two doctors give you directly conflicting advice you should ask for an explanation. If the explanation is convincing, fine. If not, you will have to get a third opinion or make up your own mind.

"Don't neglect your own health and comfort. You will be a better parent if you eat nourishing food, get enough sleep and exercise, and keep up with your friends and interests."

JOHNSON & JOHNSON
Consumer and Professional Services
220 Centennial Avenue
Piscataway, NJ 08854

The following booklets on baby care are available free from Johnson & Johnson, makers of baby care products. (MS)

FIRST-TIME PARENTS
1976, 19 pages

This good basic primer is worth writing for if it's not included in the packet you may get from the hospital. Included is a discussion of breastfeeding versus bottle-feeding as well as the options for diapering baby and common "how-to's" from bathing to safe toys to taking a temperature. Easy to read, it also includes a blank Baby's Health Record and a fairly complete list for stocking the nursery.

GETTING TO KNOW YOUR NEWBORN
1978, 18 pages

What is your crying baby "telling" you? What makes touching a baby extra special? What games make playtime more than just playtime? This little pamphlet has many good ideas about getting to know your baby. It also includes eight coupons for cents off on Johnson & Johnson baby products.

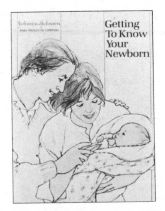

BABY CARE BASICS
1980, 50 pages

A much more complete guide than the others in this series, this pamphlet is divided into four areas of concentration: baby's eating and sleeping habits, keeping baby clean, when baby is ill, and a safe world for babies and toddlers. Considering the source of this pamphlet, the second part is understandably loaded with references to the products you may wish to use; however the rest of the pamphlet is quite factual, easy to read, and does a good job of pointing out all aspects of the choices when there are different options for caring for baby: for example, cloth versus disposable diapers. The section on diagnosing and treating illness is particularly good.

Bathing Your Baby

"During the first week, before the cord has fallen off and the navel heals, wash the baby with a cloth wrung out in warm water. The face and diaper area require frequent washing, since food, urine, and bowel movements can irritate the skin. The rest of the body may need washing only several times a week.

"After the first week or two, you may find it more convenient to give the bath in a tub or dishpan. You will need the following:

* A warm room
* A table or counter top of convenient height
* A tub or dishpan containing an inch or two of warm water. Check to be sure it is not too hot.
* You may want to put a small towel or diaper in the bottom of the tub to keep the baby from skidding on the slippery surface.
* A bar of mild soap
* A wash cloth or other soft cloth
* A full-size towel or 'receiving blanket' to dry the baby

"Wash the head and face first while the water and wash cloth are cleanest. You don't need soap for the face. Use your hand to lather the rest of the body with soap. Wash your girl's labia and your boy's penis just as you wash any other part of their body. You may find it easier to wash your baby on the table on a towel, and use the tub only for rinsing. Rinse your baby thoroughly with the wash cloth—at least two rinsings—then wrap your baby in a towel and pat dry. Wash the hair with a non-irritating baby shampoo about once a week, or more frequently if your baby has the scaly, waxy rash of cradle cap. Don't worry about the soft spot on the head—it's tough!

"Don't worry if you can't bathe your infant every day: 2 or 3 baths a week are enough for most babies. Some babies quickly learn to enjoy their bath, and it becomes a daily pleasure. Others strongly object to the bath the first 8 or 10 times it is tried. They will gradually learn to tolerate the bath and perhaps even to enjoy it.

"Use a nail clipper to keep finger and toe nails short. Cut them straight across, and try to clip them when the baby is relaxed or asleep. At other times sudden playful motions may make clipping difficult, and you might accidentally clip the skin.

"NEVER, NEVER LEAVE THE BABY ALONE IN THE WATER FOR ANY REASON WHATSOEVER!!!

"If the telephone or doorbell rings, or your 2-year-old hollers, wrap the baby (soap and all) in a towel and put the baby under your arm. The bath is *never* safe, no matter how little water you may use, until well into the second or third year of life. If there is a real crisis or emergency, put the baby on the floor. He can't fall or drown there.

"**Always check the water temperature.** Hot water causes scalds and burns! Don't leave the baby in the tub with the water running.

"**Don't try to clean the ears, nose, navel, vulva or anus with cotton-tipped sticks.** Anything you can't clean with a corner of a wash cloth doesn't need cleaning.

"**Don't use special disinfectant soap for every bath and cleansing.** Plain soap is the best. Too much soap can be almost as irritating to the skin as is dirt, food, or soiled diapers."

—Bathing instructions from *Infant Care*, distributed by the U.S. Department of Health and Human Services, see pg. 226.

Bath time is an opportunity for you and your baby to relax and remember the comfort of the womb in sound and touch and to continue bonding together. Speak softly, don't rush, and enjoy the once-every-day-or-so experience. The pamphlets listed on this page provide step-by-step instructions for safe and comfortable bathing of an infant. However, none mention the possibility of communal bathing, that is, getting into the bath tub with your baby or handling her to Daddy in the tub. While the grown-ups will have to get used to the cooler water temperature for the baby, this kind of bathing can be extra fun for all. Baby can be supported by knees, laps, chest as well as hands. It's especially nice to try this in hot weather, when you and the baby can stand a cool-off. (MS)

BATHING

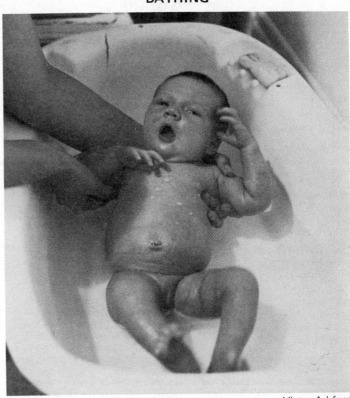
Victor Ashford

HOW TO BATHE YOUR BABY IN SAFETY AND COMFORT
brochure

from
Pansy Ellen Products, Inc.
P.O. Box 720274
Atlanta, GA 30358
free

This handy brochure illustrates sponge or tub bathing using the Pansyette Bath Aid ($7.00 plus $1.50 shipping). The Bath Aid is a formfit sponge that you can lay the baby on so s/he is comfortable and secure and your hands are free. This product can be used alone, in a baby bath tub or in the large tub until Baby learns to flip over or sit up. Pansy Ellen also makes a sponge Comfy Seat and other products.

HOW TO BATHE YOUR BABY
poster, 17" x 22"

from
Johnson & Johnson
Consumer and Professional Services
220 Centennial Avenue
Piscataway, NJ 08854

One side of this illustrated blue, yellow and white poster shows how to bathe a baby either in a baby tub or by sponge bath (although no one ever mentions the advantages of using an actual sponge rather than a wash cloth). The other side shows "How Your Baby Grows" from birth to 24 months including body, hand, speech and social development. (MS)

A GUIDE TO BATHING YOUR BABY
pamphlet

from
Newman-Fine, Inc.
P.O. Box 2004
New York, NY 10017
free

What you will need, how to test the water temperature, how much water to use, how to wash (from the top to the bottom), and how to dry are all carefully explained with cute illustrations by the makers of the Tubby inflatable baby bathtub. The Tubby supports baby's head, contains only enough water to wash without creating a hazard, and can be deflated and carried for traveling. The Tubby costs $9.95 plus $1.00 for shipping, NY residents add sales tax. (MS)

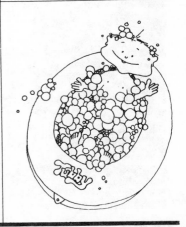

STIMULATION

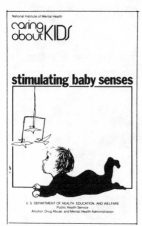

STIMULATING BABY SENSES
by Marilyn Sargent
1978, 10 pages

from
Public Inquiries
National Institute of Mental Health
5600 Fishers Lane
Rockville, MD 20857
free

Using science and common sense you can stimulate your baby's five senses with this little booklet as a first guide. It is divided into brief, thoughtful sections on each of the five senses indicating how senses function in infants and how they grow. (MS)

"Although many modern fathers and mothers are trying to free themselves from traditional sex roles, some studies show that many parents behave differently with their boy and girl babies. There seems to be a tendency for parents to imitate and re-spond to the sounds of girls more. Some researchers have wondered if this is one of the reasons little girls usually talk earlier than boys. On the other hand, parents often stimulate muscular development of boy babies more—offering thumbs to grasp, helping them to their feet when they start to pull themselves up."

100 WAYS TO ENTERTAIN YOUR BABY
by Nancy Everhart
10 page booklet

from
Nancy Everhart
Tamaqua, PA 18252
$1.00

Here is a wonderful source to spark your imagination or supplement a tired-out one. Nancy Everhart has come up with 100 ideas, divided into sections, to fit the needs of babies from birth to three years. They are usually ideas for playing *with* your child, although some instigate solo activity. None require any expensive or hard-to-find materials. Get it yourself and for a friend! (MS)

"No. 23. Blow soap bubbles for your baby to watch. . . .
No. 26. Lie the baby down and stand above him. Let a tissue, piece of cotton or feather float down and touch him. . . .
No. 46. Hang a beach ball from a tree or doorway with a piece of elastic for baby to bat."

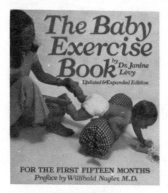

THE BABY EXERCISE BOOK: For the First Fifteen Months
by Janine Levy, translated from the French by Eira Gleasure
1975, 127 pages, Illus.

from
Pantheon/Random House
201 East 50th Street
New York, NY 10022
$4.95 pap.

"This book, which is the result of long experience, was published with the intention of offering parents and educators a method of developing self-awareness in infants and very young children through their movements," says the introduction. This book also will encourage parents to actively interact with their infants, becoming acutely aware of them and themselves as well. The book begins with a clear description of the equipment you will need (slant boards, a beachball, a roll), specific instructions for making things (including a rag doll for parents to practice on before doing exercises with baby), and a list of alternatives to the specific pieces of equipment, using ordinary things found at home. Then the book divides into chapters covering four phases from birth to fifteen months, each of which clearly describes different exercises and "gymnastics" parents can do with their baby and why they are important. Each section also contains excellent black and white photo illustrations of what to do. These exercises are not "gym" but are based on the movements that young children normally make while playing and exploring their worlds. All movements and exercises are to be done without any clothing on the infant, to allow the most freedom of movement and touch sensation. The emphasis is on relaxing, limbering and strengthening little muscles which will later be used for rolling over, crawling, lifting up the head. Dr. Levy developed both the concept and these exercises over many years while working with babies in many infant nurseries and care centers in Paris and in her special center for infant physical development. (MS)

INFANT MASSAGE
brochure

from
Monterey Laboratories, Inc.
P.O. Box 15129
Las Vegas, NV 89114
free

"Never heard of baby massage, you say? Your mother didn't massage you? Well, it's an ancient art practiced around the world. It is not only very pleasurable for the infant, but also a wholesome way to show your baby your love, as touching is the baby's first means of communication with a new environment."

Step-by-step instuctions with photographs show how to properly and enjoyably massage an infant and how to practice massage before the baby comes. It's good for the whole family! Monterey Labs make a baby massage oil with vitamin E and produces an 80-page booklet on infant massage. Write for more information. (MS)

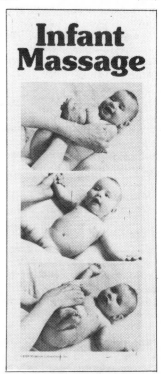

WARMTH AND YOUR BABY
2 pages

from
Weleda, Inc.
Spring Valley, NY 10977
free

How to "gentle" your newborn into the world is the topic of this little pamphlet. The warmth of natural fabrics, soft light, and soft voices in addition to warmth of temperature and temperament are discussed as necessary for healthy, happy babies. Weleda produces "natural" baby preparations including powder, cream, and oil. Write for more information. (MS)

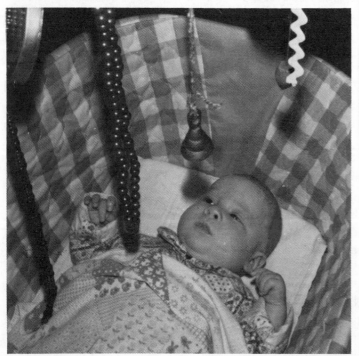

J.I.A.

IMMUNIZATION

IMMUNIZATION—Protection Against Childhood Diseases
by Jules Saltman
1978, 22 pages, Illus.

from
Public Affairs Pamphlets
381 Park Avenue South
New York, NY 10016
50 cents

This pamphlet explains in detail how immunization and vaccines work and describes the seven serious childhood diseases for which vaccines are available: diptheria, pertussis (whooping cough), tetanus (lockjaw), poliomyelitis (infantile paralysis), measles, rubella (german measles), and mumps. (JIA)

"The idea of deliberately giving people a disease in order to protect them from infection was a daring one a century and a half ago, when Dr. Edward Jenner first tried it. He had noted that milkmaids who had gone through the minor ailment caused by cowpox did not catch the much more serious disease, smallpox. The development of smallpox vaccination (the name comes from *vaccinia,* the technical word for cowpox) has been the most successful as well as being the first application of the idea. Smallpox as a naturally occurring disease has now been eradicated."

AMERICAN NATURAL HYGIENE SOCIETY
Human Rights Department
c/o Grace Girdwain
8320 S. Nashville Avenue
Burbank, IL 60459

Grace Girdwain provides assistance and support to parents who wish to refuse routine immunization for their children, particularly for those who need exemption from local laws requiring mandatory immunization for school. Ms. Girdwain has provided the following listing of further resources. (JIA)

Vaccinations Do Not Protect
by Eleanor McBean

Life Science
P.O. Box 17128
Austin, TX 78760
$1.75

The Dangers of Immunization

The Humanitarian Society
Box 77
Quakertown, PA 18951
$2.75

Parents Rights Card

National Committee for Citizens in Education
410 Wilde Lake Village Green
Columbia, MD 21044
$.10

IMMUNIZATION INFORMATION PAMPHLET
28 pages

from
Mothering Magazine
P.O. Box 2208
Albuquerque, NM 87103
$4.00

Some parents question the value and safety of mass routine immunization, particularly since immunization can occasionally have harmful side effects. In this anthology of articles from *Mothering Magazine,* nutritionist Leonard Jacobs, pediatrician Robert Mendelsohn, natural hygienist Grace Girdwain, nurses, doctors, parents and others discuss the pros and cons of immunization. (JIA)

"It is admitted by the medical profession that there are possible complications arising from the use of any vaccine. But often the family pediatrician related this to the patient by saying that the risks are hardly considerable compared to the risks of disease itself. This is misleading—actually in many instances it is false. There are many side effects from smallpox vaccine (encephalitis, eczema vaccinatum, accidental implant of vaccinia on eye, superinfection of other skin conditions), whooping cough (high fever, convulsions, encephalopathy), and measles (encephalitis, subacute sclerosing panencephalitis, ataxia, retardation, learning disability, hyperactivity, aseptic meningitis, seizure disorders, hemiparesis) that are now viewed as classic. That is, these are the more commonly seen complications as described by the medical profession. I worry about the the extent of side effects resulting from vaccination not yet questioned by doctors.

"Other interesting items with regard to assurances: 1) Today parents of school children sign a paper agreeing not to sue if complications arise from compulsory immunizations. 2) In California, there is a new law providing up to $25,000 for medical expenses for kids who have *catastrophic* reactions to mandatory immunizations. In the words of Marion Tompson, 'The fact that this law was enacted makes me feel that such reactions can't be all that rare!' "
—from *A Mother's Research on Immunization* by Patricia Savage

SCHEDULE OF VISITS

Procedures During Visit	In Hosp.	1 Mo.	2 Mos.	4 Mos.	6 Mos.	8 Mos.	12 Mos.	15 Mos.
			AGE AT VISIT					
Discussion & Questions	●	●	●	●	●	●	●	●
Examination	●	●	○	○	○	○	●	○
Measurements of Length, Weight, Head Size	●	●	●	●	●	●	●	○
Questions and Tests About Development	○	●	○	○	●	○	●	○
DTP Shot			●	●	●			
Oral Polio Vaccine			●	○	●			
Measles, Mumps and Rubella Shot								●
Blood Test for Anemia						●		

Each doctor or clinic will have its own schedule, but you should expect it to include most of the items listed above.

● usually done at this age.

○ may be done at this age.

(NOTE: The schedule above was compiled on the basis of information available as of March 1980. As new knowledge becomes available, recommendations for immunization schedules may undergo further changes.)

Immunization schedule from *Infant Care,* distributed by the U.S. Dept. of Health and Human Services, see index.

PARENTS' GUIDE TO CHILDHOOD IMMUNIZATION
U.S. Department of Health, Education and Welfare
1977, 25 pages, Illus.

from
Superintendent of Documents
Government Printing Office
Washington, DC 20402
free (DHEW Pub. No. (OS)77-50058)

The Public Health Service offers this complete guide to the immunization needed from infancy: DPT (diphtheria, pertussis, tetanus), polio, and MMR (measles, mumps, rubella). How, when and why the vaccines are given is discussed along with a description of possible side effects and how to deal with them. A blank record form for recording your child's immunizations is provided at the end of the booklet. Ask your local health service or politician for a copy. (MS)

"Vaccines work best when they are given at the recommended time and on a regular schedule. Measles vaccine, for example, is not usually given to infants before they reach the age of 15 months. When it is given earlier than that, it may not be as effective. Oral polio and DPT vaccines must be given over a period of time, in a series of properly spaced doses. Scheduling is important."

IMMUNIZATION: WHEN AND WHY
1981, brochure

from
Metropolitan
Health and Safety Education Division
1 Madison Avenue
New York, NY 10010
free

This brochure explains why immunization is valuable, gives a recommended schedule for shots, and provides a blank record for immunizations and boosters. (JIA)

"Active immunity to a disease is produced by a vaccine—either injected or swallowed—that creates antibodies. These antibodies resist specific disease germs when they enter the body. For strong resistance, it is sometimes necessary to reinforce first vaccinations with booster doses at specific intervals later on.

"Although newborn infants are susceptible to many infections, they do have a certain natural immunity to some diseases. However, this is temporary. Early vaccination is necessary so that the child will be protected as the brief, natural immunity subsides."

MISCELLANEOUS

VASCULAR BIRTHMARKS
1979, brochure

from
American Medical Association
Order Department OP-89
P.O. Box 821
Monroe, WI 53566
free

What is a birthmark? What are the three major kinds of hemangioma? What causes them and when do they go away? This pamphlet will allay your fears about your otherwise perfect baby. It was prepared by dermatology professor Victor H. Witten, M.D., of the University of Miami, Florida and explains in understandable detail the causes, types, and treatment of vascular birthmarks.
(MS)

"All parents hope for newborn infants without visible imperfections. Nevertheless, some are born with or develop them soon after birth. These surface marks or abnormalities are commonly referred to as birthmarks. Among such imperfections is the hemangioma. A hemangioma is a red mark consisting of tiny blood vessels that are bunched together. Sometimes it is called a *vascular* birthmark, vascular nevus or port-wine stain. . . .

"The nevus flammeus, frequently called the port-wine stain, is among the most common of all birthmarks. In most cases, it is present at birth and rarely fades or disappears with age. Fortunately, most of these lesions occur on the back of the scalp where they are covered with hair. Close examination shows that as many as one third of all people probably have such a birthmark."

GOOD TEETH FOR YOU AND YOUR BABY
1979, 16 pages

from
National Institute of Dental Health
Public Health Service
9000 Rockville Pike
Bethesda, MD 20205
free

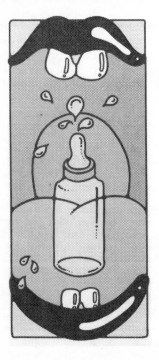

That evening bottle or reward of a cookie can do serious damage to your child's dental health! This clearly written booklet details specific things to do to keep your child's teeth clean and healthy from the first. Diet and fluoride are also discussed and the pop-art illustrations humorously help make the points.
(MS)

"Prevent Baby Bottle Tooth Decay. Many babies who go to sleep with a baby bottle may develop severe tooth decay, often in their front teeth. The problem is not the bottle, but what's in it. The sugar in milk, formula, fruit juices and sweet drinks causes the decay.

"During the day, the baby swallows these drinks quickly, so they don't damage the teeth. But during sleep, the liquid pools behind the baby's teeth and keeps them bathed in sugar for hours.

"Sometimes, these teeth become so decayed they cause severe pain and may break off or have to be pulled.

"Give your baby the last feeding before bedtime.

"Babies who need extra sucking are satisfied with a bottle of plain water, an extra bonus when the water has fluoride. Don't be upset if your baby sucks its thumb. It's usually harmless for babies and very young children."

FASCINATING FACTS ABOUT BABY'S FEET AND FOOTWEAR
16 pages

from
Fleet-Air Corporation
Ephrata, PA 17522

This little booklet describes how baby feet grow and mature, what sorts of foot coverings are needed and when, and what the proper position of the feet should be in walking. It also gives tips on footcare and provides a foot Growth Chart on heavy paper in the back of the booklet.
(MS)

"During infancy a child's foot is not a solid structure, but 52 bony masses which do not even appear united. As the child grows these little masses enlarge and assume the proper shape—gradually meeting each other. The arches then start to form, but it takes ten years before the general structure of the foot is completed. Actually, certain details of the heel bone are not completed until after the twentieth year!"

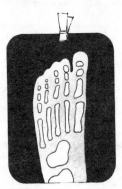

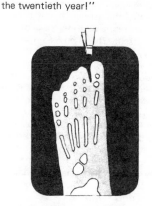

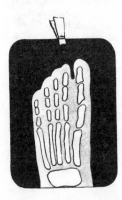

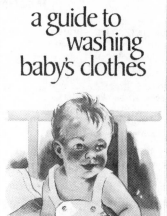

A GUIDE TO WASHING BABY'S CLOTHES
12 page booklet

from
U.S. Borax and Chemical Corp.
Consumer Affairs
3075 Wilshire Blvd.
Los Angeles, CA 90010
free

Formula, mud, grease balls, old blood, chewing gum, and flame-retardant clothing are just a few of the washing problems this booklet covers. Fairly complete and easy to read, it also covers diaper washing thoroughly and how to remedy laundry mistakes you may have made.
(MS)

THE GENTLE ART OF BABY-PROOFING
11 page booklet

from
Baby Fresh
Scott Paper Company
P.O. Box 4260
Chester, PA 19016
free

"Babyproofing is a way of thinking which enables parents to anticipate their baby's safety and comfort within the home environment and prepare accordingly for the infant's well-being. Once parents have planned for baby's safety in the nursery and throughout the entire home, they can be more relaxed and confident as they enjoy watching their baby grow."

Babyproofing involves much more than putting breakables on high shelves. Write for this well-written booklet which also includes an infant development chart and expected weight gain chart.
(MS)

TWINS

CENTER FOR THE STUDY OF MULTIPLE BIRTH
333 East Superior Street, Suite 463-5
Chicago, IL 60611
312/266-9093

The Center (formerly the Center for the Study of Multiple Gestation) cofounded by identical twins Dr. Louis Keith (an obstetrician) and Donald Keith (an engineer) provides books, factsheets, and other publications on twins. The Center's goals are to:

* Enhance early diagnoses of all multiple gestations
* Institute intensive prenatal, delivery, and postnatal care to improve chances of survival for mother and child
* Reduce the incidence of death and serious illness in the first month of life of the newborn
* Lower the risk of maternal complications   (JIA)

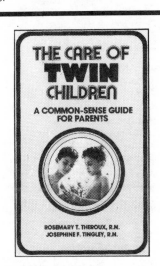

THE CARE OF TWIN CHILDREN:
A Common-Sense Guide for Parents by Rosemary T. Theroux and Josephine F. Tingley
1978, 119 pages, Illus.

from
Center for the Study of Multiple Birth
333 E. Superior Street, Suite 463-5
Chicago, IL 60611
312/266-9093
$6.75 pap.
$12.95 hd.

A large factsheet with excerpts from this book and additional resources is available free with a self-addressed, stamped envelope.

"If you have problems telling your babies apart when you bring them home from the hospital, you can leave their name bands on, put nail-polish on one baby's toenail, or use different-colored diaper pins or clothing on each baby. Among sets of identicals, one child always has a rounder or fuller face, which should help you and others tell the babies apart.

"There are many ways to foster individuality without destroying the special bond of twinship. A few are suggested here . . .

* Never call your children 'twinny' or even refer to them as 'the twins'; ask others to avoid this also. Address the children by their given names.
* Consider following the practice of many parents who use unlike sounding names for their twins, especially in the case of identicals or look-alike fraternals.
* Call both children by their names more frequently than normal to reinforce their individuality in their own minds.
* Remember and refer to dissimilarities rather than likenesses and teach others to be aware of these also.
* Assign each child different chores.
* Give both space for their own belongings and, if conditions allow, give them separate rooms.
* At a very early age, occasionally separate twins at naptime—in different rooms.
* Give each child some special time alone with you each day and, along with it, necessary love and attention to meet his particular needs.
* As they grow older and accept more responsibility, allow them to make decisions on their own, such as choice of clothing, hair style, or toys.
* Take pictures of your children separately as well as together."

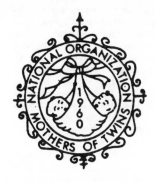

NATIONAL ORGANIZATION OF MOTHERS OF TWINS CLUBS, INC.
5402 Amberwood Lane
Rockville, MD 20853
301/460-9108

The National Organization of Mothers of Twins Clubs, Inc. (NOMTC) was founded to "provide educational materials for parents of multiples and professionals in health care and education." The national office refers the mother of twins or triplets (or more!) to the nearest local club and also provides support to the mother who lives in an area not serviced by an organized club. An introductory pamphlet called *Your Twins and You* is available free with a self-addressed, stamped envelope. The organization also produces a slide/video tape presentation on twins for childbirth educators ($100.), and sells *Special Delivery 3,*

Triplets for $1.75. A quarterly newsletter, *MOTC's Notebook* is available for $5.00 a year to non-members. Also available is *How to Organize a Mothers of Twins Club* for $1.00.
(JIA)

"HELPFUL HINTS FOR BREAST-FEEDING MULTIPLES"

* Consult your doctor or contact the local LaLeche League if you are considering breastfeeding your babies. Members of a local mothers of twins club will also be helpful with tips on successfully nursing twins or triplets.
* Evaluate your true feelings—WHY do you wish to breastfeed? Attitude and determination are keys to your success.
* Ignore outside pressures from others. Your emotions affect the success of your breastfeeding.
* Consider some of the advantages of breastfeeding your multiples: eliminated formula preparation and cost; the milk is pure, the right temperature and easy to digest.
* Drink plenty of fluids and eat a proper diet. Check with your doctor for supplemental vitamins or other dietary needs.
* Avoid drugs, alcohol, cigarettes and some foods (chocolate, highly seasoned, gas forming) while breastfeeding."

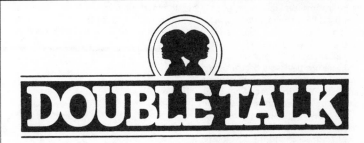

DOUBLE TALK
P.O. Box 412
Amelia, OH 45102
$4.00 a year
$7.00 two years

"Double Talk is a national quarterly newsletter which concerns itself solely with multiples and the special parenting problems they present. We, the editors, hope that we are providing a network of information and support for our readers. As far as we know, it is the only publication of its kind.

"Parenting twins is a unique experience, very different from parenting a single child. Twins' early years can be a lonely time for their mother. She is far more confined than the mother of singletons and is too tired to seek new friends with twins even if she found the time! She can, however, pick up a newsletter at two a.m., while she feeds her babies and read how others have dealt with the same problems and emotions.

"Mothers of multiples publish *Double Talk* and subscribers write most articles. We also include book reports, poems, pictures, stories, and art work submitted by our readers. An 'Order Department' featuring only twin related books and equipment completes the newsletter."

—Karen Gromada and Mary Hurlbut, editors of *Double Talk*

Also see review of *Having Twins* by Elizabeth Noble on page 27.

TO LOVE A BABY
by Sandy Jones
1981, 163 pages, Illus.

from
Houghton Mifflin
2 Park Street
Boston, MA 02107
$16.95 plus $1.50 postage, hd.

What is baby care? Does it consist of a series of methodical routines, procedures, and patterns guaranteed to ensure adequate nutrition, hygiene and order? Or is it an intimate encounter of love and close contact in which baby and parent learn each other's needs and rhythms? In *To Love a Baby* Sandy Jones argues for a style of caring which puts parental love and instinct first and "experts'" advice last—in so far as that means that parents are naturally loving and giving and frustrated by experts' admonitions to avoid "spoiling" the child. Physical closeness is of greatest importance. Jones says, "After hundreds of interviews with mothers and fathers and after examining the entire field of infant research, I am convinced that I have, indeed, found the secret of effective baby care. The answer is so simple: *respond to your baby in the physical language that she is programmed to understand.* When your baby's primal need for an intimate physical relationship is met, her life energies are free for the best possible development of her innate potential." Our culture has devised many gadgets and arrangements to keep babies and parents apart: separate bedrooms, separate beds, cribs with bars, high-chairs, strollers, walkers, playpens, clothing. Sandy Jones takes all this away and replaces it with close, bodily contact.

Jones has devised a beautiful and unusual format by which to present her ideas. The first part of her book consists of her very sensitive writing on the growth of love, beginning in pregnancy and continuing through the birth process and the developing relationship between parent and child. She speaks of "choosing the path of response" that is, of focussing on learning to respond to the baby's real needs for physical closeness rather than imposing rigid standards from without. She stresses the importance of breastfeeding as a way of strengthening nurturing attachment. There are also good discussions of relaxation techniques and massage in pregnancy, the importance of undrugged childbirth and bonding, infant massage, caring for colicky babies, and more. This section is generously illustrated with very beautiful, large black and white photographs of parents and babies, taken by Thomas Stiltz. The many photos of fathers intimately caring for their wives and babies are especially nice.

The second part of the book consists of a carefully and extensively annotated bibliography of literature in nursing, medicine, physical therapy, psychology, psychiatry, and anthropology, which substantiates Jones' ideas about loving nurturance. She includes a very helpful introduction on how to obtain copies of research papers through the reference services of your local library.

In all, *To Love a Baby* is an important and innovative book and will be of great value and interest to new parents as well as to those who are working toward more loving and responsive styles in childbearing and rearing.
(JIA)

"Your baby's head and body finally come to the outer edges of your birth canal. Her head feels hard and very large. Then, with gentle pushes controlled by your shallow breaths, her head eases out with her rubbery body slipping out behind.

"Your vagina tingles with the memory of your baby's passage. The sensation is so clear that you almost know if it's a boy or a girl. This important memory, your baby's movement from within you to the outer world, will be stored in a deep, feeling part of yourself. In the days and months ahead, this body-memory trace will help you in marrying the baby you hold in your arms with the unseen baby that you carried inside. You will come to understand that these two babies are one and the same. . . .

"Enfold your baby with your voice. Converse with him during all your actions with him. Greet him in the morning and continue a running conversation throughout your day with him. When you change his diapers, describe what you are doing. When you touch his body, name the parts for him. Tell him where you are going and what you are thinking.

"During the first year, you and your baby will carry on many marvelous communication dances with each other. Moving close in toward your baby's face, you will slow down your speech and make your voice higher. You will raise your eyebrows, exaggerate your facial expressions, and initiate a brief but satisfying encounter between the two of you.

"Your baby will respond by arresting the movement of his legs and arms. He will orient his body toward you. His eyes will dance and his face light up, and he will soon venture a smile for you. . . .

"Unfortunately, your baby doesn't understand your eight-hour-a-night sleeping ritual. She has night needs for sustenance that may continue for many months, even through the first year. If you have come to mistrust the family bed, your baby is separated from your presence by a wooden cage in a distant room. To answer her needs, you must rouse yourself to a completely awake state. You may be sleep-robbed by your own boxed-off-bedroom concept.

"The two of you sleeping with your baby through the night, besides being a form of energy conservation, can provide both the baby and you with needed 'touch time.' If you, the father, are gone during the day, in the stillness of the night you can touch the baby's head, hear her breathing, feel her closeness, and take joy in your deep sense of her nearness."

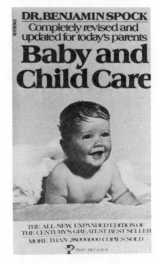

BABY AND CHILD CARE
by Benjamin Spock
1981, 666 pages, Illus.

from
Pocket Books
1230 Avenue of the Americas
New York, NY 10020
$3.95 pap.

The classic, "Dr. Spock," is still a very useful guide to the basics of baby care and illness and has been updated to include more progressive and egalitarian information on natural childbirth, parenting, the father's role, working mothers, etc. (JIA)

"Babies aren't frail. 'I'm so afraid I'll hurt her if I don't handle her right,' a parent often says about her first baby. You don't have to worry: you have a pretty tough baby. There are many ways to hold her. If her head drops backward by mistake,

"Babies aren't frail."

it won't hurt her. The open spot in her skull (the fontanel) is covered by a tough membrane like canvas that isn't easily injured. The system to control body temperature is working quite well by the time she weighs 7 pounds if she's covered halfway sensibly. She has good resistance to most germs. During a family cold epidemic, she's apt to have it the mildest of all. If she gets her head tangled in anything, she has a strong instinct to struggle and yell. If she's not getting enough to eat, she will probably cry for more. If the light is too strong for her eyes, she'll blink and fuss. (You can take her picture with a flashbulb, even if it does make her jump.) She knows how much sleep she needs, and takes it. She can care for herself pretty well for a person who can't say a word and knows nothing about the world."

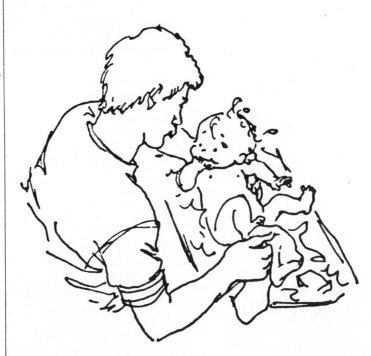

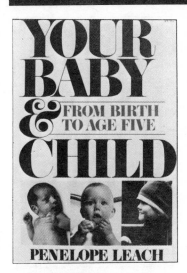

YOUR BABY AND CHILD: From Birth to Age Five
by Penelope Leach
1981, 512 pages, Illus.

from
Alfred A. Knopf
201 East 50th Street
New York, NY 10028
$9.95 pap.

This lovely book was written by an English psychologist and is intended as a companion volume to *The Complete Book of Pregnancy and Childbirth* (see index) by Sheila Kitzinger, also from England. *Your Baby and Child* is an excellent source of wise, practiced information on what babies are like and how to care for them from birth through the pre-school years. Five main sections treat the newborn, the settled baby (to six months), the older baby (six months to one year), the toddler, and the pre-school child, covering feeding, growth, sleep patterns, every-day care and toileting, crying and comforting, physical skills, learning and playing for each stage. The book is beautifully illustrated with over 650 drawings and photographs, 70 of which are in color. The text is very conveniently laid out so that the book is easy to use and a real delight to look at. Penelope Leach did her graduate work on the effects of different kinds of upbringing on personality development and her book reflects her concern with the importance of learning what babies need and responding to their needs appropriately. An "encyclopedia/index" at the back of the book makes it easy to find information fast in cases of illness or injury.
(JIA)

"The baby needs to be handled so that his new and independent life seems as little different as possible from the old dependent life in your womb. His needs are simple and repetitive. They need to be met simply and immediately. He needs food and water in combined form of milk; he needs warmth and comfort from cuddling arms and soft wrappings in a small, safe bed; he needs just enough cleanliness to keep his skin from getting sore and he needs protection. That is all he needs. The gadgets and gimmicks, the baths and changing mats, powders and lotions, brushes and bootees that tempt you in every baby store will be fun for you to buy and nice for him later. But for now he is a bundle and he should be a bundle. Wrap him warmly, hold him closely, handle him slowly, feed him when he is hungry, talk to him when he looks at you, wash him when he is actually dirty and leave him peacefully alone to come to terms with life. Unless he is actually ill and under medical care, there is absolutely nothing which it is your duty to do to him if it makes him jump or cry. Peaceful contentment means that you have got it right. Distress means that you have got it wrong. Let his reactions guide you. . . .

"Babies do not need to be kept nearly as clean as most of us keep them. It is adults who like them to smell of baby powder. The chief purpose in washing a new baby is to remove from the skin anything which might irritate and make it sore. The skin would take care of itself if it did not get drenched with urine, smeared with feces, splashed with sticky milk and lightly speckled with dust.

"Most mothers will be taught, by the hospital staff, to bathe their new babies every day. . . . But, if, like many mothers, you find that the bath is something that neither you nor the baby can enjoy just yet, you don't have to do it. You can make your baby perfectly clean by 'topping and tailing,' and what is more you can do it without frightening him or her or putting yourself through the horrors of trying to hold a slippery screaming mite safely in a bath full of water. . . .

"The topping and tailing method of washing a new baby concentrates on cleaning thoroughly the bits that really need it: the eyes, nose and ears, the face, hands and bottom. It keeps undressing (and therefore redressing) to a diaper-changing minimum and it can all be done without picking the baby up. . . .

"Babies who cry until they are picked up, stay cheerful while they are being held and then cry again when they are put down, are usually crying because they are uncomfortable without physical contact. This kind of crying for lack of 'contact comfort' is often misunderstood. Parents are told that the baby is crying 'because he wants you to pick him up.' The implication is that he is making an unreasonable demand on you and that if you 'give in' you will start 'bad habits'. In fact, the reverse is true. The baby is not making unreasonable demands, you are. . . ."

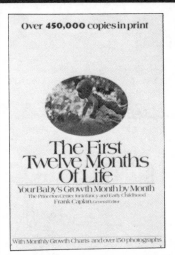

THE FIRST TWELVE MONTHS OF LIFE: Your Baby's Growth Month by Month
edited by Frank Caplan
1973, 256 pages, Illus.

from
Grosset and Dunlap
51 Madison Avenue
New York, NY 10010
$9.95 pap.

I found this book extremely useful when my first baby was born. The book devotes one chapter to each month of the baby's first year, providing a discussion of common behaviors and patterns of both baby and parents, many excellent, multi-ethnic photographs, and a very useful "growth chart" which summarizes the average baby's progress in large and small motor control, language development, mental capacity, and social skills for each month. As a new mother I didn't know much about baby behavior and development and it was very reassuring and interesting to follow along with this book's month by month descriptions.
(JIA)

"The third month of a baby's life is generally easier and more rewarding than the first two—for him and his parents. Almost magically, crying nearly vanishes by the three-month birthday. The baby's increased capacity to engage the world with vocalizing, smiling, facial expressions, and looking at people, his better physical shape and control, and his new reaching ability replace his need to cry. He is an interesting and responsive personality. He can whimper in a special way when he is hungry, chortle as he actively responds to a human being, and squeal with frustration when someone he has been socializing with leaves him. Occasionally he may stop his activity, watch his mother or father, then try a slow gurgle at the back of his throat. Some babies use an expressive face. Your baby may widen his eyes, smack his lips, and grin broadly to a new taste treat. Placed in a position he dislikes, he may stare disgruntled at the guilty party. Since he likes to play and socialize, he smiles immediately and spontaneously with his whole face at someone he recognizes. He may search your face briefly, focus on your mouth and eyes, and become more active, kick his legs, wiggle, and reach with both arms. . . .

"Like a shock absorber, the mother protects her child from too much stimulation from inside himself (like hunger or pain) or from the outside world (like cold or noise). She also enhances the positive aspects of her baby's world and directs his attention to them. Mother's sensitivity and capability in adapting the environment to her baby's characteristics actually boosts his ability to handle stress. Since he is completely dependent on you, he will need you to get him out of the binds he gets himself into and to help and protect him in periods of rage and frustration. If he propels himself to the top of his crib and wedges himself into a corner, come to the rescue and pull him to the center, even though you know he will just start all over and scream for help again. If you respond to his needs, you will enhance his and your pleasure with his learning and practice. Leaving him to his own devices may make him so fearful of situations he cannot escape from that he 'turns off.' You can also show him ways to extract himself from his frenzy and his predicament. After a few reruns, he will know how to turn around and get out of that corner."

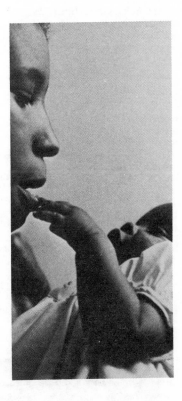

Baby Products

Mary Scott, editor

BIRTH ANNOUNCEMENTS

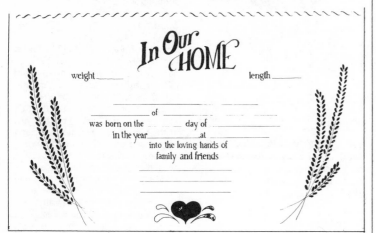

HOME BIRTH CERTIFICATES
$2.00 plus .50 postage each

from
Pam Ridling
430 St. Louis
Florissant, MO 63031

A birth at home deserves a special recognition and what better than a hand-painted 8½ x 14" certificate?

These beautiful certificates come in two designs: a floral design in brown ink on natural parchment, hand-painted in pastel tones, and an elegant Pennsylvania Dutch style in black ink on white parchment, painted in red, blue, and brown. Each is a treasure to be framed and enjoyed like the birth of the child it commemorates.

(MS)

HOME BIRTH CERTIFICATE
$1.00 each
$.50 each for 25 or more

from
Meadow Born
Lana Tazaki
9638 Helen Avenue
Sunland, CA 91040

This delightfully illustrated certificate features a place to paste the baby's photo and spaces to record birth statistics, time and date, parents, midwife or doctor's name, and birth attendants. It's printed in black ink on an 8½ x 11" sheet of tan parchment paper. Midwives might want to order a batch for their clients. (MS)

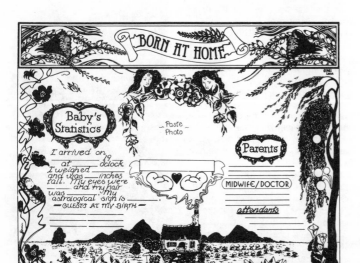

AFTERNOON GRAPHICS
P.O. Box 453
Eugene, OR 97440

Baby Cards
$.50 to .70 each
$3.00 to 3.50 for packages

Announcements, greetings, shower invitations, and thank you notes are all available in Lynn Peterson's old-fashioned designs. Inside are loving quotations and all the space you need to fill in all the details of birth or party. Printed on glossy white stock and tan parchment. (MS)

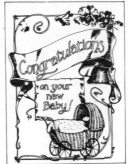

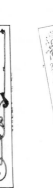

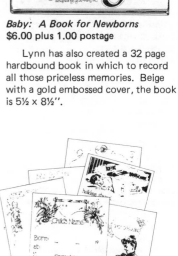

Baby: A Book for Newborns
$6.00 plus 1.00 postage

Lynn has also created a 32 page hardbound book in which to record all those priceless memories. Beige with a gold embossed cover, the book is 5½ x 8½".

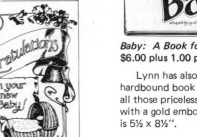

BIRTH ANNOUNCEMENTS
$4.00 per dozen plus shipping
($1.00 for first dozen, .50 each additional)

from
Barbara Wunder Black
4037 Ivy Street
Ventura, CA 93003

Having received such a favorable response to the announcement she designed to herald her own daughter's arrival, Barbara Wunder Black has now made it and three other cards available to the public as alternatives to conventional announcements. Each 4¼ x 5½" card is screen-printed in brown ink on tan parchment in one of four designs, each with an appropriate verse and space to fill in names of parents and child, birth date and weight. Orders are shipped within three days of receipt. Wholesale inquiries invited. (MS)

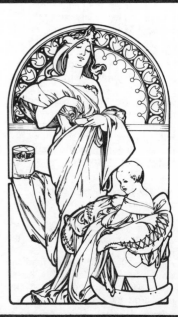

HAND LETTERED BIRTH ANNOUNCEMENTS
$25.00 for 50

from
Melodie Arterberry
675 Belmont Street
Belmont, MA 02178

Here is an extra special way to announce the arrival of that Very Important Person. These 4" x 6" cards are hand-lettered by Melodie and come with matching envelopes in your choice of blue, pink or yellow. Border designs include houses, flowers or stars and you may select a quota-tion from Shakespeare, McDonald or Barker. Please indicate Baby's name. birthdate, and birth weight when ordering as well as choice of color, border, and quotation.   (MS)

Where did you come from, baby dear?
Out of the everywhere into the here.
—George McDonald

One night as old St. Peter slept
He left the door of Heaven ajar
When through a little angel crept
And came down with a falling star.
—David Barker

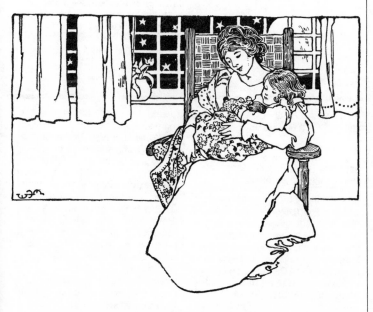

There was a star danced and under that was I born.   Shakespeare

Nicolas John Perkins

August 4th, 1980   *8 lbs. 6 oz.*

GREEN TIGER PRESS
P.O. Box 868
La Jolla, CA 92038

Green Tiger Press, in addition to their lovely illustrated children's books, sells hundreds of beautiful notecards and picture cards featuring illustrations by Jessie Wilcox Smith, Kay Nielsen, Maxfield Parrish, Arthur Rackam, Beatrix Potter, Howard Pyle, N.C. Wyeth and others. Many of these would be suitable as birth announcements. Prices range from $.25 to .75 each. Small matted prints are also available. Write for a catalog.
(JIA)

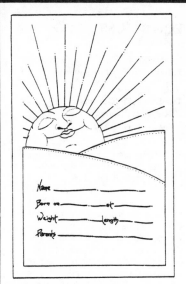

Name _____
Born on _____ at _____
Weight _____ Length _____
Parents _____

PASSAGES: Special Birth Announcements for the Newborn
$4.50 per set of 20

from
Liz Woedl-Passages
6505 Buckley Road
Oxford, OH 45056

These sunny, original designs are printed on heavy, fold-over cards you can seal, address and mail. Designs include Sprout, Fairy, Harvest, Little Bird, and Sunny Side Up, each available in your choice of blue, yellow, green, or apricot. What a lovely, light-hearted way to share your joy with friends and relatives! Indicate design and color when ordering.   (MS)

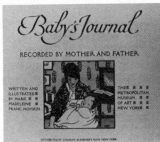

BABY'S JOURNAL
Written and Illustrated by Marie Madeleine Franc-Nohain
1978, unnumbered pages, Illus.

from
Charles Scribner's Sons
597 Fifth Avenue
New York, NY 10017
$12.95 hd.

This very lovely baby book is a reproduction of a book in the collection of The Metropolitan Museum of Art. It was first published by Bernard Grasset in Paris, in 1914. The book features two-color illustrations on each page which illustrate vignettes from baby's life. There is room to record the details of the birth and the usual milestones of growth as well as items like baby's first laugh, what the baby first notices and hears, first toys and outings, first joys and fears, favorite stories and songs, baby's first humor, and more.   (JIA)

"Passages is a home centered business that grew from my desire to stay home and raise my two daughters. I had designed their birth announcements and started doing them for others here.

"Although I will be satisfied to simply put food on the table with these earnings I look forward to expanding the efforts as my girls are older and I would have more time. I want this to be a contribution to my daughters—not take my attention from them."
—Liz Woedl of Passages

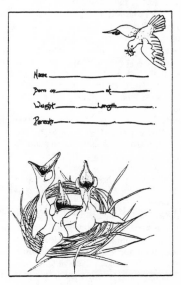

Name _____
Born on _____ at _____
Weight _____ Length _____
Parents _____

BABY BOOKS

It is a very good idea to have and use a baby book for each child. It is a convenient place to keep treasured pictures and birth certificates. Besides, when the child gets older and/or siblings arrive, it provides a real storybook to sit and enjoy together. You will thank yourself later when you re-read all the cute expressions and words of wisdom your child comes up with. A looseleaf binder or a book with blank pages will do. Just try to remember to write in it once a week. You'll be surprised how it makes you really notice your child and enjoy her or his life more. Ask your own parents about it!   (MS)

LAMBSKINS FOR BABIES

TENDER TOUCH: Washable Lambskin Infant Rugs
$44.95 plus 3.00 shipping

from
Health Care Products, Inc.
P.O. Box 26221
Denver, CO 80226

Yvonne Rosnik, of Health Care Products, began importing lambskins in 1977, among the first to introduce them in the U.S. Her Tender Touch lambskins are unshorn, have a pile depth of 1½ inches, and come in their natural, undyed color, Honey Gold. The lambskins are fully machine washable, clinically sterilized and recommended and used by the Denver Birth Center. VISA and MasterCard customers include number, expiration date, and signature. Colorado residents add sales tax. If sending as a gift, include message and address of recipient.   (MS)

"At Britain's Cambridge University a team of researchers, headed by Dr. Martin Richards, undertook a study of six pre-term low birth weight babies using lambswool as a substitute to normal cotton bedding. After checking their weight daily over a period of 16 days, alternating between lambswool and cotton bedding, the research team were astounded to find that the babies grew 50% faster on the days they spent on the lambswool. The most likely explanation for the astonishing weight gains is the security offered by the natural wool which made the babies feel far happier and show less signs of stress."

LAMBSKIN
$39.50 plus 2.50 shipping

from
The Sheepskin Company
86-07 Eliot Avenue
Rego Park, NY 11374

This 2½ x 2¼ foot pure virgin wool lambskin comes in either Sunshine Gold or Natural Fawn with a 90-day, unconditional money-back guarantee. Machine-washable, it is much better than conventional blankets in ordinary use. VISA or MasterCard customers include number, expiration date and signature. Gift orders can be sent with a card, so include the message you wish to send along with the address and your address. New York residents add sales tax.   (MS)

"The cuddly lambswool simulates the warmth and soothing environment of the womb. Research shows babies sleep longer on lambskins and more contentedly.

"The lambskin keeps your baby warm in winter yet cool in summer. The wool fleece absorbs moisture keeping baby dry and comfortable at all times.

"The tactile stimulation of the many wool fibers caress and relax your baby, reducing stress. Provides relief on colicky days."
(Editor's Note: see article by Mary Miller of the Sheepskin Company on the next page.)

KIWI KIDDIE COMFORTER:
Lambswool Baby Rug
$44.95

from
Kiwi Products International
P.O. Box 5009
Woodland Hills, CA 91365

These natural comforters come in Natural Honey, Fawn or White and are great travelers. Approximately 2½ x 2¼ feet in size, they offer year-round security and versatility. California residents add sales tax.

Also offered by the Kiwi people are "Nursery Rugs" ($49.95) which are the same size and shape as the lambskins but you have the choice of a Blue Rabbit on White, White Rabbit on Blue, Pink Duck on White or White Duck on Pink.

Sheepskin Car Seat Covers are available in beige or gray for $34.95 and anyone who travels even to the store in the summer will have a much happier baby who doesn't stick to the carseat.   (MS)

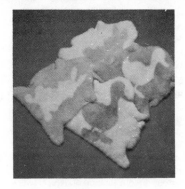

"Besides offering the ultimate in plush coziness and tactile sensation for babies, lambskin has been proven by recent medical studies to be an ideal infant care surface. Babies were found to sleep better and longer, as well as play happier and quieter on lambskin rugs. And increased baby contentment reduces worry for mother."

"The surfaces with which the baby comes into contact are very important for his physical, functional, and behavioral development. We know from experiment that rough, hard, or unyielding surfaces are experienced as unpleasant by babies, and that they prefer soft, yielding, and caressing surfaces. . .

"Clearly, both infants and mothers derive substantial benefit from the use of lambskin rugs. Indeed, the evidence of their beneficial effects is so striking, that the use of lambskins should become a routine practice in the home, not just for babies and their mothers, but also for children of older age when they are in need of special comfort."

From an article by Dr. Ashley Montagu (author of *Touching: The Human Significance of the Skin,* see index for review) published in the April-May 1979 issue of *Genesis,* the official publication of the American Society for Psychoprophylaxis in Obstetrics ASPO (see index).

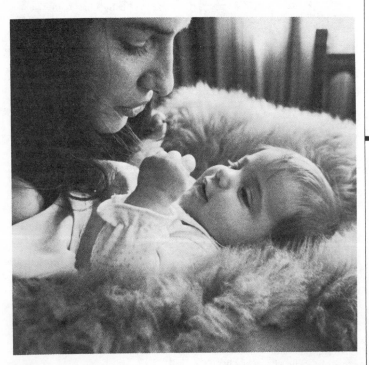

BABY-BEAUTIFUL COMFORTER
$39.95 plus 3.00 shipping

from
Imperial Sheepskins of Australia
2325 Third Street, Suite 331
San Francisco, CA 94107

Colorfast 2 by 3 foot lambskins are close-shorn and come in pink, blue, gold, and natural. Soft, sterilized and machine-washable, they meet the highest government standards. Dry indoors or out away from direct sunlight. California residents add sales tax. Call toll free for more information (800) 227-5108.   (MS)

(Editor's Note: The lambskins listed here appear to be comparable in price and quality, with the main difference being in colors available. We did not use a lambskin with either of our children—it's quite a new product—so we can't say from experience whether or not they do help to quiet colicky babies, as some sellers claim. However, we did receive a sample lambskin from Health Care Products, listed above, and we can say that it is a beautiful, soft piece of fur with a lovely thick pile and very soft chamois-like back. We all enjoy sleeping with it and touching it. If we decide to have another baby, we'll be sure to have her sleep on a lambskin.)
(JIA)

Lambskins for Babies

The special advantages of using sheepskins for babies, toddlers and school-age children.

—Mary N. Miller

"Sheepskins have long been used in nursing homes and other medical facilities as bedpads for patients. Their special qualities in preventing bedsores, absorbing moisture, distributing weight evenly and generally enhancing comfort and sleep have been appreciated by the many patients who have had occasion to use them.

"What is less well-known is that lambskins are universally used by children, especially babies, in New Zealand and Australia. Ideal for newborn babies, because the softness and comfort simulates the warmth and environment of the womb, they are non-toxic, breathable and machine-washable. Research by Dr. Martin Richards at Cambridge University in England, shows that babies grow faster and sleep better on lambswool. The researchers placed six premature babies on lambswool for one day and the next day placed them on the usual hospital bedding. They were weighed every evening. Dr. Richard's team discovered that the babies grew 50% faster each day they slept on a lambswool. While no one knows for sure why this is so, the team concluded that the babies are probably happier and less stressed when placed on natural wool.

"Imported from New Zealand and approved for infant care by the N.Z. Wool Board, the sheepskin is especially treated and sterilized so as to be safe for babies to sleep on. Wool is well-known for its warmth in winter. But it should also be remembered that the Arabs wear wool for protection against the desert sun. In hot weather the body perspires. The wool fibre attracts moisture and can absorb up to one third of its own dry weight without feeling clammy or moist. This is a quality unique to wool and enables a baby to remain warm and dry even when wet. Contrast this to a baby lying cold and damp on a wet cotton sheet placed over a rubber pad.

The dense wool of the sheep also has a resilience and springiness which allows the circulation of air. Every wool fibre has a natural wave or crimp which allows it to be stretched as much as one third and released, to spring back into place. The 'waves' and 'crimps' permit air flow and this allows the moisture from any perspiration to dissipate into the atmosphere. Because of this the summer rash, sometimes found in babies and small children, can be avoided or considerably reduced, and the lambskin assists the body's efforts to keep cool.

In winter, when it is chilly, the baby's body heat is retained by the sheepskin. The millions of wool fibres trap in air which is a poor conductor. The process of absorbing moisture vapor generates heat in the wool fibre, further assisting in keeping the body warm. Sig-nificantly, wool garments are recommended by mountain safety experts for the ever-changing conditions of alpine regions.

The circulation of air amongst the wool fibres in the lambskin also enables the baby's skin to be protected from pressure marks and helps to evenly distribute the body pressure over the lambskin. In addition, the air flow makes it impossible for a baby to suffocate. Though many parents who use baby lambskin prefer to place a cotton cloth, such as a diaper, under the baby's head to protect the cleanliness of the lambskin, it is in fact possible for a newborn to sleep face down directly on a lambskin without any risk.

Dr. Ashley Montagu, author of *Touching, The Human Significance of the Skin,* points out in articles printed in *Baby Talk* and *Genesis,* the advantages of the sheepskins in providing a soft, yielding and caressing surface for babies. He emphasizes the importance of the tactile experience for the baby and advises parents to be "aware of the softness and the feel of what [the baby] sleeps on—what he is swaddled in." Another reason the lambskin is comfortable is that it is non-static and therefore does not cling to the body. Additionally, static electricity charges actively attract dirt. The lambskin being non-static, becomes dirty more slowly and research has shown that it attracts less dust than the surrounding bed clothes.

Wool is the only common fibre which, when exposed to flame, will not readily melt, flare up or drip to cause serious burns. Firemen's uniforms are frequently made of wool for this reason. The lambskin therefore, has a natural resistance to fire and meets U.S. Consumer Product Safety Standards.

As well as being used in the baby's bassinet or crib, the lambskin can be used in the stroller, baby carriage, playpen, highchair or car seat. The infant can be rocked to sleep in it and then moved from room to room or place to place if parents are out visiting or traveling in an airplane, train, bus or other form of transportation. Insulating the baby from extremely hot or cold weather, it provides a feeling of security and enhances a restful and longer sleep—wherever the infant may be. It is conveniently machine-washable and is air-dried by hanging it from two corners. Small, slightly soiled areas can be sponged off and dried with a towel.

Although the lambskin is especially valuable for infants, who spend the better part of their day sleeping, it is not just restricted to babies. It will last years and years—its special qualities providing comfort and security for toddlers and school-age children.

Mary Miller is a New Zealander and a 'graduate' of the Maternity Center. Her newborn baby made his first trip home in a New Zealand Sheepskin. She is now marketing the Infant Care Sheepskins in the United States. For further information, write to her at THE SHEEPSKIN COMPANY, 86-07 Eliot Ave., Rego Park, N.Y. 11374.

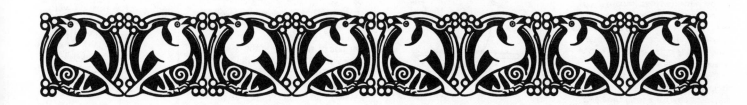

BABY CARRIERS

Mothers know that babies must be carried for longer than nine months. For thousands of years mothers have been "slinging" babies with them as they worked at home or in the fields. Modern mothers usually have more of a choice, but many are returning to the practice of carrying babies close to the body in baby carriers, in order to provide the warmth, security and intimacy so important to child/parent bonding. Baby carriers can also provide more comfort and freedom to both parents and babies than the conventional stroller or buggy. Carriers can be used on walks, hikes, and while shopping, in places where strollers are awkward or not welcome.

Parents today can find a variety of different sizes and options in carriers: front packs, back packs and pouches, with or without head support, designed according to the size of the baby and how much freedom of movement both parent and baby want. When shopping for baby carriers, think about your needs. Do you want to be able to nurse your little one while she is in the carrier? How often do you plan to use the carrier? Will you do much hiking or camping? If your baby is born in Spring or Summer, a carrier in a light-weight fabric may be more comfortable. Also remember that babies who don't sleep soundly may resent a model with lots of buckles and ties to undo when you wish to transfer them to a bed or car seat.

Listed in this section are some of the many carriers currently on the market. Talk to your friends, write for information, and take a walk through the stores before you buy so that your hard-earned money is spent on the carrier that best fits your needs.   (MS)

ANDREA'S BABY PACK
$35.00 postpaid

from
Andrea's Baby Pack
2441 Hilyard Street
Eugene, OR 97405

This hand-made, fully lined front/back carrier was designed for use from infancy through toddler years and beyond. "The contoured head support protects a tiny newborn infant and continues protecting a sleeping baby's head and neck for about two years. The sides are open to provide good ventilation but Baby cannot fall or crawl out." Made of durable fabric, Andrea's Baby Pack is easy to put on and the ring fasteners can be adjusted without help. It has an inner seat for infants which will "grow with the child." Machine washable and dryable. Specify three color choices.   (MS)

"Andrea's Baby Pack has no zippers, snaps or buckles that might fail, relying instead on straps and sturdy non-slip rings. Foam shoulder pads are provided for your comfort. . . it is made of durable fabrics fully-lined with matching prints. Each pack is made entirely by one person at home.

"Because I couldn't find any baby pack which supports the head of a sleeping baby for a long time and works equally well for the newborn and the toddler, I designed Andrea's Baby Pack around the body of my

growing baby, Emily. Emily is now almost nine years old and we have been selling the packs on a small scale, mostly through childbirth educators and related type people since Emily was two years old."
—Andrea H. Proudfoot

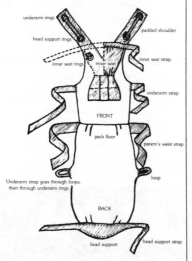

SNUGLI SOFT BABY CARRIER
$25.00 to $45.00

from
Snugli, Inc.
1212 Kerr Gulch Road
Evergreen, CO 80439

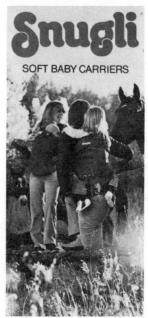

This carrier is the one most often seen in stores and has been used as a basic model for other designs. Snugli developed the first soft baby carrier fifteen years ago and now has a full line of nationally advertised carriers and other products. The original Snugli is still hand-made of corduroy or seersucker and retails for about $35 to $45. For those who find the original too expensive, there is now the Snugli 2 which is factory-made of denim and retails for about $25.

Both carriers feature an inner pouch seat with a zipper at the back for extra support for the newborn and rows of snaps at the base of the seat so it "grows" with your child. There is also a neck collar with releasable tucks for good head and neck support on the sides as well as in back of Baby's head. A newborn can be almost completely enclosed in this carrier, which is a nice feature for winter babies. Other good features include a detachable "bubble bib," a large pouch for carrying other necessary baby items, and a waistband to help distribute the weight more evenly. This type of carrier is well designed for the parent who will carry a child around for long periods of time during the day. Snugli also carries Raincapes, diaper bags, a Dolly Snugli, and New Zealand Lambskins. Write for a complete catalog. Snugli also publishes booklets of interest to expectant and new parents. *Bonding* and *Touching* are available now and others are planned.   (MS)

"In Africa, a woman uses her shawl to carry her baby everywhere she goes. Just as her mother did, and her mother before her. This age-old tradition holds an important message for today's parents.

"Babies need to be held. They need the warmth, the gentle touch that comes with close body contact. When you and your baby share this kind of time together, you develop a special closeness. It's part of a process called 'bonding' and it's essential to an infant's emotional growth and well-being."

Snugli 'grows' as your baby grows

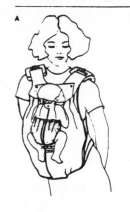

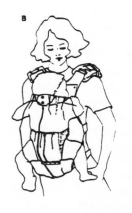

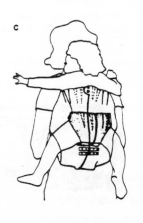

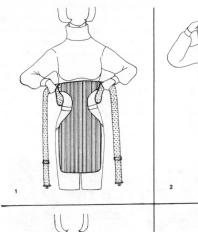

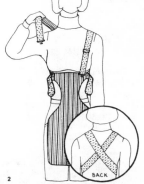

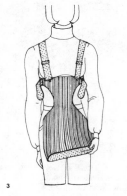

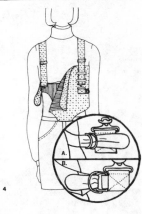

BABY, TOO
$13.95 postpaid

from
A & B House
Box 166
Gilbertsville, NY 13776

Baby, Too is a front carrier for babies 1 to 24 months. The head support for little ones folds down for older babies. This carrier is unique in that you have the option of carry-

ing your baby facing forward, so little tykes can feast on the world while still being close and secure with Mom or Dad. It comes in red and blue, is made of very good quality washable fabric and folds to fit into a purse. The straps criss-cross in back and the leg openings allow plenty of room for the chubbiest baby thighs. New York State residents add sales tax.　(MS)

BABY CARRIER PACKET (No. 410)
50 cents

from
La Leche League
Order Department
9616 Minneapolis Avenue
Franklin Park, IL 60131

Carrying your baby close to your body, just like breastfeeding, can be an extension to good mothering. La Leche League provides this packet on baby carriers which includes hints on using carriers, instructions for making your own, and flyers describ-

ing some of the commercially-available baby carriers and backpacks.　(MS)

"Whether it's a homemade rebozo or May-Tie, or an elaborate manufactured creation, a baby carrier is a wonderful way to keep baby warm and snug and close to mother where he belongs while he is little. For the first few months, while he is tiny, carry him in front. When he's older and bigger, you or Daddy will find the back carrier more satisfactory. Either way, he's cozy and safe, and in touch."

PUSHKA FRONT BABY CARRIER
$14.00 kit
$24.00 ready-made

from
Cheralin Products
P.O. Box 1018
Greeley, CO 80631

For those who like to do it themselves, this carrier can be purchased in kit form so you can tell your

friends, "I made it myself!" That also allows you the possibility of adding your own personalized options to it. Designed to promote parent/infant bonding, the Pushka is made of denim with calico lining. It is washable, easy to use, has a handy big pocket, and has nursing convenience. Cheralin also makes dolly carriers.　(MS)

BABY CARRIER KIT
$11.50 postpaid

from
CHEEKS
P.O. Box 3222
Sonora, CA 95370
$11.50 Postpaid

Cheeks offers a baby carrier kit which features removable tucks in inner and outer seat, detachable flannel bibs, double pouch- double layer construction, an outside pocket, and padded shoulder straps. You provide your own fabric (a total of about three yards) and the kit supplies the notions and hardware including shoulder pads, velcro, zippers, strap stiffener, buckles, pattern, sewing instructions, and carrier use instructions. The carrier is also available ready-made in red or blue cotton blend fabric for $34.95 postpaid.　(JIA)

HAPPY BABY CARRIERS
$17.95 to $34.95

from
Happy Family Products
12300 Venice Blvd.
Los Angeles, CA 90066

This company has designed the Happy Baby Carrier which is available in two models: the Air-Cool Napsak Carrier is made of nylon net and fabric for warm weather comfort and security; the Deluxe Vogue Carrier has double-strength seat, padded straps and leg openings, and is made of heavier fabric. Happy Family also carries two carriers by Gerry: the Cuddlepack, which has storage space for baby items, a nursing zipper in the straps, and grows with the child; and the Kiddie Pack, a metal frame backpack carrier with fold-out stand (for older babies and toddlers). Happy Dolly Carriers are also available for children who want to practice being parents. Happy Family carries a variety of other products for babies and children so their free catalog is well worth writing for.　(MS)

Baby Carrier Kit
cheeks

(Editor's Note: We used baby carriers with both our children: a soft front pack until they were about six months old and a metal frame back pack until they were too heavy to carry any longer. The carriers made it easy and enjoyable for us to go shopping, visiting and on long walks with our babies. I enjoyed holding them close to my body when they were small and the carrier seemed like a much more personable and convenient way to travel than a stroller. We found we could take our babies wherever we went, without having to worry about pushing a stroller over rough terrain or up steps and through doors. Whenever we went out with our babies in the carrier, older parents would stop to talk

to us and admire the new arrangement. Their most common comment was, "I wish they'd had those carriers when I was having my babies.")(JIA)

BABY PRODUCTS AND CLOTHING

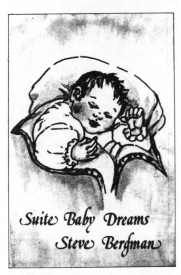

SUITE BABY DREAMS
$9.45 for each cassette

from
Steven Bergman
P.O. Box 4577
Carmel, CA 93921

Steven's *Music for an Inner Journey* has helped thousands of people to relax, so now he has put together a new cassette of music to calm and quiet mothers and babies. *"Suite Baby Dreams"* combines soothing flutes, piano and guitars with the heartbeat sounds of a pregnant mother. The effect is a soft blend of "inside and outside" sounds for the newborn. And, unlike conventional music boxes, the tape lasts 25 minutes and *you* can set the volume as loud or soft as you wish. You may also want to play it before and during the birth as an added inducement to relax. (MS)

"Music is the basic vibration on the planet. Music for new babies and parents is soothing and calming and necessary.
"Suite Baby Dreams" has been used in home deliveries, quieted nursery school children, and calmed hundreds of babies."
—Steven Bergman

SOFTSCULPTURE RAINBOWS
$4.00 cloudbow
$5.00 heartbow

from
Mary Scott
101 Stony Hill Road
Port Jefferson, NY 11777

Here is a colorful piece of art work that will last from prenatal days to grown child in use and enjoyment. Satin clouds come in white, royal blue, azure, or light blue, or navy blue with a silver lame lightning bolt. All seven colors in rainbow order in double-faced satin ribbon make it a perfect Lamaze "focal point" and then your child's first mobile. Little eyes love to "play" with the bright shiny colors whose names you can teach later. Hearts come in red and pink. Hand washable and stuffed with 100% polyester fluff, the ribbons are double-stitched to stand up to lots of love. Approximately 6" by 9", each is hand-made by the artist. Order direct or send for catalog. (MS)

(Editor's Note: Mary didn't want anyone to know that the Mary Scott who makes these beautiful rainbows is the same Mary Scott who has reviewed these sections on baby care and products. But I thought readers would like to know and should know that Mary's rainbows are special, for two important reasons: first, because these softsculptures are really lovely. I have them hanging in my children's bedrooms and enjoy looking at them every day. When Mary displays her wares at local craft fairs, she hangs the rainbows from the branches of a tree, creating a dazzling sight. Mary hand dies some of the ribbon colors to make sure that the rainbow progression is just right. But more important is the fact that Mary is legally blind, having lost a significant portion of her central vision some years ago. This makes her achievement in making the rainbows and in reviewing parts of this Catalog even more significant. JIA)

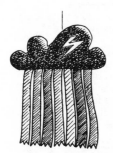 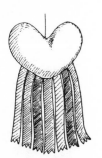 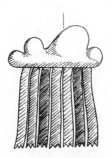

ORIGINAL HEAD SUPPORT
$7.00 postpaid

from
Little Sun
P.O. Box 22457
San Francisco, CA 94122

"We are a family operated home business. We came up with the idea for our product because our son needed head support while riding in his car seat, stroller, and infant swing."

Ideal for young infants and handicapped children who need that extra support in conventional car carriers, seats, and strollers, this soft sculptured head support cradles a little head and neck, effectively molding the seat-back to the child. Indicate red, yellow, navy, chocolate, or blue gingham or rainbow stripe when ordering. Handcrafted in machine washable cotton/polyester blend and stuffed with non-allergenic polyester fiberfill. (MS)

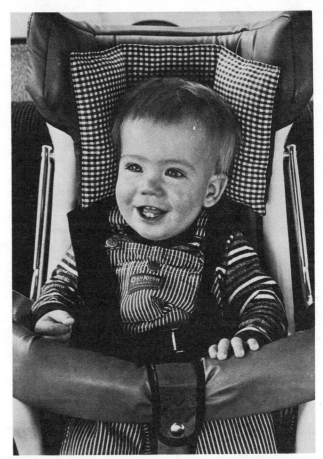

CRIBCUDDLE
$39.95 plus $2.50 shipping

from
Infacare
P.O. Box 2782
Laguna Hills, CA 92653

This yellow terrycloth hammock with a white plush sleep-area lining is designed as a transitional "cradle" for newborns. It attaches to the crib in one of three positions for back or stomach sleeping and has a white plush heart containing the heartbeat sound mechanism, Cuddle-Heart (9 volt battery not included). Between the softness of the plush and the gentle sound and vibration of the heartbeat, the newborn infant is comforted to sleep in a gentle transition from womb to more conventional crib sleeping. Safety tested and machine washable. (MS)

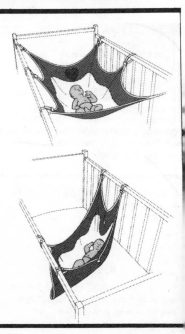

THE BABY BAG
$32.50 postpaid
(Maine residents add 5% sales tax)

from
The Baby Bag Company
2 Bisbee Street
Camden, ME 04843

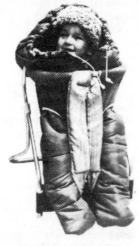

A sleeping bag with feet! This unique snowsuit is specially designed for children who ride in baby carriers. More adaptable than a bunting bag, the Baby Bag is warm and easy to use. The cotton-blend outer cloth is water repellent and its texture makes it easy for parents to grip, while the nylon inner lining makes it easy to slide the child right in. The Bag is insulated with a warm layer of Hollofil II. A velcro closure and drawstring hood make it easy to adjust the Bag for the weather or a quick diaper change. Fits babies from three months to two years, machine washable. (MS)

"The Baby Bag is too bulky to work with the smaller soft carriers

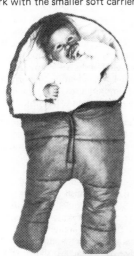

but does fit in those designed for toddlers. It works beautifully with all the back carriers, strollers and bikeseats that we have seen. In the car, the Baby Bag must be used with the particular carseat's design in mind. Some models have slippery shoulder straps and you may have to leave the bag open to prevent the straps from riding down. Of course the bag works fine with the between-the legs straps; with proper attention your child can be snug *and* safe on those chilly morning car rides.

"This is a product which I designed for my child when she turned out to hate her snowsuit. It is ideal for parents in cold climates who like to take their babies everywhere but also is so easy to use that any parent would find it useful.

"The babies are happier, too, because their hands are available (there's plenty of room inside) to use with toys, in their mouths, etc."
—Elizabeth Andrews, of the Baby Bag Company

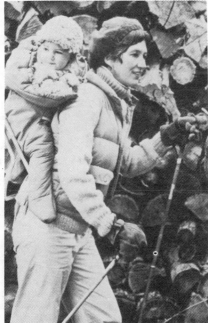

BABY BAG designer Elizabeth Andrews with daughter Jesse. At 26 months Jesse still fits in the bag, the hood now functioning as a collar.

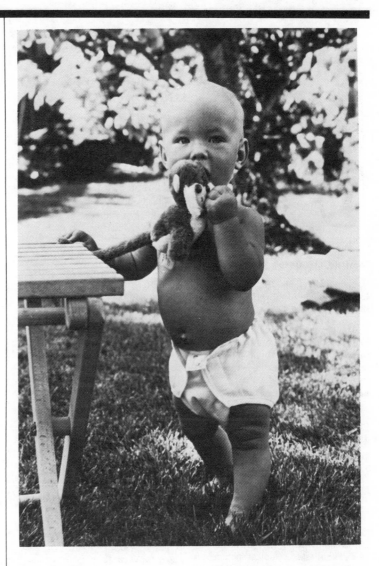

BIOBOTTOMS
$10.00 each

from
Biobottoms
P.O. Box 853
Bolinas, CA 94924

A natural fiber diaper cover, Biobottoms provide an alternative to plastic pants for mothers who choose cloth diapers. "Biobottoms, made of soft wool-felt, help prevent diaper rash and let the baby's bottom breathe. They fasten with velcro and make diaper changing a 10 second job. Biobottoms eliminate the need for any pins! Even the most timid father can diaper his squirming baby in seconds." Biobottoms come in white and are available in five sizes. A four pair supply is recommended for each child. (MS)

"This type of baby garment can be found in many varieties all over the world, except in the U.S.A. American grandmothers remember knitting soakers to place over their babies' cloth diapers. But, airless plastic and throwaway disposable diapers have taken over in the U.S.A. today. The good sense of using a pure and breathable fabric next to a baby's most sensitive area has not changed."

"Joan Cooper and Anita Dimondstein are two busy California mothers who discovered this product and decided to market it after testing it for a year on their own babies.

" 'We are 100% convinced that the American parent wants to know that there is an alternative to the ecological diaster of throwaway diapers,' states Joan Cooper. "We understand that up to one third of the garbage of an average town is the unsanitary garbage from disposable diapers. In addition, most parents think that diaper rash is an unavoidable fact of a baby's life. With fresh air circulating, rashes can be the exception, rather than the rule." —from Biobottoms

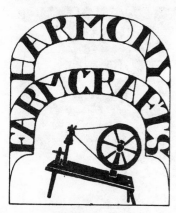

HARMONY FARMCRAFTS
Harmony Farm/Roberta Bailey
Topsfield, ME 04490

Woolen Soakers
$8.00 each, handspun yarn
$6.00 each, mill yarn

The handspun, lanolin-rich wool for these soakers is made from the Baileys' own sheep! This alternative to plastic pants comes in undyed natural wool or light color. Sizes are

small (birth to 6 months), medium (6-12 months), and large (12-18 months). (MS)

Socks and Booties
$3.00 to 7.00 a pair

Using the same handspun or quality milled yarns, these baby socks, booties and slipper socks are handknit for comfort and durability. Some have sheepskin soles, and they come in a variety of sizes and colors. Won't be kicked off by active babies. Write to Roberta for more details.

"I like to make available comfortable alternatives to plastic pants and comfortable, practical infant clothing, such as booties. I live on a small sheep farm, spinning lanolin-rich wool yarns and having some fleece processed into 'commercial' yarns at a local woolen mill. Soakers are one end product. Also socks and handspun knit booties with sheepskin soles."

—Roberta Bailey of Harmony Farmcrafts

SOFT WALKER SHOES
$7.50 to 13.00 a pair for the smaller sizes

from
Soft Walker Shoes, Inc.
2113 Manor Road
Austin, TX 78722

Handcrafting quality leather and crepe sole shoes in a variety of styles for reasonable prices is a major goal of this family business; they have succeeded admirably. Choices include one-piece upper, sandal styles, and fleece-lined boots among others and

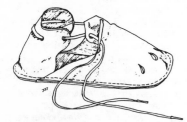

all are available in choices of leathers and color. All shoes lace to stay on comfortably. Write for their brochure which includes illustrations, a size chart, and all the information you need to order custom-made shoes for your baby. (MS)

"Soft Walker Shoes are designed to give flexible protection to children's feet from crawling through preschool development. They are made to fill the need for reasonably priced, sturdy footwear for children whose parents believe barefoot is best. Many doctors—pediatricians, chiropractors, podiatrists, and family physicians—are now advising soft shoes for early development. This is contrary to the 'support' theory because the principle involved is to strengthen the feet and ankles by allowing them to move and flex while walking rather than keeping them immobile with an artificially shaped arch. However, barefoot is preferable when it's safe."

COZY TOZ
$6.00 to 7.25 plus postage for the smaller sizes

from
BaBayit Handcrafts
P.O Box 132
Clements, MD 20624

Here are handspun, handknitted, 100% wool slippers from Grey New Zealand Romney wool. And, for the do-it-yourself folks you have a choice of a kit or the ready-made product. An elastic cord around the ankle helps keep these thick (6 ply) fleecy slippers on busy feet and each pair comes with a story about how wool yarn comes from sheep and how

Eli got his first pair of Cozy Toz. (MS)

"Cozy Toz slippers are part of our new home business: 'BaBayit Handcrafts.' BaBayit, pronounced Baba (like a sheep) and yit (it pronounced like it!) means 'at home' in Hebrew. . . . We started this home business so that I could be employed and also stay home with our 14 month old son, Eli. We had Eli at home with a midwife. It was a beautiful experience. Our goal is to have our business grow so that we can both stay home and work around our family. Family is very important to us." —Sandy Gunzburg of BaBayit.

FINGER PRINTS
17554 Hatteras Street
Encino, CA 91316

Finger Prints silk-screen their attractive designs in non-toxic, nonplastic inks on 100% cotton T-shirts in sizes from infant to adult and maternity. Prices range from $4.95 to $14.95 and distributorships are available. Write for a catalog. (MS)

"This is a family business since 1978. We have been involved in Natural Childbirth education for several years. As parents of young children, we wanted to 1) have a business centered around the home and 2) provide a quality product with 'wholesome' sayings and 3) involve a distributorship network of other parents seeking a home business, selling a product with a philosophy that supported their personal lifestyle."

—Mary Cooksey of Finger Prints

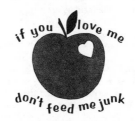

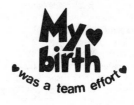

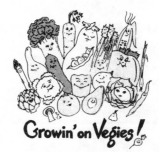

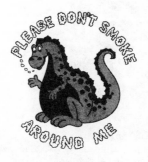

AFTER THE STORK
P.O. Box 1832
Bisbee, AZ 85603

After the Stork is a small family business with a wealth of interesting and organic products to offer, including clothes and music. Their catalog is well worth writing for. (MS)

"Parents who have cared enough to give their baby a natural birth soon find themselves faced with a new dilemma. The kinds of products they want for their child are very difficult to obtain. Local stores carry synthetic garments, disposable diapers, chemical and perfume laden powders, ointments and oils, etc. . . .

"Our goal is to help parents 'After the Stork'—to be a central source for a wide range of alternative products for infants and toddlers. Wherever the term 'natural' is meaningful, our products are of cotton, wool, or leather. A wide variety of herbal products are offered. Other products are suited to complement a New Age approach to parenting, such as carriers that encourage parent-child intimacy, a high-chair alternative that brings your child right to your table, and some excellent children's music (by real artists, not Disney robots) that the whole family will enjoy. Our decorative T-shirts feature unicorns, sunsets, hummingbirds, and rainbows, not Spiderman and the Hulk.

"In general, our products are characterized by healthfullness, quality construction, simple styling, and reasonable cost. Our service is prompt (except for occasional delays on handcrafted items) and satisfaction is guaranteed. We publish two catalogs each year, Spring/Summer and Fall/Winter. We are always looking for interesting, useful products, and encourage craftspeople and small manufacturers to contact us. Finally, rather than seeding the one-time sale we try to establish long-term relationships with parents who turn to us again and again for the finest products for their children."

—Janis Zloto and Alan Stopper of "After the Stork"

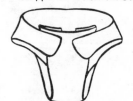

DEXTER B-29, The Finest Diapers Made

"Called the B-29 because it has wings and carries a big payload, the DEXTER is the only true form-fitting diaper on the market. Two layers of 100% cotton surround a thick, absorbent pad. The diaper is safely stitched to prevent fraying. It fits from birth to toilet training. Very durable, you'll be able to pass them on."

COTTON DREAMS
999 Laredo Lane
Sebastian, FL 32958

Cotton Dreams is a family business which sells natural fiber clothing for the whole family. The Nichols and their three attractive, young children model all the clothing in their catalog, including overalls, children's natural "loungewear" (no flame retardant chemicals), pants, tops, knickers, sweaters, skirts, underwear, socks, Chinese cotton shoes and more. (JIA)

"Our goal is to provide hard-to-find natural fiber clothing for infants and children. All three of my children were born at home with a midwife. It was a wonderful experience!"
—Cheri Nichols of Cotton Dreams

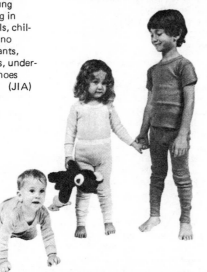

COTTON COOKIE
50 Elm Avenue
Woodacre, CA 94973

Cotton Cookie sells natural fiber clothing for children, including jackets, shirts, sheepskin hats and vests, overalls and jumpers, silk-screened shirts, and long underwear. (JIA)

"My goals in this company are to provide natural fiber clothing for infant's and children and at reasonable prices. I feel this is as much a part of a child's health care as proper nutrition—possibly a form of preventative medicine."
—Linda Ehrenberg of Cotton Cookie

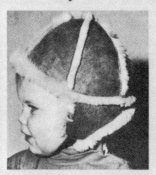

Warm and Practical for Both Boys and Girls

SHEEPSKIN HAT

INKY FINGERS
Route 1, Box 85
New Lisbon, WI 53950
608/562-3969

Inky Fingers sells infant T-shirts with a lovely "Born at Home" design on the front ($3.00 each) and with the option of printing your logo or message on the back ($3.50 each). The shirts are 100% cotton and come in long or short sleeves in 10 custom-dyed colors. Minimum order is one dozen, as these shirts are intended to be bought by birth attendants as "a very nice gift for the babies you deliver." (JIA)

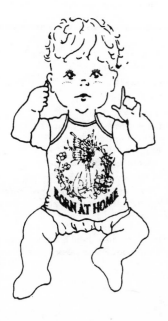

GARNET HILL
Box 262
Franconia, NH 03580

Garnet Hill began by importing and selling cotton flannel bed sheets and has gone on to include a wide variety of natural fiber products and clothing for adults (including sleep wear styles suitable for nursing mothers, and all cotton prenatal and nursing bras), and a full line of beautiful (and fairly expensive) things for babies and children, including flannel crib sheets, cotton crib bumpers, blankets, shirt sets, wrap pants and shirts, jumpsuits, sweaters, socks, booties and more. All products are beautifully displayed in their full color catalog. (JIA)

CHILDRENS SHOES (E 1225)
1971, 12 pages
$.15

BUY BY SIZE, NOT AGE (IB 19)
1971, 6 pages
$.15

BUYING CLOTHES FOR SMALL CHILDREN (S 100)
1974, 15 pages
$.25

from
Cornell University Distribution Center—WB
7 Research Park
Ithaca, NY 14850

The Cooperative Extension division of Cornell University makes available these three useful booklets on choosing children's shoes and clothing. Prices include postage. (JIA)

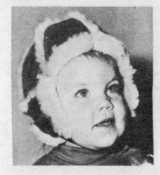

A child's first shoe should be soft and flexible and should provide plenty of toe room.

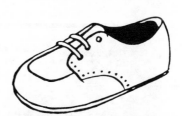

Generally, high top shoes are not needed for ankle support. If you decide to put your baby in them, be sure the tops are soft and flexible.

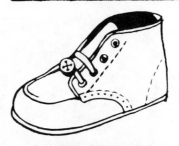

This shoe is cut too skimpily and does not provide enough toe room.

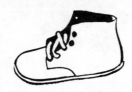

Mary Janes and similar styles are acceptable for dressy occasions but should not be worn continuously. These styles tend to be stiff and generally they provide less toe room than oxfords. Furthermore, they are often hard for the child to keep on her foot.

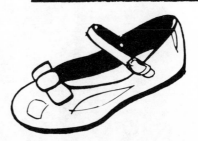

—from *Children's Shoes*

Child Health and Safety

Mary Scott, editor

YOUR CHILD'S HEALTH CARE
brochure

from
Health and Safety Education Division
Metropolitan Life Insurance Company
One Madison Avenue
New York, NY 10010
free

This fold-out brochure outlines some of the general knowledge parents need in order to oversee the health care their children receive. What is involved in a check-up, what to ask the doctor, helping children understand and participate in their own care and treatment, and going to the hospital are discussed along with questions you should ask to make informed decisions. A list of community and reading resources is included for more information. (MS)

"A doctor's care, alone, does not guarantee health. Children, like adults, need to learn to take responsibility for their health. For example:
* what foods to eat and why
* how to brush teeth
* importance of washing up before meals
* the benefits of exercise
* reasons for adequate sleep

"Children can learn much about health and safety from examples set by a parent. If you don't smoke, they might not start. Buckle up your car seat belt and they can learn to do the same. Go easy on sugar and candy and a child may follow suit."

PUBLICATIONS OF THE OFFICE OF HUMAN DEVELOPMENT SERVICES
free

from
U.S. Department of Health and Human Services
Public Health Service
National Institutes of Health
Bethesda, MD 20205

Wonder what the Government is doing to further your good health and happiness? Write for this booklet, which tells what various departments do and provides an excellent catalog which lists publications available either from HHS directly or through the U.S. Government Printing Office. These publications are interesting and usually easy to read. We have reviewed some of them here but there are lots more. (MS)

WHEN YOUR CHILD IS SICK
by Jacqueline Seaver and June V. Schwartz
1978, 24 pages

from
Public Affairs Pamphlets
381 Park Avenue South
New York, NY 10016
$.50

It may be long reading, but this common sense guide to child health will not only show you how to recognize and treat common problems, but also how to prevent them and help your child develop a healthy attitude toward bodily functions and dysfunction. The authors use anecdotes to introduce each section and apply material directly to real-life situations. To young children most illnesses and accidental scrapes are more scary than harmful and this booklet helps parents meet the emotional needs of children who are sick. (MS)

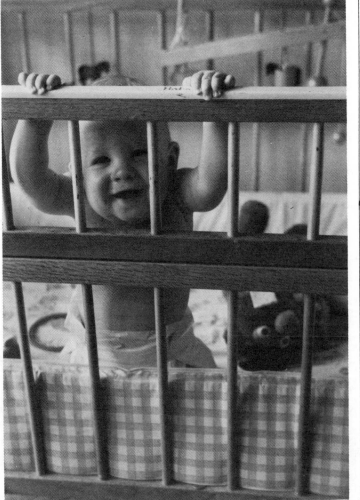

J.I.A.

HOW *NOT* TO LOVE YOUR KIDS
brochure

SECOND-HAND SMOKE
brochure

from
American Lung Association
1740 Broadway
New York, NY 10019
212/245-8000
free

These and other booklets and brochures are available from your local Lung Association, listed in the phone book. Maybe you say it's *your* life and *your* pursuit of happiness, but YOUR smoke has a direct effect on the living and unborn children around you. These brochures discuss those effects and give advice on asking people not to smoke and/or your not smoking in any social or public situation. Save some health. Get these materials. (MS)

"Everyone in the same room with you breathes in your smoke.
* When any nonsmokers—like your young children—are forced to breathe cigarette-polluted air, things happen that you can't see. Their heart beat speeds up. Their blood pressure rises. Dangerous carbon monoxide seeps into their blood.
* Babies in their first year have a higher rate of pneumonia and bronchitis if their parents smoke at home.
* In one major study, respiratory illnesses happened twice as often to young children whose parents smoked at home, compared to kids with nonsmoking parents.
* If you're pregnant and smoke, you reduce the supply of oxygen to your unborn baby and can retard its growth. You run the risk of seriously damaging its health. Even its life."

—from *How Not to Love Your Kids*

CHILDHOOD DISEASES
16 pages

from
The Prudential Insurance Company of America
Box 36
Newark, NJ 07101
free

Chicken Pox, Mumps, Scarlet Fever, Heat Rash, and other common childhood diseases are described in this little booklet which covers how to recognise and treat the diseases and when to call the doctor. A handy, quick reference. (MS)

CHICKENPOX
brochure, 1981

MUMPS
brochure, 1978

from
Center for Disease Control
Public Inquiries
Building 1-B63
Atlanta, GA 30333
free

These two single-page brochures clearly state the symptoms, dangers, treatment and prevention of each disease. Mumps is more dangerous than you may think and chickenpox breaks out 2 to 3 weeks after exposure. (MS)

HOW DOES YOUR CHILD HEAR AND TALK?
fold out chart 9'' x 16''

from
American Speech and Hearing Foundation
10801 Rockville Pike
Rockville, MD 20852
free

Catching speech and hearing problems early is the key to minimizing or eliminating them. This chart lists things to look for in your child's hearing and speaking abilities from birth to age five. If average abilities are not present, parents are advised to seek professional help. Also included are handy reminders on teaching children to speak and where to go for hearing tests. The American Speech and Hearing Foundation also produces other brochures for consumers. Write for a complete list. (MS)

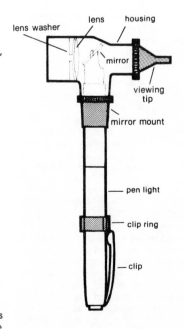

EARSCOPE
$16.95 plus 1.50 postage

from
Nash and Associates
504 Shaw Avenue
P.O. Box 300
Ferndale, CA 95536

The Earscope is a 6½ inch, tough, plastic device with a light beam and magnifying lense which lets you examine and monitor conditions in the ear canal. Much less expensive than the conventional "otoscope," the Earscope can be a useful "self-health" tool for households with young children or where there are recurrent ear problems. Lewis Nash, who designed the Earscope, wrote us this letter about it:

"I had trouble with my small daughter's ears while on a trip to Alaska and spent a lot of time and money on an emergency room and doctors' fees to find out that her 'ear problem' was merely a black-fly bite just inside the ear canal. It got me interested in otoscopes (that's what medical people call these things). Since I work at a college I had dealings with public health nurses who told me that professional units were needed in back-woods communities but were too expensive (professional otoscopes run $100. and up). I decided to try to make serviceable units myself. To everyone's surprise, these units, while inexpensive, work well indeed. A lot of the medical people here helped me develop and write a handbook to go along with the Earscope and I have sold hundreds of units to mothers of small children, nurses, family nurse practitioners, MD's and others. I took units to the American Public Health Association convention in Los Angeles last month (October, 1981), sold out in a day and a half, and had disbelieving doctors tell me, 'Hell, that's as good as my $100. unit.' Many mothers have told me that I have saved them a lot of agony and expense.

"There is no doubt in my mind that there is a real need for such units by people with ear problems. At 2 A.M. on a Sunday morning with a howling kid on your hands, you never know quite what to do—give an aspirin, take the car to the emergency room, call your doctor (maybe for nothing), etc. These units give mothers more information, allowing them to monitor the ears so that they can make better decisions about when they need medical help.

"It's nice to be working on a project that can help people so much, and yet is practical and self sustaining."

Diagram labels: lens washer, lens, housing, mirror, viewing tip, mirror mount, pen light, clip ring, clip

FLUORIDE TO PROTECT YOUR CHILDREN'S TEETH
1981, brochure

from
National Institute of Dental Health
Public Health Service
9000 Rockville Pike
Bethesda, MD 20205
free

From infancy on the use of fluoride can provide protection from cavities in children. The proper use of fluoride and the reasons for using it are discussed in this brochure. Fluoride drops, tablets, rinses, and toothpastes are all covered. (MS)

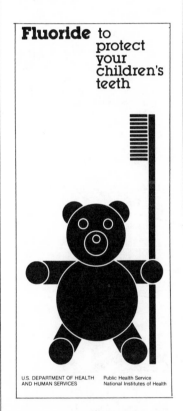

Fluoride to protect your children's teeth

U.S. DEPARTMENT OF HEALTH AND HUMAN SERVICES
Public Health Service
National Institutes of Health

CAN YOUR CHILD HEAR WELL ENOUGH TO LEARN?
by Burton L. White
1980, 8 pages

from
Baby Fresh
Scott Paper Company
P.O. Box 4260
Chester, PA 19016
free

Hearing loss may be subtle or obvious even in young infants. Often pediatricians don't recognize symptoms because normal children exhibit the same "abnormal" responses from time to time. This booklet goes over the importance of early diagnosis, danger signals to watch for, and lists step-by-step action to take and professionals to seek out once a problem has been identified. (MS)

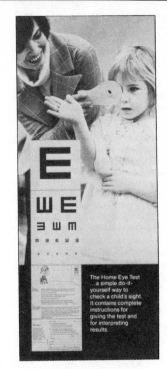

The Home Eye Test ...a simple do-it-yourself way to check a child's sight. It contains complete instructions for giving the test and for interpreting results.

HOME EYE TEST FOR PRE-SCHOOLERS
1975, fold out chart with instructions

from
National Society to Prevent Blindness
79 Madison Avenue
New York, NY 10016
free for single copies
$6.00 per 100 in bulk

Amblyopia ("lazy eye") and infant cataracts can be best cured when they are discovered early. This simple test is designed to help parents assess and take appropriate action regarding their children's vision before they start school. Any vision problems can lead to frustration not only in learning but in playing as well. The National Society to Prevent Blindness also provides a catalog of publications and teaching tools which offer further information on many rare and common eye problems and eye safety. Write for a copy. (MS)

AMERICAN ACADEMY OF PEDIATRICS
Publications Department
P.O. Box 1034
Evanston, IL 60204

The American Academy of Pediatrics (AAP) publishes a variety of public education materials, including the following: accident prevention, adolescence, adoption, asthma, child abuse, drugs, environmental hazards, government and children, handicapped children, immunization and infectious disease, learning disabilities, medical ethics and informed consent, neonatal care, nutrition, pediatric practice, physical fitness and sports, radiology, screening, and sudden infant death syndrome. Write for a free publications list. (JIA)

YOUNG CHILDREN AND ACCIDENTS IN THE HOME
1976, 28 pages

from
Superintendent of Documents
U.S. Government Printing Office
Washington, DC 20402
(Stock No. 017-091-00191-0)
free

"All young children get their share of cuts, bruises, and even sprains in the course of growing up. Minor injuries—while upsetting at the moment—can usually be treated with a gentle swab of antiseptic, a bandage, and a soothing hug and kiss.

"Serious accidents, however, are another matter. No child should experience even one such accident. The stakes are too high—brain damage, an ugly permanent scar, loss of a part of the body, or even death."

This well-written booklet discusses how to avoid the problems of falls, blows, cuts, bites, suffocation, burns, drowning, and poisoning; and how to treat them when they do

occur. It includes a pull-out First Aid Chart to hang in your medicine cabinet or other easily accessible place, a safety checklist by age of child, and lots of cute illustrations. Overall this is a handy, easy to read, quick reference for parents.   (MS)

"A baby is completely helpless and requires total protection. He wiggles, he rolls—you never know when he will roll over. His crib (with the sides pulled up) and playpen are the only safe places for the child to be left alone. *Never* let him lie unguarded on a couch, bed, changing table, or any other high place from which he might fall.

"If you have to answer the door or the telephone while you're in the middle of a diaper change, wrap the baby up and take him with you or put him back in the crib. Make it a habit to take him with you if you must reach for anything which prevents you from keeping at least one protective hand on him. Turning your back (even for a second) can be risky."

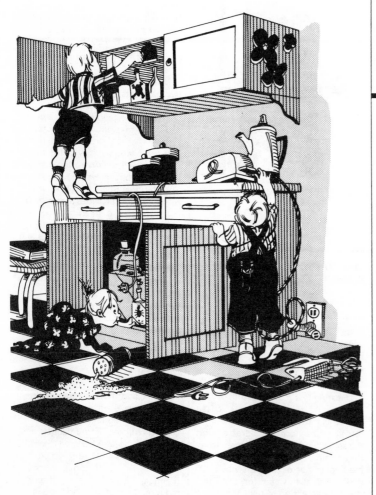

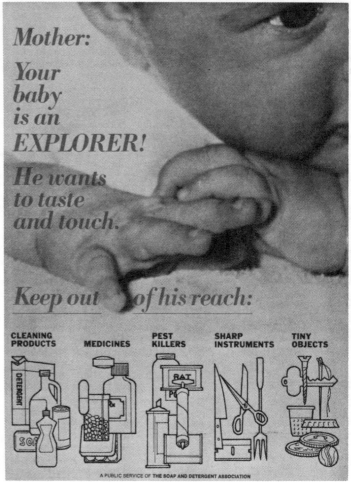

Mother:
Your
baby
is an
EXPLORER!
He wants
to taste
and touch.

Keep out   of his reach:

CLEANING PRODUCTS   MEDICINES   PEST KILLERS   SHARP INSTRUMENTS   TINY OBJECTS

PLANNING FOR SAFETY
brochure

CHILD SAFETY
brochure

from
Health and Safety Education Division
Metropolitan Life Insurance Company
One Madison Avenue
New York, NY 10010
single copies free

As an insurance company interested in minimizing claims, Metropolitan has put out these brochures as part of its "Stay Well Series." *Planning for Safety* gives some first-aid information and emergency medical I.D. information but the best part of the brochure is the Home Safety Checklist which proceeds room by room to make you aware of potential hazards and how to avoid and/or eliminate them. *Child Safety* takes a child in stages from birth to age seven, anticipating what trouble they might get into and how to avoid it, based on a knowledge of your child's physical capabilities. The emphasis is on prevention and also includes tips for babysitters. Metropolitan publishes a variety of brochures, cards, stickers, posters, and films on health and safety, most of them available free. Write for a copy of their health and safety publications catalog or ask for the

YOUR BABY IS AN EXPLORER!
poster, 8½" x 11"

from
The Soap and Detergent Association
475 Park Avenue South at 32nd St.
New York, NY 10016
single copy free

This two-color poster calls your attention to the inquisitiveness of your baby and what to watch out for. A pamphlet, *Home, Safe Home*, is also available in English and Spanish.

complete "Stay Well Series."   (MS)

"Babies soon learn to reach and grab and put things into their mouths. So clear away any sharp objects and things that are easily swallowed—buttons, pins, beads, coins, small detachable parts on toys. Avoid hanging toys on long cords that could get tangled around the baby's neck. Toys should be too large to swallow, too tough to break and should have no sharp points or edges. Keep the crib or playpen away from tables or dressers that hold perfumes, powder, cosmetics, pills, cigarettes, handbags—anything harmful that the baby might reach out and grab."
—from *Child Safety*

THE CARE AND SAFETY OF YOUNG CHILDREN
by Jay M. Arena, M.D.
14 pages

from
Council on Family Health
633 Third Avenue
New York, NY 10017
free

Dr. Arena has written another excellent booklet on child health and safety. "Most accidents to small children stem from youngster's normal, healthy curiosity and exuberance," he says on page one and goes on to discuss meeting the needs of infants, safeguarding the home for exploring youngsters, fire and traffic dangers, and "child-oriented" homes (this section is excerpted from *Child Safety Is No Accident,* opposite.) The booklet presents a positive, active approach to child safety for new parents. (Editor's Note: The Council on Family Health is a nonprofit, public service organization sponsored by the manufacturers of medicines.)　　　　　(MS)

"Hunger or fatigue makes a child more susceptible to accidents, especially an hour before feeding, late in the afternoon or just before bedtime. A sudden change in a child's environment, such as moving, going on vacation or a substitution in the person caring for him, can upset his routine and cause an accident.

"The tensions between parents are reflected in a child's behavior and often are contributing factors in mishaps. Illness or death in the family, or unusual activity in the home on weekends, distract attention from a child and may lead to accidents. A mother's pregnancy or menstrual period may reduce her stamina and possibly her alertness to impending danger, which can also spark a chain of unfortunate events. All such circumstances should be signals for parents to exercise caution."

CHILD SAFETY IS NO ACCIDENT
by Jay M. Arena, M.D.
1980, 17 pages

from
Prudential Insurance Company
Prudential Plaza
Newark, NJ 07101
free

"Be 'in tune' with your child" encourages this little booklet, which covers the potential hazards for children in stages by age as well as how to have a child-oriented home and teach discipline and respect for danger. A very positive and well-written approach to child safety.(MS)

"The basic premise of child-orienting is simply this: If a child has reached the decision, either verbally or through action, to do something, look for ways to make that decision a reality. For example, if the child is always emptying kitchen cabinets, he or she has obviously mastered the art of opening the cupboards. Instead of begrudgingly clearing away the mess and locking all the cupboards in retaliation, arrange a cabinet which contains unopened boxes and cans, pots and safe utensils. By changing the contents of this special place, parents can maintain their child's interest and, at the same time, reduce the chances that areas that are off limits will be explored. Child-orienting is an attitude, a perpetual use of the environment, not a single adjustment in the home for a short period, and it needs a commitment from parents who must continually evaluate their home environment from the point of view of the child."

A drawing by Liane Elizabeth Haynes (age 10), Madison, Alabama from the UNICEF collection of children's art, in *The Care and Safety of Young Children.*

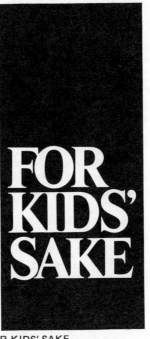

FOR KIDS' SAKE
1979, brochure

from
U.S. Consumer Product Safety Commission
c/o TOYS
Washington, DC 20207
free

This is an excellent brochure on toy safety—how to buy toys, what to look for and what to avoid—put out by that part of the federal government which is responsible for making sure that the toys on store shelves are safe. While safety standards exist, there are sometimes hazardous toys and baby products on the market and recalls sometimes occur. It's up to parents to be responsible about checking the safety features of toys they buy for their children.　　　(MS)

"Choose toys with care. Keep in mind the child's age, interests and skill level.

"Look for quality design and construction in all toys for all ages.

"Make sure that all directions or instructions are clear—to you, and, more importantly, to the child. Plastic wrappings on toys should be discarded at once before they become deadly playthings.

"*Be a label reader.* Look for age recommendations, such as 'Not recommended for children under three.' Look for other safety labels including: 'Non-toxic' on painted toys, 'Flame retardant/Flame resistant' on fabric products and 'Washable/hygenic materials' on stuffed toys and dolls."

JUVENILE PRODUCTS MANUFACTURERS ASSOCIATION

This organization of makers of children's products has taken upon itself the task of setting and maintaining product safety standards for high chairs and playpens. To meet these standards and earn the JPMA seal, a product must have no sharp edges, be well constructed of safe materials, be of stable construction, have no holes or mesh that will catch little fingers, and meet many other safety and quality control standards. Their seal provides some assurance of quality and durability in children's products. But remember to use your own careful judgment as well.　　　(MS)

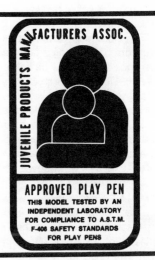

A NOTE ON THE HOME AS A FORTRESS OF CHILD SAFETY

Gates, special latches, coffee table bumpers, plastic caps for electrical outlets, etc., are just a few of the many products available to protect your things from your child and vice versa. But you will have to make common sense decisions about how far you will go to "make the house safe" for your child. Many a sleepy parent has tripped over a gate at the top of the stairs on the way to baby's room and there is always some clever two-year-old who can open that "child-proof cap" on the vitamins. In other words, passive safety devices are not always enough. You must actively teach your child how to be safe. Make the distinction between "no" and "danger," letting children know that "danger" is an always situation, while "no" may have to do with the mood of the parent at the time. Children start to understand words by about 12 months. Even before then you can use simple words to train behavior. Also get to know your own child—is she cautious or a real terror and how far can she be trusted? Remember that sometimes a *little* hurt will teach a lot, as the small scratch on one little girl's hand taught her not to pull the cat's fur. Avoid injuries *and* develop responsibility in a loving, reasonably safe environment.　　　(MS)

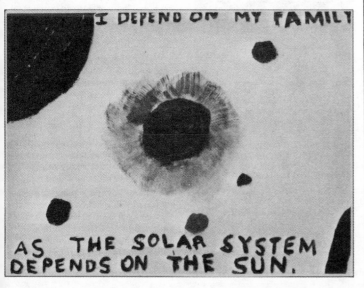

I DEPEND ON MY FAMILY

AS THE SOLAR SYSTEM DEPENDS ON THE SUN.

CAR SEAT SAFETY

Many people are as sick of the "Buckle-up" campaign as they are of the "Matter of Life and Breath" campaign. And why not? You know you are a safe driver, right? And you think you can hold on to your baby tightly if you come to a sudden stop. OH, YEAH???

If you really care about your children's safety, and your own for that matter, don't think it's enough to be a safe driver yourself. It's the OTHER GUY who will kill you or injure you and/or your family. All it takes is one drunk driver, one other parent who turns around to stop the fight in the back seat, one person stopping to read a street sign and not paying attention to the light, and you are all in BIG TROUBLE!

Over 1,500 children under age 5 die each year in auto accidents. Car accidents are the No. 1 killer in that age group, and more than half of these tragedies could have been prevented by the use of car-seats and seat belts. All infants should ride in the back seat in a safety approved carseat that faces the back window until they are 6 months old or able to sit up by themselves. After that, they may ride in the carseat that faces the front, until they are 40-50 pounds. Then they can buckle themselves into a regular belt harness. In all cases, the safest place for any child is in the back seat.

The organizations listed in this section offer newsletters and some excellent fact-sheets for comparison shopping for infant and older children's carseats. Look for the model in your price range that will fit your needs and your car. Be sure that your back seat has adult seat belts that are long enough to fit over a carseat. ALL carseats are held in the car's seat by use of the adult seat belt and usually some other fastening. Be sure that the baby is secure in the carseat, AND that the carseat is secure in the car.

There are many different models of carseats. Some are convertible from back-facing infant position to front-facing older child position. Others may be lighter-weight or useable as an infant seat as well. Decide before you buy whether you want a carseat that is easy to put in and take out of the car, or one that is installed for the duration of use. Molded seats may be easier to clean than jointed ones. "Wings" on either side of the head provide added protection and support for a sleeping child. A carseat that is on a raised base is good for long-distance travelers because the toddler can better see out the window. If the carseat you choose has a dark brown or black vinyl seat, get a cover for it or keep a light-colored towel in the car. Even in the winter, these seats can get very hot if you park in the sunshine. And, especially in Summer, always touch the metal buckles and fasteners before the baby does. We know of at least one little boy who got a bad burn on his leg from a Summer sun-heated buckle.

Many states now have mandatory child restraint laws. These include: Kansas, Massachusetts, Michigan, Minnesota, New York, North Carolina, Rhode Island, Tennessee, and West Virginia. Similar bills are pending in legislatures of many other states, and you can help pass them by writing to your local legislator. The American Automobile Association heartily endorses all these laws. Several other states also have provisions in the insurance laws whereby your auto insurance liability coverage is DOUBLED if you are in an accident and you and your passengers are all wearing seat belts. Safety pays in more ways than one.

One final note: Check how many seat belts are in *your* back seat. Never put two children in one belt. If it is that important that you all go, take more than one car. Remember, even the safest, most conscientious driver can be involved in a serious accident because another driver makes a mistake.　(MS)

PHYSICIANS FOR AUTOMOTIVE SAFETY (PAS)
P.O. Box 208[
Rye, New York 10580
914/253-9525

This national organization of American medical professionals is dedicated to the prevention of trauma on the highways through education. They recently took over the work of Action for Child Transportation Safety (ACTS) which had published a newsletter and fact sheets on carseats and issues of child safety on the highway. Write to PAS for films, pamphlets, and their newsletter which will keep you abreast of the laws and innovations in child restraint and education.　(MS)

"Adult Arms Are Not Safe

"Ordinarily, a parent's arms are a very secure place for a child, but inside a car it is the most hazardous. In a crash your body would crush the child against the dashboard and windshield. Even if you are wearing a lap and shoulder belt yourself, the child would be torn from your grasp by the violent forces of a collision.

"Never put a belt around you and a child held on your lap. Your own weight, greatly increased by crash forces, would press the belt deeply into the child's body; this could cause serious or even fatal injuries.

"Beginning with the very first car ride—the drive home from the

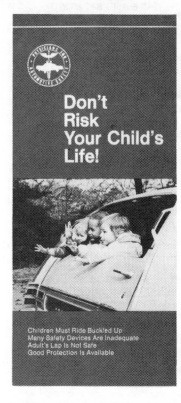

Don't Risk Your Child's Life!

Children Must Ride Buckled Up
Many Safety Devices Are Inadequate
Adult's Lap Is Not Safe
Good Protection Is Available

hospital—the baby should be secured in a crash-tested safety device." from *Don't Risk Your Child's Life*, 50 cents for single copies; bulk rates available.

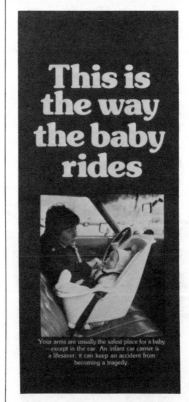

This is the way the baby rides

Your arms are usually the safest place for a baby—except in the car. An infant car carrier is a lifesaver; it can keep an accident from becoming a tragedy.

free from the Physician's for Automotive safety.

THIS IS THE WAY YOUR BABY RIDES

"Sometimes holding baby close isn't the best way to show your love. Many parents have discovered this too late, but you can safeguard your baby from the start, with an infant car carrier.

"In a crash, a baby can be torn violently from even the strongest arms. In only a 20 m.p.h. collision, for example, a 15 pound baby could be flung forward with the irresistible force of 300 pounds. Also, if *you* are riding unbelted, your own body could crush the child.

"A well-made infant car carrier is as important for your baby's fragile body as immunizations against dangerous diseases like polio and rubella. Each year more young children die in cars than from any other kind of accident. Of the tens of thousands injured, many remain permanently handicapped. You would never think of needlessly exposing your baby to disease. Don't expose him or her to injury in an auto accident.

"Being a good driver yourself isn't enough. Anyone can be the victim of an icy road or another driver's mistakes. Your best bet is to be prepared."

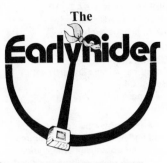

The EarlyRider

THE EARLYRIDER PROJECT
U.S. Department of Transportation
National Highway Traffic Safety
Administration
Washington, DC 20590

This project was produced in cooperation with the Michigan Jaycee Auxiliary, Action for Child Transportation Safety (ACTS), and Michigan's Motor Vehicle Occupant Protection Program. Included are four large informative booklets. All are available free. Some of the specific information on car seat models may be outdated, but the general principles outlined are still sound.   (MS)

Loan a Seat: How to Establish and Operate an Infant and Child Restraint Loan Program
An excellent guide to community participation in child auto safety and a way to save money in the bargain.

Early Rider Shopping Guide
Lists at least 19 carseats available in your local stores, prices, and illustrations

Early Rider Fact Book
Consumer advocates would be proud of this one. Lists carseats by brand name, prices, descriptions and many pros and cons for each model. An excellent, complete, easy-to-read reference.

Early Rider Publicity Handbook
Contains information on how to conduct a public relations campaign for car seat safety in your community.

This office also provides the following free brochures:
Child Restraint Systems for Your Automobile
Myths and Facts about Child Car Safety
How Many of these Fairy Tales Have You Told?

the only secure place
for a child in a car is in a crash-tested safety seat…and that's a fact!

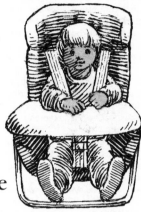

Where you can buy child safety seats: ■ Regular or discount department stores ■ Juvenile furniture or baby needs shops ■ Some new car dealers ■ Some hospital gift shops ■ Automobile parts and accessory dealers ■ Catalog sales through major retailers ■

AMERICAN ACADEMY OF PEDIATRICS
Office of Public Education
1801 Hinman Avenue
Evanston, IL 60204

The Academy provides two free brochures for parents concerned with car safety.
An Illustrated Guide to Baby's First Ride
Traveling Safely with Your Nursing Baby

THE NATIONAL CHILD PASSENGER SAFETY ASSOCIATION
c/o UNC Highway Safety Research Center
CTP-197A
Chapel Hill, NC 27514

Just getting started, this association wants to help educate the public, establish a "clearinghouse" for research and program information and set standards for loaner programs. They are also interested in helping states pass child restraint legislation, and they have a newsletter for those interested.   (MS)

You can also obtain information on car safety by writing directly to carseat manufacturers:

The Bobby-Mac Company, Inc.
95 Morris Lane
P.O. Box 209
Scarsdale, NY 10583

Offers free "buckle-up" stickers, educational and sales material including some scientific papers comparing different brands of carseats in crash tests. Interesting reading, but the photos of the tests are hard to make out.   (MS)

TRAVEL WITH BABY
11 page booklet

from
Cosco/Peterson
Subsidiary of Kidde, Inc.
2525 State Street
Columbus, IN 47201
free

Chock full of information about car safety seats, how to choose them, and how to use them. The last pages may prove to be the most interesting as they list useful tips and things to bring along to make long drives with baby relatively easy. An excellent check list.

They offer factsheets and educational materials in English and Spanish on their four models of carseats.   (MS)

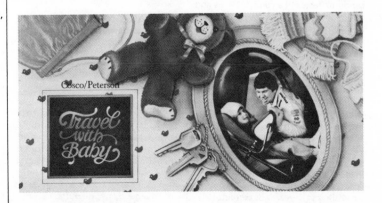

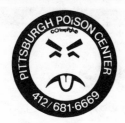

MR. YUK STICKERS
sheet of 12 self-adhesive stickers
$1.00

UNDER 5 UNDERSTANDING CARDS
packet of flash cards with parents' manual
$1.00

from
National Poison Center Network
Children's Hospital of Pittsburgh
125 De Soto Street
Pittsburgh, PA 15213

The best! The people at Children's Hospital have really done a wonderful thing by putting together these terrific durable stickers and flash card packets designed to teach you and your children how to avoid poisons and other dangers. This system really works. You might even consider increasing the donation to the Center or getting your local hospital to lay in a supply! (MS)

"Mr. Yuk stickers say 'NO!' to little children who can't read warning labels on the many dangerous products in your home. . . .
"Teach your child that Mr. Yuk means NO. Take children with you as you place Mr. Yuk stickers on dangerous products."

KEEPING POISONS AND CHILDREN APART
by Annabel Hecht
1979, 2 pages

from
U.S. Department of Health and Human Services
Public Health Service
Food and Drug Administration
5600 Fishers Lane
Rockville, MD 20857
free

"Never tell a child medicine is candy or tastes like candy." This and other do's and don't's are included in this interesting article about poison prevention which includes FDA statistics on poisonings, what to watch for based on the age and abilities of your child, and the origins of Poison Prevention Week.
"More than 15,000 2-year-olds were treated for accidentally swallowing medicines in 1976, according to FDA's figures. This was the largest number of cases in any product category and for any age group. Two-year-olds also accounted for the largest number of ingestions of cosmetics, although 1-year-olds were not far behind."

SAVE YOUR CHILD FROM POISONING
1980, 5 pages

from
Film Librarian, Corporate Communications, DA02
Aetna Life and Casualty
151 Farmington Avenue
Hartford, CT 06115

Poisonous substances are everywhere and this handy flip-up pamphlet lists common, poisonous household substances, how to properly store them, and proper first aid treatments including which poisons should *not* be treated by induced vomiting. (MS)

"If, without apparent reason, your child becomes over stimulated, drowsy or unconscious, you have good reason to suspect he has taken an overdose of drugs.
"If he develops severe stomach upset or pain or burning in the throat, he may have eaten some household cleaner or cosmetic.
"Any of these symptoms could indicate that your child has taken some pesticide or petroleum product.
"But never wait for physical symptoms to appear. If you notice unusual stains or odors on your child's skin or clothes, drugs or chemicals out of place or sudden changes in his behavior—suspect poisoning and react as if you were sure."

NATIONAL PLANNING COUNCIL OF NATIONAL POISON PREVENTION WEEK
P.O. Box 1543
Washington, DC 20013

The Council publishes, annually, a catalog of brochures, pamphlets, flyers, posters, and films and other materials from a variety of sources, designed to educate and aid people in poison prevention and treatment. Write for a copy of the current catalog or contact the Poison Center nearest you. Several of the materials reviewed in this section of the *Whole Birth Catalog* are listed by the Council. (MS)

FIRST AID GUIDE
foldout guide, 9" x 12"

from
Prudential Insurance Company
Prudential Plaza
Newark, NJ 07101
free

A very basic first aid reference, this guide covers bruises, wounds, burns, choking, and basic poisoning first aid, and provides a guide for artificial respiration. It is not illustrated. It will fit on the inside of the medicine cabinet door and has space for emergency phone numbers. (MS)

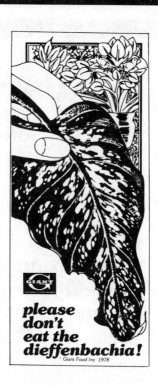

please don't eat the dieffenbachia!
Giant Food Inc. 1978

FIRST AID IN THE HOME
fold-out chart

from
Council on Family Health
633 Third Avenue
New York, NY 10017
free

This chart is very clear and easily referred to. Divided into sections on poisoning, bleeding, burns and scalds, shock, broken bones, eye contamination, and artificial respiration, it lists symptoms and proper first aid treatments as well as how to set up and keep a safe medicine cabinet. (MS)

"1. Empty out the entire contents of the cabinet once or twice each year.
2. Carefully check all items. Discard prescription drugs no longer being taken under a doctor's advice and any medication with a noticeable

BURN PREVENTION FOR 1 AND 2 YEAR OLDS
1976, brochure

from
National Institute for Burn Medicine
909 East Ann Street
Ann Arbor, MI 48104
free

Studies show that over 50% of all burn accidents involving infants could have been prevented! This pamphlet lists all the "don't's" in the kitchen, bathroom and bedroom as well as first aid and later care for minor burns. Send for it! (MS)

"IN THE KITCHEN:
1. Don't leave cords to electrical cooking appliances dangling. Your

PLEASE DON'T EAT THE DIEFFENBACHIA!
1978, brochure/chart

from
Giant Food, Inc.
Consumer Affairs Department
Box 1804
Washington, DC 20013
free

A list of over 50 common household and garden plants by common name and botanical name, indicating whether they are poisonous or not. If you have plants, this is an excellent chart to write for. Some common plants which are poisonous include: azalea, rhododendron, buttercup, castor bean, daffodil, dieffenbachia, English ivy, foxglove, fruit pits, holly, hyacinth, hydrangea, iris, jack-in-the-pulpit, lily-of-the-valley, mistletoe, mountain laurel, philodendron, privet, tomato plant (leaves only). (MS)

change in color or odor.
3. Check all medicine container labels. Discard medicines no longer in their original containers, in containers without complete label directions and in containers with labels that cannot be fully and clearly read.
4. Discard medicines safely by emptying contents of containers into sink or toilet and rinsing containers with water before placing in trash.
5. Organize contents for safe and convenient access. One suggestion is to place all internal medicines on top shelf, external medicines on center shelf and cosmetics and toiletries on bottom shelf.
6. Check to be sure medicines are safely out of reach of small children. (If necessary, find a higher storage area or use a cabinet with a lock.)

youngster can grab them and receive severe burns from the spilled hot liquids and solids.
2. Don't leave hot pans of food or liquids unattended on range, counter tops or tables. Don't leave handles extending over edge.
3. Don't let your youngster pour or serve hot food or liquids. Keep them out of reach.
4. Don't pour hot coffee, tea, soup or other fluids at the table and leave them unattended.
5. Don't drink coffee, tea or other hot fluids with your child on your lap—one slip or a sudden darting hand is all it takes to cause a serious scald burn."

UNICEF AND THE RIGHTS OF THE CHILD
1974, 23 pages, Illus.

from
United Nations Children's Fund
United States Committee for UNICEF
331 East 38th Street
New York, NY 10016
free

Illustrated with photographs of children from many nations, this booklet lists and describes the children's rights which have been established by the United Nations. (MS)

"All children, without any exception whatsoever, shall be entitled to these rights, without distinction or discrimination . . . that he may have a happy childhood, the right—from birth—to a name and nationality, the right to adequate pre-natal and post-natal care, the right to adequate nutrition, the right to adequate housing, the right to adequate medical care, the right to special care for the child who is handicapped, the right to parental affection, love and understanding, the right to an education, the right to learn to be a useful member of society, the right to develop abilities, the right to be among the first to receive relief in times of disaster, the right to enjoy full opportunity for play and recreation."

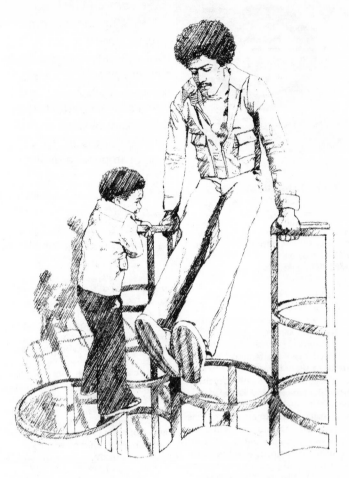

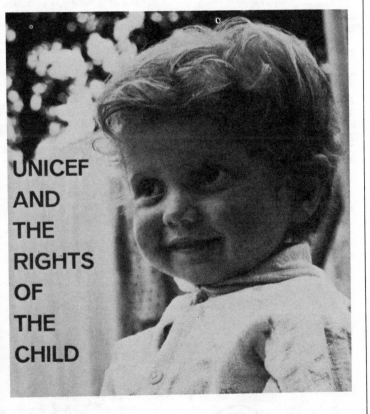

THE IMPORTANCE OF PLAY
by Constance Stapleton and Herbert Yahraes
1981, 16 pages

from
Public Inquiries
National Institute of Mental Health
5600 Fishers Lane
Rockville, MD 20857
free

One of the *Caring About Kids* series booklets, this illustrated discussion shows how play is useful and important in the physical and mental development of children from tiny infants on to school age. Tips on what to expect at each age, what behaviors mean, and what goals children have in play help to enlighten adults about how to teach rules, encourage creativity, and back off to let the child learn for herself. Get it to remind you of what it was like to be a kid. (MS)

"Play and the manipulation of objects are bases of creativity and invention later on. The creative adult retains the sense of childhood play."

CULTURAL ENRICHMENT BY MEANS OF A TOY LIBRARY
1980, 10 pages

from
Center for Studies of Child and Family Mental Health
National Institute of Mental Health
5600 Fishers Lane
Rockville, MD 20857
free

No, a "toy library" is not a tiny little library for tots to practice being quiet in. It's a wonderful concept of sharing toys to enrich the lives of many children while minimizing single family toy bills and clutter. Get this pamphlet and start one in your playgroup, if not your community! (MS)

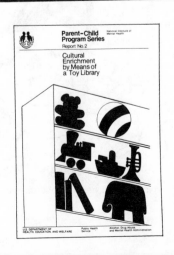

CHILD DEVELOPMENT IN THE HOME
1979, 20 pages, Illus.

from
Superintendent of Documents
U.S. Government Printing Office
Washington, DC 20402
(Stock No. 017-091-00193-6)
free

This cutely illustrated booklet discusses how to develop a healthy self-image in children, how to ease them into accepting and appreciating responsibility, and how parents help children develop problem-solving and decision-making skills and resourcefulness. Send for it, expecially if you have older small children, or ask your Senator or Congressperson to send you a copy. (MS)

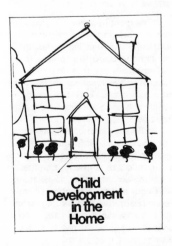

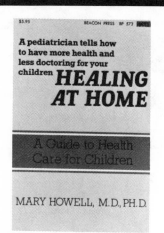

$5.95   BEACON PRESS BP 573

A pediatrician tells how to have more health and less doctoring for your children HEALING AT HOME

A Guide to Health Care for Children

MARY HOWELL, M.D., PH.D.

HEALING AT HOME: A Guide to Health Care for Children
by Mary Howell
1978, 287 pages, Illus.

from
Beacon Press
25 Beacon Street
Boston, MA 02108
$5.95 pap.

Mary Howell is a feminist, a mother of six children, and a practicing pediatrician and child psychologist. She has written *Healing at Home* with the important aim of acknowledging the mother's crucial role in her children's health care and putting skills and responsibility for health care firmly in her hands. Howell provides very useful chapters on how to take a health history, how to do a physical exam, remedies for home use, and common illnesses and injuries. But most importantly, she discusses our society's concepts of health and disease, the importance of women as health care-givers, "health promotion" (as opposed to "disease prevention") through nutrition, relaxation, and exercise, and how to deal with medical professionals. Howell works hard to "demystify" medicine and remove the awe from medical professionals and to give mothers confidence in their own judgment and skills. *Healing at Home* is a truly excellent resource and its concepts can be applied not only to children but to the health care we all receive.   (JIA)

"The most important ingredient that you bring to your assistance to your child's self-healing is your intimate knowledge of that child. In this you have information that no medical professional can match. The information and skills that you can learn for healing at home are, for the most part, fairly simple to use. This is a well-kept secret of the experts. But your store of information about your child is unique and irreplaceable. Your child's trust in you is an invaluable ingredient in healing assistance. And your ability to teach your child about healthiness and healing—from your intense desire that your child be well—is one of the most precious gifts of your mothering."

"Healing comes from within. Every culture evolves a set of remedies that are given for disease: some are thought to 'cure,' while others comfort, take away pain, overcome dysfunction or disability, or hide or improve a disfigurement. But no remedy, in and of itself, will restore good health. One's underlying good health and wish to be well do most or all of the real healing."

"All parts of the physical examination require two things of you: the practice of some fairly simple skills, and repeated, considered, and attentive focusing on your child. The skills can be practiced on yourself, other mothers and their children, and on any child who will play with you as your subject. Practice and practice until you feel confident of your eyes and hands and ears.

"Knowing your own child, in the matter of health assessments, means for the most part an organizing of what you already know as the child's mother. You have looked and listened and felt every day in the course of your ordinary caretaking. Doing a formal health assessment gives you an opportunity to pull together what you already know.

"Each of us is different from every other. Knowing one person very well —yourself, or your child—enables you to recognize changes as they occur. As a mother you are thus in a better position than a doctor to notice changes—even though you will often want professional help in interpreting those changes. If you have more than one child—or take care of children other than your own—you will learn some of the range of expected variations among children. A doctor can never know your child as well as you do—s/he can only use knowledge and experience based on some idea of 'average' or 'normal.' ". . .

"Here is a list of supplies that you might keep handy. It would be sensible if more than one household shared this store of equipment and supplies. A community center might serve as a central location, from which these items could be obtained for use.

1. Ace bandage
2. A mild steroid ointment (by prescription)
3. Aspirin or aspirin substitute
4. Bacitracin ointment
5. Betadyne or pHisohex soap (by prescription)

6. Bloodpressure apparatus—cuffs of 7, 12, and 18 centimeters width
7. Burow's Solution
8. Butterfly bandaids
9. Camomile tea
10. Centrifuge (for hematocrit)
11. Chlorpheniramine (if your family has bothersome allergies)
12. Codeine—2 tabs (by prescription)
13. Fluoresceine strips
14. Ipecac Syrup (by prescription)
15. Ipsatol Cough Remedy
16. Kerlex bandage
17. Labstix
18. Lancet, swabs, glass tubes (for hematocrit)
19. Nonallergenic tape
20. Otoscope
21. Peppermint tea
22. Rectal thermometer
23. Regular Band-Aids
24. Rosehip tea, containing vitamin C
25. Scotch tape
26. Stethoscope
27. Sterile gauze pads—small and large
28. Stresstabs—high potency vitamin B tablets
29. Telfa pads
30. Throat culture materials
31. Tincture of Benzoin
32. Uricult Kits
33. Vasoline
34. Vitamin C tablets (if this seems to help members of your family recover from upper respiratory infections)
35. Vitamin E capsules

"Good health demands the effective balance of two complex, whole-person processes that are closely related to each other. The first of these is moving and acting, focusing one's energy and strength, responding to challenge and initiating sustained and directed effort. The second is regenerative rest, the easing of mind, spirit, and body. . . .

"Nurses and social workers are very well trained to work with doctors. They know how to present information to a doctor, describing in accurate detail the patient's entire situation but leaving to the doctor the pronouncement of the diagnosis. It is far more useful for the child if you learn to act like a nurse, describing what you know by your eyes and ears and hands, than to try to beat the doctor to a diagnostic label. On the one hand, if you say, 'I think my child has a strep throat,' it is possible that your child might get a quick injection of penicillin when a careful examination and a throat culture would have been more appropriate. On the other hand, I know of one case where the same diagnostic opener led to such irritation in the doctor that no throat culture was done—the doctor unconsciously showing the mother that only he could make a diagnosis. It is far more useful for all if you begin by saying, 'Susie has had a fever of 101 to 103 degrees for the last 24 hours; she says it hurts when she swallows, and there are some lumps under her jawbone that she says are painful to push at; she has not eaten well for the last day; and her best friend at school had a throat culture two days ago that was reported to show strep.' "

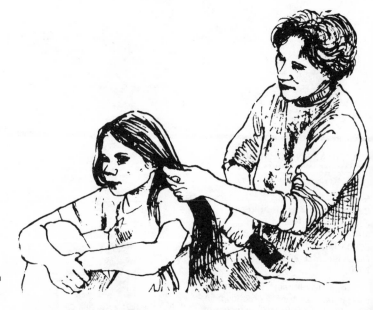

Relaxation: hairbrushing and reverie

Being Parents

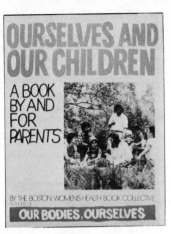

OURSELVES AND OUR CHILDREN: A Book By and For Parents
by the Boston Women's Health Book Collective
1978, 288 pages, Illus.

from
Random House
201 East 50th Street
New York, NY 10022
$7.95 pap.
$12.95 hd.

Written by some of the co-authors of *Our Bodies, Ourselves,* this book looks at the specifics of caring for children as infants, older children, teenagers, and grown-ups, and describes the way family structure and social support (or lack of support) for families affects us. The emphasis, as in *Our Bodies, Ourselves,* is on non-sexist roles, self-knowledge, self-help, social action, and community. (JIA)

"Many books, especially how-to-parent books, assume that what happens to our children is a result of what goes on between us and our children and depends almost entirely on life within the family. Our view is that it is impossible to parent alone. We parent in a context of relationships with other people; our families exist within communities, and are part of a complex web of social institutions, each of which has an impact on our parenting experience. . . .

"Attitudes toward children in public places vary from society to society. Margo tells of her travels through Europe with her husband and three-year-old daughter:
'In France, the attitude was, "What do you mean, bringing a child into a restaurant? Eating is serious business!" In Italy, the waiters would take Rachel over completely, they'd get a high chair, put a bib on her and feed her so that we could relax and enjoy our meal. Everyone seemed to really enjoy her being there.'
In this country, most of us have experienced both these attitudes and

the whole range inbetween as we go into stores, laundromats, recreational or health facilities, public meetings, etc., with our kids. Many of the day-to-day situations that we meet as parents, even those which primarily serve parents and children, seem to disregard our needs for welcome, for cooperation, for support. . . .

"One of the most formidable barriers to providing more supports for parents and children is our society's overemphasis on individualism. Self-reliance is a primary American value: each of us is expected to be able to 'go it alone,' and each family is regarded as having sole responsibility for their children, and the sense of collective social responsibility for children that is seen in many other cultures is largely missing. . . .

"The 'medicalization of the first year of childrearing' is a concept propounded by Norma Swenson, whose years of experience in the childbirth movement have convinced her that the passive role thrust upon women in medically controlled childbirth has, as one latent function, the teaching of women to be similarly dependent on doctors in their parenting. In her words:
'In other cultures, birth is just part of a woman's life in the community. In this country birth is placed in this strange medical world of the hospital and the male physician. This damages the confidence of women as individuals and as parents, gives us the notion that we're not capable of taking care of our own bodies and that body function is a deep and mysterious thing. So of course it carries over to caring for our babies.'"

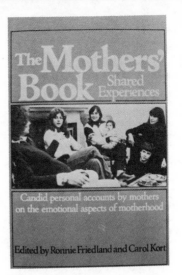

THE MOTHERS' BOOK: Shared Experiences
edited by Ronnie Friedland and Carol Kort
1981, 363 pages, Illus.

from
Houghton Mifflin
2 Park Street
Boston, MA 02107
$8.95 pap.

This is a very moving collection of stories by 64 mothers on the good and the difficult aspects of motherhood, enhanced by sensitive photographs and poetry. The subjects covered include: pregnancy, post-partum changes, breast or bottle, staying home, going to work, changes in self-concept, redefining relationships (husband, mother, friends), sexuality and motherhood, ambivalence, anger and shame, the only child, becoming a single mother, becoming a stepmother, foster, adoptive, and natural mothers, teenage mothers, feelings about surgical deliveries, mothering children with special needs, when things go wrong, dealing with death, and dealing with the future. This is the real stuff of motherhood and of life. Mothers who are caught up in the experience will appreciate the support and sense of community this book can give. And more than any book by professionals, *The Mothers' Book* can answer the prospective mother's question, "What will it be like?" (JIA)

"I often speak with other women who have also chosen to set aside career strivings temporarily for the sake of children. As in my case, they have neither been browbeaten into mothering nor are they adherents of the notion that child care is 'woman's work.' Rather, their decisions have evolved from much intensive thought, debate, and personal soul-searching. What I've gathered from them is that I haven't been alone in finding it difficult to follow my instincts and resolve to remain at home with a baby in a climate that frequently greets such a move with pure condescension. When you sense that others perceive you as

having caved in to a traditional role—that you are doing nothing particularly noteworthy or commendable—it's hard not to feel anything but insulted and defensive.

"A friend of mine told me that at a party she and her husband attended after her son was born, a woman came up to her and, after introductions, asked what sort of work she did. My friend, sick and tired of her propensity to downplay child care and dwell upon past accomplishments to elicit appropriate respect, flatly stated, 'I stay home and take care of my baby.' The woman smiled feebly and excused herself to move on. My friend felt as though she had just been given the official stamp of disapproval. Unfortunately, incidents similar to this are all too commonplace and help make the already burdensome choice to stay home even tougher."
—from "Staying Home and Liking It" by Emily L. Tipermas

"When Jessie was eighteen months old, I left her in the care of an education major from a local college, a young woman who seemed intelligent and warm. I remember telling my husband, Victor, how conflicted I was about leaving Jessie. He smiled in his low-key way and said that he had been thinking that I was a fool to have stayed home as long as I had.

"Jessica was seemingly well adjusted to her baby sitter, and I came home as early as possible that first year. But I always felt of two minds: when I was home, I wanted to be studying; when I was at school, I felt a pit in my stomach at the thought of Jessie at home. . . .

"I also began to experience the strained reactions of other women. From time to time, I would be accosted by an honest one. She would tell me straightaway, after the most cursory introduction, that anyone who would leave her child shouldn't have had one. . ."
—from "A Working Mother" by Gerri Gomperts

"As a new mother, I feel in some ways as if I have joined a new club. I can sit and discuss baby products and behavior for hours with women I would not necessarily have had much in common with before. For me, one of the most positive aspects of motherhood is that it is something shared *only* by women. Motherhood brings women together, to some degree breaking down racial and social barriers. This itself is a feminist goal, even if certain feminists downplay motherhood because it has been used against them. We do not, however, need to reject motherhood. We merely have to expand the traditional view of it."
—from "Thoughts on Friendship and Feminism" by Sarah D. Pick

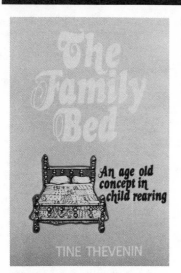

THE FAMILY BED: An Age Old
Concept in Child Rearing (2nd
edition)
by Tine Thevenin
1977, 195 pages, Illus.

from
Tine Thevenin
P.O. Box 16004
Minneapolis, MN 55416
$4.95 plus .75 postage, pap.

Most books on child care seriously
warn against letting children sleep in
their parents' bed. Tine Thevenin
wondered why and began interviewing parents and researching the literature on "co-family sleeping." The result is *The Family Bed,* a truly innovative book which has quietly sold
close to 38,000 copies since 1976.
Thevenin argues convincingly that
families sleeping together constitute
a natural, and normal phenomenon
and will not cause psychological harm;
on the contrary, the rigid separation
of babies and children from their parents at night may be the cause of
many sleep and personality disorders.

Thevenin carefully presents her
ideas by describing the experiences of
parents who use a family bed, the
questions and doubts of parents who
don't, and stresses the importance of
love and touch as expressed in sleeping together. She provides a fascinating look at the history of family sleep
customs from medieval days to the
present and provides observations
from anthropological studies. Thevenin describes how the family bed meets
the special needs of the infant for
closeness and comfort and how it
makes breastfeeding easier. She also
describes the changing needs of the
older child; siblings sleeping with each
other, and how co-family sleeping affects the marital relationship. Introductions by Niles Newton, Herbert
Ratner, and Marion Tompson and
words of praise from Margaret Mead,
Ashley Montagu, and Jane Goodall all
attest to the value of being more flexible and loving in our relationship
with our children.   (JIA)

"It is quiet. It is dark. It is night.
Somewhere a baby whimpers. His
mother stirs and pulls her infant to-
ward her. He nuzzles for her breast.
He begins to nurse and both Babe and
Mom fall back to sleep. Somewhere
in his dream Papa knows all is well.
All are asleep.

"Somewhere a toddler awakens,
and sleepily speaks, 'Mama?' Mama
stirs in her sleep, she reaches over and
takes the child's hand in her hand.
They both fall back to sleep. Papa's
dreams were not even interrupted.
All is well. All are asleep.

"Whether it be on a Japanese 'fu-
ton,' or under an arctic caribou skin,
on the bare African ground, in a large
four poster bed, or in a double-twin
size bed, whether they be poor or rich,
large or small, many families all over
the world sleep together, and have
done so since the beginning of man-
kind. . . .

"If the childrearing methods of
the past 150 years had resulted in a
great improvement over previous
methods in rearing happy, emotionally stable people, we might do well to
put great stock in it. However, I have
found no evidence of such superior
results. As a matter of fact, there
seems to be more of an indication toward the contrary. The concept of
separate sleeping arrangements is of
such new vintage that it has not yet
had a chance to stand the test of
time. The test seems to be on rather
shaky grounds. . . .

"In my reading of anthropological
studies I have found that among those
societies which seem to produce happy, emotionally stable people, co-
family sleeping, unrestricted breastfeeding, and almost constant physical
contact with the children in their
early years is the custom. . . .

"Because our beds are usually too
small and too high, and the bedroom
too crowded with the regular bedroom furniture, most families who
turn to family sleeping, have had to
improvise in making accommodations
for the whole family to sleep together.

"Some parents have been fortunate to be able to buy a larger bed or
have resorted to placing two twin-
sized beds together. . . .

"Pillows and blankets or foam
rubber pads around a low bed have
served as safety measures until the baby could crawl from the bed by himself. And some parents have resorted
to the most logical solution, namely
wall-to-wall bed made just from mat-
tresses.

"To enlarge the parents' bed, an
adjustable crib can be placed right
next to the big bed, set to the height
of the bed. Or a picnic bench can be
placed between the bed and the wall,
built up with blankets to the height
of the master bed. The slight space
between can be covered with a blanket or bed pad. Or two chairs, facing

each other, with one board bridging
the seats, will solve the problem.

"If there is room enough, another
bed can be placed in the parents'
room, either next to it, on the foot
end, or somewhere else in the room.
A side rail is another solution. Or
place the bed in a corner against the
wall, and have children sleep between
Mom and the wall. . . .

"[Our country's] strong interest
in sex may, in part, be the direct result of the minimal physical contact
which so many of the younger generation have received during infancy.
Perhaps an inner drive is attempting
to repair the damage of too little bodily stimulation during childhood. . . .

"One mother wrote, 'I feel that b
keeping children a little bit longer in
the parental bed, perhaps they will
stay a bit longer out of a premarital
bed. Maybe some of those adolescent kids who crawl into bed with
each other are really looking for Mama, except Mama was never there.'
Perhaps this mother instinctively felt
there is a connection between the
teenage search for physical contact
and a lack of sufficient infant physical contact, which could be the result of separate sleeping, bottle-feeding, schedules, and numerous mother
substitute gadgets."

SLEEP CLOSE TO ME

Fold of my flesh
I carried in my womb,
tender trembling flesh
sleep close to me!

The partridge sleeps in the wheat
listening to its heartbeat.
Let not my breath disturb you
sleep close to me!

Little tender grass
afraid to live
don't move from my arms;
sleep close to me!

I have lost everything,
and tremble until I sleep.
Don't move from my breast;
sleep close to me!

—Gabriela Mistral (1889-1957) Chile
translated from the Spanish by Dora M. Pettinella

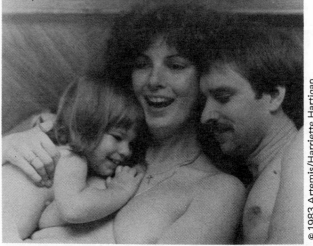

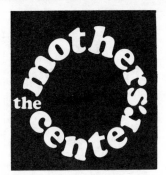

THE MOTHERS' CENTER
c/o United Methodist Church
Old Country Road and Nelson Ave.
Hicksville, New York 11801
516/822-4539

The first Mothers' Center began on Long Island—in Hicksville, New York—and is a model worth emulating around the country. The founders explain how the Center got started:

"NEW MOTHERS WANTED: Those words first appeared several years ago in a local newspaper. Fifty of us responded to that ad, which called for concerned mothers willing to assist with research on their experiences with childbirth and child-rearing.

"We met for several weeks, and during that time, were really shocked at how uninformed we were. We also learned that our own fears were not at all unusual but in fact quite common.

"When the program ended, we knew there was still much more to learn, and that most women in the community had not even begun to understand or even be aware of the problems they faced as mothers.

"We wanted to continue, and through our persistence, The Mothers' Center was formed."

Services provided by the Mother's Center include rap groups for the postpartum period, prenatal preparation, mothers of toddlers, mothers of school-age children, adoptive mothers, marriage, and sexual awareness. Also available are counseling, referrals, clothing exchange for childrens' and maternity clothing, community education events, a social action committee, child care, and peer counseling training. Activities change according to the needs of the current members. The Mothers' Center brochure says, "All our group discussions and activities at the center have three major goals: to give support to the individual women in the group, to collect information and experience, and to design new social action programs."

An important part of the Mothers' Center's activities has been postpartum discussion groups in which women have been able to air their feelings about their childbirth experience. Many women are unhappy about the treatment they have received in the

hospital and the Mothers' Center has tried to raise consumer awareness about hospital practices which may be harmful or insensitive. One of its projects was a Hospital Survey which outlined the services available at 10 local area hospitals. Fifty services items (nurse-midwives available? labor lounge? routines? early discharge?) were included.

Dr. Silvia Feldman, a Long Island psychotherapist, was instrumental in developing the Mothers' Center concept and includes a description of the model center in her excellent book *Choices in Childbirth* (see index for review). Below is a list of currently operating Mothers' Centers based on the Hicksville model. The Mothers' Center has developed a manual to help others who would like to start a mothers' center in their area. It is available from the Hicksville center for $9.90.

(JIA)

MOTHERS' CENTER OF SUFFOLK
P.O. Box 92
Holbrook, NY 11741
516/585-5587

MERRICK-BELLMORE MOTHERS'
CENTER
c/o United Methodist Church
Royle Street and St. Marks Avenue
Bellmore, NY 11710
516/781-8946

MOTHERS' CENTER OF QUEENS
c/o Bayside YMCA
214-11 35th Avenue
Bayside, NY 11361
212/229-5972

MOTHER AND CHILD CENTER
c/o YM-YWCA
175 Memorial Highway
New Rochelle, NY 10801

PENINSULA MOTHERS' CENTER
P.O. Box 337
Woodmere, NY 11598

MOTHERS' CENTER OF CENTRAL
NEW JERSEY
c/o YWCA
220 Clark Street
Westfield, NJ 07090
201/233-2833

MOTHERS' CENTER OF ST. LOUIS
516 Laughborough
St. Louis, MO 63111
314/353-1558

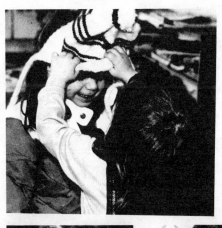
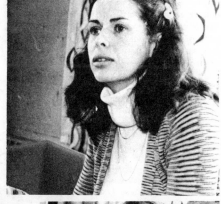
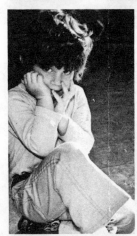
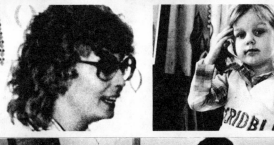
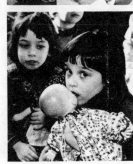
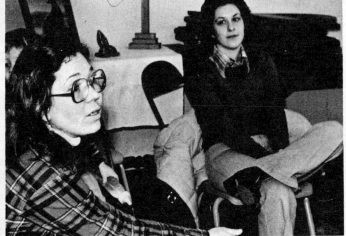

FATHERS

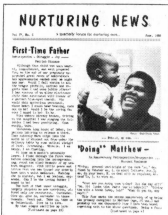

NURTURING NEWS
187 Caselli Avenue
San Francisco, CA 94114
quarterly newsletter, 10 pages
$6./year ($7. US funds for Canada)
sample copy $.50 plus 9" SASE

Nurturing News is devoted to promoting nurturing roles for men both
as fathers and as children's teachers.
The newsletter provides articles by
men who are breaking ground in these
areas, as well as resource listings, book
reviews, and letters. Editor David
Giveans is a teacher in a multi-cultural
San Francisco day care center, does
lecturing and consulting in "non-sexist learning environments and men in
nurturing roles." In addition to *Nurturing News,* Mr. Giveans has produced a 28 minute color film, *Men in
Early Childhood Education,* which is
available for rental or purchase from
Total Video, 220 E. Grand Ave.,
Suite B, South San Francisco, CA
94080.　　　　　　　　(JIA)

" 'What are you doing home to-
day? Got the day off?' 'Oh, Oh!
Looks like Dad's day to babysit!'
'Giving the wife a break today, huh?'
'What do you do, anyway?!!'

"This June marks the second anniversary of my being the primary caregiver to Matthew (age, 26 mos.) and
probably the one thousandth time I
have been asked something akin to
the above questions. Being a full-
time father is indeed a deviant role
in our society.

"I have discovered that whenever
there are two or more women with
babies in their arms (or close by),
there is an immediate affinity between them, a bonding of sorts that
occurs as the result of a mutual,
shared and recognized status—MOTH-
ERHOOD. I have also discovered
that MOTHERHOOD AND FATHER-
HOOD are not the two equivalent
components of PARENTHOOD. As
a father I am not expected to be interested in when solid foods should be
introduced. I am not expected to be
knowledgeable about creative play
or child development. I am not expected to be able to maintain an interest in spending most of my time

in the company of a child. As a
father I am not expected to enjoy
and participate in my FATHER-
HOOD to the same extent that mothers enjoy and participate in their
MOTHERHOOD. So much for expectations!"
　　—from " 'Doing' Matthew" by
Michael Robinson, *Nurturing News,*
June 1982.

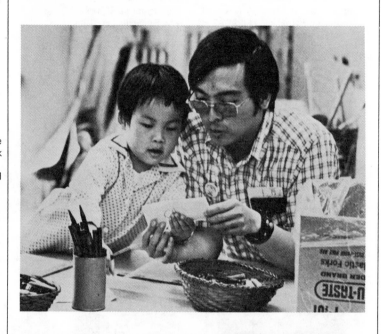

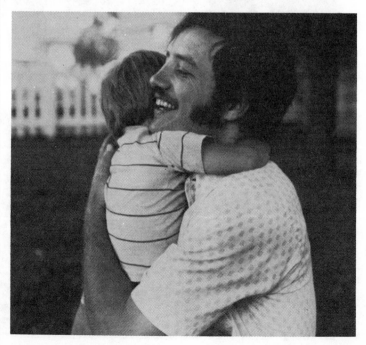

PHOTOS OF MEN IN THE NURTURING ROLE
8 photographs (8½ x 11")
1 poster (17 x 22")

from
Women's Action Alliance
370 Lexington Avenue
New York, NY 10017
$5.60 plus 15% postage

　The Non-Sexist Child Development Project of the Women's Action
Alliance has produced these photos
of men caring for their own children,
in day care and health situations.
The photos were taken by Jim Levine
of The Fatherhood Project (see this
page).

The Fatherhood Project

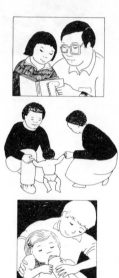

THE FATHERHOOD PROJECT
Bank Street College
610 West 112th Street
New York, NY 10025

　The Fatherhood Project is based
in the Bank Street College of Education in New York City and is directed by James A. Levine, author of
*Who Will Raise the Children? New
Options for Fathers (and Mothers).*
The Project acts as a clearinghouse
for information on men in nurturing
roles and is compiling information
for *Fatherhood USA,* a guide to innovative programs and resources. The
Project also conducts research on
policies and programs which affect
fathering (paternity leave, employment policies, custody rights, child
support, non-sexist education, male
involvement in childbirth and postpartum support, social services, and
religion). The Project's demonstration programs include the "Oh Boy!
Babies!" course in infant care for
pre-adolescent boys (it's also a book
and a film) and the "For Fathers
Only" discussion and play group for
fathers and toddlers in New York
City. Write for more information or
to contribute information on resources and programs.　　(JIA)

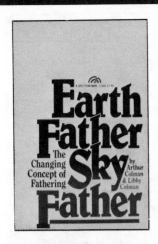

EARTH FATHER/SKY FATHER:
The Changing Concept of Fathering
by Arthur Colman and Libby Colman
1981, 206 pages, Illus.

from
Prentice-Hall
Englewood Cliffs, NJ 07632
$5.95 pap.

Arthur and Libby Colman are a husband and wife team of psychiatrist and psychologist, respectively. They have developed an interesting new framework for describing the roles which fathers play in their families. Drawing upon the "archetypes" of the father in mythology, anthropology, and the psychoanalytical literature, and also using their own work and interviews with fathers and patients, the Colmans have developed definitions of five basic types of fathering: father the creator, earth father, sky father, royal father, and dyadic father. Through these archetypes, men are encouraged to think about their own functions and feelings as fathers and to draw upon the father models to find a style of fathering which is best suited to their situation. The emphasis is on supporting and providing specific suggestions to men who want a more nurturing, intimate, "non-traditional" life as parents.   (JIA)

"Fathers and families need new images of what a father can be, images that go beyond the idea of father as outsider, father as provider, or father as intruder in the home. There is a need for images that acknowledge father as a potent nurturant force within the family as well as a creative liaison with the world outside the family. . . .

"Whether male or female, the earth parent is concerned with all the functions taking place inside the family boundary, including the intimate activities that are part of day-to-day child rearing. The sky parent, in contrast, is concerned with that which is taking place at the intersection of the family's boundary with the community, the protecting and providing functions that are essential for the family's survival.

"In our society, the mother is usually the earth parent and the father is usually the sky parent, but in theory, at least, either parent could fill one or even both functions. The father could be the earth parent and the mother the sky parent, both parents could share both functions, or one parent could do it all. Obviously, each of these alternatives would have effects on the development of the children and the development of the parents. Optimally, the two parents could choose to divide up earth and sky functions in the family in a way that was best suited to their personal needs and their competencies rather than passively accept a role in the family imposed by their sexual anatomy and social history. . . .

"It is not easy to combine the qualities of a successful working person with the qualities of a successful parent. Neither is it easy to accept work and outside activities as central to fathering, to say that one can be a better parent by being absent. And yet for the majority of men, in our own culture and others, the role of father has been defined by external action. As sky father, man is protector and provider, separator and outsider, leader and culture builder. When he feels nurturant and loving, he may think of himself as 'mother,' because his image of 'father' is so far removed from these qualities. . . .

"Sex-role stereotyping along earth and sky lines is sometimes so artificial that it becomes ludicrous. We have seen wise and gentle male pediatricians, capable of the most complex and loving behavior toward their infant patients, defer to their painfully inexperienced wives as to the best way to diaper a newborn or calm a distressed three-month-old. In the early years of our own family, Arthur, who had had months of experience with babies in emergency wards and clinics, would often watch from a distance as Libby fretted and fumbled with a sick child. Less dramatically, we have observed warm, nurturant men give up all the parenting of their children to cold, aloof wives who had little interest in or talent for the job. These are examples where stereotypes and conditioning have gotten in the way of rational decision making about who is more competent to perform one or another parenting function. . . .

"No matter how involved a father becomes in the birth experience (and we fully support his total commitment), he can only be a guide, a helper, a support to his wife. She is in the center of the stage. At the time of the birth, his role must be on the boundary of the experience. He can protect and aid, but she must do.

"For some men there is a deep hurt in this limit on the creator roles. They may still harbor an unconscious fantasy of their own totipotentiality in the sexual and reproductive realms. In men coming from special family backgrounds, this reaction is understandable. A lay midwife whose son accompanied her to several home births told us about her son's dismay when he learned that he would not be able to give birth to a baby. He cried and refused to believe the unfair fate he was told was his. Birth was highly valued in the world in which he lived. It was painful to be excluded from a central role in that act. All men share this pain to some extent, for few persons can easily accept their own limitations, especially those that are inborn. A man who is a partner in the birth experience must face his limits in the most graphic way. It is no wonder that so many men find it difficult to find a secure role at the birth. Perhaps the ambivalence of some men to partake as fully as they are allowed in the delivery of their children is not simply because of disinterest or squeamishness. Perhaps, consciously or unconsciously, they understand that only a very limited aspect of their fathering role is allowed expression at this time, one that need not represent the ultimate expression of their paternity."

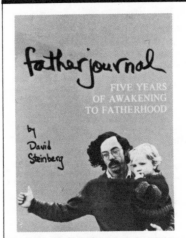

FATHER JOURNAL: Five Years of Awakening to Fatherhood
by David Steinberg
1977, 91 pages, Illus.

from
Times Change Press
Publishers Services
P.O. Box 3914
San Rafael, CA 94902
$3.00 plus .50 postage

When his first child was born, David Steinberg made a conscious decision to become fully involved in child care and fathering. He did not want to be the "second parent." This journal documents what he did and what he learned in five years of close physical and emotional care of his child.   (JIA)

"September 15, 1971 (notes at six months)
. . .When Susan was pregnant, I imagined that writing and taking care of the baby would fit together well. I figured that as long as I was home taking care of the baby I would do some writing as well. It seems incredible now that I could have so completely misunderstood what it would be like to have a baby.

"I have resisted the shift from living on my schedule to living on Dylan's. I've tried to hold on to my old patterns, failed, and built up a lot of resentment in the process. After six months I think I'm finally letting go of my old life. The task is to build a new life that I like as well or better. One day, at the ocean, I cried while trying to say goodbye to a life that I loved and had worked hard to create.
. . . "Susan and I agree that we'll both work part-time and share taking care of Dylan. That way we'll both have outside lives and both be involved as parents.

"I still get an empty feeling when people ask me what I'm doing. Most of my energy in the last six months has focused on Dylan—on taking care of him and getting used to his being here. I carry enough man-work expectations in me that I feel uncomfortable using that to identify myself to people.

"February 20, 1972
This morning I woke up feeling comfortable, warm, and solid. Then Dylan started to fuss and turned irritable right away. I wake up to a demand every morning. I'm behind before I even get out of bed. A horrible way to start the day. . . .

"March 12, 1972
Dylan is an incredibly wonderful child! . . .

"January 29, 1974
. . .Last night, in the middle of tears and confusion and frustration, sitting on the floor by the fireplace, Susan said she wanted to live apart for a while. She had made up her mind that she needed space alone to be able to see which way was up. She said she couldn't handle being together right now. She said she wanted to take Dylan. Could she take Dylan? She didn't want to talk about it, she just wanted to know if she could take Dylan.

"I was terrified. I couldn't speak. How had it come to this. Certainly there must be a way to fix things. Leave? Take Dylan?

" 'No, you can't take Dylan,' I said.
'I need him,' Susan cried.
'I need him too,' I whispered.' "

PARENTING PUBLICATIONS

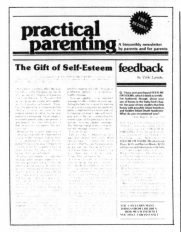

PRACTICAL PARENTING
18318 Minnetonka Blvd.
Deephaven, MN 55391
$6.50/one year (6 issues)
$12.00/two years

Vicki Lansky and YOU bring this 16 page newsletter together every other month. Each issue has question-and-answer topics which readers write and respond to. It provides dozens of practical ways to deal with growing children from emotional needs to equipment and nutrition (Vicki wrote *Feed Me, I'm Yours* and *The Taming of the C.A.N.D.Y. Monster).* Articles for fathers are excellent, and there are many humorous columns and features as well as book reviews and ads from people who work at home. Send a long self addressed, stamped envelope for a free 12 page sample. (MS)

TOTLINE NEWSLETTER
Warren Publishing
P.O. Box 2253
Alderwood Manor, WA 98036
$9.00/one year (6 issues)
$12.00/1½ years
$16.00/two years

Preschoolers will never be bored if parents use all the suggestions in this 16 page newsletter! It would also make a terrific gift for the local nursery school teacher who needs new ideas for creative play and projects using easy-to-get, free or inexpensive materials. Creative parents will appreciate it and less imaginative parents will find it an inspiration. Sample issues are $1.00 each. (MS)

GROWING CHILD
22 North 2nd Street
P.O. Box 620
Lafayette, IN 47902
$11.00/one year (12 issues)

Here is a great concept and a terrific bargain! Each month you receive a package of three publications. The 6 page Growing Child newsletter is geared to your child's age up to five years old. When subscribing, indicate the baby's birth-date, and when he or she is, for example, 5 months old, you will receive the issue which describes a five-month-old, normal baby.

Each issue provides insight, reassurance and information about the normal physical and cognitive development patterns of children, sent to you when you can *use* the information; not all at once in a book you may forget to consult after a few weeks.

Growing Parent (8 pages) is designed to help parents know themselves, understand others, and cope with parenting using practical guides. *Growing Child Store* is a catalog of excellent, educational toys and books which are presented in order by the age of the child for whom they are made to appeal.

A sample issue is free to new parents (babies under 2 years) and definitely worth sending for! (MS)

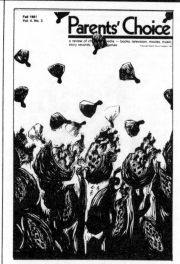

PARENTS' CHOICE
Parents' Choice Foundation
Box 185
Waban, MA 02168
$10.00/year (4 issues)

Want a good review of children's media? This small newspaper offers listings and comments on books, TV, movies, music, story records, and games, combined with articles and very attractive, large graphics. (MS)

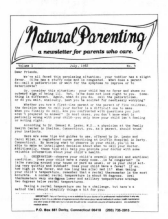

NATURAL PARENTING
P.O. Box 881
Derby, CT 06418
$12.00/year (12 issues)

Lovingly written by Carmella and John Bartimole, this small (4 page) monthly newsletter contains the basics of nutrition and natural health, including label-reading, why things like wheat germ and yogurt are good for children and you, a book review or two, and lots of helpful hints and natural recipes to save you money and avoid overly processed foods. (MS)

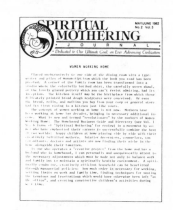

SPIRITUAL MOTHERING JOURNAL
P.O. Box 128
Dover, NH 03820
$6.00/year (6 issues)

Editor Melinda Armstrong draws on many resources to nurture the spiritual beings of parents and children in this bimonthly newsletter. The Baha'i philosophy combines with personal experiences to provide for columns of reflective, practical, and comforting thoughts on such topics as unconditional love, miscarriage, fathering, and spiritual education/home schooling, each of which has been covered in previous issues (available for one dollar apiece). Reading an issue provides a gentle break in the day. (MS)

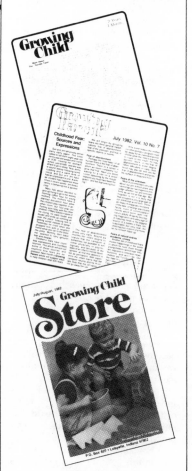

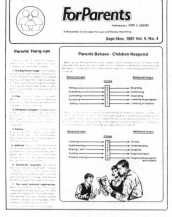

FOR PARENTS
Interpersonal Communication Services
7052 W. Lane
Eden, NY 14059
$10.00/year (5 issues)

Strategies in values-clarification and creative thinking, tips on coping with TV, and suggestions on how to approach parent-child situations are included in this 8 page newsletter in addition to reviews of resources and readers' responses. Articles are brief and thought-provoking, and they reflect editor Carolyn Shadle's training in family education and Master's Degree in Religious Education. (MS)

BUILDING BLOCKS
314 Liberty Street
Box 31
Dundee, IL 60118
$10.00/year (10 issues)

The "original edition" of this newspaper contains monthly ideas for projects and discussions with your young children in addition to a big calendar page that specifically lays out when to do each project and still have time for yourself. The pages are large (11" x 17") and laid out with large, easy-to-read, hand-written letters and illustrations. Projects are charming and inexpensive, such as how to enjoy a trip to the library or how to make placemats for a holiday by coloring the ones printed in the issue and covering them with clear contact paper.

For an extra $5.00 per year, you may want to receive the *Child Care Edition,* which contains more projects, coping resources and ideas for pre-schoolers.   (MS)

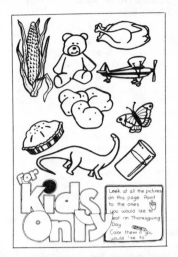

Also see review of *Mothering* magazine on page 281.

PEDIATRICS FOR PARENTS
Box 1069
Bangor, ME 04401
$12.00/year (12 issues)
$1.00/sample

"We believe that well-informed parents have healthier, happier children. *Pediatrics for Parents* was conceived to provide you with recent, practical, and important information about your children's health. There is much you as parents can do to improve your children's well-being, and we hope to help you do it." So say the editors on their masthead and indeed this excellent newsletter is full of informative, easy to understand, short articles on a whole range of topics in children's physical and mental health: from what to do before you see the doctor to how to evaluate a school sports program to what snacks are good for teeth to how to get a toddler to take medicine and on and on. All this information is presented in a lively, cheerful format with lots of very attractive and witty illustrations. The editors scan the medical literature for items of interest to parents and present the latest news and knowledge in layperson's language but always with references listed or avaliable. The emphasis is on consumer-oriented health care.   (MS)

"If your toddler's knees touch or even hit each other when she's walking, there's no need for concern.

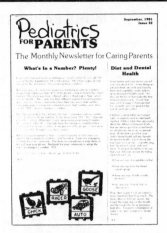

Seventy-five percent of children aged two to four and a half years have some degree of *genu valgus,* the medical term for knock-knees. One way to test your child for abnormal knock-kneedness is to measure the distance between the inside of her ankles. To do this properly, lay her on her back, put her knees together and measure the distance between the round raised portions on the inside of her ankles. If this distance is less than three inches, there's no reason to worry. A distance greater than three inches should be brought to your doctor's attention, although chances are that little, if anything, will be done. There's no evidence that special shoes, splints or exercises affect the problem."

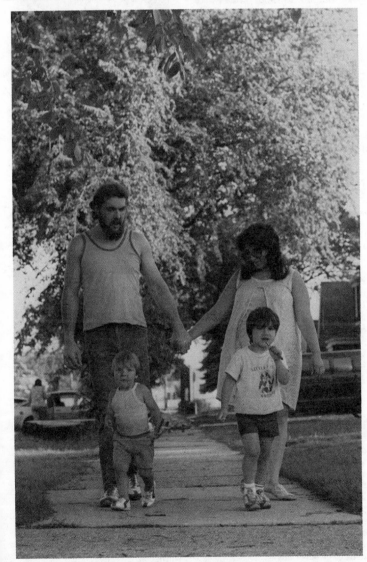

© 1983 Artemis/Harriette Hartigan
The couple in this photo are engaged in parenting their two young children and preparing for the one on the way. In fact, this mother is in labor!

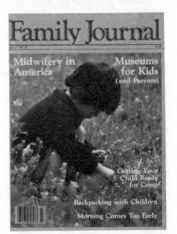

FAMILY JOURNAL
P.O. Box 118
Peterborough, NH 03458
$9.00/year (12 issues)
$11.00 in Canada
$17.00 abroad

Family Journal is geared to the consumer-oriented parent who wants information on childbirth and child-rearing with an emphasis on alternatives. The *Journal* features articles on many aspects of pregnancy, birth, baby care, parenting, children's education, family health, activities for children, products and toys, etc. Regular departments include letters, short news items, networking, com-

paring methods of childbirth preparation, family businesses, adoption, and book reviews.   (JIA)

"10 Suggestions for Better Parenting While Working Full-time

"—If your work load is uneven, and seems to be getting your child down because of too many necessary absences, compensate. For example, my son and I have created 'Pamper Peter Days.' He requests such a day when he feels the need for special attention. Then we agree upon a mutually satisfactory date for his 'Day.'

"On such a day, he may do whatever he wants (within reason, of course). He has total access to me, as he wants and needs it. My attention is focused entirely on him, and he may be given special privileges for the occasion. Often, his day may include a request as simple as taking a trip to our favorite book store to browse; or having what we call a 'story orgy'; or eating dinner in his playroom and watching one of his favorite TV programs together. Rarely does his 'Pamper Peter Day' involve elaborate activities. The secret of the day seems to lie in *his* ability to 'name the tune' and my willingness to respond."

MORE PARENTING RESOURCES

PARENTS WITHOUT PARTNERS, INC.
7910 Woodmont Avenue
Washington, DC 20014
$10-18/year dues

Parents Without Partners (PWP) is unique as the largest organization in the world devoted to the welfare of single parents and their children. It is a non-profit, educational organization. Chapters in the US and Canada hold lectures and discussions on topics of interest to single parents. They also offer many pamphlets and brochures on subjects such as custody issues, the single parent in the community, the never-married mother, raising a family alone, etc. They publish a booklist of stories and books for children from preschool to 18 years about how others have handled life situations similar to their own.
(MS)

NATIONAL ALLIANCE FOR OPTIONAL PARENTHOOD
2010 Massachusetts Avenue, N.W.
Washington, DC 20036

Perhaps this organization deserves listing in the beginning of this *Catalog*. Their purpose is "To encourage people to make informed and responsible decisions about whether or not to be parents and to work for social acceptance of the childfree choice." *Before* you decide to have children there are several brochures available which include questions to ask yourself and reflect on to make a better informed decision. Titles like *Am I Parent Material?, Are You Kidding Yourself?* and *Your Values About Parenthood* are 15 cents each and a list of publications is free.
(MS)

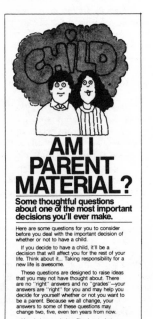

PARENTS ANONYMOUS
2230 Hawthorne Blvd.
Suite 208
Torrance, CA 90505
TOLL FREE HOTLINES
(800) 421-0353 Outside California
(800) 352-0386 California only

Parents Anonymous provides telephone counseling and mutual support from local members to help prevent or control child abuse. Parents Anonymous suggests you contact them if you answer yes to any of the following questions:

"1. Are you a troubled or nervous parent who has no place to get help?
2. When you are ready to blow up is it you and the children who bear the brunt of it?
3. Do you feel confused, guilty and frightened about your parental behavior and feelings?
4. Do you believe that you were treated indifferently or cruelly as a child and that now you're repeating some of the 'past'?
5. When you hear the words 'abuse' or 'neglect' do you end up thinking about your childhood or the parenting you're doing now?
6. Are you physically or emotionally abusing or neglecting one or more of your children?
7. Do you want your relationship with your children to be different . . . your family life more fulfilling . . . less explosive and tense . . . more loving?"
(MS)

NATIONAL COMMITTEE FOR PREVENTION OF CHILD ABUSE
332 S. Michigan Avenue, Suite 1250
Chicago, IL 60604

The Committee has local chapters and provides information on reporting suspected cases of abuse, getting help for abusing parents, and finding other ways of dealing with the stresses which can lead to child abuse.

The following materials are available free.
(MS)

YOU CAN PREVENT CHILD ABUSE
1980, 18 pages

"Understanding the Problem" is the first topic of discussion in this illustrated booklet which explains in clear brief sections the costs and effects of child abuse, who are abusers, how and why it happens, what happens when you report a suspected case, etc. It also tells what the National Committee for Prevention of Child Abuse (NCPCA) is doing in community planning to prevent child abuse and what you can do to help. Regional chapters of NCPCA are listed.

"SOME STRESS AND TENSION RELIEVERS

1. Count to 10, put the child in a safe area (crib, playpen, childproof room) and go to another room or outside for a few minutes.
2. Go into another room, close the door, and cry or scream. Then take 10 minutes to read, knit or do whatever relaxes you best.
3. Lie on the floor with your feet up on a chair; place a cool wash cloth on your face; and think of the most peaceful scene you can imagine. Stay there for 5 minutes.
4. Tell your child exactly what is making you feel angry. Be really specific about what behavior needs to be changed in order to reduce your anger level.
5. After you've put the children down for a nap, forget what you 'should' be doing. Take some time for yourself to relax—sleep, read, listen to music, take a bath—whatever makes you feel fresh again.
6. Designate a corner, chair, or some quiet spot as a 'time-out' place where you can go when you feel like losing your temper. Designate a separate one for your child. It gives both of you a few minutes to calm down, *and* it tells the other person that you are getting angry.
7. Save a special, quiet plaything to be used only at certain times. It will be a treat for your child, and will provide some quiet time for you."

—From *Families in Stress* (1979, 24 pages, HSS Pub No. (OHDS)80-30162)) available free from the National Center on Child Abuse and Neglect, Dept. of Health and Human Services, Washington, DC 20201

"To cope successfully with their roles in the family, parents and children require certain supports, training, and information. The programs that comprise the NCPCA community plan begin in the prenatal period (before birth) and the perinatal period (during and shortly after birth), continue with services and supportive programs for parents of infants and young children, and include services for children throughout the school years. . . .

"*Perinatal bonding program.* The focus of the perinatal program is on enhancing parent-infant bonding, which is the psychological attachment that usually develops between parent and child during and soon after childbirth. This bonding influences the infant's ability to relate to the outside world and depends on the kind of nurturance both parents provide to the infant. This program should emphasize childbirth procedures like rooming-in and unlimited visiting privileges for both parents with their new baby."

WHAT EVERY CHILD NEEDS
National Mental Health Association
1800 N. Kent Street
Arlington, VA 22209
free brochure

Love, Security, Protection, Acceptance, Faith, Independence, Guidance, and Control are listed and explained in this one of many useful brochures put out by the National Mental Health Association. Write for a list of other publications on parenting, child and adult mental health and its preservation.
(MS)

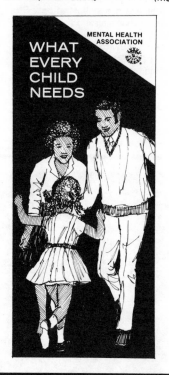

SELECTED CHILD ABUSE INFORMATION AND RESOURCES
1981, 8 pages

Besides listing NCPCA chapters by state, this reference guide gives phone numbers and addresses of organizations like Parents Anonymous and the Salvation Army as well as runaway shelters. A free literature search on the subject of child abuse can be obtained by contacting the Clearinghouse on Child Abuse and Neglect, 1700 N. Moore Street, Arlington, VA 22209, 703/558-8222. All sorts of other sources are listed for audio-visual materials, legal assistance, custody questions, etc.

CHILD ABUSE HURTS EVERYBODY
1981, brochure

This brochure describes the history, purpose and goals of NCPCA and includes a membership application ($15.00 a year regular membership).

FAMLEE (FATHERS AND MOTHERS LEARNING THROUGH EDUCATION AND EXPERIENCE)
P.O. Box 15
Telford, PA 18969
FAMLEE TALK
$8.00/year (9 issues)

"FAMLEE provides information on childbirth, breastfeeding, effective parenting and marriage enrichment. We offer childbirth, early pregnancy, cesarean birth and refresher classes. Our nursing mothers' groups and counselors give advice and encouragement to the nursing mother. The Parents' Exchange (PEX) provides speakers and workshops for parents to share their views. Our Speakers Bureau gives educational programs on childbirth, breastfeeding and parenting in schools and our community. Counselors in the Special People Committee offer support and advice to others who, like themselves, have had to deal with a high-risk pregnancy and/or delivery, or with the death of a child. Our group has the continuing support of our Professional Advisory Board, in an effort to better meet the needs of the growing family. Famlee Talk, our monthly newsletter, further enables members of our group to communicate their feelings and to offer suggestions about the various areas we cover. Through person-to-person contact FAMLEE seeks to promote individual growth and strengthening of family ties. FAMLEE is more than classes or meeting; we're an understanding ear and a helping hand."

—Barbara Myers, Secretary

THE BOOTH BUDDY EXPERIENCE
by Cathie Harvey and Mary Brett Daniels
1981, 40 pages

from
The Parenting Department
Booth Maternity Center
The Salvation Army, Inc.
City Line & Overbrook Avenues
Philadelphia, PA 19131
$3.00

The Maternity Center at Booth Hospital has created this extraordinary outreach program for pregnant couples, especially first-timers, to bring parents together for discussions and mutual support. Booth publishes this booklet and provides other pertinent information so that other hospitals or community groups may set up similar "Buddy" systems. Information includes how to target a group, what to say on the first phone call, how much a program will cost, job descriptions and training for personnel and volunteers, etc. Quite a complete package from a very successful program. (MS)

92nd STREET YM-YWHA PARENTING CENTER
1395 Lexington Avenue
New York, NY 10025

Concerts, picnics, classes, workshops and day care are but a few of the offerings of the Parenting Center. Fees for workshops vary from $5./session to $50./series and are open to all New York City members. A booklet describing all the events and programs, etc., for the coming season is available at the Young Men's-Young Women's Hebrew Association or by writing for it. You might check your neighborhood "Y" for similar programs, or start some yourself using some of the ideas in the booklet.
(MS)

NATIONAL COUNCIL ON FAMILY RELATIONS
1219 University Avenue, Southeast
Minneapolis, MN 55414

This organization publishes three journals, sells other books and publications, and also provides a computer-search service for any number of family-related topics from Adoption to Environment Space to Birth Order Difference to Marriage Customs and on and on. Write for more information and for costs of the various services, or check your local library or university to see if they have the service already. (MS)

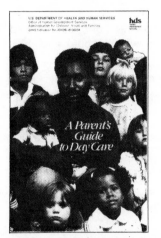

CHECKING OUT CHILD CARE: A PARENT GUIDE
28 pages

from
Day Care Council of America
711 14th Street, NW, Suite 507
Washington, DC 20005
free

"There are no set rules for selecting a child care program. What's good for one child and one family may not be the best choice for another. However, there are some general issues relating to caregiver competency and the program environment that indicate quality child care and are applicable to all programs, whether they are home-based or center-based."

So begins this excellent, brief guide to check out what child care situation is best for your needs. Where to look, how to evaluate what you find, danger signals, and a suggested reading list are all included in this booklet.

"Any of the following 'Danger Signals' should automatically rule out a center or home from your final choice:

* The caregiver does not want you to visit the program or ask specific questions about what your child will do during the day.

* The children move about at the program without any guidance from the caregiver for 30 minutes or more. They have no apparent involvement with anything or anyone.

* The caregiver does not respond to the children. He or she looks past them when talking to them and gives the general impression of not caring about or responding to the children's presence.

* The caregiver's voice often sounds angry or cross.

* The caregiver seems overwhelmed with the work and responsibility of caring for children.

* The caregiver is physically rough and abuses the children.

* The house or center is dirty and/or unsafe. The caregiver is messy or sloppy in physical appearance.

* Your child appears unhappy and suddenly doesn't seem to be eating or sleeping well and doesn't have much enthusiasm for playing with you, other children and her/his toys."

Does Your Child's Caregiver...

	Yes	No
Appear to be warm and friendly?	☐	☐
Seem calm and gentle?	☐	☐
Seem to have a sense of humor?	☐	☐
Seem to be someone with whom you can develop a relaxed, sharing relationship?	☐	☐
Seem to be someone your child will enjoy being with?	☐	☐
Seem to feel good about herself and her job?	☐	☐
Have child-rearing attitudes and methods that are similar to your own?	☐	☐
Treat each child as a special person?	☐	☐
Understand what children can and want to do at different stages of growth?	☐	☐
Have the right materials and equipment on hand to help them learn and grow mentally and physically?	☐	☐
Patiently help children solve their problems?	☐	☐
Provide activities that encourage children to think things through?	☐	☐

	Yes	No
Encourage good health habits, such as washing hands before eating?	☐	☐
Talk to the children and encourage them to express themselves through words?	☐	☐
Encourage children to express themselves in creative ways?	☐	☐
Have art and music supplies suited to the ages of all children in care?	☐	☐
Seem to have enough time to look after all the children in her care?	☐	☐
Help your child to know, accept, and feel good about him- or herself?	☐	☐
Help your child become independent in ways you approve?	☐	☐
Help your child learn to get along with and to respect other people, no matter what their backgrounds are?	☐	☐
Provide a routine and rules the children can understand and follow?	☐	☐
Accept and respect your family's cultural values?	☐	☐
Take time to discuss your child with you regularly?	☐	☐
Have previous experience or training in working with children?	☐	☐
Have a yearly physical exam and TB test?	☐	☐

from *A Parent's Guide to Day Care*

A PARENT'S GUIDE TO DAY CARE
1980, 74 pages

PARENTS' CHECKLIST FOR DAY CARE
1981, 12 pages

from
Day Care Division
Administration for Children, Youth and Families
U.S. Dept. of Health and Human Services
Washington, DC 20201
free

Here we have an example of tax dollars well spent. This illustrated booklet clearly describes the different types of day care available, from "in home" care to day care centers and provides guidelines on how to choose a caregiver, a setting, and all the "What to do if . . ." possibilities that arise about safety, clothing, behavior, etc. Included are checklists and information sheets to fill out to help you evaluate any particular day care situation so that it fits your needs and those of your child. Once a setting is chosen, there is a step-by-step guide to solving any problems that may arise. Interestingly, the guidelines given for evaluating day care can also be used to evaluate yourself as a parent and your home as a child care "setting." All in all, this booklet is an excellent, well-organized, well-written, complete guide to day care and a must for working parents. (The *Parents' Checklist for Day Care* is a reasonably good, short version of the longer Guide.)

Family Planning

Susan Ritchie, editor

Family planning is not just for families who want only a certain number of children spaced a certain number of years apart. It can also be relevant for a teenager, a man of 45 considering sterilization, a couple who want children but haven't been able to have them, or anyone in between. Family planning encompasses all the issues and information about birth control including contraception, abortion, sterilization, infertility and adoption.

When you are considering a birth control method, both partners need to think through these points:

1) How important is it that pregnancy be avoided? If it's very important, protect against it with the best possible method for you.

2) How often will you need birth control? (Once a day/once a week/once a month/variable?)

3) Do either of you have medical problems which might be a contraindication for use of one or another method?

4) Have you just had a baby and/or are you breastfeeding?

5) What is your personal/religious philosophy about birth control? about each method?

6) Can you be supportive of your partner's birth control method? Will you both take the responsibility or will only one of you be responsible for birth control?

Birth control needs will probably change throughout your life. Reconsider the options when your body, lifestyle or circumstances change.

Birth control methods or contraception involve using one or more of the following:

1) Natural family planning
2) Chemical barriers (foam, cream, jelly or suppositories placed in the vagina to chemically prevent live sperm from entering the uterus)
3) Mechanical barriers
   a) condoms
   b) diaphragm or cervical cap
   c) IUD (intrauterine device)
4) Hormonal intervention: the pill (oral contraceptive)
5) Surgical intervention
   a) therapeutic abortion
   b) male sterilization (vasectomy)
   c) female sterilization (tubal ligation)

The first two methods listed (natural family planning and chemical barriers) along with condoms are available to anyone without a doctor's prescription. Those methods which require medical consultation and follow-up are diaphragms, IUD's, the pill, and surgical intervention.

CONTRACEPTION: Comparing the Options
1980, chart

from
Public Health Service
5600 Fishers Lane
Rockville, MD 20857
free

This fold-out chart lists the six common birth control options plus male and female sterilization along with an outline of effectiveness, advantages/disadvantages, side effects, health factors to consider and long-term effect on ability to have children. Chart indicates briefly how the method works and whether or not a prescription is required. (SR)

"Women who use The Pill are strongly advised not to smoke because smoking increases the risk of heart attack or stroke.

"Other women who should not take The Pill are those who have had a heart attack, stroke, angina pectoris, blood clots, cancer of the breast or uterus. Women who have scanty or irregular periods should be encouraged to use some other method.

"A woman who believes she may be pregnant should not take The Pill because it increases the risk of defect in the fetus.

"Health problems, such as migraine headaches, mental depression, fibroids of the uterus, heart or kidney disease, asthma, high blood pressure, diabetes or epilepsy may be made worse by use of The Pill.

"Risks associated with The Pill increase with age."

FAMILY PLANNING: Today's Choices
by Dorothy Millstone
1980, 28 pages, Illus.

from
Public Affairs Pamphlets
381 Park Avenue South
New York, NY 10016
$.50

This pamphlet discusses the available birth control methods with statistics on effectiveness and major side-effects (current to May, 1980) and also includes a few pages on sterilization, abortion and infertility, and a section on teenage pregnancy and sexuality. (SR)

"The perfect birth control method would be effective, wholly free of side effects, administered at a time separate from the sex act, reversible, inexpensive, and aesthetically acceptable. This method does not exist. Scientists in many laboratories are working on it, and development of a 'perfect' method is expected in the next few years. But despite the limitations of present technology, today's options are sufficiently broad to permit the realization of a new era in human freedom: women in control of their reproductive destiny; wanted babies born to joyful parents."

CONTRACEPTION
1980, 30 pages

from
U.S. Dept. of Health and Human Services
Bureau of Community Health Services
Rockville, MD 20857
free

This booklet reviews the six major methods of birth control in a self-instructional format, including step-by-step instructions and diagrams. The six methods are oral contraceptives, intrauterine device, diaphragm, condom, contraceptive foam, and "natural" methods. (SR)

"First, foam is often confused with 'feminine hygiene' products. So, in purchasing it, a man or woman should be sure that the label specifically says that it is for CONTRACEPTION. Second, a couple should always be prepared with an extra container of foam, since it's often difficult to tell when the can is almost empty. And, finally, if a particular brand of foam is irritating to the sex organs, the couple should try another brand."

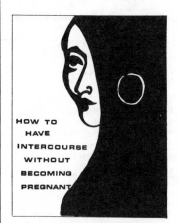

HOW TO HAVE INTERCOURSE WITHOUT BECOMING PREGNANT

HOW TO HAVE INTERCOURSE WITHOUT BECOMING PREGNANT
1979, 18 pages, Illus.

from
Alliance for Perinatal Research and Services
P.O. Box 6358
Alexandria, VA 22306-0358
$2.00
bulk rates available

Simple but effective line drawings and descriptions of the male and female bodies are used to explain how pregnancy occurs and describe birth control methods.

LIBERATED WOMAN'S CANVAS
needlework, 1972-1973

from
Ita Aber
One Fanshaw Avenue
Yonkers, NY 10705

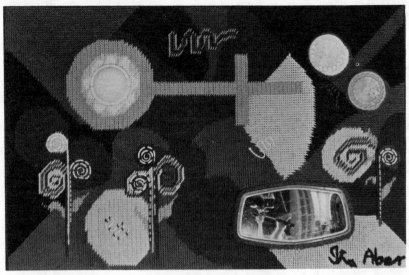

Ita Aber has worked as an art historian, textile conservator, and embroiderer in a variety of institutions including Yeshiva University Museum, the Cooper Hewitt Museum, and the Hudson River Museum. Her work has been exhibited widely since 1975 and has been reproduced in many publications. (JIA)

"The idea of a 'Liberated Woman's Canvas' is taken from the needlework term 'liberated canvas' which means to do exactly as one pleases. Here, in showing these women's contraceptive methods, we are saying that every day women worry that they are pregnant and that they are not pregnant. How liberated can they be until the child bearing years are over?

"In the upper left a diaphragm is worked into a reclining feminine symbol. In the lower left, Dr. Margolies intrauterine loops are separated by a

Dr. Lippy loop which has five yellow cords attached that everyone tries to pick up out of the embroidery only to find out that they are attached. In the upper right are 2 birth control pill packs—one empty, one partly used—worked into a dragonfly which

is also phallic. The lower right has a mirror held on with needle weaving in which the viewers image is caught while observing the piece. The idea is for the viewer to see how they fit into the picture. The colors are vibrant reds, oranges, light and dark

blue. The edge is velvet ribbon."

"I have recently removed my name from the front of the work so as not to detract from the work. Interestingly, the diaphragm has dried out and is crumbling.

THE BIRTH CONTROL BOOK: A
Complete Guide for Men and Women
by Howard I. Shapiro
1978, 356 pages, Illus.

from
Avon Books
959 Eighth Avenue
New York, NY 10019
$3.50 pap.

Howard Shapiro is a gynecologist and serves as a medical advisor for the National Organization for Women and his local Planned Parenthood chapter. In this book he describes the reproductive system (including how to examine yourself with a speculum) and evaluates in detail the risks and benefits of the different methods of birth control, including birth control pills, IUDs, diaphragms, spermicides, and condoms, coitus interruptus and rhythm (including the sympto-thermal method of natural birth control), postcoital contraception, abortion, vasectomy, tubal ligation, hysterectomy, and methods still being developed. Presented in a question-and-answer format, this book is intended to provide women with the consumer-oriented information they need to make their own informed decisions about birth control. (JIA)

"1. The Pill and the IUD are relatively safe when compared with the risk of death from pregnancy and childbirth when no fertility control method is used.
2. The risk of death increases significantly after the age of forty when birth control pills are used.
3. The use of traditional contraception, such as the diaphragm and condom backed up by early induced abor-

tion of all unwanted pregnancies that result from contraceptive failure, is the safest method of birth control. . . .

"Perhaps the greatest obstacle against reducing pregnancy rates is the maturity and motivation of the couple using the diaphragm. Although all methods of contraception require a certain degree of motivation, it is especially true of the diaphragm. Too often a 'diaphragm failure' really means that it was never used. The best diaphragm success rates are in those women who insert the diaphragm every night before going to bed, and remove it the following morning. When intercourse is spontaneous at other times during the day, a considerate, mature man patiently waits while his partner inserts the diaphragm. A woman is not the only one who can insert the diaphragm, and active participation by a man in this act can represent both a sensual and a mature expression of his feelings."

THE DOCTORS' CASE AGAINST
THE PILL
by Barbara Seaman
1980, 240 pages

from
Doubleday/Dolphin
245 Park Avenue
New York, NY 10017
$6.50 pap.

The first edition of this book in 1969 brought controversy over the safety of the contraceptive pill into the public spotlight and led to Senate hearings which resulted in the adoption of mandatory patient package inserts for birth control pills. Ms. Seaman is credited with having introduced the concept of patient labeling for drugs. In this new, revised edition, Seaman continues to describe the medically documented harmful side-effects of the Pill, which include blood-clots, heart disease, strokes, cancer, diabetes, reduced sex drive, sterility, genetic changes, miscellaneous health effects (including jaundice, thyroid function changes, weight gain, urinary infections, arthritis, skin and gum problems, etc.), depression, irritability, and altered nutrition. Seaman uses many case histories of women who have suffered these side effects to illustrate the statistics and includes a long list of notes and references. There is also a very good chapter on alternatives to the Pill. (JIA)

"The Food and Drug Administration now admits that several hundred otherwise healthy young women die each year from Pill-caused clots that travel to the lung. The federal agency also advises women

to stop taking the Pill for at least a full cycle before surgery. Because the Pill increases the risk of postoperative clotting complications, patients should also stay off the Pill for at least two weeks after any operation. . . .

"Of all the methods a woman can initiate, the diaphragm and cervical cap are the most effective alternatives to the Pill. In some ways these methods are better than the Pill, for the woman controls them more if she is conscientious. In actual use the Pill is not quite the 99 percent effective method manufacturers boast of. A national fertility survey showed that during the first year they took it, 6 percent of Pill users got pregnant. After that the figure declined. Doctors and manufacturers used to blame these 'breakthrough' pregnancies on missed pills, but there is recent evidence that certain common drugs sometimes block the contraceptive action of the Pill. These include some antihistamines, barbiturates, and other drugs: specifically, Amytal, Nembutal, phenobarbital, Seconal, Butazolidin, Dilantin, Equanil, Miltown, Rimactane.

"Backed up by legal abortion in those rare cases of failure, the motivated woman can feel safe and not sorry, protected by the diaphragm, the same old 'rubber parachute' that helped her mother keep a family down to size. Women—and men—are newly aware of the diaphragm's efficiency and the safety record of abortions. But many still trust the diaphragm too little and the Pill and IUD too much."

MONTREAL HEALTH PRESS, INC.
P.O. Box 1000, Station G
Montreal, Quebec
H2W 2N1, Canada
514/272-5441

The Montreal Health Press does an impressive job in producing their books and posters. They publish newsprint handbooks on birth control, venereal disease and sexual assault which are well-organized, have useful graphics and give essential information. They also produce two poster kits (male and female anatomy and birth control). The soft line drawings are beautiful as art works in themselves as well as conveying medically accurate information. Because of the soft tones and light lines, these posters might be difficult to use in a large group situation, but for small groups, in clinics, and for individual viewing these are the best graphics I have seen on these subjects.
(SR)

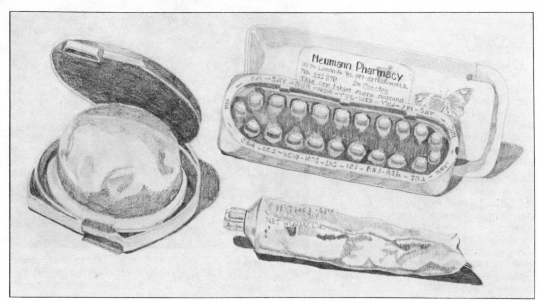

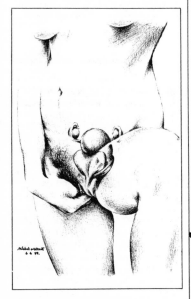

Poster Kit No. 1:
Female and Male Anatomy
includes
Female Anatomy
Male Anatomy
Prediction of Fertile Period
Bi-manual examination
Speculum examination

Poster Kit No. 2
Birth Control Methods
includes
Condom/Foam
Diaphragm
Pill/IUD
Abortion
Vasectomy/Tubal ligation

"Each kit contains five (16 x 24") posters. Printed in brown on white, they are carefully conceived to be medically accurate, non-sexist, and aesthetically appealing. The cost of $10. per kit includes postage and handling." (Canadian funds)

BIRTH CONTROL
Pencil drawing, 8" x 12"
1973
Janet Isaacs Ashford

"In 1973, after five years continuously on the Pill, I decided to stop. The Pill had been very convenient during my college years, but I began to worry about the reports of bad side effects I was hearing. When I began taking pills in 1968, I was not told of any side effects, but looking back I wonder whether the mild depression I often suffered during those years may have been caused by the pills. At any rate, I did know that my menstrual flow had become very scant, even after switching to a lower dosage pill, and that worried me. I had just started living with my husband and I was thinking about having children. I decided to go off the Pill to get my body ready for pregnancy. I went to a local ob/gyn doctor for a diaphragm. He was really reluctant to fit me for a diaphragm and said, "What's wrong with the pill?" I had to argue with him for a while before he finally relented and showed me how to insert the diaphragm properly. Some time later I made this drawing of my birth control methods: my last package of pills, which I never took, and my brand new diaphragm and tube of spermicidal jelly. I'm still using a diaphragm."
(JIA)

PLANNED PARENTHOOD
810 Seventh Avenue
New York, NY 10019

Planned Parenthood provides many services to help promote and provide family planning and birth control and to maintain access to safe, legal abortion. Planned Parenthood, from its national headquarters in New York City, directs almost 200 local affiliates and over 700 local clinics. Clinics provide contraceptive services and counseling and related medical services including pregnancy tests, diagnosis and treatment of venereal disease, tests for cancer of the breast and uterus, and vasectomies. (See your local phone book for the Planned Parenthood clinic nearest you.) Planned Parenthood works on projects to provide sex education in schools and to help reduce the high rate of teenage pregnancy. PP's public affairs program lobbies on behalf of increased government support for family planning services and to restore Medicaid funding for abortion. The international program also works in 102 nations to provide family planning services. The follow-

ing publications are available from Planned Parenthood in single copies (at prices listed) and also at bulk rates.
(JIA)

PUBLICATIONS

Basics of Birth Control. No. 1253
All the methods in chart form. Explains each and allows easy comparison. Gives use, effectiveness, acceptibility, where obtained and average costs. Revised 1981. 8 pp. 4"x 9"
Single copy $.50

Ways to Chart Your Fertility Pattern.
No. 404
How Temperature, Calendar and Mucus Methods work. Menstrual cycle explained. Need for professional instruction and supervision stressed, revised 1980. 8 pp. Includes charts and tables. 3½ x 7¼"
Single copy $.50

Fertility Awareness Chart. No. 900
Chart simplifies recordkeeping and provides a filled-in sample. Pub. 1980.
Two sides, 8½ x 11"
100 for $6. (Available in multiples of 100 only.)

Can Smokers Take the Pill? No. 1609
Facts about the effects of combining smoking and taking contraceptive pills, showing who is at risk and how seriously. Explains the health risks involved and the need for some women to find alternatives. Written in easy-to-understand language suitable for all educational levels. Revised 1981. Illustrated. Six-panel folder, two colors. 8½ x 3½"
Single copy $.50

Daughters of DES Mothers. No. 1568
Questions and answers for women who may be family planning patients. Booklet discusses degree of risk, possible symptoms, examinations, stresses need for continuing checkups. Revised 1981. 8-panel folder. 6½ x 3¾".
Single copy $.50

About Childbirth. No. 1583
The scope of the content is broad, including important facts for mothers and fathers-to-be relating to the birth experience before, during, and after delivery. Easy to read; appropriate for all age groups. Pub. 1978. 16 pp. Illustrated. 5½ x 8"
Single copy $.50

PATIENT INFORMATION LIBRARY
PAS Publishing
345-G Serramonte Plaza
Daly City, CA 94015
415/994-1150

This company provides many booklets and posters on a variety of health subjects from the *Back Owner's Manual* to *Understanding Nasal Surgery* and *The Gallbladder Book*. The materials are designed to supplement physician instructions and serve as office hand-outs. Bulk rates are available on publications and single copies may be ordered for review at a nominal cost. Request a complete catalog.

PAS publications especially relevant to birth control are listed below: (SR)

CONTRACEPTION?: Facts on Birth Control
by Howard E. Selinger, MD
1980, 16 pages, Illus.

Written in a very lively and funny comic book style, this booklet reviews currently available birth control methods and discusses their effectiveness, effects on sexual habits, health effects and risks, and provides instructions for use.

"The sharing of love ideally includes the sharing of responsibility for contraception. Today, more and more men are participating in contraceptive decision-making.

"Choosing a method of contraception should be based on knowing the various methods available, their current use, relative effectiveness, and particular advantages and disadvantages. The reported health risks of some of the more effective methods are of some concern and require careful consideration. These must always be weighed against the increased risk of pregnancy associated with the 'safer,' less effective methods of contraception—the complications of pregnancy itself carry overall greater and more frequent risks to your health.

"It is important to remember that attitudes, situations, needs, and desires change—what is right for you today may not be tomorrow. *The best method of contraception will be the one you and your partner are most comfortable with and will use correctly each and every time you have sexual intercourse.*"

TUBAL OCCLUSION: Facts About Female Sterilization
by Carl J. Levinson, MD
1981, 8 pages, Illus.

This booklet focuses on laparoscopy and minilaparotomy. It underscores the permanency of the procedure and assists with informed consent requirements. Pre- and post-operative anatomy are illustrated in full color.

POPULATION CRISIS COMMITTEE
1120 Nineteenth Street NW
Suite 550
Washington, DC 20036
202/659-1833

"The Population Crisis Committee seeks to increase worldwide support for international population and family planning programs through public education, population policy analysis, liaison with international leaders and organizations, and support of innovative, cost-effective family planning projects in developing countries."

The Population Crisis Committee publishes *Population Briefing Sheets* (issued 2-3 times yearly) and the *Draper Fund Report* (issued twice yearly). Copies are available free in limited quantities. Write for a listing of topics discussed. Several papers of special interest are: (SR)

1. June 1981 issue (No. 11) of *Population Briefing Sheet* discusses worldwide use of natural family planning (NFP), the different methods, advantages, and the issue of birth defects related to pregnancies which result from failure of NFP.
2. September 1979 issue (No. 10) of *Population Briefing Sheet* lists private organizations in the population field, with descriptions of activities and services.
3. Issue No. 9 of the *Draper Fund Report* (October, 1980) specifically deals with "Improving the Status of Women":

"The continuous cycle of pregnancy and breast-feeding is particularly damaging to those whose nutritional status is marginal. Studies have indicated that in many areas of the developing world women gain little or no weight during pregnancy and often lose weight during lactation. Maternal malnutrition and anemia, conditions usually associated with frequent pregnancies, attenuate resistance to infectious diseases and increase the probability of complications or even death during childbirth.

"By freeing women from unwanted fertility and by promoting their physical health, family planning also permits women to reach out beyond their traditional roles. In so doing, it enhances their own sense of social and psychological well-being and the contribution they are able to make to the well-being of their families and communities. While women remain the principal beneficiaries of family planning services, there are few other programs which are more far-reaching in scope or longer-range in their impact."

—from "Family Planning: Improving the Health of Women and Their Children" by Nafis Sadik, in the *Draper Fund Report,* No. 9, October, 1980.

METHODS OF CONTRACEPTION
Prepared by Planned Parenthood Federation of America
1980, flip-chart, Illus.

from
Public Health Service
Bureau of Community Health Services
Rockville, MD 20857
free

This is a sturdy cardboard flip chart (11" x 15") on female and male anatomy and birth control methods. Clearly-drawn, large, black and white graphics make it a useful tool for patient education in classes and clinics. Details about each graphic are printed on the back of each page, so the instructor can glance over the information and present it while the clients view the pictures. Discusses sterilization and natural family planning as well as the "usual" contraceptive methods but lists them under "methods that are rarely effective." Otherwise, this is a very informative booklet, especially for low-level readers. The booklet is available in English and thirteen other languages, including Spanish, Vietnamese, Italian, Chinese, Laotian, and Cambodian. (SR)

"The diaphragm is easy to use, and it offers excellent contraceptive protection. When the diaphragm size is correct and when the diaphragm is properly in place, the woman cannot feel the diaphragm. Her partner cannot feel the diaphragm during intercourse, since it is difficult for the penis to feel the material out of which the diaphragm is made. The diaphragm is considered to be one of the most effective contraceptive methods. It also has no known ill effects. It is therefore a method that can be used by any woman as long as she is willing to insert it properly and remembers to leave it in place for six hours after intercourse has ended."

CAROLINA POPULATION CENTER
University of North Carolina at Chapel Hill
University Square, 300A
Chapel Hill, NC 27514
919/966-2152

The Carolina Population Center provides a variety of educational materials (booklets, pamphlets, audiovisuals) and publications (books, monographs, journal reprints) on birth control and related topics for consumers and professionals. Topics include birth control methods, sexual counseling, teenage pregnancy, birth control for the retarded, abortion, population trends, and socioeconomic factors in family planning. Write for a complete publications list. (SR)

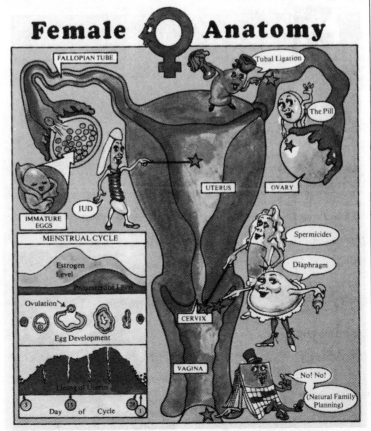

from *Contraception: Facts on Birth Control*

Natural Family Planning

Natural family planning involves finding out when a woman is going to ovulate (release a ripe egg) and then abstaining from intercourse or using an alternate form of birth control (diaphragm or condom) during this "fertile time" of each monthly cycle. The method can be used also to *achieve* a pregnancy, by planning to have intercourse during the time when conception is most likely to occur. The method can also help women become more aware of their bodily cycles.

There are several different "schools of thought" on how the natural family planning method should be used, but all are based on the observation of one or more of three basic body signs: temperature, cervical mucus, and length of menstrual cycle. The method is probably most effective when all three components are used together. These include:

1. Basal Body Temperature: The woman takes her temperature each morning before getting out of bed and records it on a graph or chart. She uses a special thermometer which indicates temperature in tenths of degrees. There is usually a slight drop in body temperature of from 2 to 3 tenths degrees 24-36 hours before ovulation and then a rise of from 7 to 8 tenths degrees 24-48 hours after ovulation. The temperature then remains elevated until menstruation begins.

2. Cervical Mucus: the woman observes and charts the changes in the cervical mucus which normally flows from the cervix (neck of the uterus) down through the vagina. Cervical mucus is usually dry just after menstruation, becomes stretchy and slippery around the time of ovulation and becomes sticky, thick and cloudy after ovulation. (Secondary signs of ovulation may also be noted by some women and give further clues as to when the fertile period is. These include Mittelschmertz ["middle pain," a slight pain felt in the area of the ovary when the egg is released], physical changes of the cervix, slight bloody staining, swelling of the vulva, abdominal bloating and increased sex drive.)

3. Calendar Method: by keeping track of when each menstrual cycle begins, one can estimate when the fourteenth day before menstruation occurs. This is the "average" time of ovulation.

Though it sounds complicated at first, many good books, pamphlets, and articles are available on natural family planning which can make the method self-instructional. Classes and counseling sessions on the method are also available through many sources, some of which are listed in this section.

Natural family planning is seen by many advocates as an egalitarian or non-sexist method of birth control because it requires the cooperation of both partners. It is also completely free of harmful health side effects. In addition, the method satisfies the proscriptions of some religious or moral views because it does not require any mechanical or "artificial" methods of birth control. So natural family planning is endorsed by a diverse range of groups ranging from feminist women's health advocates to Catholic anti-abortion groups.

The more conservative groups involved with natural family planning feel that the couple should refrain from sexual intercourse entirely during the fertile period, finding other ways to show their affection and love for each other. These "other ways" may or may not include oral sex or mutual masturbation, depending upon the moral viewpoint of the group concerned. However, it is interesting and important to note that the fertile time for a woman may be the time in her monthly cycle when her greatest sexual needs and desires surface. Using natural family planning to determine the fertile period and then using a barrier method (diaphragm, condoms, or foam) for intercourse during this time would allow the couple to enjoy the woman's increased sexual energy with very little fear of pregnancy. Such a combination of methods might also be useful if there was some question about whether or not the woman was fertile, because of an unexpected temperature variation (due to illness, fatigue, etc.) or a questionable mucus "reading."

Information is also available on how to use the natural family planning method after the birth of a baby, before the menstrual cycles have become reestablished, as well as on how to use the method with very irregular cycles and when approaching menopause.

The effectiveness rate of natural family planning is still being studied. As with other birth control methods, effectiveness is dependent on how correctly the method is used. If only the calendar method is used, effectiveness is anywhere from 50 to 85%. Using the basal body temperature method only, effectiveness ranges from 80 to 99%. Using the mucus method alone, rates of 75 to 99% effectiveness have been found. Combining all three methods leads one to believe that effectiveness rates would fall in the 80 to 99% range. If barrier methods or extended abstinence are used to cover any "questionable day," one would expect effectiveness rates to be higher.

The necessity for daily observation of temperature and mucus may be seen as "disadvantages" of this method. They can, however, become part of the daily routine, just as taking a pill, checking for an IUD string, or putting in a diaphragm must become routine for users of those methods. Also, many couples welcome the opportunity to become more closely aware of the woman's body rhythms. No health factors, such as diabetes or high blood pressure, need be considered before using this method and there is no long-term effect on one's ability to have children. The one consideration which has been cited statistically in preliminary epidemiologic studies is that there is an increase in congenital anomalies such as Down's syndrome and anencephaly among infants born after failure of the natural family planning method. A possible explanation is that conception has taken place late in the fertile period when the egg has aged. This finding will need more study and further scrutiny, especially with the increasing popularity of natural family planning.

(SR)

THE MAINSTREAM

> All one's actual apprehension of what it is like to be a woman, the irreconcilable difference of it—that sense of living one's deepest life underwater, that dark involvement with blood & birth & death . . . [is lost in our society.]
> —Joan Didion, *The White Album*

That time of month.
All day long I am under
water in anticipation.
My stomach slogs and sloshes
like milk in a jug carted
over a rocky road.
The sullen moon pulls out
the balance;
the monthly tide returns.

Swaddled in water, cradled in salt,
we lived nine months in the current
before that first swim,
the gush and run
of the birthing flood,
when the water broke
on boulders and we fell
into the alien air.
Not fish out of water,
we survived, grew older,
watched the grass swish and eddy.

But once each month,
our quivering gills remember.
We swim again in the mainstream,
touching the current.
We know what is real:
birth water, bathwater, milk & manna.
My woman's hair
rivers out behind
like tributaries
seeking the sea.

Barbara Crooker

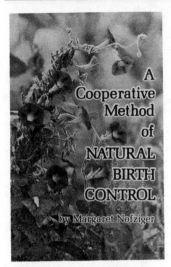

A COOPERATIVE METHOD OF
NATURAL BIRTH CONTROL
(3rd Ed.)
by Margaret Nofziger
1979, 121 pages, Illus.

from
The Book Publishing Company
156 Drakes Lane
Summertown, TN 38483
$5.00

BASAL TEMPERATURE AND
MUCUS CHART
8½ x 11", monthly chart
$5.00 per 100
$20.00 per 500

This is a very clear and simple guide to natural birth control and probably the best handbook available for learning the sympto-thermal method. Margaret Nofziger explains the basics of menstrual cycles and how conception occurs and then launches into a detailed description of calendar rhythm, cervical mucus, and basal body temperature, the three observations upon which her method is based. She includes lots of sample fertility charts, which help a great deal in understanding how to interpret the three different "readings." There are also special sections for nursing mothers with no periods, women approaching menopause, coming off "the Pill" and "if you wish to conceive." An appendix covers reproductive physiology and endocrinology in more detail. Included is an unmarked sample "Basal Temperature and Mucus Chart" as used in the book. Additional copies can be ordered from the publisher.

(SR)

"The front cover is a spray of flowers—morning glories. The title is put in between the flowers in such a way that the title doesn't run over any of the flowers. We thought that it was a medium-message of what the whole thing is about. It's about how to do it without running over the flowers."

—Stephen

"I want to put in a word for love here, before we get into details of this method. This is the only form of birth control that is a *cooperative*

venture. Neither husband nor wife has to bear a health burden or do it alone. It is the only non-sexist form of birth control, requiring the love and understanding of both.

"The basis of this method is the *agreement* to pay close attention and lovingly abstain for a bit in order to not conceive at this time. This way, when you do make love, it is complete and open to all the life force energy there is. And when you are not prepared to conceive, you don't do what causes conception. Now, don't give up loving altogether. There are many ways to show your love besides the usual way. With love and imagination, those few days a month can be as fulfilling and repairing as the rest. Learning how to cooperate on this issue tends to draw a couple closer together. . . .

"In order for pregnancy to occur, a fresh, live sperm from the man must meet and fertilize a live egg from the woman. This can only happen during a few days in a woman's fertility cycle. Pregnancy can happen if you make love at the exact time of ovulation. You can also get pregnant by making love up to 72 hours before or 24 hours after ovulation. This is because:

THE EGG ONLY LIVES FOR 12-
24 HOURS and
SPERM CAN FERTILIZE AN EGG
FOR 3 DAYS (PERHAPS UP TO 5)

"So in order to avoid pregnancy, a couple needs to abstain from making love for 3 days preceding ovulation and 1 day after.

"This would be very simple if we could pinpoint the exact time of ovulation. But at this stage of fertility research, we can only estimate the approximate time of ovulation and allow some extra leeway for error. . . .

"You need to take your temperature every morning after at least three hours of sleep and before getting out of bed, eating, drinking, or getting up to pee. (Shake your thermometer down the night before.) You should take your temperature rectally or vaginally rather than in your mouth because it is more accurate, and accuracy is certainly what we need. Don't ever take it orally one half of the month and rectally or vaginally the other half because there is about a degree difference between the two and that would really mess up your chart. Don't wash the thermometer in hot water. Just wipe it with a tissue.

"A very important aspect of this method is keeping good charts and records. Write your temperature on a graph to make a curve you can look at. It won't do to just write some numbers on your calendar. You won't be able to see what's happening. Write your mucus changes down on the same chart. You will be glad you

did when you can compare several months of charts and see exactly how your mucus lined up with your temperature. Put a lot of value in your charts. Keep them neat and clear to read. This is like taking a course in YOU. You are studying your body at a very detailed level, and should study it as carefully as you would a scientific course. . . .

"If you should slip up, or miscalculate, or just do it anyway, and end up pregnant with a baby you don't want, you can give the baby to me."

—Margaret

"The Farm Midwives also make this offer:

If you or anyone you know is thinking about getting an abortion, here is an alternative: We will deliver your baby by natural childbirth, for free. If you decide to keep the baby, you can; or we will raise it for you. If you ever decide that you want the baby back, you can have it. (We offer this alternative to the limit of our ability to provide good care.)"

(Editor's Note: For more information on The Farm, see page 110.)

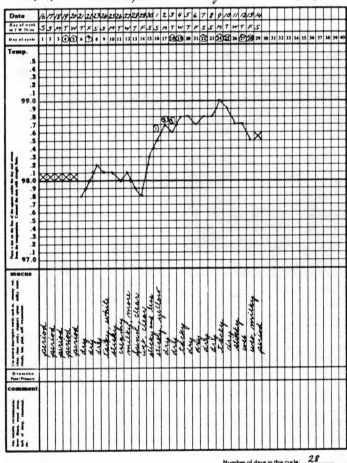

Number of days in this cycle: 28
Shortest previous cycle: 28

COUPLE TO COUPLE LEAGUE
3621 Glenmore Avenue
P.O. Box 11084
Cincinnati, OH 45211
513/661-7612

The Couple to Couple League (CCL) is a Catholic-oriented non-profit organization devoted to teaching the full sympto-thermal method of natural family planning, which involves observation of all the practical signs of fertility. The organization is morally opposed to abortion, sterilization, and the use of contraceptive drugs and devices and supports efforts to restrict access to these methods of birth control. The CCL method advises total abstinence from intercourse (or other genital sexual activity) during the fertile period. The League emphasizes the need for communication in marriage and "creative continence."

CCL provides a variety of publications and services to promote the use of natural family planning. The *Basic Materials List* describes books, pamphlets, and reprints available on natural family planning, Christian marriage and sexuality, breastfeeding and "natural" mothering, and on the medical and moral disadvantages of contraception and abortion. CCL also sells a workbook, daily observation charts, and Ovulindex Basal Temperature thermometer, for use with their official manual *The Art of Natural Family Planning* (see review below). A monthly newsletter is included with membership ($10.00 a year).

Local CCL chapters offer a series of classes for couples interested in the sympto-thermal method, taught by couples who have completed a certification program. The national office can provide assistance in locating a local CCL chapter. (JIA)

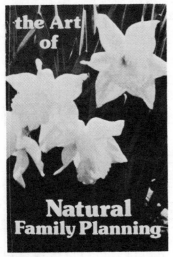

THE ART OF NATURAL FAMILY PLANNING
by John and Sheila Kippley
1979, 258 pages, Illus.

from
Couple to Couple League
$5.95 plus .75 postage

Written by co-founders of the Couple to Couple League, this book teaches the full sympto-thermal method using basal body temperature readings, checking cervical mucus, observing changes in the cervix, secondary signs of ovulation and previous cycle history. Careful reading is necessary to fully understand the method, but the authors have provided many examples (with sample charts) and question/answer sections which are useful. The first four chapters of the book review the Couple to Couple League's philosophy about morality in family planning and marriage. Even if your views differ from the authors' in these areas, the "how-to" chapters will be valuable. (SR)

"During the infertile phases of the cycle, the cervix remains firm, closed, and is easy to reach. As ovulation approaches, the following changes take place:

1. The os opens enough to accept a fingertip.
2. The portion of the cervix protruding into the vagina becomes softer attaining a rubberiness and softness similar to the walls of the vagina.
3. The cervix rises and becomes more difficult to reach.
4. There is an abundance of mucus.
5. The mucus makes the cervix feel more slippery.

"Does the mucus-only system provide positive proof that ovulation has actually occurred?

'No. Only the elevated basal temperatures provide positive proof that ovulation has occurred. Rather, the mucus indicates a time of overall fertility. It is a possible though an infrequent occurrence to observe the mucus sign without a subsequent ovulation even when a woman is having regular cycles."

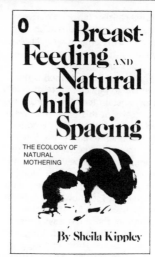

BREAST-FEEDING AND NATURAL CHILD SPACING:
The Ecology of Natural Mothering
by Sheila Kippley
1979, 197 pages, Illus.

from
Penguin Books, publisher
Also available through Couple to Couple League
$3.50 plus .75 postage

Breastfeeding on a restrictive schedule, providing a pacifier, and "letting the baby cry it out" have no place in the "natural mothering" process that Sheila Kippley describes in this book. She presents, through her own experiences and those of others, the benefits of providing the baby's nourishment *and* the greater part of its other sucking and security needs at the breast, with an almost guaranteed side effect of natural infertility. She includes discussion on night feedings, social life, weaning, nursing the older child and a short review of research on breastfeeding and its relation to concurrent infertility. Her emphasis is on the benefits of breastfeeding and closeness of skin-to-skin contact, and secondarily on natural child-spacing. (SR)

"Another physical aspect that is often forgotten in our busy world is the tranquilizing effect that nursing has on a woman. It provides brief rests during the day, and this form of relaxation can be a 'plus factor' for the mother who tends to be tense and nervous. In addition, her body is producing prolactin, a 'mothering' hormone that bottle-feeding mothers don't have. Thus, the nursing mother is not only *thinking* of being a good mother, but her body is producing the mood and she is *feeling* it as well. . . .

"The first sign of the future return of fertility is generally what we have been talking about, the return of menstruation. I say 'future return,' because ovulation does not usually occur before the first period following childbirth. Many nursing mothers have relied successfully on breastfeeding during amenorrhea, and some mothers have experienced some infertile cycles after the return of menses. On the other hand, some nursing mothers have conceived without a return of menses. Present research seems to indicate that the risk of pregnancy prior to the first menses is about 6 percent.

"The absence of menstruation provides a sense of security for the nursing mother who would like to avoid an immediate pregnancy following childbirth. This feeling of security can be lost if any bleeding or spotting occurs. Some mothers experience spotting or bleeding in the early months, but then increase the nursings to hold back menstruation once again. Spotting may also be a warning that menstruation or ovulation is just around the corner. Indeed, a few mothers have conceived after a spotting and without having had a regular menses. For mothers who do not desire another pregnancy and are concerned about the risk of pregnancy prior to the return of menstruation, proper information about the mucus discharge that occurs prior to ovulation or the first postpartum menses can be extremely valuable."

"Many nursing mothers have relied successfully on breastfeeding during amenorrhea, and some mothers have experienced some infertile cycles after the return of menses. On the other hand, some nursing mothers have conceived without a return of menses."

THE HUMAN LIFE AND NATURAL FAMILY PLANNING FOUNDATION
205 South Patrick Street
Alexandria, VA 22314
703/836-3377

This foundation is the national headquarters for about 500 Catholic diocesan-related natural family planning programs. These programs are presented via family life agencies, parishes, Catholic social services agencies, Catholic hospitals or health care agencies, and service programs at Catholic colleges and universities. The foundation endorses the teaching of the Ovulation Method, the Basal Body Temperature Method and the Sympto-Thermal Method (a combination of the first two) and encourages Catholic couples to make an informed choice among the natural planning methods.

The foundation provides publications on natural family planning and fertility awareness, instructor training materials, and an instructional series for learners. The learner booklets are available in English, Spanish, Vietnamese, and Chinese. (SR)

OVULATION METHOD TEACHERS ASSOCIATION
P.O. Box 14511
Portland, OR 97214

The Ovulation Method Teacher's Association (OMTA) is a non-profit public service organization which works to: make fertility awareness information more available; train teachers in the Ovulation Method (OM); and serve as a public resource for information on OM.

Services include:

* referral for OM classes
* teacher training and certification
* newsletter
* statistics
* speakers and conferences
(SR)

"We would like every woman to have the information which the Ovulation Method of fertility awareness has to offer her, whether or not she should use this information for avoiding or achieving pregnancy. It is our hope that we will be able to reach many men and women, with the aim of enabling them to make more informed choices regarding their bodies, birth control, and their lives."

THE OVULATION METHOD:
Cycles of Fertility
by Denise Guren and Nealy Gillette

Published by the Ovulation Method Teachers Association
Order from:
Denise Guren
4760 Aldrich Road
Bellingham, WA 98225
$2.95
bulk rates available

"The Ovulation Method: Cycles of Fertility is a detailed, practical introduction to this method. The female fertility pattern and reproductive anatomy and physiology is presented in layperson's terms. Scientific and clinical studies are included, along with a comprehensive bibliography."

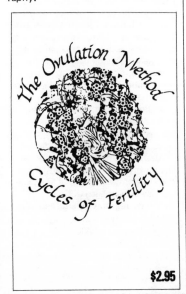

$2.95

NATURAL FAMILY PLANNING
1980, brochure

from
Bureau of Community Health Services
Public Health Service
Rockville, MD 20857
free

There are three often-used methods for determining a woman's fertile period—the BBT (basal body temperature) method, the ovulation method, and the sympto-thermal method. The basics of these three are explained in this pamphlet published by the federal government. Effectiveness rates, and the advantages and disadvantages of natural family planning are discussed. (SR)

"Calculation of the fertile time in the menstrual cycle is based on three scientifically acceptable assumptions: (1) that release of the egg (ovulation) occurs approximately 14 days before the beginning of menstruation; (2) that the egg (ovum) survives for 24 hours; and (3) that the male sperm is capable of fertilizing an egg for 48-72 hours."

WORLD ORGANIZATION OVULATION METHOD-BILLINGS
1750 S. Brentwood
St. Louis, MO 63144

World Organization Ovulation-Method-Billings (WOOMB) was formed at the request of Drs. John and Evelyn Billings who initially described the "Billings Method" or Ovulation Method of natural family planning. The goal of WOOMB is "to certify teachers and spread the message of the Ovulation Method all over the world."

Write for a list of WOOMB publications. The WOOMB office can also send a list of regional/local coordinators of WOOMB services and classes.
(SR)

"Theoretically, the Billings Ovulation Method's rate of effectiveness is roughly that of the pill. But this rate is achieved *only* by couples who know the Method thoroughly and who follow it carefully.

"Most so-called 'failures' are people-failures, in that the couple chose to disregard the rules. So each couple using it should understand that in this Method, unlike contraception, the potential of human creativity is always preserved."

NATURAL FAMILY PLANNING TEACHERS, INC.
700 NE 47th Avenue
Portland, OR 97213

This organization provides direct services in natural family planning, primarily to teachers and couples in the Northwest, but also supplies publications and educational materials by mail throughout the country. Emphasis is on the Billings "Ovulation Method."

"NFPT, Inc. exists to help people avoid or achieve pregnancy naturally. We help sub-fertile couples know when they are most likely to succeed in conceiving. Many who have used the temperature change to indicate ovulation have been frustrated until they talk to us.

"We teach breastfeeding women to know about the basic infertile pattern which means intercourse will not lead to pregnancy. We help people who want to plan to achieve a son or daughter to know how to increase their chances from about 50% to 85%.

"We provide general health education, especially to women, since understanding their cycles can help them understand more about the effects of light, stress, diet, and infections on their health, comfort, and fertility.

"We promote the idea that since healthy men are always fertile, they need to share in the motivation and

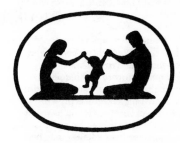

responsibility for combined fertility."

Services available include:

* class instruction for women and couples in natural family planning methods
* counseling in the use of NFP
* guest speakers on NFP
* bimonthly newsletter, *The Chart*
* supply house of books and publications on NFP and related subjects
* teacher training and certification
* education and training workshops
* supportive services for teachers
(SR)

"We promote the idea that since healthy men are always fertile, they need to share in the motivation and responsibility for combined fertility."

THE NATURAL BIRTH CONTROL BOOK
by Art Rosenblum
1976, 156 pages, Illus.

from
Aquarian Research Foundation
5620 Morton Street
Philadelphia, PA 19144
215/849-3237 or 1259
$4.95

With increased interest in avoiding the problems and side-effects of currently available contraceptive devices, the area of "natural" birth control has become more popular. This book discusses four methods which people are exploring—mental control over conception, astrological birth control, the ovulation method (checking vaginal mucus, basal body temperature, and the calendar) and lunaception. The author suggests combining some methods for increased effectiveness (e.g. astrological birth control and the ovulation method). There is at present no large scale scientific evidence on these methods, other than the ovulation method, which is considered to be quite effective. Read about the other three methods with a dose of healthy skepticism, realizing that there are no apparent side-effects but the possibility of pregnancy might be higher than you would wish. (SR)

"Here we shall meet a method of birth control which has been more fully researched and tested than mental control of conception. This is the Jonas-Rechnitz method sometimes called 'Astrological Birth Control' because it is based on the discovery that most women can have a fertile time in addition to the usual ovulation time and that this fertile period is related to the position of the sun and the moon at the woman's birth time. . . .

"The essential idea of Lunaception is that by the use of light on certain nights of the month and total darkness on other nights, many women can so regulate their ovulation times that they are able to predict ovulation accurately to the very day. Together with that, they use the Ovulation Method and temperature charting to confirm the accuracy of the predictions."

Sterilization

There are several methods of birth control which are considered *permanent* and *irreversible.* With new micro-surgery techniques, the possibilities of reversing sterilization are increasing but at the present time the probability is still low that reversal will be successful and the cost (greater than $4000.) may be prohibitive.

Several important issues surround the use of sterilization at present:

1. sterilization being performed without knowledgeable informed consent
2. discrimination in sterilization in matters of age, spousal consent, number of children, etc.
3. the potential physical long-term effects of sterilization for both men and women

If you or your partner is considering sterilization, find out all you can about the procedures, find a doctor who will discuss the procedures with you and who routinely performs this procedure, and ask about the latest information on long-term side effects. If you aren't able to obtain this information from a doctor, check with the Association for Voluntary Sterilization (see listing in this section), a local family planning clinic, or the local health department. Don't make this important decision without knowing as much as you possibly can about sterilization and feeling comfortable with your decision.   (SR)

IMPORTANT FACTS ABOUT POSTPARTUM STERILIZATION
1979, 11 pages, Illus.

from
American College of Obstetricians and Gynecologists
600 Maryland Avenue, SW
Washington, DC 20024
free

This booklet discusses the advantages of having sterilization done when you are in the hospital after the birth of a baby. A brief description of tubal ligation is given, but there is no discussion of the different types of "tubals." A short outline of discomforts and risks is included.
          (SR)

"In general, the operation is done within three days of delivering your last baby, although many factors influence the exact time to do a postpartum tubal ligation: the health of the mother just after delivery, the health of the baby, the availability of operating room personnel and time for the procedure, and so on. In some situations it can be done a few minutes after delivery, using the same anesthesia as was used for the delivery. If a Caesarian Section is done, tubal ligation can easily be carried out at that time."

INFORMATION FOR WOMEN: YOUR STERILIZATION OPERATION
1978, 12 pages

from
U.S. Dept. of Health and Human Services
Public Health Service
Rockville, MD 20857

This pamphlet is the one given to women who will be having sterilizations paid for through federal funds. It includes the regulations for sterilization operations when funded by the government and discusses the four types of tubal sterilization, their benefits and risks/discomforts. This pamphlet emphasizes that *no one can force a woman to be sterilized* or take away federal benefits if she refuses sterilization. The required written consent forms for sterilization are included.   (SR)

"Sterilization must be considered permanent. For nearly all women, once this operation has been done, it can never be undone. Some doctors try to undo a sterilization by rejoining the tubes. This is a difficult and expensive operation and it doesn't work very often. Some people call sterilization 'tying the tubes.' But don't think the tubes can be untied! They can't. So it's not a good idea to think your sterilization can be undone.

"To have this operation paid for with Federal funds, you must be at least 21 years old. If you are married, you should discuss the operation with your husband. However, his consent is not required if Medicaid or any other Federal Government program is going to pay for your operation. Your consent to sterilization cannot be obtained while you are in the hospital for childbirth or abortion....

"A woman can have a sterilization operation right after having a baby.

This means that a woman may want to be sterilized while she is in the hospital for the delivery. A woman should think about this early in her pregnancy because in order for the sterilization to be paid for with Federal funds she must sign the consent form at least 30 days before the baby is due."

INFORMATION FOR MEN: YOUR STERILIZATION OPERATION
1978, 12 pages

Same source as above.

This is the equivalent male version of the female sterilization pamphlet described above. It discusses vasectomy—how it is done, the benefits, risks, and discomforts.   (SR)

"The surgical method of birth control is called a vasectomy. It is done in a doctor's office or clinic. Under local anesthesia, the doctor closes off the sperm ducts (tubes) so that sperm cannot get through these ducts into the semen (the fluid ejected at climax)... When there are no sperm in the semen, you cannot cause a pregnancy. Only the sperm are blocked, not the liquid part of the semen. You will still ejaculate (eject fluid) as before. Vasectomy will not change your hormones. (NOTE: Vasectomy is not castration. The testicles are not removed.)"

ASSOCIATION FOR VOLUNTARY STERILIZATION
708 Third Avenue
New York, NY 10017
212/986-3880

The goal of this association is "to make voluntary sterilization readily available to all adults regardless of parenthood, marital status or income." The association maintains a roster of over 2000 cooperating physicians in the U.S. who will perform sterilizations.

A selection of educational brochures and fact sheets are available free in single copies. Request a complete list.   (SR)

"According to the 1973 National Survey of Family Growth, sterilization has become the number one method of choice for married couples where the wife is 30 years of age or older and over 9 million Americans have already chosen sterilization for contraceptive reasons. AVS estimates that the number has increased about one million each year since 1970."
—from *Questions and Answers on Voluntary Sterilization for Men and Women,* 1979.

"Men are not sterile immediately following vasectomy. It usually requires from 10 to 15 ejaculations to clear the ducts of residual sperm. A temporary form of birth control must be used until the doctor reports that laboratory tests show the semen to be sperm-free."
—from *Voluntary Sterilization: Your Right to Know, Your Right to Choose,* 1979

SECOND THOUGHTS ABOUT STERILIZATION
by Karen Wynn
1977, 4 pages, Illus.

from
SISTER
250 Howard Avenue
New Haven, CT 06519
$.25 each
bulk rates available

The question of whether sterilization is really a "no-risk" procedure is discussed in this article. Personal experiences as well as results of a 1975 British study are included.

The motivations and understanding of federal policy makers about sterilization also come under scrutiny. Wynn concludes that "like all other birth control methods available today, sterilization has liabilities, some still unsuspected."   (SR)

"The principle involved in laparoscopic sterilization is not very elegant: cauterization is the medical term for burning, and the tubes are burned shut. What makes some people uneasy about the procedure is that healthy tissue is deliberately destroyed, a contradiction of the usual philosophy of surgical practice. But what is unclear is how much surrounding tissue is destroyed. Because earlier laparoscopic techniques resulted in a high number of subsequent pregnancies, the techniques tended to become more destructive year-by-year. Many gynecologists now suspect that the ovaries may be damaged during sterilization leading to premature menopause."

Abortion

The right to safe, legal abortion is fundamental to women's self-determination. As Margaret Sanger said, "No woman can call herself free who does not own and control her own body. No woman can call herself free until she can choose whether she will or will not be a mother." Every effort should be made to prevent unwanted pregnancies, through education for sexuality and family planning. But when abortion is necessary, it must be provided freely to all women, with medical safety, and with respect for individual judgment and choice.

(JIA)

KEEPING ABORTION LEGAL

The following organizations are among those working to keep abortion legal and safe. Write for information on membership, making contributions, and on how you can help promote reproductive freedom for all women.

NATIONAL ABORTION RIGHTS
ACTION LEAGUE (NARAL)
825 15th Street, NW
Washington, DC 20005
202/347-7774

AMERICAN CIVIL LIBERTIES
UNION
22 East 40th Street
New York, NY 10016
212/944-9800

RELIGIOUS COALITION FOR
ABORTION RIGHTS
100 Maryland Avenue, NE
Washington, DC 20002
202/543-7032

CENTER FOR CONSTITUTIONAL
RIGHTS
853 Broadway, 14th Floor
New York, NY 10003
212/674-3303

NATIONAL ORGANIZATION
FOR WOMEN (NOW)
425 13th Street, NW, Suite 1048
Washington, DC 20004
202/347-2279

A sheet of fifty stamps to help promote the concept of safe, legal abortion is available for $5.00 per sheet from NYS-NARAL (New York State Affiliate of the National Abortion Rights Action League), 20 West 40th Street, New York, NY 10018.

NATIONAL ABORTION
FEDERATION
110 East 59th Street
New York, NY 10022
212/688-8516
800/233-0618 (Consumer Hotline)

The National Abortion Federation (NAF) provides training workshops and seminars for its institutional members, has a review system to check providers' services, provides a data collection system about abortions, publishes educational materials, and provides other educational services for the public.

The NAF provides the only national, toll-free Hotline for guidance and information about pregnancy and abortion. The number is 800/223-0618 and calls are taken from 10 A.M. to 6 P.M. Eastern Standard Time.

Publications available from NAF include:

Facts about the NAF, free
Guidelines on How To Choose an Abortion Facility, free for abridged self-mailing pamphlet

Write for a complete publications list.

(SR)

"In 1973, the United States Supreme Court ruled that abortion should be a legal choice made between a woman and her physician. Previous to this decision, women with unwanted pregnancies were forced into parenthood, into the hands of illegal abortionists, into fear, pain, exorbitant expenses and sometimes death."

IN NECESSITY AND SORROW:
Life and Death in an Abortion
Hospital
by Magda Denes
1977, 247 pages

from
Penguin Books
625 Madison Avenue
New York, NY 10022
$2.95 pap.

This is a powerful book, written by a psychologist who herself decided to have an abortion when she became pregnant by mistake at age 37 after having had two children. The experience was difficult and prompted Magda Denes to return to the same hospital where she had her abortion to interview patients, staff, parents and others involved in the abortion process. She includes many case histories and interviews on both first and second trimester abortions, using both the D&C and saline techniques. The moral and emotional complexity of the abortion experience is strongly conveyed and we are reminded that, because of their fertility, women often have to make very difficult decisions.

(SR)

"On rereading it, my book appears to me booby-trapped. It seems a mined object ready to explode in utter destructiveness at the slightest corrupt or careless touch. For in fact I am for abortions. My rage throughout these pages is at the human predicament. At the finitude of our lives, at our nakedness, at the absurdity of our perpetual ambivalence toward the terror of life and toward the horror of death.

"Abortions I think should be legal throughout the world. They should be at the mother's will, on demand, safe, dignified, provided free by the state, supported with mercy by the church.

"And that, just exactly that, would make abortions more problematic than they have ever been before. For if we remove them from the category of forbidden acts whose commission is the embodiment of risk and the embodiment of self-assertion in the face of coercive forces, if we permit them to be acts of freedom as they should be, their meaning, private and collective, will inescapably emerge in the consciousness of every person."

" 'In the beginning I was mixed up because I was taught by the Hippocratic oath not to take a life. But I mixed up my feelings about the fetus as an entity versus just as a procedure, and when life begins. Does life begin at the moment of conception or does life begin at viability, which is twenty-eight weeks? Or does it begin at the moment of birth? So, with that in mind, I had to resolve my feelings. And I resolved it like this. That since I've been in practice for more than ten years and seen what criminal abortion can do, people have forgotten what criminal abortion can do, in those ten years I've seen everything. From crippled patients, to infections, to death. Directly traceable to criminal abortions. So long as there is a money factor and criminal abortions exist, and they don't do it at an established hospital, by certified and competent doctors, you're going to have that tragedy occur over and over again. I felt that this was detrimental to good medical practice, and it was also a condemnation against women. Since women are the ones that get pregnant and not men, I feel this way: I don't think women should be a second minor sex. I think they have just as much right to their bodies as men do. If men could get pregnant they would have had abortion on demand ten centuries ago.' "

—from an interview with a male physician working on the D&C floor.

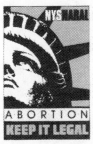
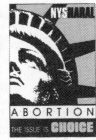
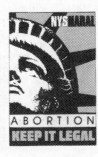
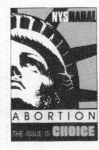
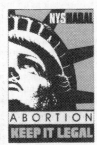
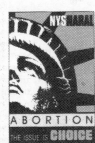
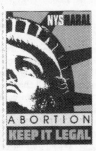

Infertility

SUPPORT GROUPS

RESOLVE
Box 474
Belmont, MA 02178
617/484-2424

RESOLVE is a national support, information, and referral organization with over 35 local chapters. These groups provide a place for people with infertility to learn about themselves and infertility, to share their feelings with others in the same situation, and to learn how to cope with their problem. Services include telephone counseling, referral to medical services or alternatives, support groups for infertile people, public education, and literature.
—Abby Pariser

THE AMERICAN FERTILITY SOCIETY
1608 13th Avenue South
Birmingham, AL 35256

The American Fertility Society is composed of physicians and scientists for whom infertility is a concern. The Society provides booklets for physicians and patients and refers patients to specialists.

UNITED INFERTILITY ORGANIZATION
51 Carey
Maropac, NY 10541
914/723-1687

This consumer group maintains an infertility hotline, offers support groups, and provides medical information and publications.

THE FERTILITY QUESTION
by Margaret Nofziger
1982, 104 pages, Illus.

from
The Book Publishing Company
156 Drakes Lane
Summertown, TN 38483
$4.95

Margaret Nofziger's first book, *A Cooperative Method of Natural Birth Control,* describes how to use awareness of a woman's natural body cycles to avoid getting pregnant (see index for review). This new book turns the table, showing couples how to use the techniques of natural family planning to achieve a pregnancy. Margaret provides very clear explanations of how to use and combine the observations of basal body temperature, cervical mucus, and menstrual cycles to determine the time of maximum fertility. Couples who have had difficulty conceiving are encouraged to keep a chart of the woman's basal body temperature, which will indicate when and if she is ovulating. By making love during the four most fertile days of each cycle, the chances for conception are greatly increased. Many sample temperature charts and question-and-answers are included along with a sample, an unmarked basal temperature chart which readers can photocopy and use. Charts are also available from the Book Publishing Company for $5.00 for 100.

Margaret also discusses other factors which may reduce fertility or be causes of infertility. These include scarred fallopian tubes, problems with sperm count, post-Pill amenorrhea (lack of periods), incompatible mucus, hormonal imbalance, anovulatory cycles, amenorrhea, endometriosis, inadequate cervical mucus, and dietary deficiencies.

Margaret Nofziger herself is the mother of two children. Her first child was born after eight years of apparent infertility, and the second after three years of trying. She knows whereof she speaks. (JIA)

"There are really only about four days each cycle when conception can occur. Obviously, you could conceive on the day of ovulation (if the fallopian tubes are open, sperm abundant, etc.). But the egg only lives for 12 to 24 hours after it pops out of the follicle. If it popped at 6:30 AM and lived until 7:30 PM, and you made love at 10:00 PM, it would be too late for that whole cycle. . . .

"If scheduling intercourse is ruining your sex life, making you feel pressured, unspontaneous, desperate, turned off . . . DON'T DO IT! Believe me, it's not worth it if it causes tension or friction. You might do better to let nature take its course once you have established ovulation by the basal temperature method.

"But if you both want to try to have intercourse at optimum times, and avoid it sometimes for an increased sperm count, then good luck on your cooperative journey. . . .

"Whether you are coping with established subfertility factors, coming to peace with medically confirmed infertility, or just wondering why the expected conception hasn't happened yet, you will gain many personal benefits from monitoring the signs of your own reproductive cycle. Even if you only watch your mucus changes and/or chart your temperature for a few months, you will be surprised at how familiar and 'in charge' you will feel with your body. It's a liberating feeling to be able to observe ovulation approach and pass, and to accurately predict one's periods."

INFERTILITY: A Guide for the Childless Couple
by Barbara Eck Menning
1977

from
NACAC
3900 Market Street, Suite 247
Riverside, CA 92501
$3.45

INFERTILITY!! Who would ever think of it before it becomes an ever-present partner in your marriage? First you give up your contraception and try to get pregnant. After a few months you don't even suspect infertility. Six months to a year later you begin to think about seeing your regular Ob/Gyn doctor. "Perhaps there's some small problem," you say to yourself, hiding from reality. By the time you've had a few tests, you or the doctor begins to talk about "infertility" and an infertility specialist. Mostly we assume and hope that we can be "cured."

By this time basal body temperatures, charts, post-coital tests, semen analyses, and any number of blood and urine tests are a normal part of your life. You forget that you used to take your body's functioning for granted. Now your mind is full of estrogens, follicle stimulating hormone, luteinizing hormone, prolactin, cervical mucus, laparascopy, hysterosalpinograms, and D&C's. Does anyone ever ask how you feel: scared, angry, frustrated, outraged, despairing? Can you ever talk about IT to your spouse? Will there ever be a baby in your arms, in your house, in your life?

Fifteen to twenty percent of American couples experience infertility. Of these, half can achieve a pregnancy and live birth, mostly through medical intervention—surgery and/or medication ("fertility drugs"). Five percent have spontaneous pregnancies.

The best book on infertility is written by an infertile woman. Barbara Eck Menning covers the medical aspects: infertility in the male and female, medical investigation and treatments, and miscarriage. She also covers the psychological aspects of infertility, providing chapters on infertility as a life crisis and discussing the common feelings of surprise, denial, isolation, anger, guilt and unworthiness, depression, grief, and resolution. Other important sections include "Sexuality, Self Image, and Self Esteem," "Infertility and the Bedroom," and the alternatives of adoption and artificial donor insemination. There is a good glossary, a small pre-1977 bibliography, and a short list of organizations and resources.

Barbara Eck Menning is a founder of Resolve, a support group for infertile people (see above).
—Abby Pariser

"Infertility hurts. I know . . . I am an infertile woman. There was a time, some years ago, when I was not able to say those words at all, much less think of myself as an infertile *woman.* The words seemed mutually exclusive. I could be either infertile or a woman but not both. The time of my infertility investigation and attempted treatment were filled with turmoil, both physical and mental. I did not understand what was happening to me, in spite of an advanced degree in Maternal-Child Health and Nursing. I did not understand my feelings, in spite of the fact that I had counseled others extensively. I did not understand why my husband could not understand my pain, in spite of a marriage blessed with good communication. Most of all I could not understand why infertility HURT so much. After all, I had a career to pursue if I couldn't have children. I was born of a generation who are doing such liberal things as choosing to cohabit instead of marry, choosing to form open marriages, and choosing not to have children at all. The key word here is CHOICE. I had *chosen* to marry; I had *chosen* a traditional relationship; and I had *chosen* to have children. Infertility robbed me of my right to choose to have my own genetic children.

"The infertile couple who earnestly desires to have a family deserves respect and attention. The couple should be seen to have a legitimate health problem, that is not stigmatized by myths, superstitions, or misinformation. It is true that infertility rarely proves fatal and usually does not render people incapable of performing their other functions in life. But infertility extracts a heavy toll on the quality of life and the emotional well-being of those affected. Infertility may be invisible in society, but its pain is real."

> "The infertile couple who earnestly desire to have a family deserve respect and attention. . . . Infertility may be invisible in society, but its pain is real."

Adoption

BEATING THE ADOPTION GAME
by Cynthia D. Martin
1980

from
Oak Tree Publications
11175 Flintkote Avenue
San Diego, CA 92121
$9.95

This is by far the most useful adoption book available. If you want to adopt, this book will tell you how to do it. Martin covers every aspect of adoption today in thoroughly researched chapters full of vital information, yet with real personal details of her own and others' adoption experiences.

Martin's message is that adoption today takes lots of hard work by you, the pre-parents. There is a baby out there for you but you have to actively find it. Because of declining birth rates and because more teenage mothers are keeping their babies, the situation is very different from what it was eight to ten years ago when it was quite easy for a couple to get a newborn from an adoption agency. Now adoption agencies meet the needs of just a few families. "Where Have All the Babies Gone?" and "The Adoption Agency Game" chapters explain this and help you go past this barrier.

Part of the adoption process is making the decision to adopt, rather than produce, a baby. The decision usually comes after dealing with your infertility medically and emotionally and even exploring the alternatives to standard baby-making: artificial insemination by donor (AID), test tube babies (in vitro fertilization), and surrogate mothering.

The core of *Beating the Adoption Game* is its in-depth explanation of private adoption (non-agency adoption) and the many creative and clever ways Martin suggests for you to search for your baby. Legal and medical issues for the pregnant woman and her (your) baby are explained. Other sections help you through agency processes (if you are lucky enough to be chosen by an agency), how to enhance your chances with agencies, foreign adoptions, special kids (older, non-white, physically, emotionally, and mentally handicapped, siblings) and special parents (older, handicapped, single, gay).

If you are like many infertile couples wanting to adopt, you have probably read every book at your library. Many first-hand family stories and how-to books are available, but *Beating the Adoption Game* is the one book to buy and keep while you look for and adopt your children.
—Abby Pariser

ADOPTION: The Grafted Tree
by Laurie Wishard and William Wishard
1979, 198 pages

from
Avon Books
959 Eighth Avenue
New York, NY 10019
$3.50 pap.

This comprehensive book provides information on many of the important issues in adoption, covering the concerns and decisions to be made by birth parents, adoptive parents, and adoptees. It describes the legal process of adoption and agency, non-agency, and intercountry adoption. There are chapters on how the adopting family fares, on "birthparents through the years," and on the rights of adoptees to know of their origins. Included is a listing of state agencies and adoption organizations and of state adoption requirements. (JIA)

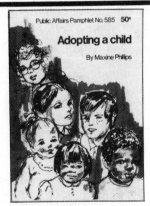

ADOPTING A CHILD
by Maxine Phillips
1980, 30 pages, Illus.

from
Public Affairs Pamphlets
381 Park Avenue South
New York, NY 10016
$.50
bulk rates available

This pamphlet explains what adoption is, and describes the steps involved in finding a baby or child through an adoption agency. The legal issues are explained and advice is given on telling the adopted child about her adoption and birth parents. There are sections on transracial adoption, handicapped children, the older adopted child, and foreign adoptions. Adoption by relatives, and non-agency adoption are discussed. Public issues in adoption, concerning open versus sealed birth records, are discussed and an extensive list of books and organizations is included. (JIA)

FOR CHILDREN

FAMILIES GROW IN DIFFERENT WAYS
by Barbara Parrish-Benson
illustrated by Karen Fletcher
undated, 28 pages, Illus.

from
Before We Are Six, publisher
The Women's Press, distributor
280 Bloor Street West, Suite 313
Toronto, Ontario
M5S 1W1, Canada
$2.50 pap.

Best friends Sara and Jamie are both expecting a new baby in their family. Jamie's mother is pregnant and Sara's parents are planning to adopt a baby. This gentle book tells of the two new arrivals, with nice line drawings. (JIA)

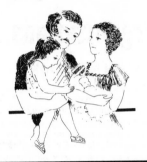

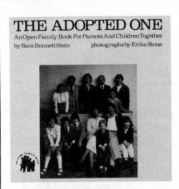

THE ADOPTED ONE
by Sara Bonnett Stein
1979, 48 pages, Illus.

from
Walker and Company
720 Fifth Avenue
New York, NY 10019
$6.95 hd.

Part of the *Open Family* series, this book is written with a dual text (one for children, one for parents) and explains some of the conflicts of the adopted child who is becoming aware of his status. Excellent photographs. (JIA)

FOR BIRTHPARENTS AND ADOPTEES

CONCERNED UNITED BIRTHPARENTS
P.O. Box 573
Milford, MA 01757

Concerned United Birthparents (CUB) provides support and advocacy for women who have given up a child for adoption, provides support for women facing an untimely pregnancy, and helps birthparents find their children. CUB publishes a newsletter and provides many other services for its members, including CUB Sister support for pregnant women, family advocacy, liaison for reunion contacts, media resources, meetings, penpal/search buddies, personal problem-solving, a reunion registry, and search referrals. An extensive list of literature is also available. (JIA)

"CUB Sister Program—with the decline of federally funded programs, and implementation of the Adolescent Family Life Bill which seeks to 'encourage' teens to surrender their children for adoption, many parents are at risk of adoption abuse. This CUB program links jeopardized parents with members who have 'been there,' ensuring disclosure of all alternatives and a free choice."

ADOPTEES' LIBERTY MOVEMENT ASSOCIATION
P.O. Box 154, Washington Bridge Sta.
New York, NY 10033

Adoptees' Liberty Movement Association (ALMA) was founded by a woman who was adopted as a child and spent 21 years searching for her birthparents. ALMA maintains a computerized International Reunion Registry Databank and works toward "open records" adoption laws. ALMA also provides a search committee and "buddy" system, a newsletter, and search workshops. (JIA)

"Our name is derived from the Spanish word 'alma' which means 'soul.' The denial of an adult human being's right to 'the truth of his origin' creates a scar which is imbedded in his soul forever. So ALMA has a very special meaning to all of us, for we have each been hurt in the same way."

Working for Change

Being a careful consumer of maternity care will help the couple achieve a safe, satisfying birth experience. And each time *one* person asks for family-centered services and insists on her rights as a medical consumer, the medical community is affected and *all* of us benefit. But even more organized effort is needed to make sure that every birth is safe and satisfying, whether the parents are "consumer-oriented" or not. Right now, only parents who are very well-informed and motivated and who have the time and resources to pursue their goals are able to get the childbirth alternatives they want. But these alternatives should be available to everyone.

Some parents find that their interest in childbirth and childbearing rights continues even after their own babies are born and are growing up. These are the people who become parent advocates, consumer health activists, childbirth educators, and midwives. There are many such women and men working around the country, almost always as unpaid volunteers, to help make childbirth in America a better experience for everyone. They are working on a community level and are also members of large national organizations. Altogether they are "the childbirth movement" which is part of the women's health movement, which in turn is part of the larger network of social change organizations working toward consumer rights, social justice, a clean environment, and world peace.

All of us are working against formidable odds, for our "opposition" (for instance, the medical profession) has tremendous resources in money, power, and public influence. Most of us see the struggle for childbearing rights as a life-time commitment and in this sense, we are joined with women throughout history who have moved slowly and surely toward freedom.

Women's Health Organizations

NATIONAL WOMEN'S HEALTH NETWORK

NATIONAL WOMEN'S HEALTH NETWORK
224 Seventh Street, SE
Washington, DC 20003
202/543-9222

Memberships
$25. individual
$35. women's health or consumer group
$50. business or institution
$100. sponsor
(no one will be denied membership for lack of funds)

"The National Women's Health Network is a consumer advocacy organization and informational clearinghouse on women's health issues. We are the only national consumer organization committed exclusively to women and health. The Network monitors federal policies which affect women's health issues, especially in the areas of reproductive rights, environmental and occupational health. Additionally, the Network provides a national Speakers Bureau, publishes a bimonthly newsletter and emergency Newsalerts for members, and has publications on a wide range of topics."
—Belita Cowan, Executive Director

Publications available from the Network are listed below.

MATERNAL HEALTH AND CHILDBIRTH: Resource Guide 4 by the National Women's Health Network
1980, 86 pages, Illus.

The Network publishes a series of *Health Resource Guides,* including this one on childbirth. This guide includes two essays on birth and politics by Norma Swenson (of *Our Bodies, Ourselves);* "Can Natural Childbirth Survive Technology?" by K.C. Cole; a home birth story; a description of the Maternity Center's birth center; and a reproduction of the "Pregnant Patient's Bill of Rights." Included is an extensive bibliography and list of references in pregnancy, birth, breast-feeding, child care and a listing of general resources on women and health, including health centers, advocacy groups, periodicals, books, and films.

The Network also publishes *Resource Guides* on breast cancer, hysterectomy, DES, self help, abortion, and sterilization. The complete set of seven guides is available for $16.00.

"The diverse elements of the [childbirth] movement have thus far focused on the practices of individual physicians, midwives, or institutions, in the interests of the improved experiences of individual women, couples, and families through education and preparation. Little or no attempt has been made to mobilize the hundreds of thousands of members of the different groups for political action or policy initiatives around these issues. However, there are signs that this may happen in the future. . . ."

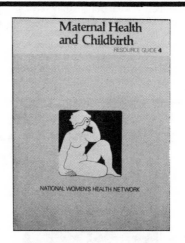

Maternal Health and Childbirth
RESOURCE GUIDE 4

NATIONAL WOMEN'S HEALTH NETWORK

"The movement to change hospital childbirth practices and bottle-feeding has been growing and diversifying since the early 1950s, the point at which virtually 100 percent hospitalization was achieved. But the hospital as the proper place of birth and the physician as the rightful attendant was not questioned by most parts of this movement until the mid 1970s. Primarily parents, with some professionals, the movement has been characterized rightly as pro-natalist, though including those who accept fertility control in some if not all its forms. While often present in the past, open anti-abortion, anti-ERA, and other right-wing sentiment has recently become a significant force in the movement toward alternatives to conventional births in hospitals. The diverse elements of the movement have thus far focused on the practices of individual physicians, midwives, or institutions, in the interests of the improved experiences of individual women, couples, and families through education and preparation. Little or no attempt has been made to mobilize the hundreds of thousands of members of the different groups for political action or

policy initiatives around these issues. However, there are signs that this may happen in the future, since most of the major groups have now presented position papers on planning, some of them together.
—from "Procreation Politics" by Norma Swenson, in *Maternal Health and Childbirth*

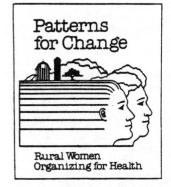

Patterns for Change

Rural Women Organizing for Health

PATTERNS FOR CHANGE: Rural Women Organizing for Health
$5.50

Prepared by the Network's Rural Health Issues Committee, this handbook covers health issues for rural American women, organizing for change (community outreach and volunteer recruitment and training, fundraising, public relations and media, health advocacy and law), case studies, and resources and references.

HOW SAFE IS "SAFE"? How the FDA Determines the "Safety" of Drugs
by Doris Haire
$1.00

See reviews on pages 10 and 75.

BOSTON WOMEN'S HEALTH BOOK COLLECTIVE

**BOSTON WOMEN'S HEALTH
BOOK COLLECTIVE**
Box 192
West Somerville, MA 02144
617/924-0271

The Boston Women's Health Book Collective is the group of eleven women who wrote *Our Bodies, Ourselves,* bringing the philosophy, knowledge, and skills of the women's health movement to thousands of women around the country. *OBOS* was first published in 1970 by the New England Free Press as a 112-page, newsprint book and sold 250,000 copies through the women's "underground" before Simon and Schuster published it in two editions in 1973 and 1976, selling millions of copies. The Collective has very conscientiously used their royalty money to fund women's projects ever since and their work on behalf of freestanding birth centers, midwifery, and other childbirth alternatives has been especially good. The Collective now maintains an office and staff to continue its work and is a vital and practical resource for those working in the women's health movement as well as an inspiring model of what women can achieve in "taking our bodies back." (An excellent description of the Collective, its history and work appears in *Networking: The First Report and Directory* by Jessica Lipnack and Jeffrey Stamps, reviewed on page 297).

Listed below are some of the publications of the Boston Women's Health Book Collective. The Collective also answers inquiries and maintains information and referral files on women's health organizations and issues. Contact them for more information.

**OUR BODIES, OURSELVES: A
Book By and For Women**
(Revised Edition)
by the Boston Women's Health
Book Collective
1976, 383 pages, Illus.

from
Simon and Schuster
630 Fifth Avenue
New York, NY 10020
$8.95 pap.
(discounts available to clinics and other groups providing health-counseling and information services)

The "classic" women's self-health resource, this book has given me and many others the courage and information needed to take charge of our own health care and shrug off dependence on the (male) medical establishment. Included are sections on our sense of self, anatomy and physiology, sexuality, nutrition, exercise and health habits, rape, self-defense, venereal disease, birth control, abor-

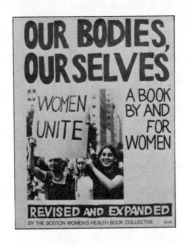

tion, childbearing, menopause, and women and the health care system. Sound, practical advice, researched by women, is interspersed with personal comments from many women which convey a real sense of community and sisterly caring. (Editor's Note: As I write this, the Collective is in the process of writing a new, third edition of *Our Bodies, Ourselves* which will be published in Spring, 1983. The new edition will provide more emphasis on older women, women with disabilities, and women of color. The section on childbearing will provide more information on what normal birth is like including the importance of creating a "climate of confidence" for birth through careful attention to prenatal care and nutrition, acknowledging feelings and fears, carefully choosing supportive birth attendants, and learning to "let go" during labor. The use of nurse-midwives and lay midwives for birth ["women caring for women"] will be emphasized, the concept of childbirth preparation will be expanded to include planning for the place and attendants for birth, and different birth options will be discussed, while recognizing that not all women have access to the alternatives they need and want.)

**NUESTROS CUERPOS, NUESTRAS
VIDAS:** Un Libro Por Y Para
Las Mujeres
$5.00 plus 1.00 postage
bulk rates available
order from the Collective office

This Spanish language edition of *Our Bodies, Ourselves* has been funded by the Collective through royalty monies and grants and is available directly from the Collective.

**INTERNATIONAL WOMEN &
HEALTH RESOURCE GUIDE**
Preliminary Draft Edition
July, 1980, 177 pages, Illus.
$5.00 surface mail
$8.00 air mail
order from the Collective office

This guide is a joint project of the Women's International Information and Communication Service (ISIS) and the Boston Women's Health Book Collective. It represents four years of information gathering from sources all over the world. The book provides resource listings for organizations and publications dealing with women's health in general, reproductive issues, drugs, food, childbearing, menopause and aging, environmental and occupational health, self-help, and audio-visual resources. Annotations are provided in English and one other language (French, Spanish, Italian, or German). This preliminary edition was prepared for the Mid-Decade Conference on Women held in Copenhagen in July, 1980. Feedback and additions for future editions are welcome.

MENSTRUATION
Compiled by Esther Rome and
Emily Culpepper
1981, 10 pages

**SEXUALLY TRANSMITTED
DISEASES AND HOW TO AVOID
THEM**
by Peggy Lynch and Esther Rome
1980, 8 pages

Single copies of these two pamphlets are available free from the Collective if you include a self-addressed, stamped envelope with your request.

**OURSELVES AND OUR
CHILDREN: A Book By and For
Parents**
by the Boston Women's Health
Book Collective
1978, 288 pages, Illus.

from
Random House
201 East 50th Street
New York, NY 10022
$7.95 pap.
(discounts available to clinics and groups providing health-counseling and information services)
See review on page 253.

**CHANGING BODIES, CHANGING
LIVES: A Book for Teens on Sex
and Relationships**
by Ruth Bell and other co-authors of *Our Bodies, Ourselves* and *Ourselves and Our Children,* together with members of the Teen-book Project
1980, 242 pages, Illus.

from
Random House
201 East 50th Street
New York, NY 10022
$7.95 pap.
(discounts available to clinics and health services which serve teenagers)
See review on page 64.

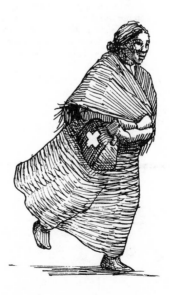

"REMEMBER THE DIGNITY OF YOUR WOMANHOOD. DO NOT APPEAL, DO NOT BEG, DO NOT GROVEL. TAKE COURAGE, JOIN HANDS STAND BESIDE US, FIGHT WITH US...."

CHRISTABEL PANKHURST ENGLISH SUFFRAGIST, (1880-1958)

—from the *International Women & Health Resource Guide.*
drawing by Karen Nomberg

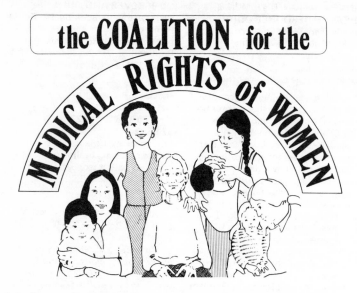

the COALITION for the MEDICAL RIGHTS of WOMEN

THE COALITION FOR THE MEDICAL RIGHTS OF WOMEN
1638-B Haight Street
San Francisco, CA 94117

The Coalition for the Medical Rights of Women is "an organization of activists—consumers and providers—working together to make the health care system more responsive to women's need." The Coalition engages in public policy and political action work, organizes workshops and conferences, provides educational materials, and maintains a resource center. Listed below are some of the Coalition's publications. Others are available on pap smear labs, DES, the morning-after-pill, the "right-to-life" movement, estrogen replacement therapy, radiation hazards, and reproductive rights.

SECOND OPINION
monthly newsletter, 8 pages
$15. to $40./year ($50. for organizations), includes membership

THE ROCK WILL WEAR AWAY:
Handbook for Women's Health Advocates
1980, 61 pages, Illus.
$2.75

This booklet "shares our experiences and suggests ideas for changing the health care system" including information on how the Coalition was founded and funded, and what some of their projects have been.

SAFE NATURAL REMEDIES FOR DISCOMFORTS OF PREGNANCY
30 pages
$1.50

See review on page 34.

THE MEDIA BOOK: Making the Media Work for Your Grassroots Group
48 pages, 8½ x 11"
$8.50

WOMEN AND HEALTH CARE:
Your Legal Rights
brochure
$.10 each in bulk

"When you pursue legal remedies, you remind industry and the medical profession that the law imposes a duty upon them to provide products and practices that are reliable."

WOMEN'S INTERNATIONAL NETWORK
Fran P. Hosken, director
187 Grant Street
Lexington, MA 02173

Women's International Network (WIN), headed by women's rights activist Fran Hosken, publishes books and a quarterly newsletter devoted to women's health and political status and particularly to documenting and preventing the practice of female circumcision or genital mutilation. Recently, WIN has published the *Childbirth Picture Book* series to help describe the healthy processes of pregnancy and childbirth to women around the world.

WIN NEWS
$20.00 a year for individuals
$25.00 a year for institutions
(add $3. for postage abroad, $9. for air mail abroad)
back issues available for $5. each or $15. for one volume year (four issues)

WIN NEWS provides international news and networking in the areas of women and their relations to the United Nations, international affairs, development, human rights, health, genital and sexual mutilation, violence, and media. Also included are regular reports from around the world (Asia and Pacific, Africa and the Middle East, Europe, and the Americas). *WIN News* is 'an open, participatory, worldwide network by, for, and about women . . . You are invited to subscribe and participate."

THE UNIVERSAL CHILDBIRTH PICTURE BOOK
by Fran P. Hosken, with illustrations by Marcia L. Williams
1981, 72 pages, Illus.
$7.00 postpaid
(air mail overseas add $3.00)
bulk rates available

Addressed to the community health worker/educator worldwide as a flexible, adaptable, multi-ethnic teaching aid, the *Universal CBPB* has 34 drawings, illustrates the female body and genital organs, menstruation, the male body, fertilization, implantation and beginning of growth, cell division, development of embryo/fetus, changes during pregnancy, nutrition and food, the birth process, afterbirth, breastfeeding, family planning and much more. The cover of the *Universal CBPB* is removable and all the inside pages are hole-punched so that drawings and teaching materials can be used separately. Includes a separate text, teacher's discussion guide, picture glossary and international reading and resource list. Additions on prevention of excision and infibulation including drawings and text are available in English and French, free of charge, for Africa and the Middle East.

Translations in French and Spanish are available with the same contents and at the same price as the above.

THE CHILDBIRTH PICTURE BOOK
by Fran P. Hosken
illustrations by Marcia L. Williams
1981, 60 pages, Illus.
$7.00 postpaid

Adapted for use in the U.S., this version of the *CBPB* has the same illustrations as the Universal prototype. Also includes a text, picture glossary, short discussion guide, reading and resource list of USA publications, and multi-ethnic photographs.

See illustrations from the CBPB on pages 4, 6 and 27.

THE CHILDBIRTH PICTURE BOOK FLIP CHART
34 pages, 17 x 22", ringbound
$19.50 plus 2.00 postage

For use in larger groups, the flip chart contains all the *CBPB* illustrations plus a separate text and leader's guide/discussion points.

THE CHILDBIRTH PICTURE BOOK SLIDE PROGRAM
34 slides
$48. per set

The slides show the same drawings as in the *CBPB* but with color added. Includes a separate text and discussion guide.

FEMINIST HEALTH WORKS
325 Spring Street, Room 227
New York, NY 10013
212/929-7886

The Feminist Health Works, a women's health center in New York City, provides booklets and fact sheets on a variety of health topics including natural birth control, contraceptives, radiation hazards, pregnancy, and herbal and home remedies. Write for a complete publications list.

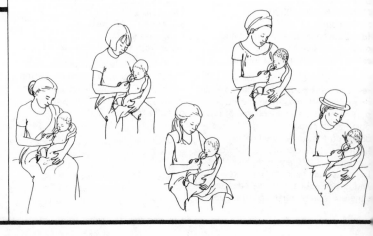

WOMEN'S HEALTH PUBLICATIONS

HEALTHSHARING: A Canadian
Women's Health Quarterly
Box 230, Station M
Toronto, Ontario
M6S 2T3
Canada

$6.75 a year for individuals
$13.50 a year institutions and groups
$25.00 a year sustaining
$8.00 a year, foreign individuals
$15.00 a year, foreign institutions
and groups

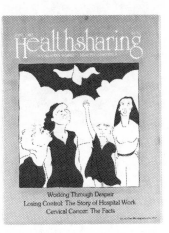

Working Through Despair
Losing Control: The Story of Hospital Work
Cervical Cancer: The Facts

Healthsharing is an excellent, 24-page news magazine which features articles on women's health and alternative medicine, regular short medical updates, and regional reports on women's health activities in the provinces. Recent issues have included articles on nuclear war, cervical cancer, hospital workers, diabetes, doing your own medical research, herpes, pregnancy, natural birth control, and infertility. *Healthsharing* is professionally produced, with lively illustrations, by a collective of women with a clear, feminist perspective.

Regulatory Body Against Home Birth

"Recently the Ontario College of Physicians and Surgeons has published a notice in their bulletin that may have implications for midwives and physicians involved in homebirth in Ontario.

"The January, 1982, Issue No. 3 of the College Notice under a headline entitled "Nurse Midwives" stated: 'Current interest in home birth has created an opportunity for certain individuals to offer their services as home birth attendants. Non-medical practitioners are not entitled to provide obstetrical services which are clearly within the practice of medicine. It is professional misconduct for a member to permit, counsel, or assist any person not licensed as a physician to engage in the practice of medicine.

" 'Some physicians have been urged by their patients to attend them at home when they go into labour. The College would discourage this practice because it does not consider home birth to be safe or in the patient's best interest.' "

"There has been no further interpretation of what this notice means in actuality. Recently the Alberta College of Physicians and Surgeons prohibited physicians from attending home births. Is Ontario following the trend of other provinces?"
—from *Healthsharing*

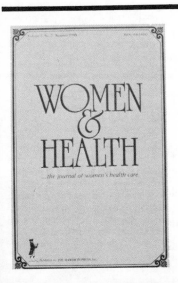

WOMEN AND HEALTH
c/o The Haworth Press
149 Fifth Avenue
New York, NY 10010

$24.00 a year individuals
$48.00 a year libraries
$42.00 a year other institutions

Women and Health began as a project of the Biological Sciences Program at SUNY/Old Westbury and is now published as a scholarly journal by the Haworth Press. Past articles have included:
* "Nausea of Pregnancy: An Historical Medical Prejudice"
* "Evaluation of Outcomes of Non-Nurse Midwives: Matched Comparisons with Physicians"
* "The Alternative Birth Center: Option or Cooptation?"

WOMENWISE: The New Hampshire
Feminist Health Center Quarterly
38 S. Main Street
Concord, NH 03301

$5.00 a year individual
$10.00 a year organizational
$25.00 a year supporting subscriber

WomenWise began as a special project of the New Hampshire Feminist Health Center in 1978 and is an excellent 12 page quarterly newsletter (pages are large, 11 x 17") with articles on health care, personal stories, nutrition, and featuring poetry, book reviews, health briefs, and letters. Past articles have included:
* "One C-Section May be Enough"
* "A Consumer's Guide to Cervical Cap Providers"
* "Controlling Nausea in Pregnancy"
* "Resource Guide to Home Birth in New Hampshire"
* "Vaginal Health Remedies"
* "Women and the Nuclear Mentality"
* "The Speculum Gateway to Cervical Health"

"[Valmai] Elkins, as wrap-up speaker, was to talk directly to the major theme of the conference: the impact of medical technology on the birth experience. I expected a grim forecast replete with rising statistics on increasing medical intervention in childbirth through greater and greater reliance on fetal monitors, IVs, use of forceps, episiotomies, drugs, and cesarian deliveries. But Elkins surprised me with her optimism for the 80s. Referring to 'the plague of cesarians' she stated: 'I see them as a bubble that is about to burst.' Why? Because of both 'well-prepared parents' and the 'tremendous expansion of (childbirth) alternatives' where the goal will be for parents to get 'the birth of their choice.'

" 'Well-prepared parents don't want c-sections and they usually don't get them' she said, referring to her years of experience as a childbirth preparation teacher. According to Elkins, prepared women avoid induction of labor, choose not to have an IV, will remain upright and move around during labor, usually won't choose epidurals, and will avoid a supine position and a fetal monitor.

" 'Consumerism is the key to change,' she said. 'Prepared parents are changing hospitals and the obstetrical community.'

"Elkins predicted that the concept of birth as a normal physiological event will grow in favor during the next ten years.

" 'I see a tremendous increase in information where parents will choose the least intervention while those needing it will get it,' she said."
—from "Childbirth in the '80s", Alice Downey, editor of *WomenWise,* reporting on the 1981 eastern regional conference of ICEA held in Portsmouth, New Hampshire.

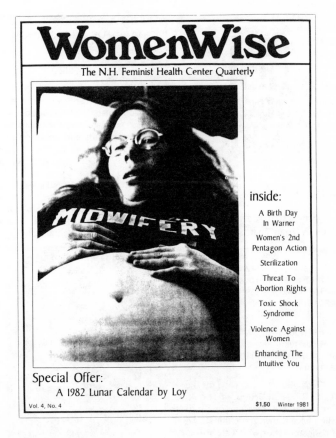

WomenWise
The N.H. Feminist Health Center Quarterly

MIDWIFERY

inside:

A Birth Day
In Warner

Women's 2nd
Pentagon Action

Sterilization

Threat To
Abortion Rights

Toxic Shock
Syndrome

Violence Against
Women

Enhancing The
Intuitive You

Special Offer:
A 1982 Lunar Calendar by Loy

Vol. 4, No. 4 $1.50   Winter 1981

CONSUMER HEALTH RESOURCES

The following health organizations also provide information and resources which may be of use for those working for change in childbirth.

NATIONAL SELF-HELP CLEARINGHOUSE
Graduate School and University Center
CUNY
33 West 42nd Street, Room 1227
New York, NY 10036
212/840-7606

The Clearinghouse provides a newsletter and other resources for lay people interested in starting a self-help group.

HEALTH RESEARCH GROUP
2000 P Street, NW
Washington, DC 20036

The Health Research Group of Public Citizen (founded by Ralph Nader) lobbies for public health issues in Washington and provides a variety of publications on food and drugs, health care delivery, medical devices and product safety, and occupational safety and health.

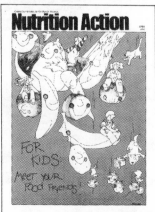

PILLS THAT DON'T WORK: Prescription Drugs That Lack Evidence of Effectiveness
by Sidney M. Wolfe, M.D., Christopher M. Coley and The Health Research Group founded by Ralph Nader
1982

from
Warner Books
75 Rockefeller Plaza
New York, NY 10019
$3.95 pap.

Originally self-published by the Health Research Group, this book describes over 600 prescription drugs which have shown to be ineffective or dangerous, but which are still on the market.

HEALTH/PAC
Health Policy Advisory Center
17 Murray Street
New York, NY 10007

Health/PAC is "an independent, non-profit, public interest center concerned with monitoring and interpreting the health system to change-oriented groups of health workers, consumers, professionals and students."

Publications include:

HEALTH/PAC BULLETIN
bimonthly magazine, 32 pages
$15./year individuals
$30./year institutions

WOMEN'S HEALTH PACKET
$6.00 plus .90 postage

Collected back issues of *Health/PAC Bulletin* covering women's health.

CONSUMER COALITION FOR HEALTH
P.O. Box 50088
930 F Street NW, Suite 617
Washington, DC 20004
202/638-5828

The Consumer Coalition for Health is "a national alliance of labor, civil rights, and public interest organizations dedicated to expanding consumer control over the health care system." The organization publishes a bimonthly newsletter and provides other services.

CENTER FOR SCIENCE IN THE PUBLIC INTEREST
1755 S Street NW
Washington, DC 20009
202/332-9110

The Center for Science in the Public Interest is "a non-profit organization that provides the public with reliable up-to-date information about the effects of science and technology on society. CSPI's major focus is on food and health."

CSPI publishes an excellent monthly newsletter, *Nutrition Action*, and a variety of books, pamphlets, T-shirts, and posters, including items on breastfeeding (see index).

HEALTHY MOTHERS, HEALTHY BABIES

Healthy Mothers, Healthy Babies (HMHB) is a public information program designed to help lower U.S. infant mortality and morbidity rates by fostering education efforts for pregnant women. The HMHB Coalition consists of government, professional, and voluntary organizations which cooperate to share resources and plan activities. Members include the American Academy of Pediatrics, American College of Obstetricians and Gynecologists, American College of Nurse-Midwives, La Leche League, March of Dimes, ICEA, ASPO, and NAPSAC. The coalition is inviting new members among national organizations and is working on a directory of educational materials and the development of new materials.
For further information contact:
Elaine Bratic
Office of Public Affairs
Public Health Service
U.S. Department of Health and Human Services
200 Independence Ave., SW, Rm. 740-G
Washington, DC 20201
202/245-6867

FRIENDS OF THE EARTH
530 Seventh Street, SE
Washington, DC 20003
Attn: Erik Jansson
202/543-4312

Friends of the Earth, an environmental advocacy group, has proposed legislation which would "establish a national policy on human reproductive health, birth defects, and the health of young children," with a stated purpose being to "promote efforts which will prevent or eliminate the adverse impact of hazardous substances." The draft legislation outlines many factors which Friends of the Earth feel have an adverse effect on fetal and child health, including:

1. Contamination of human sperm with hazardous substances.
2. Prematurity and low birth weight.
3. Contamination of human mothers' milk.
4. Use of high-risk techniques and equipment for low-risk pregnancies.
5. Poor medical care delivery and inadequate programs for prevention.
6. Inadequate recognition of parents as primary influence on child health.
7. Inadequate programs for nutritional counseling.
8. Lack of opportunities for parent/infant bonding at birth (which may be a factor in child abuse).

Friends of the Earth is actively seeking help from organizations which would like to co-sponsor this legislation. For more information or to receive a copy of the proposed legislation (please include $2.00) contact Friends of the Earth.

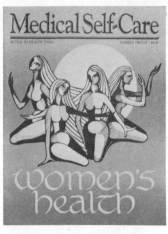

MEDICAL SELF-CARE
P.O. Box 717
Inverness, CA 94937
$15.00 a year
$27.50 two years
$36.00 three years

Medical Self-Care, edited by Tom Ferguson, M.D. (also medical editor for the *Whole Earth Catalog*), is a very good resource for "self-health," providing articles, book reviews, news updates, letters, abstracts, and access reports all designed to help consumers take control of their own health care. Issue No. 12 (Spring, 1981) was devoted to "Women's Health" and Issue No. 10 included an article on home birth. Back issues are available for $4.00 each. Write for a complete list of back issue contents.

HEALTH ADVOCACY PROGRAM
Sarah Lawrence College
Bronxville, NY 10708
914/337-0700
Contact: Joan Marks

In the Fall of 1980, Sarah Lawrence College began the nation's first graduate program in health advocacy. The master's program is designed to train graduates to act as patient advocates and to organize advocacy programs in hospitals and other health care institutions. The curriculum involves 36 course credits and 600 hours of field work. Applications for admission can be requested from the College.

HEALTH WRITERS, INC.
306 N. Brooks Street
Madison, WI 53715
608/255-2555

Health Writers is a non-profit organization which works to improve health care and patient's rights by providing educational materials, in-service training and consultation, community organizing, and health advocacy. Write for a complete list of publications and services.

Childbirth Advocacy Publications and Groups

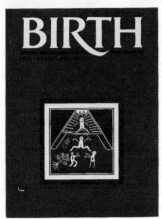

BIRTH: Issues in Perinatal Care and Education
110 El Camino Real
Berkeley, CA 94705

$12.00 a year, individuals
$15.00 a year, foreign individuals
$18.00 a year, institutions
$4.00 for single issues

BIRTH (formerly *Birth and the Family Journal*) has changed its name and expanded its format, attesting to a growth in readership and a tremendous growth of interest in consumer-oriented information on childbirth. *BIRTH* is sponsored jointly by ICEA and ASPO, and while childbirth educators make up the largest group of subscribers, parents, nurse-midwives, medical libraries, nursing schools, and physicians also find it an invaluable resource. Editors Madeleine Shearer and Nenelle Bunnin have said, "The two words that best describe the activities and aspirations of our readers, judged from their letters, conferences, and papers, are *independence* and *autonomy*. They have some control over their practice and are independent in their evaluation of ideas and data. Although many of our readers are members of professional groups and receive those publications, by subscribing to *BIRTH* they look outside their own professional group for a broader range of information and assistance."

Each quarter *BIRTH* provides four to six original papers, a roundtable discussion, an editorial, childbirth news updates (prepared by the editors of the *APRS Federal Monitor*), letters, book and film reviews, a calendar of conferences and events, and abstracts and an index to the current literature. Issues cover virtually everything of interest in the areas of childbirth education, childbirth, and maternal/child health, including home birth, midwifery, family-centered maternity care, obstetrical practices, drugs and devices, nutrition, breastfeeding, psychological aspects of childbearing, family planning, childbirth preparation methods, and birth in cultural or historical perspective. For parents and providers who want to really keep in touch with ideas and events in the childbirth movement, *BIRTH* is perhaps the best single source.

Following are the titles and abstracts of articles appearing in the Spring, 1982 issue of *BIRTH*.

A COMPARATIVE STUDY OF WOMEN CHOOSING TWO DIFFERENT CHILDBIRTH ALTERNATIVES
by Richard L. Cohen, M.D.

"Abstract: This is a report of the differences and similarities between two groups of 30 women each who selected widely divergent types of childbirth care. One group chose to deliver their babies in a tertiary university hospital obstetric service, the other in an out-of-hospital alternative birth center staffed by nurse-midwives.

"Women choosing the birth center were not demographically different from those choosing the tertiary hospital except that they were somewhat older. However, women choosing the birth center planned to emphasize autonomy and independence rather than intimacy in their child rearing, and they described their partners as much more supportive and involved in the birth, and were much more adaptive in preparation for the birth and the baby's care."

NEW MOTHERHOOD: A TIME OF CRISIS?
by Beverly Celotta, Ph.D.

"Abstract: Twenty-three women who sought out prenatal (22) and parenting (23) classes scored in the normal range for physical complaints, ego strength, depression, anxiety, and the lie scale of the Minnesota Multiphasic Personality Inventory (MMPI) at an average of 3.5 months postpartum, and had improved scores overall when tested again six weeks later. It is suggested that for this group of women new parenthood may not be as great a crisis as some studies have indicated."

THE RISKS AND BENEFITS OF EPISIOTOMY: A REVIEW
by David Banta, M.D. and Stephen B. Thacker, M.D.

"Abstract: A review of the medical literature shows that episiotomy is done in about two-thirds of births in the U.S., and routinely in many settings, especially in primiparas. While episiotomy can be clinically justified in specific circumstances such as impending laceration of the perineum, the literature does not support its routine use, since it is associated with significant risks of pain and infection, and the benefits claimed for routine episiotomy have not been subjected to randomized controlled trials."

EDUCATION FOR VAGINAL BIRTH AFTER CESAREAN
by Elizabeth Conner Shearer, M.ED, M.P.H.

"Abstract: Childbirth education for parents who elect to attempt a vaginal birth after cesarean (VBAC) has many of the same elements of traditional childbirth education, including the imparting of knowledge and confidence, training in breathing and relaxation techniques, and helping parents to arrange for the most supportive environment and caregivers. Special differences in VBAC parents include the need to mourn the previous loss of an ideal birth, to analyze why they want a VBAC, and to understand the reason for the previous cesarean and realistically assess the chance of recurrence. The fear of uterine rupture or scar separation afflicts both parents and physicians, but has been shown to occur no more frequently than in repeat cesarean. By one analysis the elective repeat cesarean is a higher risk procedure than is a trial of labor."

AN ANSWER TO CHILDBIRTH EDUCATOR BURN-OUT
by Carolyn Hecht, R.N., A.C.C.E.

"Abstract: A childbirth educator describes burn-out as having been due to boredom, frustration and exhaustion. She overcame burn-out by changing focus in her classes, and by introducing skills learned in courses in teaching the adult learner, group dynamics, and assertiveness training. Many new books were added to her lending library, and she joined two new organizations in the childbirth field. She drew up a Prepared Childbirth Preferences form to help couples talk to their doctors during pregnancy. Finally, she devised an evaluation system for her classes, and helped begin a teacher enrichment series within her local chapter."

Back issue copies are available for $4.00 each going back to Volume 2, 1975. Write for information on reduced prices for purchase of complete volumes. *BIRTH* also publishes glossy, bound reprints of important articles, which are listed below.

REPRINTS

Caldeyro-Barcia (three articles): Some Consequences of Obstetrical Interference; The Influence of Maternal Position on Time of Spontaneous Rupture of the Membranes, Progress of Labor, and Fetal Head Compression; and The Influence of Maternal Bearing Down Efforts during Second Stage on Fetal Well-being.
24 pages, $2.00

1981 Cesarean Update
Enkin: Having a Section is Having a Baby
Conner Shearer: Teaching about Cesarean Birth in Traditional Childbirth Classes
Cohen: Minimizing the Emotional Sequelae of Cesarean Childbirth-plus referenced charts of complications of cesarean to mother and baby
Conner Shearer: NIH Consensus Development Task Force on Cesarean Childbirth: The Process and the Result
36 pages, $2.50

Devitt: The Transition from Home to Hospital Birth 1930-1960
16 pages, $1.50
Stevens: Psychological Strategies for Relief of Childbirth Pain (Parts I and II)
16 pages, $1.50
Faber and Rothermel: Drugs in Breastfeeding: A Consumer's Guide
12 pages, $1.50
Shearer: The Effects of Regionalization of Perinatal Care on Hospital Services for Normal Childbirth
16 pages, $1.50
Shrock: Instructional Materials in Childbirth and New Parent Education I-VI
48 pages, $3.00
Stratmeyer: Research in Ultrasound Bioeffects: A Public Health View
12 pages, $1.50

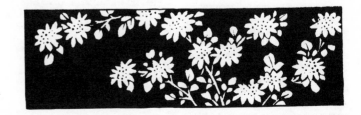

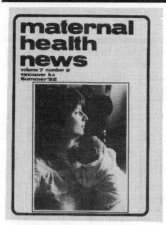

MATERNAL HEALTH NEWS
Box 46563, Station G
Vancouver, British Columbia
V6R 4G8
Canada
$7. to $10. a year
quarterly, all subscriptions begin
with the first issue of the volume
year
$.50 each for back issues, also
available in bulk

Maternal Health News is an excellent newspaper from Canada which covers hospital news, midwifery, cesarean section, breastfeeding, family planning, child-rearing, and women's health. Articles are outspoken, lively, and feminist-oriented and will be of interest to readers in the U.S. as well as in Canada. Regular features include a calendar of events, a sharing network, book reviews, letters, and news updates.

"From the *Parents for Positive Beginnings,* comes word on the cesarean situation at Lions Gate Hospital. The Dept. of General Practice would like to see a policy allowing fathers to be present for elective cesarean sections. They sent letters to the Dept. of Ob/Gyn, Dept. of Anesthesia, Dept. of Pediatrics making their position known. A return letter states: 'After considerable dis-

cussion and review by all depts., it has been decided that *no change* in the present policy *prohibiting* mother-conscious, father-present c/s, will be made at Lions Gate Hospital.' *PARENTS MUST BOYCOTT LIONS GATE FOR BIRTHING!!!...*

"From the women who have been doing labour support at GRACE HOSPITAL comes praise for the nurses working in the caseroom. Over the past few months there appears to be a definite change in the attitudes toward the women in labour and toward their labour support people. Although we still receive the looks and comments of, 'Oh, here comes another one of those!', we generally have been shown respect and consideration while the nurses do an excellent job of monitoring labouring women (often no easy task with extra people around).

"Women attempting a vaginal delivery after a previous c/s are wanting all the support and love that they can get. Over and over they express their appreciation of having people of their choice with them—someone that they can share the experience with long after the actual birth.

"Granted there are still many traditional nurses who are having a difficult time understanding and supporting true family directed maternity care. The belief in the importance of the comfort and satisfaction of the birthing women is sometimes difficult to incorporate into practical nursing routines, especially when hospital policies were written years ago.

"It is not easy to bring about changes—not for any of us. We are thankful, however, for those caseroom nurses who are sincerely trying—who struggle with differing values, attitudes and beliefs, who try to accomodate the varying wishes of women in labour. *The Grace seems to be the best hospital in Vancouver in which to have a baby.*"

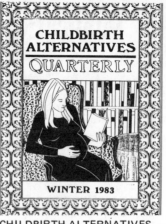

CHILDBIRTH ALTERNATIVES QUARTERLY
c/o Janet Ashford
BIN 62, S.L.A.C.
Stanford, CA 94305
$10. a year
$18. two years
$2.00 back issues and samples

Childbirth Alternatives Quarterly is the newsletter I edit myself. It started in 1979 as a publication for Long Island Childbirth Alternatives, our local NAPSAC member group, and since moving to California I am now putting it out as an independent publication. Each 20-page issue includes original articles and reprints on childbirth alternatives, midwifery, and related issues plus our regular features: childbirth news, calendar, birthing network resources, and letters. Recent issues have included articles on the practice of midwifery, effects of labor drugs, electronic fetal monitoring, amniocentesis, nutrition in pregnancy, hospital birthing rooms, vaginal birth after cesarean, and much more. The *Quarterly* is a good resource (I think) for news and information on childbirth alternatives and it will be the source for updates and additions to the *Whole

Birth Catalog until the next edition is published.

"I'm not hostile about doctors. I'm trying to educate some of them because I think it's needed. I think that the changes that are needed in obstetric treatment in this country are not due to malice of the doctors but to ignorance. When we were in the early days of the country, we had midwives but we didn't have communication, so the midwives were

". . . it's one of our most precious freedoms—that you get to choose how you want to have your own baby, that you're well-informed enough that you make a wise choice. . . ."

not able to organize in any fashion. Then when there were plenty of doctors there was a natural enough sort of competition. And it was easy to see, maybe, why we had such a high infant mortality rate compared with the European countries. It's natural enough to see why women would like to start going to hospitals. We would like to keep hospitals. Everybody does not want to have a home birth. But I think it's just as important that we keep home birth as an alternative because it's one of our most precious freedoms—that you get to choose how you want to have your own baby, that you're well-informed enough that you make a wise choice, and that we don't have the two professions at odds with each other."
—from "Practicing Midwifery: A Talk by Ina May Gaskin" in the Summer, 1981 issue of *Childbirth Alternatives Quarterly.*

THE APRS FEDERAL MONITOR
Alliance for Perinatal Research and Services, Inc.
P.O. Box 6358
Alexandria, VA 22306
$10. a year
$18. two years
(8 issues each year)

The *Federal Monitor* was started by childbirth activist Ann Gray and later taken on by the Alliance for Perinatal Research and Services, Inc. (APRS), under the editorship of Rae Grad and Deborah Bash. The *Federal Monitor* is "a news alert on legislative and regulatory activities relating to the health of women and children" and is issued eight times a year, irregularly, depending on what's happening in the news. It's an invaluable resource for people who want to keep abreast of what's

happening in the courts, in the states, in Washington, DC, and in the news. The *Monitor* provides very useful access information on new government publications, public hearings, conferences, regulations, legislation, and programs affecting childbirth and women's health.
"BLUE CROSS/BLUE SHIELD ALLOWS FOR FEDERAL EMPLOYEES TO RECEIVE 100% REIMBURSEMENT FOR HOME DELIVERIES BY NURSE-MIDWIVES."

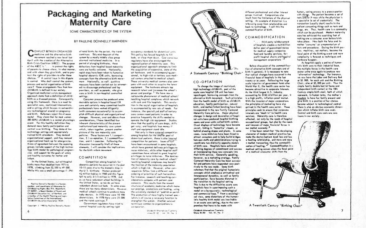

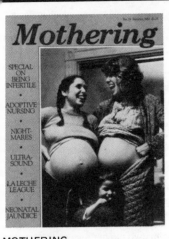

MOTHERING
P.O. Box 2208
Albuquerque, NM 87103
505/867-3110
$10. a year (quarterly)
$18. two years
add $3.00 for non-USA addresses
$2.25 for sample issue

Though *Mothering* is in theory a magazine about nurturing skills, I read it for its excellent coverage of alternative birth and midwifery. For instance, the Summer, 1982 issue contained articles on ultrasound in obstetrics, neonatal jaundice, infertility, postpartum hemorrhage, adoptive nursing, and the new Midwives Alliance of North America. *Mothering* articles are usually written by mothers (!) and midwives and are very consumer-oriented. Their book reviews, letters from readers, news tidbits, and even the advertisements provide an excellent means of staying informed about the alternative birth movement. (There are also regular sections on parenting, children's activities, family health, nutrition, family businesses, and alternative schooling.) *Mothering* is usually about 122 pages long and includes lots of good photographs.

Mothering Publications also pro-

PERINATAL PRESS
The Perinatal Center
Sutter Memorial Hospital
52nd and F Streets
Sacramento, CA 95819
$15. a year
$27. two years
$20. a year, U.S. currency, for Canada and Mexico
$25. a year, U.S. currency, for other foreign subscribers

The *Perinatal Press* is "a non-affiliated, non-profit publication designed for those dedicated to improving the health care of the pregnant woman, fetus and newborn." Edited by a team of doctors, the Press provides articles and abstracts with an emphasis on the more technical aspects of maternity care. There is also information on childbirth education and parent programs and a calendar of meet-

vides the following reprints. See the index for reviews in this *Catalog.*

Lay Midwifery and the Law, 1982
34 pages
$3.50
Circumcision Information Pamphlet
21 pages
$3.50
Immunization Information Pamphlet
27 pages
$4.00

"There is a growing casualness about the administration of ultrasound scans. One study found that the most important factor in determining who received a scan was the availability of an ultrasound machine. If it is there, it will be used. (Today virtually every hospital and 35,000 private offices and genetic counseling centers have ultra sound equipment.) Some doctors allow waiting patients to entertain themselves by listening to their babies' hearts with a handheld scanner. Some use a Doptone stethoscope to listen to the fetal heart after the twentieth week when a normal stethoscope will do the same job. Many prefer ultrasound to palpation. As some say 'Why palpate when you can sonocate?' Some women request a scan to learn the sex of their baby, to watch 'the baby grow' or to relieve pangs of anxiety about the baby's well-being. In light of the unknown risks of ultrasound it seems as if these uses may represent misuses. . . ."

"A mother who knows the dangers of radiation might protest violently about the use of an x-ray as part of a yearly dental exam but agree to an x-ray if her child breaks an arm. In deciding whether or not a real benefit will be gained from a scan, women should ask their doctors or midwives the following two questions: 'What information will the scan provide that is not available through other means (stethoscope, palpation)?' 'Will this information affect prenatal care? If so, how?' "

ings sponsored by consumer and professional groups. (Members of the National Perinatal Association, 1311 A Dolley Madison Blvd., Suite 3A, McLean, VA 22101, receive a discount on subscriptions to the *Perinatal Press.* Write for more information.)

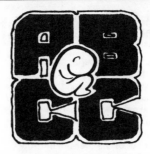

ALTERNATIVE BIRTH CRISIS COALITION
P.O. Box 48371
Chicago, IL 60648
312/625-4054

The Alternative Birth Crisis Coalition (ABCC) was formed in 1981 by a group of physicians and alternative birth activists to provide support and legal defense aid to doctors, midwives, and parents who are harrassed for their home birth activities. Perceiving a "conspiracy" by the medical establishment to persecute those involved in birth alternatives, the ABCC has pledged to end the isolation and lack of adequate defense counsel for those being constrained or harrassed by hospitals, medical licensing boards, nurse practice boards, insurance companies, and courts of law.

Marian Tompson, a founding mother of La Leche League, is Executive Director of the Coalition and the board of directors is made up of Hai Abdul, M.D. (a California birth center physician who left the state when his license to practice medicine was suspended), Mary Jean Abdul, Gail Roy Fraties, J.D. (an attorney who specializes in cases concerning childbirth), Marjie and Jay Hathaway (directors of the American Academy of Husband-Coached Childbirth), David and Lee Stewart (directors of the National Association of Parents and Professionals for Safe Alternatives in Childbirth [NAPSAC]), Robert S. Mendelsohn, M.D., William D. Matviuw, and Gregory White, M.D. Unfortunately, this board represents what may be called the "traditionalist" part of the alternative childbirth movement, which has aligned itself against abortion rights, the Equal Rights Amendment, and other women's concerns. At present there is no representation of feminist women's health organizations or concerns on the board of ABCC, though the women's health movement has been an important force in working for women's rights in childbirth. This "split" in the alternative birth movement points up a dilemma with which many birth activists are struggling: whether freedom of choice for women in childbirth can be obtained without a parallel commitment to women's rights and freedom to choose in all areas of reproductive health, including the right to make their own decision about whether or not to terminate a pregnancy.

AMERICAN FOUNDATION FOR MATERNAL AND CHILD HEALTH
30 Beekman Place
New York, NY 10022
212/759-5510

"The American Foundation for Maternal and Child Health, Inc. is a non-profit foundation for interdisciplinary research in maternal and child health whose main focus is on the perinatal period and its effect on infant outcome and child development.

"The foundation acts as a clearinghouse for information from various national and international medical and social science disciplines concerned with the perinatal period and sponsors medical research designed to shed light on the effects of various perinatal influences on infant outcome and child development."

This foundation, directed by Doris Haire, provides funding for selected projects and sponsors a yearly conference in New York City on obstetrical management and infant outcome, designed to alert medical professionals to childbirth practices which may have an adverse effect on children's later mental and physical development. Doris Haire served as president of the International Childbirth Education Association (ICEA) from 1970-72 and has worked for many years focussing public attention on harmful and unproven obstetrical practices. For more information on Haire's work see *The Cultural Warping of Childbirth, How Safe is 'Safe'?* and "The Federal Government Investigates Obstetrical Practices" (see index for listings).

FOR MORE INFORMATION

For more resources and information on working for change in childbirth also see the index for the following organizations.

INTERNATIONAL CHILDBIRTH EDUCATION ASSOCIATION (ICEA)

MATERNITY CENTER ASSOCIATION

COOPERATIVE BIRTH CENTER NETWORK

MIDWIVES ALLIANCE OF NORTH AMERICA

NATIONAL ASSOCIATION OF PARENTS AND PROFESSIONALS FOR SAFE ALTERNATIVES IN CHILDBIRTH (NAPSAC)

International Childbirth Movement

England

At the beginning of the home birth movement, in the late 1960's, many people looked to England as a model for good home birth care. Trained English "domiciliary" midwives attended home births with back-up from emergency "flying squads" and instructions for "home confinement" were always included in English midwifery texts. Unfortunately, over the last decade England has become "Americanized" to the extent that its home birth rate is now the same as ours, only about 2%, and the use of drugs and technology for birth is very high. In addition, many people feel that English midwives have lost their sense of autonomy and become nothing more than obstetrical nurses.

In response, many English parents and midwives are now protesting the state of maternity care in the United Kingdom. In London, on April 4, 1982, 5000 people marched to protest a recent ban on natural childbirth at the Royal Free Hospital. The following groups are among many which are working to restore natural childbirth and home birth and to promote the midwife as the guardian of healthy childbearing.

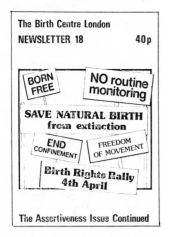

THE BIRTH CENTRE, LONDON
16 Simpson Street
London, SW11
England
Telephone: 01-223-1052

The Birth Centre, London, was founded in 1977 and publishes an excellent newsletter and a series of information leaflets on alternatives in childbearing. Write for prices.

"The Birth Centre London gives support to those people who seek an alternative to the ever increasing 'mechanisation' of birth. Our intention is to encourage those who want a more natural labour for the mother, a calmer, less traumatic birth for the baby, and full participation for the father in an atmosphere of loving and caring, whether at home or in hospital.

"Whilst recognising the advances and contributions of orthodox medicine, we are very concerned about routine medical intervention and the many side-effects, particularly for the baby, of the over-use of drugs during childbirth.

"We believe in the promotion of 'good health' (ideally before conception) as the best form of preventive medicine and are very interested in the contribution of alternative forms of health care. For example: alternative medicine—homeopathy, herbal remedies, acupuncture, etc., the practise of yoga during pregnancy as a way of promoting physical, mental and spiritual well-being; the importance of a healthy diet. We are also concerned about environmental pollution and the ways it is affecting our children before and after birth."

THE NATIONAL CHILDBIRTH TRUST
9 Queensborough Terrace
London W2
England

A non-governmental organization, the Trust promotes natural childbirth and childbirth preparation, provides teacher training and classes in Sheila Kitzinger's Psychosexual Method, and provides study days and publications for midwives, physiotherapists, and antenatal teachers.

INTERNATIONAL WOMEN'S COUNCIL ON OBSTETRICAL PRACTICES
c/o Patricia A. Barki, Chair
149 Pratts Mill Road
Sudbury, MA 01776
U.S.A.
and
c/o Beverly A. Beech, International Coordinator
21 Iver Lane
Iver, Bukinghamshire
England

"The International Women's Council on Obstetrical Practices is an organization that has been in existence for six years, and the greatest goal of the Council is to reach women and give them the information and answer the questions that can, in some cases, make for a better situation. We act as a referral and resources agency and have several publications available for women, in order to give them a tool to secure that their rights and wishes are respected during their birthing experience. On November 5, 1982, the Council launched a publication called the "Maternal and Child Health Consumer Informed Consent Handbook.' The purpose being that the definition of informed consent varies so from person to person, state to state, that in order for consumers to get the birth they want, and in order to avoid unwanted and unnecessary drugs and procedures, consumers need a tool to enable them to take back the rights over their lives and births."

(Patricia Barki)
Write to Patricia Barki for more information on this handbook.

ASSOCIATION FOR IMPROVEMENT IN THE MATERNITY SERVICES (AIMS)
c/o Beverly A. Beech
21 Iver Lane
Iver, Buckinghamshire
England

"AIMS is responsible for many of the major changes that go on in England for the betterment of women's health care, and supply counsel and support for anyone who needs them. One of the joint projects that the International Women's Council of Obstetrical Practices and AIMS undertook is a petition to the House of Parliament to establish a patient's bill of rights. It is hoped to be presented during 1982. There are thousands of British women signed onto the petition and hopefully this will have a favourable outcome." (Patricia Barki)

ASSOCIATION OF RADICAL MIDWIVES
Harcourt House
8 a The Drive
Wimbledon
London SWR
England

"Our overall aim is to restore the role of the midwife for the benefit of the childbearing woman and her baby. We don't see this as going back but rather as going forward . . . Our objectives are:
1) to re-establish the confidence of the midwife in her own skills.
2) to share ideas, skills and information.
3) to encourage midwives in their support of a woman's active participation in childbirth.
4) to reaffirm the need for midwives to provide continuity of care.
5) to explore alternative patterns of care.
6) to encourage evaluation of development in our field."

SOCIETY FOR THE SUPPORT OF HOME CONFINEMENTS
c/o Margaret Whyte
19 Laburnum Road
Durham City,
England

BIRTH RIGHTS
c/o Yvonne Baginsky
2 Forth Street
Edinburgh 1
Scotland

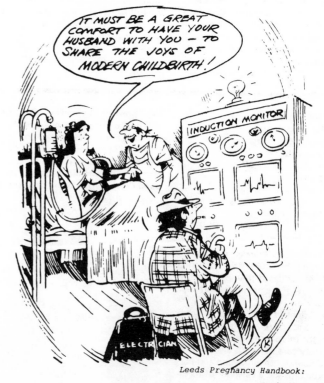

Leeds Pregnancy Handbook:
England

"One of the main things that is involved in getting what you want is persistence. What we call the broken record technique. You just keep saying the same thing over and over, and amazingly enough it frequently works.
(Nancy and Hilary did some role playing. Nancy is the obstetrician, Hilary the pregnant woman.)

H. O.K. We'll do 'setting up a drip.' I've come into hospital, I'm in labour and the first thing that you want to do, shave and enema of course, is to set up a drip and plug me in.

N. Hello, how are you doing?

H. Fine thank you, I think.

N. Well you're going to have a fine time I'm sure. Now if you can just lie still I have this drip here, it's just to give you some fluid so that you won't need any fluids by mouth during your labour. I'll be getting this set up, you just . . .

H. That's just fluid is it?

N. Oh yes, it's just in case you might need something else later.

H. Well I think I'd rather not have that now, thanks.

N. Well of course you don't need it now, but you never know, later on you might need something else and it might be too late to set it up then, so we really need to do it now.

H. I can understand, I might need it later, but since I don't need it now, I'd rather not have it now.

N. Well, it'll be too late later, (much laughter from group). I think we need to do this *now.*

H. I understand what you mean, but I don't want to have the drip set up now.

N. It is routine policy in this hospital. We do this for all our mothers and it has very good results. I'm sure it will cause no discomfort to you whatsoever. It doesn't hurt, it's no more than a little prick, you won't notice a thing.

H. I understand that it's routine but I don't want it done to me.

N. It does work very well, we've had very good results with doing this. I'm sure you'll find it's fine—don't worry about it.

H. I'm sure it has had, well, I'm sure that some people think it has had good results, but I don't want it done to me anyway, thanks (winning and assertive smile).

N. I understand that some people have reservations about this. You don't want people bothering you at this point, that's perfectly understandable, but later on, you know, for instance you might go into post-partum haemorrhage and by the time we get something to you it's going to be too late. You could die in just a few minutes. It takes 2 minutes of bleeding and we could have you dead. Now we don't want that to happen, do we? (more laughter)

H. I realize I'm taking responsibility on myself for the outcome of my labour by refusing the drip. It's a risk I think I know a bit about and it's a risk I'm willing to take.

N. Well really it's my responsibility since I am in charge of this hospital. It's my responsibility to set up the policies which I know are safest for the mothers and babies in my care. Therefore I do feel responsible for insisting that you have this drip.

H. Yes, I understand that you think it's a good idea, but I don't want it done to me at this time.

N. Would you be willing to sign a paper that you refuse my advice and . . .?

H. O yes I would, certainly.

N. All right.

—Excerpt from a talk given by Hilary Ratna on "Assertive Training and Its Relevance to Childbirth" transcribed in The Birth Centre London Newsletter 18, Winter 1982.

"In countries which are 'less technologically advanced,' the thrust in building up health systems generally involves constructing hospitals and bringing health issues as much into the attendant 'medical sphere' as possible. If birth is to become a technological procedure along the lines of the USA and other Western countries, it will be detrimental to women.
"The movement towards home birth in Western countries may seem an indulgent luxury to women in countries or regions where there is no choice but to give birth at home, without adequate hygiene or simple sterilizing equipment, and where mortality rates are high. But the answer here is not necessarily to turn to hospitals which are going to be expensive in one way or another, and ultimately harmful in many cases. Rather it is to provide access to good food, simple hygienic conditions and sterilizing equipment. Above all, it is a question of women everywhere having access to information which will enable them to make choices, or, where those choices do not exist, to be empowered to make their own alternatives."

—from the *International Women & Health Resource Guide,* preliminary draft edition July 1980, available through the Boston Women's Health Book Collective.

Canada is one of only nine countries in the world which do not legally recognize the practice of midwifery. However, Canada has a strong childbirth movement and underground network for midwifery and home birth. Listings for Canadian resources and organizations are included throughout the Catalog.

Australia

BIRTH RITES, BIRTH RIGHTS: Childbirth Alternatives for Australian Parents
by Judith Lumley and Jill Astbury
1980, 325 pages

from
Thomas Nelson Australia (publisher)
19-41 Jeffcott Street West
Melbourne, Victoria
Australia 3003

Available from:
Birth and Life Bookstore
P.O. Box 70625
Seattle, WA 98107
$6.95 plus 1.00 shipping within U.S.A. and 1.50 outside

In this book an obstetrician and a clinical psychologist take a critical look at obstetrical practices and alternatives in childbirth, in order to aid Australian parents in choosing the kind of care they want. However, readers everywhere will be interested in the authors' excellent discussion of woman's nature, sexuality, and emotions in childbearing and their comments on bonding, babies, breastfeeding, sex after birth, grief and loss, and postpartum adjustment. A long list of Australian resource organizations is included.
"The number of medically attended home births is still very small (less than 0.5 percent of all births in Australia in 1978), but informal estimates are that in Victoria the number has doubled in each six month period since the beginning of 1975. This recent trend is at first surprising, since hospital confinement has been the only accepted pattern of care here for thirty years and there is no tradition of home care by midwives as there is in areas of Europe. Moreover, in Australia, as elsewhere, professional medical opinion is almost totally opposed to the practice. Nor is there an informed and organised lobby of other professionals (psychologists, paediatricians, sociologists and educators) to support home confinement such as exists in the United Kingdom. Why, then, in the face of wholesale condemnation, are women choosing home birth?
"The commonest reason given by Melbourne women interviewed by one of us in 1977 was that they had previously had a hospital birth. . . ."

The following organizations provide referrals and information for home birth and alternative childbirth in Australia.

CANBERRA HOMEBIRTH ASSOCIATION
C1-Box 88
PO O'Connor
Australian Capital Territory
Australia 2601

HOMEBIRTH
1-A Shoalwater Road
Shoalwater, W.A.
Australia 6169

MIDWIFERY CONTACT CENTRE
7 North Road
Shoalwater, W.A.
Australia 6169

ORGANIZATION OF AUSTRALIAN MIDWIVES
P.O. Box 305
Strathfield, New South Wales
Australia 2135

PARENT CENTRES AUSTRALIA
83 Albert Drive
Killara
Australia 2071

NEW ZEALAND HOMEBIRTH ASSOCIATION
P.O. Box 7093
Auckland
New Zealand

For More Information

Ina May Gaskin, author of *Spiritual Midwifery* and head midwife for The Farm in Tennessee, toured Great Britain during the Spring of 1982, speaking and visiting with childbirth reform groups. Her reports on this trip are published in *The Practicing Midwife,* beginning with the Fall 1982 issue. For more information, consult the listing for "The Farm Midwives."

ICEA INTERNATIONAL DIRECTOR
Jan Cornfoot
P.O. Box 115
Belmont, Western Australia
Australia 6104

ICEA (the International Childbirth Education Association) regularly covers international childbirth news in its newsletter and its International Director, currently based in Australia, provides information on ICEA, other members, and local childbirth options to all ICEA members living outside of North America. See listing for ICEA for more information.

For further information on international women's health issues, see the listings for the Boston Women's Health Book Collective, WIN News (Women's International Network News), or contact:

ISIS (Women's International Information and Communication Service)
Case Postale 301
1227 Carouge
Switzerland

Political Action Skills

Social change activists have been working toward their goals for a long time and have developed many tools and skills for political action. Many of these can be used to good advantage by childbirth activists, so we don't have to "start from scratch" on every project. How do you organize a rally? publish a newsletter? arrange a press conference? lobby the legislature? run a group meeting? raise money? The resources listed in this section can provide many of the answers; some are geared especially for childbirth groups, some for women's rights groups, and some for the larger social action community.

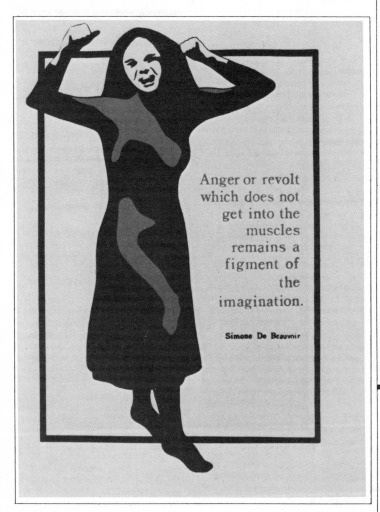

Anger or revolt which does not get into the muscles remains a figment of the imagination.

Simone De Beauvoir

Silk-screened poster, 18" x 24", 1975. Janet Isaacs Ashford

Public Relations

MEDIA KIT
20 pages

from
League of Women Voters
1730 M Street, NW
Washington, DC 20036
$2.00 plus .50 handling

This media kit, from the League of Women Voters, includes five of their factsheets on public relations, each of which is available separately and in bulk. Included are:

Projecting Your Image: How to Produce a Slide Show. How to decide if a slide show is the medium for your message: guidelines for getting your story on the screen. $.40

Speaking Out: Setting Up a Speakers Bureau. A step-by-step guide to getting League speakers heard in your community.

Reaching the Public. The role of public relations in whatever you do.

Breaking Into Broadcasting. Guidelines for approaching media and for producing radio spots, TV spots, films.

Getting into Print. Tips on working effectively with the print media.

Write to the League for a free copy of their *Citizen Participation Catalog* which lists other useful publications.

"A good *letter to the editor* signed by a well known name may be more effective than an editorial. A few tips. Take sides on issues but avoid personalities. Tie the letter to the news or editorial coverage that moved you to write. Be brief—you're less likely to be cut. Decide whether an official letter from your organization, or letters from individuals or *both* would be best. Letters, like feature stories, are a good device for maintaining interest in your group's issues and for communicating something not suited to a press release or feature story."

PUBLIC RELATIONS: Making the Media Work for You.

Ms. Magazine, April 1974
pps. 107-110, Vol. II, No. 10

This article provides an excellent, brief introduction to public relations, written specifically for women who will be representing feminist concerns and who have no prior experience with the media. Prepared with help from the Women's Action Alliance (see index), it provides information on dealing with different media (newspapers, radio, TV), how to write a press release (includes a sample), and how to organize a press conference. Look for this back issue of *Ms.* at your local library or ask for a photocopy of the article through your inter library loan system.

"The follow-up phone call should be short, informative, and cheerful. Humor jumps hurdles. As a public relations person, you can't be so solemn that you forget that you're trying to make friends with another person. But you should not be afraid to press beyond politeness if courtesy threatens to leave your group out in the cold. (For example, if a reporter tells you to wait for her call, don't—if you feel your event or group has been forgotten.)

"In the first phone call, you might explain a bit about the group and say, 'I've read your publication (or listened to your show), and I notice that you do such-and-such (interview politicians with new ideas, or report local news events). I have several ideas about how you could use our group. Shall I tell you now, or put them in writing, or would you like to have a cup of coffee some afternoon when you have the time.' "

HOW TO GET IN THE PAPER

One of our local newspapers recently ran an article on "How to Get in the Paper," for all the many public interest groups, businesses, wedding parties, etc., which are continuously competing for the editor's time and the paper's space. Briefly, their guidelines are these:

* KEEP IT SHORT
* SEND A PROFESSIONAL, HIGH QUALITY, BLACK AND WHITE PHOTO
* MAIL IT EARLY
* DO IT REGULARLY

* DON'T THREATEN
* DO SOMETHING WORTH PUTTING IN THE PAPER
* TYPE IT

EFFECTIVE LOCAL PUBLICITY:
A Guide to Increasing the Visibility of Birth Alternatives for Local Childbirth Education Groups
Edited by Deb Pike
1979, 54 pages

from
NAPSAC
P.O. Box 267
Marble Hill, MO 63764
$2.75 postpaid

This booklet was prepared by the NAPSAC Committee to Increase Local Visibility of Birth Alternatives (see index). It is especially geared to groups which are working to promote local acceptance of home birth, midwifery and other childbirth alternatives while also raising public awareness of harmful obstetrical practices. The booklet provides an introduction to public relations skills and includes an excellent selection of sample Public Service Announcements (short announcements for radio and television) and longer press releases which can be taken right from the book and used by local groups. Topics include informed consent, freedom of choice in childbirth, nutrition in pregnancy, safety of home birth, hazards of oxy-tocic drugs, unphysiologic birth practices, obstetrical medication, fetal monitors, home vs. hospital birth statistics, smoking in pregnancy, and rising cesarean rates. There is also a section on getting "equal time" access to the media to balance coverage of the medical profession in your area. Sample equal time "slots" are included for state lay midwifery legislation and home birth.

A PUBLIC RELATIONS HANDBOOK for childbirth education groups

A PUBLIC RELATIONS HANDBOOK for Childbirth Education Groups
by Elaine Levine
1977, 48 pages, Illus.

from
ICEA Bookcenter
P.O. Box 20048
Minneapolis, MN 55420
$3.50 plus 1.25 shipping

This booklet provides an introduction to media and public relations skills, especially geared to childbirth educators and groups who want to become more visible in their communities, attract more students to childbirth education classes, and effect change in the policies of local hospitals and health care providers. Topics include how to get class referrals from the local medical community, how to work with medical professionals who are not supportive of the work of childbirth educators (patience, persistence, strategy, compromise), how to effectively advertise your classes or group (brochures and posters, film showings, newsletters, local health fairs, etc.), how to work with the media (press releases, feature news, interviews and press conferences, broadcast media, etc.) and consumerism in health care (writing letters to health care providers, letters to the editor, evaluating and becoming aware of local alternatives in maternity care). This material was prepared by the Outreach committee of the Child-birth Education Association of Greater Minneapolis/St. Paul and includes excellent samples and examples of their own effective public relations work.

"Post-birth letters can be used to exert influence on maternity care practices. These letters can give those people charged with the major influence over people's birth experiences a knowledge of the parents' concerns. Letters serve to draw attention to the factors that are acting as positive and negative aspects of people's birth experiences so that these factors can be evaluated. . . .

"Tell your students that a letter that begins and ends with positive comments is more likely to be read and considered seriously than a letter that is angry or hostile. Hostile letters are generally categorized as 'crank' letters and tend to be disregarded. The beginning statement could acknowledge and thank the people involved in the birth for the things that they did to make the experience a good one. If the parents have only good things to say, so much the better. Remind your class members that the positive aspects of care they experienced will only be present for others if the medical community feels it is worthwhile for them to continue to offer these services.

"If there were aspects of the care/experience that were less than ideal, the parents should go on in the next paragraph to discuss these points. They can mention the disturbing factors and explain why they found them unpleasant. If the people feel very strongly about a negative aspect of their care, they could state that unless the situation improves they will seek alternative care for any subsequent pregnancies. They should express their reluctance to do this in view of their satisfaction with other aspects of their care, while emphasizing that the issue is important enough for them to seek other care to satisfy their requirements."

"SAMPLE PUBLIC SERVICE ANNOUNCEMENT

From: Aimed at: Expectant and new parents

NAME OF ORGANIZATION

Person to contact: To be aired anytime.
Title
Address
City
Phone Number

Time: 60 seconds

Words: 164

"Physicians and nurse-midwives are legally obligated to obtain a pregnant parent's informed consent before administering any treatment during the course of pregnancy and childbirth. Knowledge of this fact is of great importance to all women about to give birth, since evidence is rapidly being accumulated demonstrating the potential hazards of obstetric interference in childbirth.

"Informed consent, according to the American College of Obstetricians and Gynecologists, consists of an explanation of the treatment being considered, the risks and hazards of the treatment, the chances for recovery, the treatment's necessity, and the feasibility of alternative methods. The health care provider has the responsibility of presenting this information in language that the patient understands.

"*(Name of organization)* advocates the observance of 'The Pregnant Patient's Bill of Rights and Responsibilities' as set forth by the International Childbirth Education Association, in order to encourage the physician and the pregnant parent to work together to ensure the safest and healthiest childbirth possible. For more information call *(Name of Organization)* at *(phone number)*."

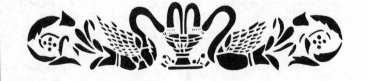

EFFECTIVE PROMOTION: A Guide to Low Cost Use of Media for Community Organizations
by Michelle Cauble
1977, 22 pages, Illus.
$.65, bulk rates available

HOW TO PUBLISH COMMUNITY INFORMATION ON AN IMPOSSIBLY TIGHT BUDGET
by Vic Pawlak
1976, 24 pages, Illus.
$.65 / bulk rates available
from
Do It Now Foundation
P.O. Box 5115
Phoenix, AZ 85010

These two useful and cheap booklets are published by the Do It Now Foundation, a non-profit organization which provides information and publications on drug abuse, venereal disease, health, and birth control. The booklets are written to help other

DUSTBOOKS
Box 100
Paradise, CA 95969
free catalog

Dustbooks keeps track of what's happening in the world of small presses and little magazines and also provides a mail-order catalog of books on self-publishing, ranging from brochures to books. It's a useful resource for groups which will be producing their own teaching manuals, handbooks, newsletters, etc.

"small belt-tightening organizations who wish to reach as wide an audience as possible" on a limited budget. *Effective Promotion* is a simple and realistic guide to media and public relations. *How to Publish* helps lay people understand the offset printing process and how to get the most for your time and money when working with printers.

"Each office should get LETTERHEAD stationery and envelopes as soon as possible. This is not for 'flash,' but simply to establish credibility with the media. It looks official, and assures the media that they are not being asked to deal with a one-shot, fly-by-night group of amateurs. All releases and written contracts with the media should be on letterhead and typed double-spaced. If your group is incorporated as a non-profit organization, your letterhead should say so: this is particularly key in getting free speech or public service time. Names of LOCAL officers and contacts on the letterhead are more important to the working media than State or National supporters, though later when you have accumulated some big-name endorsers you can run a list of them down the side. Adopting a LOGO for your group, used somewhere near the top of the page, is also graphically attractive."

HOW TO PRODUCE A SMALL NEWSPAPER: A Guide for Independent Journalists
by the Editors of the Harvard Post
1978, 158 pages, Illus.
$8.95 pap.
$11.95 hd.
from
The Harvard Common Press
The Common
Harvard, MA 01451

This book helped me a lot in setting up and running *Childbirth Alternatives Quarterly,* the newsletter I edit and publish (see index). It includes excellent chapters on content, printing, typography, pasteup, design and layout, advertising, financial matters, circulation and distribution, and deadlines, which provide really useful tips and information. It all comes from an experienced team of three bright young people who produce the alternative *Harvard Post* in Cambridge. This book is detailed enough to be useful for those who are publishing a good-sized community newspaper, but scaled down a bit, will also help anyone who is producing a 4-page, typewritten newsletter.

"If you are considering a very smallscale publishing enterprise and you have absolutely no money to

start out with, you may want to try setting your copy on an IBM typewriter. The IBM, with its unusually even striking impression and with the blackness of the characters it can produce with a carbon ribbon, is one of the few kinds of typewriter that can generate acceptable copy for offset reproduction. Moreover, the IBM Executive employs a system of modified proportional spacing based on a 2-to 5-unit range—lowercase 'i,' for example, is 2 units wide, whereas upper-case 'M' is 5 units—and this makes the type considerably more attractive than that produced by a conventional typewriter. Many small, cheaply-produced newsletters are set on the Executive for this reason.

"IBM typewriter type should not be reproduced full-size for newspaper use; it will look much better on the page if your printer photographically reduces it to about 80 percent of its original size. You can simply type your copy and lay out complete pages that are 125 percent as large, in every dimension, as you want the finished pages to be. If the finished page is to be 10 inches wide and 14 inches deep, for instance, the layout you give the printer should be 12½ inches wide and 17½ inches deep—with the instruction to shoot it at 80 percent."

Printing It
By Clifford Burke

Here is everything you need to know to produce anything by offset — from a poster or a handbill to a complete book — with style and beauty, and without expensive equipment. PRINTING IT is already the standard guide for the novice and judging from the growing number of printers and publishers who keep it on their reference shelves, it is destined to become a classic. Burke is a poet and master printer and book designer with many awards to his credit. Since 1966 he has been conducting a one-man campaign to take the mystery out of printing and to restore common sense to the craft.

Wingbow Press. $4.95/paper

Publishing How-To

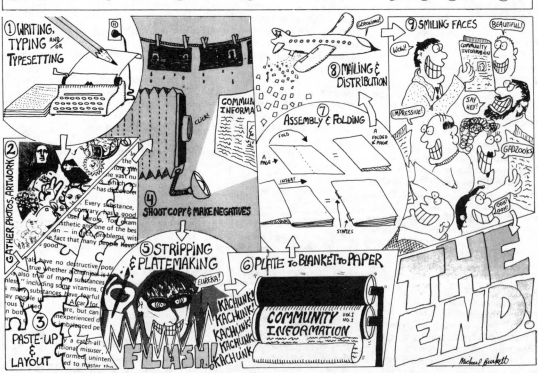

From *How to Publish Community Information on an Impossibly Tight Budget.*

GRAPHICS SUPPLIES

The following companies provide free mail-order catalogs with useful art supplies, graphics, and other materials you'll need to produce your own printed brochures, newsletters, posters, etc.

GRAPHIC PRODUCTS CORPORATION
3601 Edison Place
Rolling Meadows, IL 60008

Manufacturers of Formatt and Formaline graphic products, including transfer type, self-adhesive clip art, Border Boards, art tapes, and more.

CHARRETTE
31 Olympia Avenue
Woburn, MA 01888

Retails a complete line of art supplies and pressure graphics.

DOVER PICTORIAL ARCHIVE SERIES
Dover Publications
180 Varick Street
New York, NY 10014

Dover publishes a line of over 300 moderately priced books ($3.00 to $5.00) with collections of copyright-free art, most of it compiled from 19th Century sources. A tremendous source of handsome, black and white illustrations for virtually any purpose.

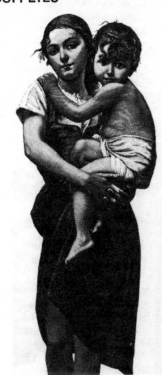

from *Women: A Pictorial Archive from Nineteenth-Century Sources,* selected by Jim Harter, Dover Publications, 1978.

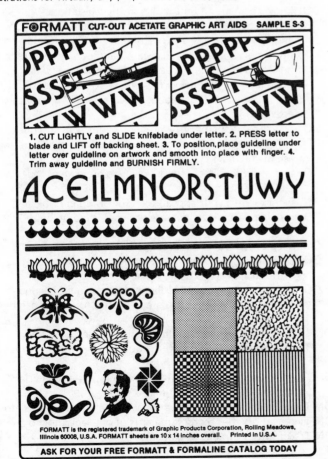

FORMATT CUT-OUT ACETATE GRAPHIC ART AIDS   SAMPLE S-3

1. CUT LIGHTLY and SLIDE knifeblade under letter. 2. PRESS letter to blade and LIFT off backing sheet. 3. To position, place guideline under letter over guideline on artwork and smooth into place with finger. 4. Trim away guideline and BURNISH FIRMLY.

ACEILMNORSTUWY

FORMATT is the registered trademark of Graphic Products Corporation, Rolling Meadows, Illinois 60008, U.S.A. FORMATT sheets are 10 x 14 inches overall.   Printed in U.S.A.

ASK FOR YOUR FREE FORMATT & FORMALINE CATALOG TODAY

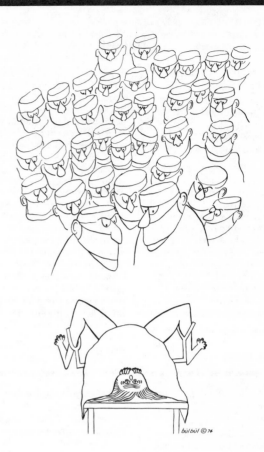

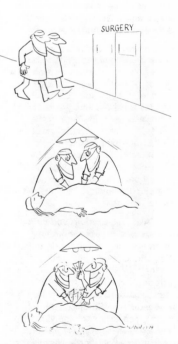

DISSECTING DOCTOR MEDICORPSE
by Bulbul
1974, 48 pages, Illus.

from
Arachne Publishing
P.O. Box 4100
Mountain View, CA 94040
$1.25 plus .35 postage

Cartoonist Bulbul has created these pointed and funny cartoons exposing the anti-woman bias of the medical profession. In the introduction she says, "We give doctors too much power over us. We are mystified by his technical virtuosities and overlook the abuse of power. I feel the sacred doctor should be demystified by a good burst of laughter. While we're laughing we can redefine healer and make health care a patient controlled right." Also available from Arachne Publishing at the same price are Bulbul's *Sugar Daddy's a Sticky Myth!* and *I'm Not for Women's Lib . . . but.*

PERIODICALS OF PUBLIC INTEREST ORGANIZATIONS:
A Citizen's Guide
June, 1979, 58 pages

Commission for the Advancement of Public Interest Organizations
1875 Connecticut Avenue, NW
Washington, DC 20009
$5.00

This guide lists the best of the public interest newsletters and journals, including a category on health-related publications. Each listing features a photo of the publication's cover with subscription information and a description. It's useful to compare your subscription rates, content scope, and cover artwork with what others are doing.

Lobbying

GUIDE TO PUBLIC AFFAIRS
1971, 22 pages

from
Planned Parenthood
810 Seventh Avenue
New York, NY 10019
$.25 plus .20 postage

The Public Policy unit of Planned Parenthood has produced this guide to public policy which explains how to find out who makes and affects health policy on the local, state and federal levels and how you can affect them. The booklet describes how to organize and run a public affairs committee and also how individuals can affect public policy through personal letter writing and lobbying. One person can make a difference!

"It is important to be able to identify accurately which elected or appointed public official or officials are key to development of a particular policy. The approach and the course of action will be different, for example, in a situation where the key official is receiving negative or inaccurate information from his staff, from one where the official is overruling the supportive recommendations of his associates or department. Resistance to policy change may stem from lack of knowledge about its beneficial effects, fear of stepping on a superior's toes, or "rocking the boat," or, occasionally, to unreasoned hostility. The approach and appropriate course of action will, of course, differ accordingly. In order to create a good climate for public policy decisions regarding family planning, it is necessary to educate and inform public officials. In order to educate, one must know who needs information and what facts are likely to be persuasive."

MAKING AN ISSUE OF IT: The Campaign Handbook (No. 613)
1976, 12 pages

from
League of Women Voters
1730 M Street, NW
Washington, DC 20036
$.75 plus .50 handling

This booklet provides a very useful and no-nonsense guide to building a political/legislative action coalition to work toward passage of particular legislation. Especially helpful for those who are working to legalize lay midwifery in the states, this booklet describes coalition structure and function, campaign techniques, how to lobby effectively, testifying at public hearings, monitoring the opposition, a suggested calendar of action, and more.

"Ask *organizations and opinion leaders* who have, or should have, an interest in the legislation to participate. Contact state and local counterparts of national endorsers, but don't ignore a local organization just because its national affiliate has not endorsed. Similarly, do not ignore organizations or individuals merely because you disagree on other issues: *a coalition is formed for one purpose—to secure legislation.* All other agreements or disagreements can and should take a back seat. Once the prime goal is achieved, the members of the coalition go their own ways (though you may have found interesting new allies on other fronts). . . .

"If your coalition is effective, it should produce these results:

* Lobbyists know whom to talk to on what issues.
* Legislative attitudes are reported (particularly changes), and proper action results.
* Communications go to the right people in the right districts on the right issues at the right time.
* Visibility is promoted by a unified, cooperative campaign.
* Proponents *act* instead of reacting.
* The opposition is pinpointed and out-maneuvered.
* Everyone who wants to work has something useful to do.
* People and organizations with specific talents can use them most effectively.
* With constant interaction among committees (via task forces), no effort is wasted and action is directed effectively.
     And 'with a little bit of luck' it *should* also get that legislation passed."

Also available from the League of Women Voters is:

PUBLIC ACTION KIT (PAK). How to organize and gain support for public action goals. The ingredients necessary to PAK political wallop from city hall to Washington. Approximately 130 pages, No. 629, $4.00 plus .50 handling.

HOW TO WRITE TO YOUR REPRESENTATIVES

Senators:

The Honorable _____
United States Senate
Washington, DC 20510

Dear Senator _____
(Telephone: 202/224-3121)

Representatives:

The Honorable
House of Representatives
Washington, DC 20515

Dear Representative/Mr./Ms. _____
(Telephone: 202/224-3121)

Some do's and don'ts for lobbyists

DO: recognize the legislator and the legislative staff as human beings; respect and *listen* to their views.

DO: get to know legislative staff and treat them courteously—their cooperation can make or break your chances to reach the legislators themselves.

DO: identify yourself immediately at each contact; public officials meet too many people to remember everyone.

DO: know the issue and the status of the legislation.

DO: know your legislator—past record on related legislation and/or votes; party and position in the legislative and political power structure; legislative and outside interests; how long he or she has been in the legislature; what kind of a personal interview will be most effective (sensitivity to legislative attitudes about appearance and approach is *essential*).

DO: be aware of any prior favorable commitment to your cause; enlist such a legislator to promote support among colleagues; ask his/her advice.

DO: commend legislators for actions you approve of, but don't feel as free to criticize.

DO: be brief with your appeal, then follow up periodically.

DO: give legislators succinct, easy-to-read literature with important facts and arguments highlighted.

DO: *keep off-the-record comments confidential.*

DO: keep the door open for further discussion even if legislator's attitude appears to be negative.

DO: report all contacts immediately to headcount headquarters so that appropriate district and capitol follow-up can be carried out.

DON'T: be arrogant, condescending or threatening.

DON'T: back recalcitrant legislators into a corner where they take a definite position against you.

DON'T: overwhelm legislators with too much written material, which they won't have time to read.

DON'T: make notes of a conversation while talking to a legislator.

DON'T: repeat off-the-record comments of one legislator to another.

DON'T: get into protracted arguments.

—from The League of Women Voters

COMMON CAUSE CITIZEN'S ACTION GUIDE
brochure

from
Common Cause
2030 M Street, NW
Washington, DC 20036
free

Common Cause, the "citizen's lobby," provides a good, brief introduction to personal lobbying in this brochure. It covers writing to your representatives, how a bill becomes law, and other public relations ideas for making your voice heard.

"Here are some tips on writing to your representatives:

1. Write on personal or business letterhead (if you have it), and sign your name over your signature if you have typed the letter.
2. Put your return address on the letter. Envelopes get thrown away.
3. Identify your subject clearly, giving the name of the legislation you are writing about, and the bill number if you know it.

4. State your reason for writing. Your own personal experience is the best supporting evidence. Tell how the issue would affect you, your family, community, or livelihood—or the effect you believe it would have on your community or state, or on our country.
5. Be as brief as you can without losing the message you want to convey.
6. Use your own words, and avoid stereotyped phrases that sound like form letters.
7. Be reasonable. Don't ask for the impossible or engage in threats.
8. Ask your legislators to state their positions on the issue in their replies. You are entitled to know.
9. Time the arrival of your letter so it reaches the Capitol *before* legislation is acted upon in the committee or on the floor. (See the section, 'When To Write Your Representatives.')
10. Be sure to thank your legislators if they have done something you think is right on a particular issue."

Group Organization

ICEA FORUM
c/o International Childbirth
Education Association
P.O. Box 20048
Minneapolis, MN 55420
612/854-8660

ICEA Forum is a newsletter for member groups of ICEA, published three times a year. Each issue contains useful information on group organization and function. Subscriptions are available to ICEA members only at the time of joining or renewing. Write for more information. Back issues are available for $1.00 postpaid from the address above. Below is a selection of back issue contents.

JUNE, 1982
conducting meetings
motivating people

MARCH, 1982
writing bylaws
group development
publicity

NOVEMBER, 1981
public relations ideas
using the board of consultants
incorporation and tax information

JUNE, 1981
resource network
board liability
group dissension
fundraising

OCTOBER, 1980
the treasurer's role
IRS tax filing revisions

JUNE, 1980
understanding bylaws
annual financial reports
recruiting and retaining volunteers

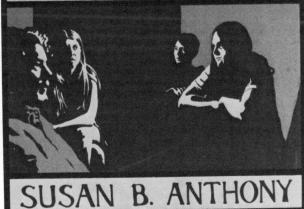

Silk-screened poster, 18" x 24", 1975. Janet Isaacs Ashford

SIMPLIFIED PARLIAMENTARY PROCEDURE (No. 138)
1979, 12 page pamphlet

from
League of Women Voters
1730 M Street, NW
Washington, DC 20036
$.30 plus .50 handling

Based on *Robert's Rules of Order,* this pamphlet provides the basic, conventional rules for governing an organization and conducting a business meeting.

"Order of business

A minimum number *(quorum)*, as prescribed in the bylaws, must be present before business can be legally transacted. The presiding officer should determine that there is a quorum before beginning the meeting. Every organization is free to decide the order in which its business will be conducted, but most agendas follow a standard pattern:

1. Call to order.

2. Minutes are read by the secretary

and corrections requested. The presiding officer says: *If there are no corrections the minutes stand approved as read.*

3. Treasurer's Report is given and questions called for: *The Treasurer's Report will be filed.*

4. Reports of officers, the board and standing committees. Recommendations in reports should be dealt with as motions at this point.

5. Reports of special committees.

6. Unfinished business. Items left over from the previous meeting are brought up in turn by the presiding officer.

7. New business: *Is there any new business?*

8. Program. The program chairperson is called upon to introduce a speaker, film or other presentation.

9. Announcements.

10. Adjournment: *Is there any further business?* (pause) *The meeting is adjourned.''*

MIDWEST ACADEMY
600 W. Fullerton
Chicago, IL 60614
312/975-3670

Midwest Academy is "an independent, non-profit, tax-exempt (501(c)(3)) educational institution dedicated to training leaders and organizers of membership-based citizen action groups working for social and economic justice." The Academy provides literature on direct action organizing, fundraising, research, and meetings which will be of interest to consumer health activists. Titles include:

Strategy Planning
Why Organize?
Organizing Rallies
Fundraising How-to's
Checking on Elected Officials
Write for a complete literature list.

WOMEN'S ACTION ALLIANCE

370 Lexington Avenue, Room 603
New York, NY 10017
212/532-8330

The Women's Action Alliance provides a variety of publications and services to help women who are working toward equality through women's programs and issues. The Alliance operates an information service, a resource library (open to the public in New York City—staff will answer questions by letter or phone), a women's centers project and a non-sexist child development project. Four of the Alliance's publications are listed below. Order the first three directly from the Alliance and add 10% to your order for postage and handling.

How to Organize a Multi-Service Women's Center

A guide to organizing a women's center that is responsive to a wide range of community needs and involves community women in planning and implementing its services. Intended as a working guideline rather than a set of rules, this booklet is divided into three sections: "Organizing the Center" (community outreach, goals, staff training, legalities and the like); "Services and Special Projects" (including information and referral, newsletters, speakers' bureau, divorce, employment, rape counseling); and a list of women's centers.
35 pages, 8½" x 11", $3.00

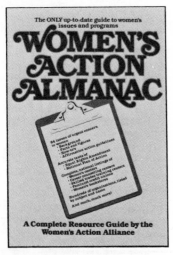

WOMEN'S ACTION ALMANAC

Each day the Women's Action Alliance receives hundreds of requests: What is the text of the ERA? How many women work? Whom do I call to make a Title IX complaint? What can I do about sexual harrassment on the job? What can I do if my husband isn't keeping up with child support payments? The *Women's Action Almanac* is a quick reference handbook to answer these questions and many more—designed to do in print and in one place what the Alliance does every day. Ninety alphabetical subject entries provide

a wealth of background information on each issue and list pertinent books, magazines, and organizations. A separate directory of national organizations describes the goals and activities of each group.
448 pages, 6½" x 9¼", $7.95

Getting Your $hare: An Introduction to Fundraising

Designed to take non-professional grant seekers through all the steps of foundation fundraising—from writing a proposal, researching foundations and making contact with the foundation, to what to do when you do (or do not) receive a grant. Includes a proposal checklist, an annotated resource listing of helpful groups, and publications, and a list of (self-described) change-oriented foundations.
36 pages, 4" x 9", $2.00

Women Helping Women: A State by State Directory of Services

1981, 179 pages

from
Neal-Schuman Publishers, Inc.
23 Cornelia Street
New York, NY 10014
$14.95 plus 1.00 postage

This book "documents the network of nontraditional counseling and shelter services across the country which offer help to women. These services deal with problems ranging from unemployment through health to physical abuse. All share one vital characteristic: they are provided by women for women to meet women's needs. Because many are small, new, and nontraditional, they are not included in standard social service directories and are often difficult to locate.

INCORPORATION

For information on becoming incorporated as a non-profit organization, contact your state government (department of state, bureau of corporation, etc.). Also contact your state for information about becoming tax-exempt from state taxes.

For information on obtaining federal tax exempt status (you need this to get a special non-profit, tax-exempt bulk mailing permit) contact the Internal Revenue Service.

If you have trouble getting the information you need, it's a good idea to ask your local state or federal representative for assistance. S/he will not only be glad to help you, but will be interested to know of the formation of your group and its goals.

MORE RESOURCES

TECHNICAL ASSISTANCE BIBLIOGRAPHIES
Fundraising (6 pages)
Organizational Development (4 pgs)
Public Relations/ Communications (2)

These annotated bibliographies cite useful books and pamphlets with source and address information and are available free from the Alliance, though a contribution of $3.00 would be appreciated to cover costs. A selection of resources from these bibliographies is listed below:

THE GRANTSMANSHIP CENTER
1015 W. Olympic Blvd.
Los Angeles, CA 90015

This organization publishes a bimonthly newsletter, and reprints on fund-raising through grants.

AMERICAN ASSOCIATION OF UNIVERSITY WOMEN
AAUW Sales Office
2401 Virginia Avenue, NW
Washington, DC 20037

AAUW publishes several useful publications including *Foundation Fund-Raisers, Community Action Tool Catalog: Techniques and Strategies for Successful Action Programs* and *Techniques for Organizational Effectiveness.*

NATIONAL WOMEN'S POLITICAL CAUCUS
1411 K Street, NW
Washington, DC, 20005

The Caucus publishes *Fundraising Events: Making Womanpower Profitable* and *The How-To Press and Public Relations Handbook.*

THE GRASS ROOTS FUNDRAISING BOOK: How to Raise Money in Your Community
by Joan Flanagan
Swallow Press, 1977

Available from
The Youth Project
1000 Wisconsin Avenue, NW
Washington, DC 20007

MAKING THE MOST OF SPECIAL EVENTS
by Harold N. Weiner
National Communications Council for Human Services, 1977

Available from:
Public Relations Society of America
845 Third Avenue
New York, NY 10022

TAX-EXEMPT STATUS FOR YOUR ORGANIZATION
Publication 557
by
Department of the Treasury
Internal Revenue Service

Available from
Superintendent of Documents
U.S. Government Printing Office
Washington, DC 20402

HOW TO DO LEAFLETS, NEWSLETTERS AND NEWSPAPERS
by Nancy Brigham

Available from
New England Free Press
60 Union Square
Somerville, MA 02143

TELLING YOUR STORY: Ideas for Local Publicity
edited by Kate W. Jackson

Available from
National Center for Voluntary Action
1214 16th Street, NW
Washington, DC 20036

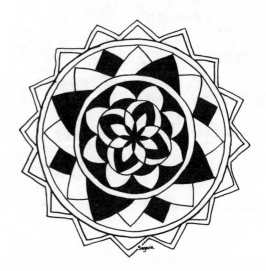

Fund Raising

THE DOLLARS AND SENSE OF FUND-RAISING
by Virginia Kerr
Ms. Magazine, June, 1973
pps. 120-124, Vol. I, No. 12

This article provides an excellent introduction to fundraising for women's interests organizations. It covers tax exempt status, writing a grant proposal, government resources, researching grant-giving foundations, individual contributions, direct mail fundraising, organizing special events, and getting backing from corporations. Look for this back issue of *Ms.* in your local library or ask for a photocopy of the article through your interlibrary loan system.

"Women are not accustomed to making direct demands, and men are not accustomed to assertive women with strong opinions and fundable talents. But we are beginning to recognize that our egos are not so crushable or inflatable that we cannot take the good and the bad in fundraising with equanimity, good sense, and a minimum of gloom. In short, we can raise money for our own projects and we can also do the job with integrity, sincerity, and professionalism."

LARRY FOX
Box M
Valley Stream, NY 11582
516/791-7929

Larry Fox specializes in producing custom printed buttons, bumperstickers, T-shirts, and many other items which can be made with your logo or message and used in fundraising efforts. He often works with childbirth education and other social action groups. Write for a catalog and a price list.

Local printers in your area will also be able to produce many custom-printed items. Here are some slogans others have used on bumperstickers and buttons:

SUPPORT YOUR LOCAL MIDWIFE

SUPPORT YOUR LOCAL PERINEUM!

FREEDOM OF CHOICE IN CHILDBIRTH

HOME BIRTH IS BETTER

MIDWIVES DO IT AT HOME

ASK ME ABOUT MY HOME BIRTH

EINSTEIN WAS BORN AT HOME!

SQUATTER'S RIGHTS IN CHILDBIRTH

STAND AND DELIVER!

MIDWIFERY IS CATCHING

MAILING LISTS AND MISCELLANEOUS

Mailing lists of people and organizations who may be sympathetic to your cause can help if you are doing a direct mail fundraising campaign, trying to boost circulation of your newsletter or just trying to get the word out about a special idea or event. The following organizations sell mailing lists which may be helpful for people working in maternal/child health issues.

INTERNATIONAL CHILDBIRTH EDUCATION ASSOCIATION (ICEA)
P.O. Box 20048
Minneapolis, MN 55420

ICEA, a national organization with thousands of childbirth educator and parent members, announced in February, 1982 that it would rent its membership list as a means of earning money for the organization. The following guidelines have been adopted:

The membership list will be rented:
* Not to organizations or businesses offering competitive services or espousing goals in conflict with those of ICEA.
* Not to organizations for the purpose of influencing opinions on social or political policies, except when in concert with ICEA goals and positions.
* Not to bookstore operations.
* Not to events within an 800 mile radius of an ICEA event six weeks prior or six weeks following.
* Not for ICEA campaign purposes.
* No mention of ICEA as the source of the mailing list may be stated or implied.

CONTEMPORARY HISTORY ENTERPRISES
2315 Westwood Blvd.
Los Angeles, CA 90064
213/386-1543

David Dismore, a feminist activist, provides this research and clipping service. His goal is "to provide activists, non-profit organizations, and concerned individuals with an up-to-date, careful monitoring of key publications in the areas of family life, feminism and family planning, and to do so at minimal cost. In addition to current articles clipped, we also have historical archives going back to the turn of the century in many subject areas." Topics available under Family include childbirth, midwifery, motherhood, and pregnancy. Other subject areas are abortion rights, contraception, equal rights amendment, gay/lesbian rights, new right, non-parenthood, population and environment, sexual exploitation, and women and employment. Rates are about $2.00 a month plus .07 a page. Write for a descriptive brochure.

RESOURCES
Box 134, Harvard Square
Cambridge, MA 02238
617/876-2789

Richard Gardner, of Resources, provides mailing lists which are printed on 3.5" x 15/16" self-sticking labels (or cheshire labels on request). Many different lists are available, including women's health care organizations, human potential movement, health care organizations and publications, communities, alternative schools, etc. Be sure to ask when the list was last updated. Resources also provides services in list automation and subscription fulfillment (data entry, labels, editlisting, etc.) for small publications.

WOMEN'S ACTION ALLIANCE
370 Lexington Avenue, Room 603
New York, NY 10017

The Alliance has up-to-date, comprehensive mailing lists available on pressure-sensitive labels:
National Women's Organizations: 500 professional, service, education, and political organizations for women
Women's Media: 350 national and local women's magazines, newspapers, newsletters, and journals
Women's Centers: 300 programs offering services to women on the local level, nationwide

Write for current prices.

SMALL-TIME OPERATOR: How to Start Your Own Small Business, Keep Your Books, Pay Your Taxes, and Stay Out of Trouble!
by Bernard Kamoroff
1976, 192 pages, Illus.

from
Bell Springs Publishing
P.O. Box 640
Laytonville, CA 95454
$8.95 plus $1.00 shipping

In many ways a childbirth organization is like a small business. If you are raising and spending money you'll need to keep track of it. If you are incorporated you'll have to file tax returns. *Small-Time Operator* can help. Written by an "alternative" accountant in northern California, the book is geared toward small businesses (there's no information specifically for tax-exempt groups) but can be very useful for any group large enough to need a bank account. The book clearly explains such esoteric subjects as bookkeeping, payroll, incorporation, taxes, accounting, and includes sample blank ledgers and worksheets for a whole year.

Lesbian Mothers

Edited by Cheri Pies and Cheryl Jones

Over the past few years, a growing number of lesbians have decided to become parents. Of these women, a large percentage have had their children through AID (Artificial Insemination by Donor) either through a doctor or on their own. Others have adopted children or had sexual relations with men to become pregnant. Lesbians who have helped to raise their lover's or friend's children are also increasingly considering themselves parents.

Because the process of becoming parents is usually very conscious for lesbians, there is the opportunity to really explore, before actually having a child, all of the issues relevant to parenting and come to concrete decisions of choice about whether children are right for us. Several books and articles have been developed to help women in this process and to educate them about various methods of becoming parents. Other resources include films, support groups, and information networks. Although some of the work included here is still in the process of being produced, the sources we have listed can give women a start in thinking about this important decision in their lives.

It is important to remember that a "woman's right to choose" applies not only to a decision not to parent but also to the option to have children in our lives. Choosing to parent must be considered separately from issues of sexuality. Children who are planned for as these children are, will be, by definition, wanted children. This gives us a head start in dealing with the complex and often stressful issues which face all parents.

WOMAN CONTROLLED CONCEPTION

WOMAN CONTROLLED CONCEPTION
by Sarah and Mary Anonymous
1979, 23 pages, Illus.

from
Union WAGE
P.O. Box 40904
San Francisco, CA 94140
out of print (check Women's Centers for copies)

Woman Controlled Conception was written by two women who have had children by AID (Artificial Insemination by Donor). It describes, often in a very personal way, the methods these two women used, why they chose these methods and what helped them to succeed. The mechanics they describe are very similar to those found in other books on the subject. The personal context in which the book is written, however, is helpful in getting a feeling for what the options are and what their advantages and disadvantages might be. This book also helps to demystify the process because its authors share the trial and error process which eventually ended in success for both of them.

The personal focus and political framework of *Woman Controlled Conception* is evident in its conclusion:

"We would like to end with a photograph of our beautiful children and our friends with their big bellies. Although nothing we've done is illegal—yet—people in power don't want women to have this kind of control over their lives. This means we must protect our anonymity. The beauty of artificial insemination is that we can do it ourselves, no matter what laws they might pass. But we're still up against the problems of how to survive and raise healthy children. Though often we feel we are barely surviving, our goal is to find ways to fight back."

The bibliography included focuses on sources specifically for lesbians considering parenthood.
(CP and CJ)

ARTIFICIAL INSEMINATION:
An Alternative Conception
1979, 19 pages, Illus.

from
Lesbian Health Information Project
3543 18th Street
San Francisco, CA 94110
$2.00 for single copy
$1.50 each for bulk orders

Written by a lesbian attempting to become pregnant and her gay male liaison, *Artificial Insemination* lays out the basics to become pregnant through insemination. The bias clearly favors anonymous donation with a liaison making the choice of donor and transporting sperm for the inseminating woman.

The book is divided into three basic sections: Lesbians—The Donee; The Liaison—The Go-Between; and Gay Men—The Donor. For each of the three, the authors review what will be expected of that person, what their rights are and what their responsibilities are. Methods of calculating ovulation time and how to inseminate are discussed in detail. The appendix also includes sample medical questionnaires which donees might want donors to fill out. A short bibliography focuses on books which aid women in calculating the time of ovulation. (CP and CJ)

"As more gay women are considering having children by means of artificial insemination, there are many problems and much information to be shared. Although much confidentiality is required for all our security, people involved in this process do have a relationship to each other. Understanding each of our roles in this process may help."

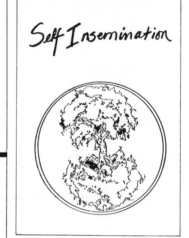

SELF INSEMINATION
by The Feminist Self Insemination Group
1979, 47 pages, Illus.

from
Self Insemination
27 Clerkenwell Close
London WC1
England
write for price

Written by a group of women who participated in a support group while trying to become pregnant, *Self Insemination* is an excellent resource for lesbians who want to become more aware of the feelings they will experience while self inseminating. It is full of personal accounts describing every stage of the process and also includes entries by a lover/co-parent of one inseminating woman.

This book would be a particular comfort for women who are having trouble becoming pregnant, as several members of this group inseminated for a long time before succeeding. It also offers a valuable perspective on the emotional aspects of the process, from coming to a decision to finally becoming pregnant.

The lesbians in this group devised an unusual donor system consisting of a group of gay men who all donated to them at various times. This helped ensure an adequate supply and a degree of anonymity. This unique approach helps the reader to expand her thinking in terms of possible methods for insemination.

It is encouraging that many of the personal and political issues being discussed by American lesbians who are choosing to parent can also be found in this British book. Although the technical information on insemination is covered very thoroughly, this book is certainly most interesting for its broad personal perspective and its information on the emotional aspects of trying to self-insemination conceive. (CP and CJ)

"Self insemination has political significance because it widens the choice women have about how to conceive, and gives women more choice about the type of relationship they have with a biological father. It challenges the idea of biological links as the basis for a relationship between the adult and child. It separates conception and reproduction from a sexual relationship, allowing us the choice to have a child and the freedom to have the sexual relationships we choose."

"Self insemination has political significance because it widens the choice women have about how to conceive and gives women more choice about the type of relationship they have with a biological father."

LESBIAN HEALTH MATTERS
1979, 101 pages, Illus.

from
Santa Cruz Women's Health Center
250 Locust Street
Santa Cruz, CA 95060
$3.95

The chapter on Alternative Fertilization in *Lesbian Health Matters* presents, in a clear and straightforward manner, the physical and emotional aspects of alternative conception for lesbians. It lists advantages and disadvantages of various sources for sperm donation as well as outlining what medical questions are useful to ask potential donors.

In discussing the emotional factors associated with the decision to have children, the article lists several issues which are crucial to consider in the process, then leaves in-depth consideration of these matters to the reader.

The writing is clear and concise and would be a good choice for a brief overview of the issues involved in lesbian insemination. In addition, "Conception Comix" by Mary Wings offers a lighter look at the issues and decisions facing the prospective lesbian parent. (CP and CJ)

"The Women's Movement has strongly supported the right of women to decide if and when they want to have children. We see this section on alternative fertilization as giving support to women who want to choose how to conceive their children. Believing in the power of lan-

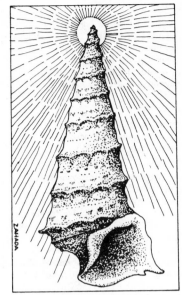

guage to reflect and define norms, we are using "alternative fertilization' instead of 'artificial insemination.' Although 'inseminate' can be used accurately to describe the act of putting semen into one's vagina, we find it lacking when combined with 'artificial' to describe the overall concept at hand. Alternative fertilization gives us more of a sense of woman controlled conception rather than medical profession controlled insemination."

ROCKING THE CRADLE: Lesbian Mothers: A Challenge in Family Living
by Gillian E. Hanscombe and Jackie Forster
1981, 153 pages

from
Alyson Publications, Inc.
P.O. Box 2783, Dept. B-17
Boston, MA 12208
$5.95

Although *Rocking the Cradle* explores all aspects of lesbian parenting, it is especially valuable to lesbians who want to become parents. Much of the book is based on intensive interviews with lesbian parents, many of whom had children as lesbians, through AID, adoption, or by sleeping with a man. A chapter entitled "Where There's a Will, There's a Way" describes both the methods individual lesbians have used to have children and the issues, emotional and political, surrounding insemination. However, discussion of AID is not restricted to this section, and the whole book would be worthwhile reading for the future lesbian parent.

Through this book, future parents will gain a perspective on many different kinds of gay families and how they fit into the overall picture of gay parenting. Since, in the end, how we

had our children will matter less than how we parent, the information offered in *Rocking the Cradle* is as valuable for its broad focus as for its specific information about how to become a parent. (CP and CJ)

"I shall always be honest with my children, right from the start. Our love is simply a variation on a theme and is equally as good and true as any other love. If something seems *right* to a person then it *is* right, no matter who says otherwise. We are just *one* part of a world which has many worlds within it. I shall be truthful with my son when he asks. He was more 'thought out,' planned and discussed beforehand than the 'average' child, and the choice to go ahead against all social odds makes him very much a wanted child. AID and adoption should be more available to single women as well as gay women."

FEMINIST SPERM BANK

SPERM BANK OF NORTHERN CALIFORNIA
Oakland Feminist Women's
Health Center
2930 McClure Street
Oakland, CA 94609
415/444-5676

The Sperm Bank of Northern California is designed to meet the needs of a variety of groups: women choosing donor insemination to have a child, the increasing number of men wishing to store samples of their semen for future procreation, medical personnel in need of prompt and efficient delivery of semen for use with their clients, and women who already have their own donors. The program features donor insemination for single women and couples, comprehensive medical and genetic screening of donors, a wide variety of donor types, confidentiality, short and long term semen preservation, quick specimen retrieval and delivery for doctors and clients. A sliding scale is charged for all services. For further information and a brochure, please write or call.
(CP and CJ)

ARTICLES ON INSEMINATION

LESBIAN INSEMINATION
by Susan Stern
(Summer 1980 issue)

CoEvolution Quarterly
P.O. Box 428
Sausalito, CA 94965
$3.00 each for back issue copies

"Lily jumped out of her van and charged up the steps to Gaea's flat, ... clutching the precious brown paper bag. She rang the bell and waited impatiently for the answering buzz that would open the wrought iron gate. Sometimes she wondered what the neighbors thought if they noticed her going into Gaea's house every other day for three days, every month for six months, with the brown bag. They probably thought it was some sort of drug deal. That made Lily laugh; because what she was doing was really so much more ordinary and so much more revolutionary."

In this highly informative and thorough article the author provides the reader with an actual description of the "go-between" process of one San Francisco midwife who specializes in assisting lesbian women in the process of insemination. The narrative is interspersed with facts and figures about lesbian parenting, information on lesbian insemination, and the psychological and demographic data about lesbian mothers. Throughout the narrative the reader is given a sensitive and gentle glimpse into the thoughts and feelings of both the lesbian who is inseminating and the donor who has donated his sperm. This article is highly recommended for its comprehensive look at the phenomenon of lesbian insemination. Some legal information is covered, but for further legal advice the author suggests consulting an attorney. (CP and CJ)
(Editor's Note: An article by Susan Stern entitled "Amateur Insemination" appears on page 345 of *The Next Whole Earth Catalog* (1980, Random House), edited by the same editors as *CoEvolution Quarterly*.)

SPEAKING WITH LESBIAN MOTHERS
by Lesbian Mothers Group

PLEXUS
(December 1982, Vol. IX, No. 10)
545 Athol Avenue
Oakland, CA 94606
415/451-2585
$1.00 for back issue copies

This is a brief yet extremely timely article discussing the need for sensitivity and thoughtfulness when seeking information about alternative fertilization from lesbian mothers. Helpful suggestions are given for ways in which to ask lesbian mothers about alternative fertilization without their having to reveal their own process.

"Women we don't even know ask us questions like: 'Is that a turkey baster baby?' or 'Did you use artificial insemination?' How we conceived our children is a personal matter."

LESBIAN SELF-INSEMINATION: Life Without Father?
by Jean Horan

in
off our backs
(January 1982, Vol. XII, No. 1)
1841 Columbia Road NW, Room 212
Washington, DC 20009
202/234-8072
$1.00 for back issue copies

This excellent article is an interview with three women who are part of a Philadelphia based support group of women considering self-insemination. The thoughts and feelings expressed in this interview give meaningful and poignant insight into the variety of issues needing discussion when considering self-insemination and parenthood. The women also speak in a moving and sensitive manner to the issue of knowing versus not knowing the donor.
(CP and CJ)

RIGHTS OF LESBIAN PARENTS

For Children

LESBIAN MOTHERS' NATIONAL DEFENSE FUND
P.O. Box 21567
Seattle, WA 98111
206/325-2643

Newsletter subscription $5.00/year
Membership (includes newsletter)
$15-$50/year, sliding scale
All contributions are tax deductible

The Lesbian Mothers' National Defense Fund (LMNDF) was founded in July 1974 by twelve women. Through the years they have assisted over 1000 women and their attorneys with information, financial assistance, and emotional support. Many women decide to fight for custody/visitation after reading of other cases and being referred to this organization. Each time a lesbian mother wins custody or visitation it is encouraging to us all. Each win brings this group closer to the goal of LMNDF: for the courts to decide custody matters in the best interest of the child(ren). "We believe that sexual orientation has no bearing on effective parenting and is an irrelevant point when deciding matters of custody."

Several services are offered to both lesbian mothers and their attorneys facing custody battles: educational materials, support services, both emotional and financial whenever possible, and a quarterly newsletter, "MOM's Apple Pie," which discusses new cases, updates old cases and reports on current trends. The articles for the newsletter are written for the most part by lesbian mothers. Beginning in Summer 1982, a "Kidz Korner" was added, written by the youngest member of LMNDF.
(CP and CJ)

"Raising our children is a right, not a heterosexual privilege."

LESBIAN PARENTING AND CHILD CUSTODY STRUGGLES: Community Organizing and Legal Defense Networks
by Wendy J. Cutler, Yasmin A. Sayyed, and Jeane Vaughn
1982

from
Jeane Vaughn
217 Palo Verde Terrace
Santa Cruz, CA 95060
$2.50

The writing of this pamphlet grew out of the Susan Parker Defense Committee in Santa Cruz, California, a group which was formed to aid a lesbian mother in a legal custody battle for her daughter. The pamphlet is divided into three sections: a brief history of lesbian child custody cases in the context of the legal system, a "how-to" section that talks about the practical aspects of how to start and maintain a lesbian child custody support group, and a discussion of the authors' vision of a national network for lesbian parenting and child custody.

The pamphlet also contains a complete resource listing of legal projects and services. The authors have taken careful attention to include a glossary of legal terms which will be useful to lesbians unfamiliar with "legal-eze." (CP and CJ)

WHEN MEGAN WENT AWAY
by Jane Severance, illustrated by Tea Schook
1979

from
Lollipop Power, Inc.
P.O. Box 1171
Chapel Hill, NC 27514
request price information

Lollipop Power is "a feminist collective that writes, illustrates and publishes books to counteract sex-stereotyped behavior and role models presented by society to young children." The dedication of *When Megan Went Away* reads: "This story is for all children of lesbian mothers, for the special hardships they may face, and for the understanding we hope they will reach." The story portrays Shannon's (the young girl and main character) feelings and adjustment to Megan's (her mother's lover) absence from the household. Not only does this story fill a void of children's stories about lesbian households, but it deals with the aspect of change in partners that is true for all families. The illustrations are delightful. Most importantly, the perspective in the story is the child's. This book is an important resource and reasonably priced.
(Wendy J. Cutler)

LESBIAN RIGHTS PROJECT
1370 Mission Street, 4th Floor
San Francisco, CA 94103
415/621-0675

The Lesbian Rights Project provides legal services for lawyers and consumers on issues related to lesbian mothers and child custody. Publications by this group include a *Litigation Manual for Lawyers* concerning lesbian mothers and child custody, an Annotated Bibliography of legal and psychological materials related to lesbian mothers and their children, and an informative pamphlet discussing the *Legal Issues of Donor Insemination*. (CP and CJ)

LESBIANS CHOOSING MOTHERHOOD: Legal Issues in Donor Insemination
by Donna Hitchens
1980, 20 pages

from
Lesbian Rights Project (above)
$2.50

This is an excellent and informative paper on the legal aspects of the various insemination options available to lesbians choosing to become pregnant. Also attached are sample legal contracts between the woman and any individual with whom she intends to raise the child, in the event that they separate or the biological mother becomes incapacitated or dies. (CP and CJ)

"The purpose of this article is to share the results of our legal research and work with lesbians who are conceiving children through donor insemination. It is our hope . . . we will alert women to potential legal problems that can be avoided through careful planning."

LESBIAN MOTHERS AND THEIR CHILDREN: An Annotated Bibliography of Legal and Psychological Materials
Edited by Donna J. Hitchens, J.D. and Ann G. Thomas, Ed. D.
1980, 45 pages

from
Lesbian Rights Project (above)
$2.00

This is a well-researched and well-written bibliography of articles which will be useful to both lawyers and mental health professionals working with lesbian mothers and their families. A revised edition is currently in progress, to be completed in 1983. (CP and CJ)

"If the best interests of children are truly to be served in cases where the mother is a lesbian, the decisions of judges must be based upon factual data instead of on unsubstantiated assumptions. It is in this spirit that this booklet has been prepared. The materials annotated in this bibliography include published cases, law review articles and psychological research on the rights and abilities of lesbians to be active parents."

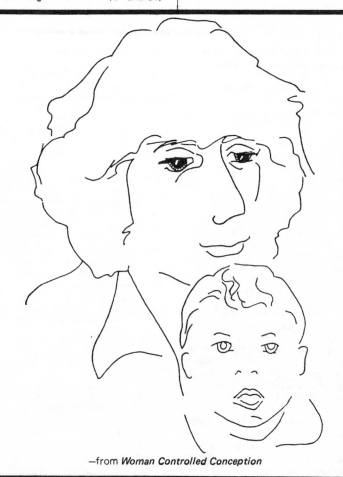

—from *Woman Controlled Conception*

MORE RESOURCES

GROUPS FOR LESBIANS CONSIDERING PARENTHOOD
Cheri Pies, M.S.W.
P.O. Box 3173
Oakland, CA 94609

These groups are designed to assist lesbians in the process of deciding whether to become a parent. The group generally meets for six weeks with a group leader and then continues on its own as a support group for members. Issues covered include: how does a child fit into your life, alternative fertilization, legal issues of donor insemination, relationships with family, friends, lovers, co-workers, the decision-making process, the image of lesbian mothers in the lesbian community. Contact Cheri Pies for more information.

WOMEN'S CENTERS AND WOMEN'S HEALTH CENTERS

All women's centers and women's health centers in major cities can be a valuable networking resource enabling women to contact other lesbian mothers and lesbians considering parenthood. If you are unable to locate any resources in your immediate area, check with a women's bookstore near you, a women's newspaper or even the YWCA.   (CP and CJ)

LESBIAN AND GAY PARENTING PROJECT
Katherine English, attorney
408 SW Second Street
Portland, OR 97204
503/295-2456

FILMS

IN THE BEST INTERESTS OF THE CHILDREN: A Film about Lesbian Mothers and Child Custody
1977, 16 mm color film, 53 minutes

from
Iris Films/Iris Feminist Collective, Inc.
Box 5353
Berkeley, CA 94705
415/835-9118
$70. rental
$660. sale

This excellent film portrays in a sensitive and poignant manner the struggle of lesbian mothers and their children, especially concerning the issues of child custody. "The film is a direct challenge to the prevailing myths about the lesbian as mother." Well done and useful for audiences in a variety of settings including classrooms, medical facilities, legal centers, and childcare centers. The filmmakers are available to speak with this film.   (CP and CJ)

"Eight Lesbian mothers talking of their experiences as Lesbians and mothers. They make statements that show them both to be the same as, and different than other mothers. Their children are shown in interaction with their mothers, and in a rap group with each other discussing how their mothers are different, how they feel about the court's right to decide where they will live, and what they think about their own sexuality. Also presented are an attorney and a clinical social worker, both of whom have done extensive work with Lesbian mothers. They offer their professional opinions around the issue of a Lesbian's right to maintain custody of her children."

SQUARE PEG PRODUCTIONS
46 Bay State Avenue, No. 2
Somerville, MA 02144
617/776-6759

Square Peg Productions is producing a 30 minute color documentary film about lesbians who decide to have children after they have come out. Featuring interviews with lesbians, their lovers and children, the film raises questions about how to conceive or adopt and how having a child affects a lesbian's lifestyle. For more information contact Square Peg Productions at the address or phone number above.
(CP and CJ)

WORKS IN PROGRESS

LESBIAN PARENTING ANTHOLOGY

Jeane Vaughn, co-author and source for *Lesbian Parenting and Child Custody Struggles* (see this section) is soliciting materials intended for publication, including: essays, stories, poems, letters, interviews, critiques, reviews, visual art, tapes, etc. The anthology is to reflect the diversity of experience of lesbian parents: race, class, culture, ethnicity, age, able-bodiness, nationality. To contribute send work before August 1983 to:
ANTHOLOGY
c/o Jeane Vaughn
217 Palo Verde Terrace
Santa Cruz, CA 95060

ALTERNATIVE CONCEPTIONS:
A Workbook for Lesbians Considering Parenthood
by Cheryl Jones and Cheri Pies

This upcoming publication is a workbook designed to assist lesbians in exploring the various issues involved in considering parenthood. The book includes exercises for decision-making to enable the lesbian to clarify her concerns, questions and feelings. Topics covered include different parenting alternatives, alternative fertilization, legal issues of donor insemination, family structures, financial questions, relationships with family, friends, lovers and co-workers, birthing choices and an annotated bibliography of related literature with an eye toward its applicability and appropriateness for lesbians. The work-

book will be approximately 200 pages in length and includes interviews with lesbian mothers, lesbians considering parenthood and those who have decided not to parent. For more information regarding publication or if you would like to complete a questionnaire about your experience considering parenthood send a self-addressed stamped envelope to C.P. Jones, P.O. Box 3173, Oakland, CA 94609.

LESBIAN PARENTING AND CHILD CUSTODY ANTHOLOGY
Wendy Judith Cutler
c/o History of Consciousness Program
U.C. Santa Cruz
Santa Cruz, CA 95064
408/426-9777

"I am a lesbian feminist writer who is seeking contributions (written, oral, visual) and people to serve as resources for an anthology on lesbian parenting and child custody.

"Lesbians are particularly vulnerable when faced with a legal child custody challenge. The assumption that lesbians are unfit to raise children (viewing lesbianism and motherhood as contradictions) threatens all lesbians with loss of custody of their children. . . .

"Major topics to be covered are:
* Winning, Losing, Relinquishing Custody
* Legal Strategies in the Courtroom
* Formation of Defense Funds and Support Networks
* Organizing Community Support
* Expert Witness Testimony
* Settlements Out of Court
* Current Studies and Research
* Anti-racist and Anti-sexist Childrearing
* Coming Out to Children/Family
* Raising Male Children
* Co-Parenting/Single Parenting
* Alternative Fertilization
* Dealing with Ex-Husbands

"Included will be an up to date Resource Directory including lists of support groups, attorneys, law projects, expert witnesses and summaries of cases and current literature concerned with lesbian parenting and child custody.

"You are encouraged to share your knowledge, experiences, and visions by submitting your work. All stages of work are acceptable. Anthology is intended for publication. Send submissions and correspondence before December 1983."
—Wendy Judith Cutler

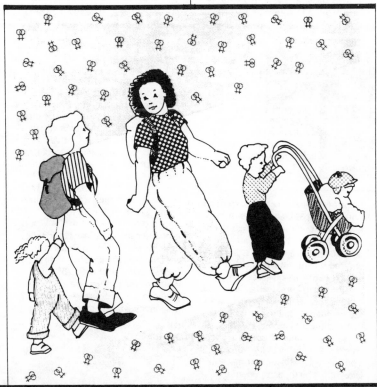

Important Books and Statements

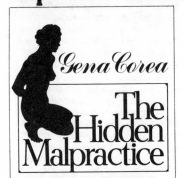

Gena Corea
The Hidden Malpractice

How American Medicine Treats Women as Patients and Professionals

THE HIDDEN MALPRACTICE:
How American Medicine Mistreats Women
by Gena Corea
1977, 309 pages

from
William Morrow
105 Madison Avenue
New York, NY 10016
$10.00 hd.

Gena Corea describes the male stranglehold on women's health care and how it harms us. In Part I she presents the historical background on how women have been barred from healing. In Part II, she discusses "How the Male Domination of Medicine Affects the Health Care Women Receive." Again drawing from history and adding many present day examples, Corea systematically reveals how birth control, treatment of venereal disease, abortion, sterilization, male contraception, childbirth, and common female health concerns have all been severely influenced and research and development in these areas delayed by male/doctor domination. In the epilogue Corea describes what has been done (and how) by women to regain control over their bodies and their health care. She traces the history of the women's health movement and describes the important programs of its three major components—health organizations, women's clinics and self-help groups. An appendix lists women's health groups, publications and films; Corea's extensive source notes provide invaluable information for those interested in further research and action.
—Susan Ritchie

"Taking responsibility for your health, I had learned during my research, was often essential to maintaining it. As I saw in the case of drugs like the Pill, you endanger yourself when you assume that every physician, clinic, drug company and federal regulatory agency places your welfare above all other considerations.

"It is safer to assume that no one cares about your life quite as much as you do. . . .

"*During delivery, the woman is laid on her back, solely for the obstetrician's convenience, in a position which creates a need for an episiotomy. Since the birth canal is curved upward, she is thus forced to give birth uphill.*

"Before men took over midwifery in the United States, a woman used to sit upright, sometimes on a birthing stool, and deliver a child while the female midwife coaxed and encouraged her. When male doctors became the birth attendants, they adopted the lithotomy position (back flat, knees drawn up and spread apart by stirrups) for their own convenience and not for any medically valid reason. . . .

"Today, while in many American hospitals doctors perform episiotomies on 70 percent of mothers, there is only a 6 percent rate in Sweden, the country which also has the lowest infant mortality rate. Mothers and babies there appear to be doing just fine without this operation."

"By acting together, we can certainly take back control of our bodies. I see it happening now. And as I attend feminist health conferences, talk with committed activists . . . and read the newsletters of various health groups—full of energy, outrage and fierce self-respect—I feel so proud of what we women are doing."

"*The Exclusion of Male Medical Students from Obstetrics and Gynecology:* When medical writer Barbara Seaman made this proposal at the woman's health conference in Boston in 1975, it did indeed seem radical to me. It does not today. The truly radical proposals, I now see, were advanced in the 17th century when men took over midwifery, and in the 19th century when 'gynecology' was created as a speciality in which only men—with very few exceptions— engaged. Women did not like that situation then, as numerous physicians of the time testified, and many do not like it now. If enough of us feel this way, we must decide what we will do about it. It may not be enough to simply increase the number of female gynecologists because, as Seaman points out, the few men remaining in the field will rise to the top, controlling hospital departments, research laboratories and population agencies. This has already happened in socialist countries where many, if not most, gynecologists are women.

"We could deal with this and other health issues if each of us did one or all of the following:
1. Launched a local health group, using some of the 'Resources for Change' listed in the Appendix.
2. Helped form a Coalition for the Medical Rights of Women, modeled after California's, in our own states.
3. Join the National Women's Health Lobby Network.

"By acting together, we can certainly take back control of our bodies. I see it happening now. And as I attend feminist health conferences, talk with committed activists like Doris Haire and Kay Weiss, and read the newsletters of various health groups—full of energy, outrage and fierce self-respect—I feel so proud of what we women are doing."

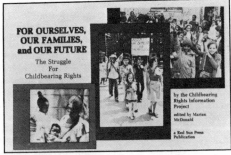

FOR OURSELVES, OUR FAMILIES, AND OUR FUTURE: The Struggle for Childbearing Rights
by the Childbearing Rights Information Project
1981, 140 pages, Illus.

from
Red Sun Press
P.O. Box 18178
Boston, MA 02118
$4.95 plus 1.00 postage
40% discount for 5 or more

This book, the work of a Boston-area collective, covers the whole range of childbearing rights from abortion to genocide, and is one of the few books to directly address the concerns of minority women and the need for political action. Subjects covered include abortion rights, population control, sex education, the health care system, welfare and social services, occupational hazards, teenage pregnancy, gay parents' rights, disabled parents' rights, sterilization abuse, and women prisoners. The chapter on childbirth includes discussions of regionalization of maternity care, home birth, and midwifery.

"Malnutrition, poor housing and sanitation, unsafe working conditions, lack of facilities in the community, and the tensions of racism and poverty, all contribute to the poor health conditions of most minority communities. This can be seen in the infant mortality rates (the rate at which infants die within their first year) for minorities. Oakland, California, recently protested the alarming infant mortality rate in that Third-world community: 26.3 infants per 1,000 births, double the infant mortality figure for white babies in California. This is directly linked to the lack of prenatal care facilities. Nationally, only 52% of pregnant Black women get any prenatal care in the first trimester, compared with 75% of all white women. They are much more likely to develop diseases of late pregnancy such as toxemia."

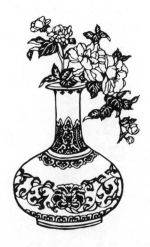

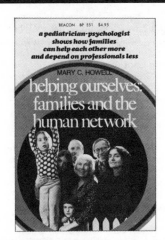

HELPING OURSELVES: Families and the Human Network
by Mary C. Howell
1975, 231 pages

from
Beacon Press
25 Beacon Street
Boston, MA 02108
$4.95 pap.

Mary Howell has written an extraordinarily "activating" book on how families can learn to "help each other more and depend on professionals less." And unlike some other books on this subject, Howell's book is very *gentle* and compassionate in leading readers to explode the myths that keep them dependent on "experts." As a pediatrician and psychologist, Mary Howell knows that much of the special knowledge possessed by doctors and other professionals is not so special after all, and shows us how the professions have "mystified" their activities and skills in order to maintain their control over those they serve. Howell talks about how we can demystify institutions and empower ourselves in the areas of family life, employment, child care, education, and health care. This is a very valuable book and an essential tool for those working to regain the people's control of childbirth.

"The strategies proposed, alternatives to reliance on professionals for direction, are simple in outline, although they may take years of struggle and effort to work into the reality of our lives. I believe that our families could thrive by:
1. Working to develop trusting relationships with a wide human network of kin, friends, neighbors, and others with whom we feel a sense of community;
2. Insisting that 'experts' share with us the knowledge and skills that we need to conduct our own affairs;
3. Utilizing the paid services of professionals at our own convenience—that is, only when we wish to do so, and on *our* terms. . . .

"It is becoming increasingly clear to many that to continue to strive for absolute mastery and control of everything in the natural world, and to expect 'perfect' and 'unflawed' lives, is to risk the further disintegration of our affinity with the world of nature. . . .

"We have been robbed, by our conventional arrangements for professionalized medical care, of our competence to promote the good health of our families and to provide skilled home-based care. We have even been 'relieved' of our participation in birth and death. We have allowed ourselves to hope that the 'science of medicine' will, if we give it enough rope, keep us all alive forever—for fighting death has been the physician's major goal. We have almost forgotten that there is more to health care than the application of chemicals and technology. Physicians have been taught *not* to take care, and to be not servants but masters of those they take care of. Medical care has focused on 'being alive,' as a product; health care demands attention to the quality of life, a process. As patients, we have forgotten how to claim what should be ours: the ability to take good care of ourselves and those we love and trust, in sickness and in health. . . .

"I propose that a model for transactions of *mutual* trust, the source of a kind of magic we are only beginning to rediscover, is to be found in the assistance provided by a midwife at birth. At a home birth the midwife, fortified with transportable oxygen, suction, intravenous solutions, and a rapid transport system that permits hospitalization in case of unforeseen disaster, comes to attend when labor pains begin to be regular. Assisting in the preparations, instructing family members in their part in the event and their collaborative support of the delivering mother, the midwife encourages and coaxes the birth in its *own due time*. The process builds to the peak of the moment of the crowning head, but the midwife's assistance continues—to clean up after the delivery of the afterbirth, return the house to order, support the exhilarated and exhausted participants and observers, assist in the feeding of the new family member, and share in the rejoicing. The midwife informs, teaches, and allows the magical powers of trust and caring to envelop the family, the mother, and infant. The root of caring is to respect the rhythms, needs, and abilities of another. The family's trust in the midwife, and the midwife's trust in the competence of family members, are the basis of caring that has the power of magic."

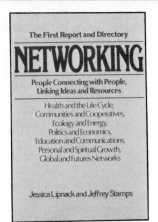

NETWORKING: The First Report and Directory
by Jessica Lipnack and Jeffrey Stamps
1982, 397 pages

from
Doubleday
245 Park Avenue
New York, NY 10017
$15.95 pap.

Jessica Lipnack is a journalist who has often written on the women's health movement. Her husband, Jeffrey Stamps, has written on human systems theory. Together they have researched and written this book on networking which includes introductory essays and listings of organizations, publications, etc., on each of the eight subject areas covered: health and the life cycle, communities and cooperatives, ecology and energy, politics and economics, education and communications, personal and spiritual growth, and global and futures networks. There is also a special section on the Boston Women's Health Book Collective, its history and function, and much information on how networks function to connect the people and resources of "alternative America." The alternative childbirth movement is one of the many interconnected networks of people working to improve life on our planet.

"In this book, we are describing and documenting networks spontaneously created by people to address problems and offer possibilities primarily outside of established institutions. . . .

"The history of the Collective offers a valuable insight into how networks form, jell, and persist over time without elaborate planning, self-conscious statements of purpose, or long-term goals. The Boston Women's Health Book Collective, one of the oldest and most successful of the networks we have learned about, just happened.

" 'We never set out to do anything,' Vilunya recalls. 'You don't plan to bring a group of twelve women together, enlist the help of hundreds of others, write a book that sells 250,000 copies over 2 years through "underground" distribution with a price that is *lowered* from $.75 to $.30, face the choice of *which* major publisher to sign with, and then find your book on the New York Times best-seller list for 3 years.'

" 'Everything flowed organically from one thing to another,' she says. 'And it's still growing.'. . .

"In his now-classic essay *The Structure of Scientific Revolutions,* Thomas Kuhn brilliantly described the chaos that exists just prior to and during periods of transition between 'old' and 'new' scientific worldviews, a recurrent pattern in the evolution of scientific thought. Dominant scientific models reach a certain peak of success in being able 'to explain everything' just when anomalies—odd fragments of experiments and theories that do not fit the prevailing view—become numerous and troublesome. Adherents of new viewpoints—generally younger, uncommitted scientists—attack the dominant model and promote a profusion of alternative models.

"A 'clash of worldviews' between scientific perspectives creates a period of confusion and tension that is suddenly resolved by the presentation of a new synthesis. The new paradigm invariably incorporates the now-apparent partial truths of the older model, provides consistent explanations for the precipitating anomalies, and opens up new territory for scientific exploration. In time, the 'new synthesis' becomes the 'established model' and begins to reach its exploratory limits, as a new cycle of challenge, chaos, and transformation ensues. . . .

"Practiced networkers move with delicacy and humility, knowing that waiting to be asked is more appropriate than imposing help where it is not wanted. In their cores, networkers are generous; they are able to give without keeping score. One vital exemplary network expresses this idea, as well as its attitude toward the world, in its one-word title: PLENTY. . . .

"In this nourishing role, networkers become like parents. In an impromptu interview with Hazel Henderson, she said, 'Being a networker is just like being a mother. You're constantly giving out, sending things, making new matches, writing letters, increasing the size of your phone bill. But you don't count how many letters you've written or total up the hours that you spend networking. You just do it because it has to be done, just the way you do with children.' "

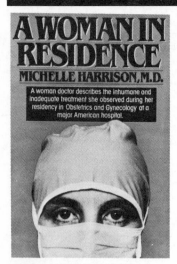

A WOMAN IN RESIDENCE
by Michelle Harrison, M.D.
1982, 264 pages

from
Random House
201 East 50th Street
New York, NY 10022
$13.95 hd.

Michelle Harrison was in family practice and attending home births when she became frustrated at not being able to care for her mothers in the hospital when transfer was necessary. So at the age of 35, after a decade in practice, Harrison began a part-time residency in obstetrics/gynecology, hoping to gain the specialized skills she wanted and also be able to care for her 5-year-old daughter as a single parent. *A Woman in Residence* is her record of a harrowing six and a half months training at a major, "progressive" metropolitan hospital; a residency which Harrison did not complete.

Harrison's account alternates between her very detailed descriptions of her training and participation in surgery and other procedures and her difficulties in arranging and maintaining adequate child care for her daughter. Through her diary, recorded daily into a tape recorder, we are able to see how very damaging and dehumanizing the medical system is both to its patients and practitioners. We follow Harrison as she learns to perform dilation and curettage (D & C), laparoscopy, tubal ligation and other gynecological procedures in situations which will make potential patients cringe. Many factors other than sound medical judgment and skill influence the conduct of surgery, including interprofessional rivalries, research needs, needs for "teaching material," sleep deprivation, etc. On her labor and delivery rotation, Harrison witnesses many unnecessary cesareans and sees normal labors routinely distorted by unnecessary drugs and procedures: all this in a hospital which does contain an "alternative birth service" and is well known for its progressive care.

Several things become clear in the course of this book: first, the

hospital is simply *not* a safe place in which to have a baby and physicians are not safe birth attendants. Second, women doctors are just as dehumanized by their training as men and end up practicing in a way which is no different from their male colleagues. It is clear that hospital reform and bringing more women into obstetrics will not solve the problems of poor obstetrical care.

Some reviewers have criticized Harrison's "inflammatory rhetoric" and accused her of exaggeration. Based on what I know about hospital practice, though, Harrison's accounts are *under*stated, if anything. I would urge any potential hospital patient, whether a woman scheduled for a D & C or a couple expecting a baby, to read this book *first.*

"My first delivery at DH was with Dr. HIlda Cameron, a physician, I hadn't met until I was taking care of her laboring patient. I told her I was new here, but I don't think she heard me. Just before the delivery I took the woman back to the delivery room and had her prepped and draped by the time Hilda got there.

" 'I think you should do the episiotomy on the next contraction,' she told me.

"I was not used to doing episiotomies, since at home births I had learned to deliver babies without cutting the perineum. I asked her, 'Do you routinely do episiotomies?' She had just commented on how much

room there was for the baby, since the woman had a loose perineum, so I had hoped we might leave it alone.

"She responded brusquely, 'Nothing is routine in obstetrics. Now do the episiotomy.'

"My hand was shaking as I took the scissors and tried to make a very small cut.

" 'Deeper! Deeper!' she said and then angrily took the scissors from my hand and made a large cut in the woman's perineum and extended the cut into the vagina. We delivered the baby on the next contraction."

* * *

"Yesterday Murray Avery gave a conference on fetal monitoring where he discussed the presumed mechanisms of control of fetal heart rate. I suddenly realized that these doctors are not obstetricians—i.e., people who take care of pregnant women—but pre pre-birth pediatricians, or what I call 'feteotricians.' The doctors have set up a relationship between themselves and the unborn child that does not include the mother. If these doctors don't care whether a woman uses natural childbirth or has epidural anesthesia, it is only because she has been written off, and her experience, whether she is awake or asleep, is irrelevant. She is the maternal environment. They are frustrated only that they cannot control her more."

* * *

"The birthing woman plays in an orchestra of her body, her soul, her baby, her loved ones, her past and her future. And we do not know who leads the orchestra.

"Doctors can't lead the orchestra, because they are not within the process. Unable to hear the music, trained only in modalities of power and control, they can only interfere with the music being played.

"What should they be able to do? They should stand ready to help the player in trouble to get back into the rhythm. Instead, they take over Instead of supporting the mother, they say, 'Okay, you have failed. It's our piece now.'

"How do you get a 30 percent Caesarean-section rate? You orchestrate it. You write a piece in which the third movement is a Caesarean, then build the first two with that in mind. You write in a different language; you write in terms of centimeters of dilation, external fetal monitor, internal fetal monitor, pH, scalp electrodes, Caesarean-birth experience, arrest of labor, protracted labor, fetal distress, episiotomy, prolapse, cephalo-pelvic disproportion, ultrasound waves, amniocentesis, 'premium baby,' post-mature (when the baby stays too long in utero) and 'maternal environment' (formerly known as the mother). Those are the words, the notes, while the piece is played to the rhythm of fear."

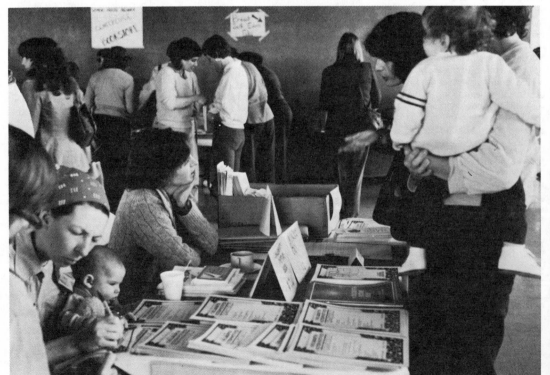

Members of the Long Island Childbirth Alternatives present options at a women's health fair.

J.I.A.

CLOSING STATEMENTS

I close the *Whole Birth Catalog* with two statements on childbirth reform. The first is an excerpt from *Changing Childbirth: Family Birth in the Hospital,* an excellent new book which is reviewed in the section on Family-Centered Care. The excerpt is reprinted here with the kind permission of the author, Diony Young, and the publisher, Jamie Bolane of Childbirth Graphics. The second statement is an excerpt from a speech given by Gena Corea, author of *The Hidden Malpractice.* Reprints of this speech are available from H.O.M.E., as listed.

These two statements offer examples of two contrasting approaches to the reform of childbirth practices. Young argues, in effect, that we can change and improve childbirth by working to change the medical system which provides maternity care. Corea argues that this approach has never worked and that women must create and control their own health care systems. I leave it to the reader to ponder and evaluate these statements, choose a course of action, and act.

"SCIENTIFIC" OBSTETRICS ATTACKS THE HOME BIRTH MOVEMENT
by Gena Corea
1981, 9 pages

from
H.O.M.E.
511 New York Avenue
Takoma Park, MD 20912
$2.00

Gena Corea is the author of *The Hidden Malpractice* (see review in this *Catalog*) which contains excellent material on the way male control of childbirth and the suppression of midwives has distorted the birth process. In this transcript of a speech given by Corea in 1981, she goes into even more detail on the abuses of modern obstetrical technology and attitudes and on the efforts by the obstetrical profession to suppress home birth. Speaking before a sympathetic audience of women's health movement activists, Corea doesn't compromise in her language and outrage.

"The new childbirth movement challenges consumers and professionals alike to become involved actively in changing and renewing the maternity care system. Every pregnant woman must learn to become responsible for her body, her health, and her newborn. Every childbirth group must assume a role of advocacy for the childbearing population. Changing childbirth is the responsibility of us all, consumers and providers, and we must work both together and separately to make sure that families inherit the benefit of our efforts.

"This is not to say that confrontation can or should always be avoided. There are times when it may be necessary and appropriate, leading to constructive action. But those consumers involved in urging change and those providers involved in implementing it must be flexible and willing to examine all sides of an issue so that solutions can be worked out. Refusal to listen and consider the other's viewpoint and suggestions is inexcusable, whether the person be a consumer or a provider. Consumers should also bear in mind that their mere presence, their temerity in raising questions, can be threatening to some health providers. Joint consumer-provider discussion about obstetrical practices may be an entirely new experience for some health professionals.

"Parental anger and distress about an unhappy birth experience can become a constructive tool for creating change. Through communication with the health providers and hospital administration, the consumer can focus personal anger and direct it in positive ways to promote among providers a new sensitivity to family needs and a decision to improve services and care. Sometimes all it takes is one letter to start the ball rolling.

"Consumers must be willing to put forth the necessary effort to persuade health providers of the need for change, using all the many avenues available to them. If the door is closed and no action forthcoming after using one strategy, they must move on to the next strategy, and the next, until they stand before the hospital Board of Trustees, or, if necessary, outside the hospital itself, picket in hand! It all boils down to the fact that if something is wrong, find the way to fix it! All the childbearing families who follow will benefit from the constructive use of consumer power, and hospitals will have moved one step further toward offering a system of care that supports and strengthens the families in their community."

Diony Young

"If, years after women have repeatedly pointed out the problems with obstetrical care and written reams of articles and pounds of books carefully documenting those problems, physicians finally respond by placing potted plants around the Electronic Fetal Monitor, then I, for one, am giving up on them.

"Let's just walk away. They can go on fiddling with their machines. One day they will look up and notice there are no longer any female bodies to which they can attach those machines.

"We cannot reform obstetrical practices for any length of time within the present medical system. This is one of the facts which makes me so pessimistic about obstetrical reform: The first expose of American childbirth practices I read was written in 1836 and the abuses described, though different in form, are essentially the abuses which are still occurring today.

"Instead of spending all our energy defending ourselves from obstetricians then, and negotiating with them (May I do this? Will you allow me to forgo that?), let's withdraw and meet our own needs ourselves. Women are already beginning to do so. We can certainly set up our own midwifery schools, birth centers and health centers—all independent of physician control.

"Physicians will try to stop us. They will oppose the legalization of lay midwives. They will oppose the opening of midwifery schools which do *not* teach that the midwife is an integral part of the obstetrical team, operating immediately below the physicians' foot.

"In opposing us, physicians will continue to present themselves to state and national legislatures as the protectors of woman's health and the articulators of her needs.

"We must challenge their right to speak for us. We must give the lie to the assertion that the obstetrician's interests and the woman's are one and the same thing. . . .

"We women need to inform law-makers that it is not obstetrician-gynecologists, members of an almost exclusively male professional group, who are the experts on our bodies and our welfare.

"*We* are the experts."

Gena Corea

Index